ANTIBIOTIC AND CHEMOTHERAPY

ANTIBIOTIC AND CHEMOTHERAPY

BY

LAWRENCE P. GARROD

M.D. (Camb.) Hon. LL.D. (Glasgow) F.R.C.P.

Emeritus Professor of Bacteriology,
University of London
Hon. Consultant in Chemotherapy,
Royal Postgraduate Medical School,
Formerly Bacteriologist, St. Bartholomew's Hospital

AND

FRANCIS O'GRADY

T.D., M.D. (Lond.) M.Sc. (Lond.) M.R.C.Path.

Professor of Bacteriology,
University of London
Bacteriologist, St. Bartholomew's Hospital

THIRD EDITION
Reprint

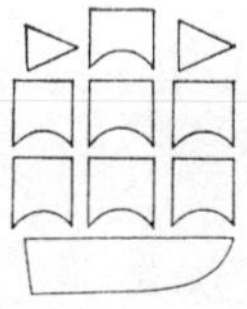

CHURCHILL LIVINGSTONE
EDINBURGH AND LONDON
1972

PREFACE TO THIRD EDITION

THE study of anti-microbic chemotherapy is still expanding at such a pace that when the second edition of this book was exhausted within eighteen months of publication a third edition rather than a reprint was clearly necessary. The incorporation of much new material has necessitated extensive revision, and two new chapters have been added. We are grateful to our publishers for enabling us to make further additions even in proof, and some of the publications quoted ante-date this edition itself only by months.

We are again indebted to many colleagues for advice, and to Miss J. Allen, F.P.S., for her help with the subject of Table XL. Cultures or data for filling gaps in Table XXXVIII were kindly provided by Professor B. W. Lacey, Dr. G. C. Blake and Dr. P. G. Mann. The much expanded final chapter on technical methods has been the work of Miss Pamela M. Waterworth, who also did the experiments embodied in Table II, provided most of the new data in Table XXXVIII, and has contributed to our work in many other ways, including the preparation of the index.

L.P.G.
F.O'G.

London, 1971.

PREFACE TO FIRST EDITION

THIS book is mainly about antibiotics, but embraces sulphonamides and other synthetic drugs employed in the chemotherapy of the microbic infections of temperate climates. That of malaria and most other protozoal infections, helminthiases and malignant disease is excluded. The first part describes the properties of antibiotics and other drugs, with emphasis on their degree of activity against different bacterial species. The large body of detailed information on this presented in a series of tables, some of it hitherto unpublished, provides one essential basis for rational prescribing, since the first requirement of any drug is an adequate and preferably high degree of activity against the species responsible for the infection.

The second part is concerned with chemotherapy in its practical aspects, in infections which are classified by systems. As professional bacteriologists who have had no clinical responsibilities for many years we are fully conscious of our temerity in invading the sphere of therapeutics. Nevertheless each of us has been so frequently consulted by clinical colleagues about the treatment of individual patients that we can claim a knowledge of this subject in its practical as well as theoretical aspects, and feel justified in writing of what we have learned. The treatment we describe is solely that directed against the microbe. We are well aware that other kinds of treatment, quite outside our sphere, are sometimes an important element in success, and moreover that circumstances may exist, again beyond our ken, which can modify the usual indications for chemotherapy. The clinician must be the ultimate judge: our aim has been to provide him with as much factual information as possible, and accounts of the results achieved by previous competent observers. We believe that this information may be found useful at all levels in the profession; to both junior and senior members of hospital staffs and to consultants as well as general practitioners. We trust also that laboratory workers may find the book helpful.

We are indebted to many colleagues for advice, mainly on clinical matters, among whom we would particularly mention Miss J. Allen, F.P.S., Professor J. W. Crofton, Mr. H. G. Dixon, Dr. S. C. Gold, Dr. D. A. Mitchison, Dr. C. S. Nicol, Professor J. G. Scadding, Mr. W. H. Stephenson and Dr. J. P. M. Tizard. They have not actually read our text, and should not be held responsible for the views expressed, or for any errors. Our special thanks are due to Miss Pamela M. Waterworth, who has served both of us as a research assistant. She performed most of the experiments on which our original observations are based: among those hitherto unpublished are numerous data in Tables XI and XXII, and the findings illustrated in Figures 6 and 9. Some of her other contributions to the subject are referred to in the text. We are also indebted to her for advice about Chapter XXVII and for preparing the index.

London, 1963.   M. B.
                                                   L. P. G.

ACKNOWLEDGMENTS

I_N addition to the figures acknowledged in the text, we are indebted to the following authors and editors for permission to reproduce original material:

to Dr. G. H. Hitchings and *Trans. N.Y. Acad. Sci.* for Fig. 3,
Prof. R. Kirkpatrick and *Lancet* for Fig. 2,
Brit. med. J. for Table XI,
Dr. T. D. Brock and *Experimental Chemotherapy* for Fig. 8 and Table XXIII,
Dr. M. L. Koch and *Antibiot. Chemother.* for Table XXI,
Dr. P. R. McCurdy and *Blood* for Fig. 9,
Dr. M. Finland and *Amer. J. med. Sci.* for Fig. 14,
Dr. E. B. Herr and *Antimicrob. Agents Chemother.* for Table XXVII,
Mr. W. R. Maxted and *J. clin. Path.* for Table XXVIII,
Miss M. Barnett and *Brit. J. Pharmacol.* for Table XXX,
J. med. Lab. Technol. for Figs. 17 and 28A,
Dr. A. W. Mathies and *Antimicrob. Agents Chemother.* for Table XLII,
Dr. I. H. Leopold and *Invest. Ophthal.* for Table XLV,
Office of Health Economics for Fig. 24.

CONTENTS

PART I

Chapter		Page
I	THE EVOLUTION OF ANTI-MICROBIC DRUGS	1
II	SULPHONAMIDES	12
III	OTHER SYNTHETIC ANTIMICROBIAL AGENTS	34
IV	PENICILLINS 1. NATURAL	53
V	PENICILLINS 2. SEMI-SYNTHETIC PENICILLINS AND CEPHALOSPORINS	70
VI	STREPTOMYCIN	98
VII	THE NEOMYCIN GROUP	115
VIII	CHLORAMPHENICOL	132
IX	TETRACYCLINES	147
X	THE ERYTHROMYCIN GROUP (MACROLIDES)	166
XI	PEPTIDE ANTIBIOTICS	182
XII	VARIOUS ANTI-BACTERIAL ANTIBIOTICS	202
XIII	ANTI-FUNGAL ANTIBIOTICS	235
XIV	DRUG RESISTANCE	248

PART II

Chapter		Page
XV	GENERAL PRINCIPLES OF TREATMENT	263
XVI	DOSAGE	276
XVII	SEPTICAEMIA AND ENDOCARDITIS	284
XVIII	INFECTIONS OF SKIN, SOFT TISSUES AND BONES	302
XIX	BACTERIAL MENINGITIS	323
XX	INFECTIONS OF THE AIR PASSAGES	336
XXI	INFECTIONS OF THE ALIMENTARY TRACT	347
XXII	ANTIBIOTICS IN OBSTETRICS	359
XXIII	URINARY TRACT INFECTIONS	368
XXIV	INFECTIONS OF THE EYE	385
XXV	TUBERCULOSIS	400
XXVI	VENEREAL DISEASES: SPIROCHAETOSES	420
XXVII	VIRUS DISEASES	440
XXVIII	LABORATORY CONTROL	451
	INDEX	487

Chapter I

THE EVOLUTION OF ANTI-MICROBIC DRUGS

No one recently qualified, even with the liveliest imagination, can picture the ravages of bacterial infection which continued until little more than thirty years ago. To take only two examples, lobar pneumonia was a common cause of death even in young and vigorous patients, and puerperal septicaemia and other forms of acute streptococcal sepsis had a high mortality, little affected by any treatment then available. One purpose of this chapter is therefore to place the subject of this book in historical perspective.

This subject is chemotherapy, which may be defined as the administration of a substance with a systemic anti-microbic action. Some would confine the term to synthetic drugs, and the distinction is recognized in the title of this book, but since some all-embracing term is needed, this one might with advantage be understood also to include substances of natural origin. Several antibiotics can now be synthesized, and it would be ludicrous if their use should qualify for description as chemotherapy only because they happened to be prepared in this way. The essence of the term is that the effect must be systemic, the substance being absorbed, whether from the alimentary tract or a site of injection, and reaching the infected area by way of the blood stream. 'Local chemotherapy' is in this sense a contradiction in terms: any application to a surface, even of something capable of exerting a systemic effect, is better described as antisepsis.

THE THREE ERAS OF CHEMOTHERAPY

There are three distinct periods in the history of this subject. In the first, which is of great antiquity, the only substances capable of curing an infection by systemic action were natural plant products. The second was the era of synthesis, and in the third we return to natural plant products, although from plants of a much lower order, the moulds and bacteria forming anti-biotics.

1. ALKALOIDS. This era may be dated from 1619, since it is from this year that the first record is derived of the successful treatment of malaria with an extract of cinchona bark, the patient being the wife of the Spanish governor of Peru. Another South American discovery was the efficacy of ipecacuanha root in amoebic dysentery. Until the early years of this century these extracts, and in more recent times the alkaloids, quinine and emetine, derived from them, provided the only curative chemo-therapy known.

2. SYNTHETIC COMPOUNDS. Therapeutic progress in this field, which initially and for many years after was due almost entirely to research in Germany, dates from the discovery of salvarsan by Ehrlich in 1909. His successors produced germanin for trypanosomiasis and other drugs effective in protozoal infec-tions. A common view at that time was that protozoa were susceptible to chemotherapeutic attack, but that bacteria were not: the treponemata, which had been shown to be susceptible to organic arsenicals, are no ordinary bacteria, and were regarded as a class apart.

The belief that bacteria are by nature insusceptible to any drug which is not also prohibitively toxic to the human body was finally destroyed by the discovery of Prontosil. This, the forerunner of the sulphonamides, was again a product of German research, and its discovery was publicly announced in 1935. All the work with which this book is concerned is subse-quent to this year: it saw the beginning of the effective treat-ment of bacterial infections.

Progress in the synthesis of anti-microbic drugs has continued to the present day. Apart from many new sulphonamides, perhaps the most notable additions have been the synthetic compounds used in the treatment of tuberculosis.

3. ANTIBIOTICS. The therapeutic revolution produced by the sulphonamides, which included the conquest of haemolytic streptococcal and pneumococcal infections and of gonorrhoea and cerebrospinal fever, was still in progress and even causing some bewilderment when the first report appeared of a study which was to have even wider consequences. This was not the discovery of penicillin—that had been made by Fleming in

1929—but the demonstration by Florey and his colleagues that it was a chemotherapeutic agent of unexampled potency. The first announcement of this, made in 1940, was the beginning of the antibiotic era, and the unimagined developments from it are still in progress. We little knew at the time that penicillin, besides providing a remedy for infections insusceptible to sulphonamide treatment, was also a necessary second line of defence against those fully susceptible to it. During the early 'forties resistance to sulphonamides appeared successively in gonococci, haemolytic streptococci and pneumococci: nearly twenty years later it has appeared also in meningococci. But for the advent of the antibiotics, all the benefits stemming from Domagk's discovery might by now have been lost, and bacterial infections have regained their pre-1935 prevalence and mortality.

The earlier history of two of these discoveries calls for further description.

Sulphonamides

Prontosil, or sulphonamido-chrysoidin, was first synthesized by Klarer and Mietzsch in 1932, and was one of a series of azo dyes examined by Domagk for possible effects on haemolytic streptococcal infection. When a curative effect in mice had been demonstrated, cautious trials in erysipelas and other human infections were undertaken, and not until the evidence afforded by these was conclusive did the discoverers make their announcement. Domagk (1935) published the original claims, and the same information was communicated by Hörlein (1935) to a notable meeting in London.

These claims, which initially concerned only the treatment of haemolytic streptococcal infections, were soon confirmed in other countries, and one of the most notable early studies was that of Colebrook and Kenny (1936) in England, who demonstrated the efficacy of the drug in puerperal fever. This infection had until then been taking a steady toll of about 1,000 young lives per annum in England and Wales, despite every effort to prevent it by hygienic measures and futile efforts to overcome it by serotherapy. The immediate effect of the adoption of this treatment can be seen in Figure 1: a steep fall in mortality began in 1935, and continued, as the treatment became universal and better understood, and as more potent sulphonamides were introduced, until the present-day low level had almost been reached *before penicillin became generally available*. The effect of penicillin between 1945 and 1950 is perhaps more evident on incidence: its widespread use tends completely to

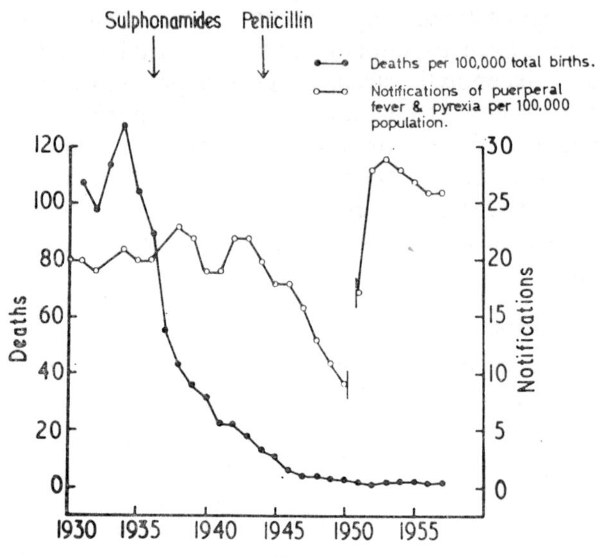

FIG. 1

Puerperal pyrexia. Deaths per 100,000 total births and incidence per 100,000 population in England and Wales, 1930-1957.

N.B. the apparent rise in incidence in 1950 is due to the fact that the definition of puerperal pyrexia was changed in this year (see text).

(Reproduced from Barber (1960), *J. Obstet. & Gynaec.* **67,** 727, by kind permission of the editor.)

banish haemolytic streptococci from the environment. The apparent rise in incidence after 1950 is due to the redefinition of puerperal pyrexia as any rise of temperature to 100·4° F., whereas previously the term was only applied when the temperature was maintained for 24 hours or recurred. Needless to say, fever so defined is frequently not of uterine origin.

Prontosil had no anti-bacterial action *in vitro*, and it was soon suggested by workers in Paris (Tréfouel *et al.*, 1935) that it owed its activity to the liberation from it in the body of *p*-amino-benzene sulphonamide (sulphanilamide); that this compound is so formed was subsequently proved by Fuller (1937). Sulphanilamide had a demonstrable inhibitory action on streptococci *in vitro,* much dependent on the medium and particularly on the size of the inoculum, facts which are readily understandable in the light of modern knowledge. This explanation of the therapeutic action of prontosil was hotly contested by Domagk. It must be remembered that it relegated the chrysoidin component to an inert role, whereas the affinity of dyes for bacteria had been a basis of German research since the time of Ehrlich, and was the doctrine underlying the choice of this series of compounds for examination. German workers also took the attitude that there must be something mysterious about the action of a true chemotherapeutic agent: an effect easily demonstrable in a test tube by any tyro was too banal altogether to explain it. Finally, they felt justifiable resentment that sulphanilamide, as a compound which had been described many years earlier, could be freely manufactured by anyone.

Every enterprising pharmaceutical house in the world was soon making this drug, and at one time it was on the market under at least 70 different proprietary names. What was more important, chemists were soon busy modifying the molecule to improve its performance. Early advances so secured were of two kinds, the first being higher activity against a wider range of bacteria: sulphapyridine (M and B 693), discovered in 1938, was the greatest single advance, since it was the first drug to be effective in pneumococcal pneumonia. The next stage, the introduction of sulphathiazole and sulphadiazine, while retaining and enhancing anti-bacterial activity, eliminated the frequent nausea and cyanosis caused by earlier drugs. Further developments, mainly in the direction of altered pharmacological properties, have continued to the present day and are described in Chapter II.

ANTIBIOTICS

' Out of the earth shall come thy salvation.'—S. A. Waksman.

Definition

Of many definitions of the term antibiotic which have been proposed the narrower seem preferable. It is true that the word ' antibiosis ' was coined by Vuillemin in 1889 to denote antagonism between living creatures in general, but the noun ' antibiotic ' was first used by Waksman in 1942 (Waksman and Lechevalier, 1962), which gives him a right to re-define it, and his definition confines it to substances produced by micro-organisms antagonistic to the growth or life of others in high dilution (the last clause being necessary to exclude such metabolic products as organic acids, hydrogen peroxide and alcohol). To define an antibiotic simply as an anti-bacterial substance from a living source would embrace gastric juice, antibodies and lysozyme from man, essential oils and alkaloids from plants, and such oddities as the substance in the faeces of blowfly larvae which exerts an antiseptic effect in wounds. All substances known as antibiotics which are in clinical use and capable of exerting a systemic effect are in fact products of micro-organisms.

Early History

The study of inter-microbic antagonism is almost as old as microbiology itself: several instances of it were described, one by Pasteur himself, in the seventies of the last century. Therapeutic applications followed, some employing actual living cultures, others extracts of bacteria or moulds which had been found active. One of the best known products was an extract of *Ps. aeruginosa,* first used as a local application by Czech workers, Honl and Bukovsky, in 1899: this was commercially available as ' pyocyanase ' on the continent for many years. Other investigators used extracts of species of *Penicillium* and *Aspergillus* which probably or certainly contained antibiotics, but in too low a concentration to exert more than a local and transient effect. Florey (1945) gave a revealing account of these early developments in a lecture with the intriguing title ' The Use of Micro-organisms as Therapeutic Agents ': this was amplified in a later publication (Florey, 1949).

The systematic search, by an ingenious method, for an organism which could attack pyogenic cocci, conducted by Dubos (1939) in New York, led to the discovery of tyrothricin (gramicidin + tyrocidine), formed by *Bacillus brevis,* a substance which although too toxic for systemic use in man, had in fact a systemic curative effect in mice. This work exerted a strong influence in inducing Florey and his colleagues to embark on a study of naturally formed anti-bacterial substances, and penicillin was the second on their list.

Penicillin

The present antibiotic era may be said to date from 1940, when the first account of the properties of an extract of cultures of *Penicillium notatum* appeared from Oxford (Chain *et al.*, 1940): a fuller account followed, with impressive clinical evidence (Abraham *et al.*, 1941). It had been necessary to find means of extracting a very labile substance from culture fluids, to examine its action on a wide range of bacteria, to examine its toxicity by a variety of methods, to establish a unit of its activity, to study its distribution and excretion when administered to animals, and finally to prove its systemic efficacy in mouse infections. There then remained the gigantic task, seemingly impossible except on a factory scale, of producing in the School of Pathology at Oxford enough of a substance, which was known to be excreted with unexampled rapidity, for the treatment of human disease. One means of maintaining supplies was extraction from the patients' urine and re-administration.

It was several years before penicillin was fully purified, its structure ascertained, and its large-scale commercial production achieved. That this was of necessity first entrusted to manufacturers in the United States gave them a lead in a highly profitable industry which was not to be overtaken for many years.

Later Antibiotics

The dates of discovery and sources of the principal antibiotics are given chronologically in Table I. A few, including penicillin, were chance discoveries, but ' stretching out suppliant Petri dishes ' (Florey, 1945) in the hope of catching a new antibiotic-producing organism was not to lead anywhere. Most further discoveries resulted from soil surveys, a process from which a large annual outlay might or might not be repaid a hundred-fold, a gamble against much longer odds than most oil prospecting. Soil contains a profuse and very mixed flora varying with climate, vegetation, mineral content and other factors, and is a medium in which antibiotic formation may well play a part in the competition for nutriment. A soil survey consists of

TABLE I

Date of Discovery and Source of the More Important Antibiotics

Name	Date of Discovery	Microbe	Source
Penicillin	1929-1940	*Penicillium notatum*	Air, London
Tyrothricin { Gramicidin / Tyrocidine }	1939	*Bacillus brevis*	Soil, New York
Griseofulvin	1939	*Penicillium griseofulvum Dierckx*	
	1945	*Penicillium janczewski*	Soil, Dorset
Streptomycin	1944	*Streptomyces griseus*	A chicken's throat
Bacitracin	1945	*Bacillus licheniformis*	Contaminated wound
Chloramphenicol	1947	*Streptomyces venezuelae*	Mulched field, Venezuela
Polymyxin	1947	*Bacillus polymyxa*	Soil, Britain and U.S.A.
Framycetin	1947-1953	*Streptomyces lavendulae*	Damp patch on wall, Paris
Chlortetracycline	1948	*Streptomyces aureofaciens*	Soil
Cephalosporin C, N and P	1948	*Cephalosporium sp.*	Sewage outfall, Sardinia
Neomycin	1949	*Streptomyces fradiae*	Soil, New Jersey
Oxytetracycline	1950	*Streptomyces rimosus*	Soil
Nystatin	1950	*Streptomyces noursei*	Farm soil, Fauquier County, Va.
Erythromycin	1952	*Streptomyces erythreus*	Soil, Island in Philippines
Novobiocin	1955	*Streptomyces spheroides*	Pastureland, Vermont, U.S.A.
		Streptomyces niveus	
Cycloserine	1955	*Streptomyces orchidaceus*	Soil, Indiana
		Streptomyces gaeryphalus	Soil, Guatemala
Vancomycin	1956	*Streptomyces orientalis*	Soil, Borneo and Indiana
Kanamycin	1957	*Streptomyces kanamyceticus*	Soil, Japan
Paromomycin	1959	*Streptomyces rimosus*	Soil, Columbia
Fusidic acid	1960	*Fusidium coccineum*	Monkey dung, Japan
Lincomycin	1962	*Streptomyces lincolnensis*	Soil, Lincoln, Nebraska
Gentamicin	1963	*Micromonospora purpurea*	Soil, Syracuse, N.Y.

obtaining samples from as many and as varied sources as possible, cultivating them on plates, subcultivating all colonies of promising organisms such as actinomycetes and examining each for anti-bacterial activity. Alternatively the primary plate culture may be inoculated by spraying or by agar layering with suitable bacteria, the growth of which may then be seen to be inhibited in a zone surrounding some of the original colonies. This is only a beginning: many thousands of successive colonies so examined are found to form an antibiotic already known or useless by reason of toxicity.

It will be noticed from Table I that antibiotics have been derived from some odd sources other than soil. Although the original strain of *Penicillium notatum* apparently floated in through a window at St. Mary's Hospital, that of *P. chrysogenum* now used for penicillin production was derived from a mouldy Canteloupe melon in a market at Peoria, Illinois. Perhaps the strangest derivation was that of helenine, an antibiotic with some anti-viral activity, isolated by Shope (1953) from *Penicillium funiculosum* growing on ' the isinglass cover of a photograph of my wife, Helen, on Guam, near the end of the war in 1945 '. He proceeds to explain that he chose the name because it was non-descriptive, non-committal and not pre-empted, ' but largely out of recognition of the good taste shown by the mold . . . in locating on the picture of my wife '.

Those antibiotics out of thousands now discovered which have qualified for therapeutic use are described in chapters which follow.

FUTURE PROSPECTS

All successful chemotherapeutic agents have certain properties in common. They must exert an anti-microbic action, whether inhibitory or lethal, in high dilution, and in the complex chemical environment which they encounter in the body. Secondly, since they are brought into contact with every tissue in the body, they must so far as possible be without harmful effect on the function of any organ. To these two essential qualities may be added others which are highly desirable, although sometimes lacking in useful drugs: stability, free solubility, a slow rate of excretion, and diffusibility into remote areas.

If a drug is toxic to bacteria but not to mammalian cells the probability is that it interferes with some structure or function peculiar to bacteria. When the mode of action of sulphanilamide was elucidated by Woods and Fildes, and the theory was put forward of bacterial inhibition by metabolite analogues, the way seemed open for devising further anti-bacterial drugs on a rational basis. Immense subsequent advances in knowledge of the anatomy, chemical composition and metabolism of the bacterial cell should have encouraged such hopes still further. This new knowledge has been helpful in explaining what drugs do to bacteria, but not in devising new ones. Discoveries have continued to result only from random trials, purely empirical in the antibiotic field, although sometimes based on reasonable theoretical expectation in the synthetic.

Not only is the action of any new drug on individual bacteria still unpredictable on a theoretical basis, but so are its effects on the body itself. Most of the toxic effects of antibiotics have come to light only after extensive use, and even now no one can explain their affinity for some of the organs attacked. Some new observations in this field have contributed something to the present climate of suspicion about new drugs generally, which is insisting on far more searching tests of toxicity, and delaying the release of drugs for therapeutic use, particularly in the United States.

The Present Scope of Chemotherapy

Successive discoveries have added to the list of infections amenable to chemotherapy until nothing remains altogether untouched except the smaller viruses. On the other hand, some of the drugs which it is necessary to use are far from ideal, whether because of toxicity or of unsatisfactory pharmacological properties, and some forms of treatment are consequently less often successful than others. Moreover microbic resistance is a constant threat to the future usefulness of almost any drug. It seems unlikely that any totally new antibiotic remains to be discovered, since those of recent origin have similar properties to others already known. It therefore will be wise to husband our resources, and employ them in such a way as to preserve them. The problems of drug resistance and policies for preventing it are discussed in Chapters XIV and XV.

Adaptation of Existing Drugs

A line of advance other than the discovery of new drugs is the adaptation of old ones. An outstanding example of what can be achieved in this way is presented by the sulphonamides. Similar attention has naturally been directed to the antibiotics, with fruitful results of two different kinds. One is simply an alteration for the better in pharmacological properties. Thus procaine penicillin, because less soluble, is longer acting than potassium penicillin: the esterification of macrolides improves absorption: chloramphenicol palmitate is palatable, and other variants so produced are more stable, more soluble and less irritant.

Most of these changes are produced by additions to the drug molecule, but modifications in its essential structure can alter its anti-microbic properties as well—usually for the worse, but sometimes with advantage. The outstanding success here has been achieved by synthetic manipulation of the molecule of penicillin, since new penicillins have thus been obtained with three desirable properties: resistance to acid, resistance to penicillinase, and enhanced action on some Gram-negative species. Derivatives of cephalosporin C and rifamycin now in clinical use have been obtained in the same way. The present complexity of choice among antibiotics for some types of infection is an embarrassment, resulting largely from these efforts, of which it would be ungrateful to complain.

REFERENCES

ABRAHAM, E. P., CHAIN, E., FLETCHER, C. M., FLOREY, H. W., GARDNER, A. D., HEATLEY, N. G. & JENNINGS, M. A. (1941). *Lancet* **2**, 177.
CHAIN, E., FLOREY, H. W., GARDNER, A. D., HEATLEY, N. G., JENNINGS, M. A., ORR-EWING, J. & SANDERS, A. G. (1940). *Lancet* **2**, 226.
COLEBROOK, L. & KENNY, M. (1936). *Lancet* **1**, 1279.
DOMAGK, G. (1935). *Dtsch. med. Wschr.* **61**, 250.
DUBOS, R. J. (1939). *J. exp. Med.* **70**, 1, 11.
FLOREY, H. W. (1945). *Brit. med. J.* **2**, 635.
FLOREY, H. W. (1949). *Antibiotics,* chap. I. London: Oxford University Press.
FULLER, A. T. (1937). *Lancet* **1**, 194.
HONL, J. & BUKOVSKY, J. (1899). *Zbl. Bakt.* Abt. I. **26**, 305. (See Florey, 1949.)
HÖRLEIN, H. (1935). *Proc. R. Soc. Med.* **29**, 313.
SHOPE, R. E. (1953). *J. exp. Med.* **97**, 601, 627, 639.
TRÉFOUEL, J., TRÉFOUEL, J., NITTI, F. & BOVET, D. (1935). *C.R. Soc. Biol.* (*Paris*) **120**, 756.
WAKSMAN, S. A. & LECHEVALIER, H. A. (1962). *The Actinomycetes,* vol. 3. London: Baillière.

CHAPTER II

SULPHONAMIDES

THE discovery and early history of the sulphonamides are described in Chapter I. The introduction of further compounds has now continued for over 30 years, representing advances in the following directions:—

1. Better tolerance. The frequent nausea and cyanosis caused by sulphanilamide and sulphapyridine were eliminated by the introduction of sulphathiazole and sulphadiazine.
2. Higher anti-bacterial activity. The two compounds just named reached a peak of activity little exceeded by any introduced since.
3. Greater solubility. Some compounds and their derivatives formed in the body are more soluble in urine and thus reduce the risk of renal blockage.
4. Lesser solubility. At this other extreme are compounds relatively so insoluble that they are little absorbed and so act mainly in the bowel.
5. Slower excretion. These latest introductions are the long-acting compounds which enable the frequency of doses to be much reduced.

It no longer seems necessary to include a full account of all these numerous drugs in a work of this kind, particularly since the scope of their therapeutic use has been much diminished by the substitution of antibiotics.

ANTIBACTERIAL ACTIVITY

Sulphonamides have what in an antibiotic is now called a broad spectrum. Among Gram-positive organisms, group A streptococci and pneumococci are highly sensitive, staphylococci and *Cl. welchii* moderately so (other clostridia are more resistant), but *Str. faecalis* is resistant. The most sensitive Gram-negative species are the *Neisseria*, but the list includes many enterobacteria. Thus in the early days sulphonamide treatment was successful in all forms of streptococcal sepsis, pneumococcal pneumonia and other infections, gas gangrene, gonorrhoea and cerebrospinal fever, and some enterobacterial infections of both gastro-intestinal and urinary tracts. Of these uses only the last is now common.

All sulphonamides act alike, and an organism sensitive to one will be sensitive in some degree to all others. Much has been written about the relative degrees of activity of different sulphonamides against individual species. Such findings are difficult to evaluate, because comparisons have rarely been made with more than a few other drugs. A greater difficulty is the strong dependence of the result of any *in vitro* test on the composition of the culture medium and on the size of the inoculum. Because of the magnitude of these effects it is impossible to state the minimum inhibitory concentration (M.I.C.) of a sulphonamide for a given organism with anything approaching the precision such as is possible, for instance, with penicillin, which is little affected by either of these factors.

The results of tests of therapeutic activity in mice are also difficult to interpret in comparative terms, since they also are much affected by the conditions of the experiment. As an example, single doses or doses given only once daily strongly favour long-acting compounds, whereas had they been administered at the usual clinical intervals, a more rapidly eliminated compound might have performed as well or better.

Rather than attempting to review the voluminous and sometimes contradictory literature on the relative *in vitro* activities of different sulphonamides, we have felt it necessary to make our own comparison. The following tests were carried out recently and the results are here published for the first time.

Determinations of the M.I.C. of Different Sulphonamides for Strains of More Important Susceptible Pathogens

DRUGS. Sulphacetamide was chosen as a representative of the earliest and less potent compounds, since alone among them it is still in use. The remainder include the more widely used short-acting compounds and nearly all the recently introduced long-acting. Compounds of low solubility administered only for their effect on the bowel flora are excluded. The drugs were dissolved by adding the minimum necessary amount of NaOH.

BACTERIA. These were mostly recent clinical isolates with approximately normal sulphonamide sensitivity. Some had been kept at −70°C. for varying periods of time.

METHOD. A single batch of Oxoid DST Agar was used throughout. Freshly lysed horse-blood was added in a concentration of 5 per cent, and 14 ml. of medium was mixed in plates with 1 ml. of drug dilution to give final concentrations varying two-fold and based on 1 μg./ml., the whole range used for different organisms varying from 128 to 0·12 μg./ml.

The plates were inoculated with a 32-prong replicator from approximately 1 in 200 dilutions of overnight broth or blood broth cultures. Ditches were cut to isolate areas inoculated with swarming *Proteus*. Plates were read for the presence or absence of growth on the following day. Each organism was tested against the whole range of drugs in a single experiment, always controlled by the inclusion of a standard strain of *Esch. coli* (N.C.T.C. 10418).

The results are given in Table II. They confirm the low activity of sulphacetamide and of sulphadimidine, and the high activity of sulphadiazine, which is equalled and in a few instances exceeded by that of several other compounds, including sulphafurazole and sulphamethoxazole. They conflict in innumerable particulars with the results of others. As an example Neipp (1964) in tests of which the results were quoted (Table III, p. 15) in the last edition of this book, credits sulphadiazine with an incredibly low degree of activity against *Str. pneumoniae*, the M.I.C. being forty times greater than that of sulphamethoxazole. This test was done with a single strain: those in Table II were done with six. For two of these strains the M.I.C. of sulphadiazine and sulphamethoxazole were the same; for the other four they differed only two-fold. Various claims for the superior activity of individual sulphonamides against particular species are not confirmed. We venture to suggest that the findings reported here are more dependable than some comparisons in the literature, because they relate to a wide range of representative sulphonamides, all of which were tested together in one experiment, they were done with multiple strains of all the more important bacteria, and particularly because they were all carried out in the same way on a single batch of a suitable medium.

The main conclusion to be drawn is that there is very little indeed to choose between the antibacterial activities of the more potent sulphonamides. Choice among them should rather depend on their pharmacological properties, and when these are similar it is almost indifferent.

Mode of Action

Woods (1940) postulated that sulphonamides compete with the structurally similar para-aminobenzoic acid for the same enzyme. Para-aminobenzoic acid is incorporated into the co-enzyme folic acid (Hutner *et al.*, 1959) and considerable evidence has accumulated to show that sulphonamide-inhibited organisms exhibit the metabolic signs of folic acid deficiency.

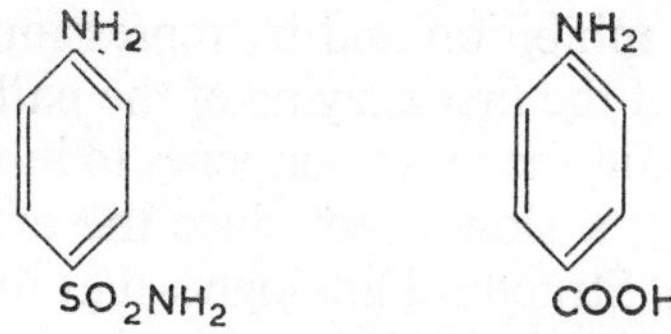

Synthesis of folic acid and its inhibition by sulphonamides has been demonstrated in living *Esch. coli,* and convincing confirmation of Woods' hypothesis has come from the demonstration that purified tetrahydropteroic acid synthetase—the enzyme which condenses para-aminobenzoic acid with 2-amino-4-hydroxy-tetrahydropteridine to form tetrahydropteroic acid, a step in the synthesis of folic acid—is competitively inhibited by sulphonamide (Brown *et al.*, 1961). There is also some evidence that sulphonamides can be incorporated into folic acid-like compounds (Brown, 1962).

Richmond (1966) has argued that for structural analogues to be successful antimicrobial agents, they must function as something more than simple competitive inhibitors. A compound may strongly inhibit an isolated, purified enzyme *in vitro,* but conditions *in vivo* are quite different. In the living cell, substrate is continuously supplied to the enzyme by the previous enzyme in the metabolic pathway, and its product removed by the next enzyme. In this balanced system a steady state is reached in which the quantities of substrate are insufficient to saturate the enzymes. If a competitive inhibitor is added to such a system, the competitor is taken up by the enzyme, and the natural precursor, of which the supply continues, accumulates. In time, the concentration of natural substrate becomes sufficiently high to reverse the effect of the inhibitor and the normal process is resumed—with the ' steady state ' concentration of substrate at a higher level. A successful competitive inhibitor has, therefore, either to have a much higher affinity for the enzyme than has the natural substrate (a very unusual state of affairs since the enzyme has evolved to handle the natural substrate—but evidently the case with sulphonamides) or it must act in some other way.

Control over microbial enzymes is exercised in two main ways: by feed-back inhibition and by repression. The product inhibits the activity of the first enzyme of the pathway—a rapid effect—and also acts on the repressor genes to inhibit the formation of new enzymes, a slow effect since the existing enzymes continue to function. Structural analogues may mimic this effect, which cannot be overcome by increasing the concentration of the natural product, the supply of which is, in any case, cut off by this kind of inhibition. There is some evidence that sulphonamides may owe their action in part to such a mechanism (Richmond, 1966).

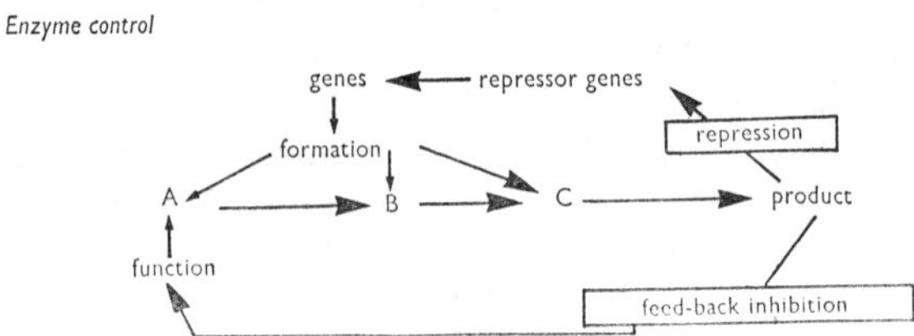

Acquired Bacterial Resistance

Bacteria can be slowly trained to sulphonamide resistance *in vitro,* and every important pathogenic species has sooner or later been found resistant *in vivo.* This change occurred earliest and most rapidly in gonococci, which nevertheless have reverted to sensitivity during the many years which have elapsed since sulphonamide treatment for gonorrhoea was abandoned. A further quarter-century elapsed before it was seen in the closely related meningococcus (Millar *et al.*, 1963). Resistant strains of *Str. pyogenes* and pneumococci began to appear in the early 'forties, and but for the advent of the antibiotics there might by now be no effective specific treatment for the important infections caused by these organisms. Resistance in all enterobacteria is now common, and in *Sh. sonnei* almost invariable. Needless to say, resistance to any sulphonamide is accompanied by resistance to all others.

Some mutants owe their sulphonamide resistance to the synthesis of a folic acid synthetase with a lowered affinity for sulphonamide. Some other mutants appear to owe their resistance to changes in the feed-back mechanism. Some overproduce *p*-aminobenzoic acid (Pato and Brown, 1963), an effect which could result from ' switching off ' the feed-back control, thereby making the organism insusceptible to sulphonamide interference with enzyme production and function (Richmond, 1966).

Combined Action with Other Antibacterial Drugs

Although the effect of sulphonamides is purely bacteristatic, it does not, like that of some similarly acting antibiotics, antagonize the bactericidal effect of penicillin. This is not to say that such a combination is often indicated. With one antibiotic, polymyxin, sulphonamides may act synergically (Herman, 1959; Russell, 1963). By far the most important combination is with trimethoprim, which is so much more effective than a sulphonamide alone that we ventured even in the previous edition of this book to say: " the possibility arises that trimethoprin should also be given whenever sulphonamides are used ". This drug is described in Chapter III.

PHARMACOLOGY

Absorption

Most sulphonamides are well absorbed after oral administration, reaching a peak concentration in the blood after 2-4 hours, which after a dose of 2 g. is of the order of 100 μg./ml. Parenteral preparations of some are available, usually sodium salts, which with the exception of sodium sulphasomizole are strongly alkaline and can only be given intravenously.

Conjugation

After absorption a proportion of the drug is conjugated, usually with acetate, this proportion varying considerably with different compounds. The lower this is the better, since the conjugates are inactive therapeutically and the acetyl derivatives are rather more toxic than the free drug. Their solubility in the urine is also a factor to be considered.

Plasma Binding

Of sulphonamide in the blood a proportion, varying considerably with different compounds, is contained in the red cells, some is free in the plasma, and another proportion, again varying greatly, is bound to plasma albumin. This bound drug is usually considered to be antibacterially inactive (Newbould & Kilpatrick, 1960; Anton, 1960), but the findings of Bøe (1966) suggest that this may be an over-simplified view. He compared the effects of adding different amounts of protein on the activity of sulphadiazine and of sulphadimethoxine, which at the same concentration in plasma are respectively 45·1 per cent and 98·7 per cent protein-bound, and found discrepancies inexplicable on this basis. In this and in a previous paper (Madsen, Øvsthus and Bøe, 1963) it is pointed out that a drug of which 98 per cent is inactive cannot be expected to have much therapeutic effect, and suggested that " the strength of the binding is more important than the extent ".

It will be seen from Figure 2 that the percentage bound varies, although not directly, with the total drug concentration in the blood. It is also affected by the albumin concentration: in hypoalbuminaemia the percentage is much decreased (Anton, 1968). This author also found that the administration of various drugs diminished the bound percentage of sulphadimethoxine, particularly when several were present together. He suggests that such factors operating to reduce the binding of normally highly bound sulphonamides may account for adverse reactions to them.

There is a striking increase in the proportion of drug bound with increase in *p*H, and a fall with increase in sulphonamide concentration (Fig. 2). Protein-bound drug is distributed as protein, and binding consequently affects the concentration of drug entering the tissues from the capillaries. Access to the C.S.F. for example, is normally limited to the unbound drug but with increasing capillary permeability and the passage of protein into the C.S.F. in inflammation, protein-bound sulphonamide enters and the total concentration of sulphonamide in the C.S.F. rises.

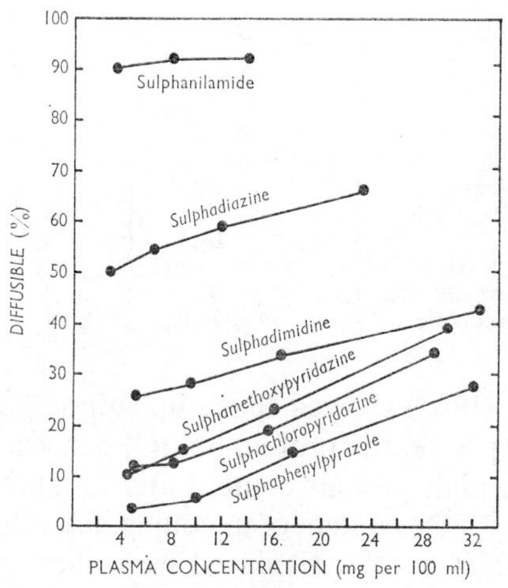

Fig. 2

Effect of increasing concentration of various sulphonamides on binding of sulphonamide to plasma-proteins at pH 7·4.

Redrawn from Newbould and Kilpatrick (1960).

It will be seen from Table III that the very large differences in the extent of protein binding shown in Figure 2 are reflected in the relationships between concentrations attained in the C.S.F. and those in the blood.

While the effective concentration of sulphonamide at any instant is represented only by the unconjugated, diffusible fraction, it must not be supposed that the protein-bound fraction plays no part in antibacterial action. If this were so, sulphonamides like sulphamethoxypyridazine which are very strongly bound to protein would have very little therapeutic effect. The erythrocyte and protein-bound fractions of the drug are in equilibrium with the unconjugated diffusible drug in the plasma and as this is utilized, more drug is released from binding.

TABLE III

	Approximate Concentration in C.S.F. when Concentration in Plasma is 1·0	Percentage of Drug bound to Plasma Proteins
Sulphanilamide	1·0	5-20
Sulphapyridine	0·5 -0·8	10-45
Sulphathiazole	0·15-0·4	55-80
Sulphadiazine	0·4 -0·8	20-60
Sulphamerazine	0·3 -0·8	60-80
Sulphadimidine	0·3 -0·8	60-80
Sulphafurazole	0·3 -0·5	
Sulphasomidine	0·2 -0·5	
Sulphamethizole	<0·1	
Sulphamethoxypyridazine	0·1	90
Sulphadimethoxine	0·1 -0·15	
Sulphamethoxydiazine	0·3	75
Sulphamethoxazole	0·3 -0·5	60-70

Madsen *et al.* (1963) showed that sulphadimethoxine, of which more than 90 per cent is protein-bound, penetrates readily into exudates with high protein content and its antibacterial effect corresponds with the content of unconjugated drug.

Sulphonamides can be displaced from their protein binding sites by a variety of compounds including phenylbutazone and ethyl-bis-coumarin, and simultaneous administration of these substances produces higher concentrations of diffusible sulphonamide (Anton, 1961). This competition for plasma albumin binding sites is also responsible for the effect of sulphonamide in displacing albumen-bound bilirubin (see p. 25).

PASSAGE THROUGH PLACENTA. Sulphonamides pass readily through the placenta into the foetal circulation and the possible dangers of this to the foetus must be remembered when treating pregnant women with sulphonamides (p. 25).

Excretion

The plasma level of free sulphonamide depends on the rate of absorption, the rate and extent of conjugation, and above all, on the rate of excretion. Sulphonamides are excreted mainly in the urine, the free drug and its conjugates being frequently excreted at different rates and by different mechanisms. As a result, the peak plasma concentrations of free drug and conjugate may occur at different times and the proportion of free drug to conjugate may be very different in the plasma and urine.

As with isoniazid (p. 403), the capacity to inactivate sulphadimidine is bimodally distributed in the population, those who acetylate most (62-90 per cent) of the drug being clearly different from those who acetylate only 40-53 per cent (Evans and White, 1964). Active acetylators of sulphadimidine correspond with rapid inactivators of isoniazid. Sulphanilamide and PAS appear to be so readily acetylated that no similar polymorphism is apparent in the population. Studies with liver from rapid and slow acetylators (Evans and White, 1964) showed that the polymorphism lies in the activity of hepatic acetyl transferase, the enzyme which transfers the acetyl group from acetyl-coenzyme 1 to the drug. Whether rapid acetylators possess more enzyme or a more active enzyme is not yet established. Genetically, the capacity for rapid acetylation is an autosomal dominant character, *i.e.* is transmitted by a single gene. The distribution of this character varies greatly in different populations.

Sulphonamides are partly filtered through the glomeruli and partly secreted by the tubules, where some of the excreted drug is reabsorbed. The extent of these processes differs amongst the sulphonamides and may differ markedly for the free drug and its conjugates. For example, 50 per cent of sulphamethoxazole is reabsorbed by the tubules whereas its acetyl derivative is actively excreted. The sum of the effect of glomerular filtration, tubular secretion and readsorption, is seen in the plasma clearance values which vary from <10 to >200 ml./min. Substances with high clearances like sulphafurazole are rapidly eliminated from the plasma and achieve high concentrations in the urine. Substances with low clearances are slowly excreted, plasma levels are maintained for long periods, and low concentrations appear in the urine. With substances like sulphadimethoxine and sulphamethoxypyridazine, which have clearance values around 10 ml. per minute, therapeutic levels are present in the plasma for about 24 hours, and it is not necessary to give the drug more than once a day. If renal function is impaired, excretion may be still further delayed and therapeutic levels may persist for considerably longer. Equally, if such drugs are given repeatedly, high and possibly toxic levels may develop. Naturally no protein-bound drug escapes through the kidney, and therefore highly protein-bound compounds are in general long-acting, but correspondence between the two properties is far from exact because of differences in the degree of tubular re-absorption, which may be a major factor in maintaining the plasma level.

Excretion in Bile. Less than 1 per cent of the dose of the older sulphonamides is excreted in the bile but the proportion is greater (2·4-6·3 per cent) for the new long-acting compounds (Neipp *et al.*, 1961).

TOXICITY

There has been a tendency recently to exaggerate the ill effects produced by these drugs. Proper choice of compound and reasonable dosage can ensure that such effects will be uncommon.

The cyanosis frequently caused by the earliest compounds is now almost never seen, and such effects as nausea and vomiting, headache and dizziness have become very exceptional. Several other distinct types of possible effect require separate consideration.

Renal Blockage

The first edition of this book (Barber & Garrod, 1963) contained a full page table of the solubilities of 17 sulphonamides and of their conjugates in urine at 4 different ranges of pH. It is now perhaps enough to say that all are more soluble in alkaline than acid urine, that long-acting compounds present little danger because of their slow rate of excretion, and that among others only sulphapyridine (no longer used), sulphathiazole, sulphadiazine and sulphamerazine have dangerously low solubilities. The risk of giving even these and even in maximum doses can be much diminished by giving alkali and enough fluid to ensure a good output of urine, although sulphamerazine may be an exception to this. Triple mixtures containing them render the risk almost negligible. Failing such precautions crystals deposited in the urine may block either the renal tubules or the upper orifice of the ureter. Haematuria is a common early sign.

Hypersensitivity Reactions

Protein-bound sulphonamide can function as a haptene, and the usual result of antibody formation is moderate fever with a urticarial or maculo-erythematous rash occurring on about the ninth day of a course of treatment. Repetition after an interval will elicit the reaction immediately. No one can say why this occurs in some patients and not in others, nor is it clear that the degree of protein binding is a direct determinant, but some compounds, particularly sulphathiazole, are much more liable to produce the reaction than others.

'Polyarteritis nodosa'. Sulphonamides have frequently figured amongst the drugs administered to patients who subsequently developed polyarteritis nodosa. While the role of the drug is not settled (Rose and Spencer, 1957) it is possible that allergy to sulphonamide-modified protein is implicated in the auto-sensitizing process believed to underly the condition.

Stevens-Johnson syndrome. This fortunately rare but frequently fatal variety of erythema multiforme has been described as an occasional complication of sulphonamide therapy (Salvaggio and Gonzales, 1959). The etiology of the condition is unknown, but it has been supposed that like polyarteritis nodosa it may sometimes result from allergy to sulphonamide-modified endogenous protein. The relative dangers of different sulphonamides cannot be accurately assessed but those which persist in plasma for prolonged periods present a double hazard. They are extensively bound to plasma proteins—and to this extent are more liable to function as haptenes—and their persistence means that toxic manifestations may continue to develop for days after cessation of therapy. A number of reports have described the condition following treatment with long-acting sulphonamides (Beveridge *et al.*, 1964) and the F.D.A. collected 116 cases in which it was believed these drugs were implicated (Carroll, Bryan and Robinson, 1966). The majority (79) were under the age of 15 and there were 20 deaths. Of the 37 adults, 9 died. The time of onset varied from 2 to 24 days, sometimes as long as 6 days after discontinuing the drug.

2

It was estimated that there had been about 1 or 2 cases per 10 million doses distributed.

EFFECTS OF APPLICATION TO THE SKIN. Local treatment of skin conditions with sulphonamides is now recognized as contra-indicated because a very intractable type of sensitization may result, manifested at first by a local dermatitis, later by extension of this to other areas, and sometimes by fever, and persistence of the reaction long after the treatment has been stopped.

TESTS OF SULPHONAMIDE SENSITIVITY. Patients who have developed eczematous dermatitis after local sulphonamide therapy usually react to a simple patch test, in which 50 per cent sulphonamide powder in hydrous lanoline is applied to the skin after light scarification. Patients who have developed hypersensitivity after internal administration show no reaction to skin tests with sulphonamides alone but usually show a typical immediate allergic reaction when tested by the intradermal injection of serum from a patient containing at least 20 μg. per ml. of the appropriate sulphonamide.

In keeping with the role of delayed hypersensitivity in contact dermatitis, Caron and Sarkarny (1965) claimed that lymphocytes from a sulphonamide-sensitive patient when cultured *in vitro* and exposed to sulphonamide, underwent transformation and mitosis similar to that seen when tuberculin-sensitive cells are exposed to tuberculin.

Blood Dyscrasias

AGRANULOCYTOSIS. The commonest effect of sulphonamides on the bone marrow is a depression of leucopoiesis, and this rarely proceeds to agranulocytosis. Modern sulphonamides seem less liable to have this effect than the earlier (Yow, 1953). Before concluding that a sulphonamide is responsible, the prescription sheet should be reviewed. Discombe (1952), having seen necropsies on three patients from one surgical unit within a month where deaths from agranulocytosis were attributed to sulphapyridine, found that each of them had also been given a proprietary sedative which, unknown to the prescriber, contained amidopyrin. It seems possible here that two marrow depressants had acted synergically.

Haemolytic anaemia

Sulphonamides, like a number of other drugs, tend to oxidize haemoglobin to methaemoglobin, and this effect is normally combated through the activity of glucose-6-phosphate dehydrogenase. In patients with inherited deficiency of this enzyme, treatment with sulphonamides may cause denatured haemoglobin to accumulate in the red cells in the form of Heinz bodies, and intravascular haemolysis and haemoglobinuria to occur.

Jaundice

Jaundice resulting from liver damage is a very rare complication of sulphonamide treatment in the adult.

Bilirubin is transported in the blood bound to plasma albumin and a number of drugs, including some sulphonamides (O'Dell, 1959), compete for the binding sites and so interfere with bilirubin excretion. Sulphonamides administered to pregnant women cross the placenta and may circulate in the foetus for several days or even weeks (Sparr and Pritchard, 1958; Lucey and Driscoll, 1961). Interference with bilirubin transport during this period may increase the free plasma bilirubin level and result in kernicterus. For this reason, sulphonamides should not be given to pregnant women where there is a possibility of rhesus incompatibility, premature delivery, or any history of previous neo-natal jaundice. Sulphonamides should not be given to neonates and this is especially important in premature infants in whom bilirubin conjugation is particularly imperfectly developed.

Embryopathy

There have been several reports of teratogenic activity in experimental animals by some long-acting sulphonamides (Paget and Thorpe, 1964), but in a retrospective study, Cahal (1965) found no evidence of embryopathy in man.

CLINICAL APPLICATIONS

Sulphonamides have a wide antibacterial range, yet they do not produce the troublesome disturbances of gut flora which frequently occur with other broad spectrum agents, notably the tetracyclines. They are active not only against staphylococci, haemolytic streptococci, pneumococci and meningococci, but also against many enterobacteria including some species resistant to common antibiotics. It has also been claimed—though the evidence for this is not particularly good —that sulphonamides may usefully augment the action of antibiotics in the treatment of a variety of infections.

Although severe toxic manifestations have been described and some authors (Murdoch, 1964) have condemned sulphonamides on this account, severe reactions are uncommon and treatment for 14 days with conventional doses of current sulphonamides rarely gives rise to trouble. From amongst the thousands that have been synthesized a sulphonamide can be chosen which possesses almost any desirable pharmacological attribute: free absorption from the gut with high blood levels, wide distribution in the body, and ready penetration into the C.S.F.; little or no absorption from the gut; rapid excretion with high urinary concentrations; or very slow excretion with prolonged blood levels. In addition to all this, sulphonamides are cheap and very stable.

In short, except for the fact that they are not bactericidal, sulphonamides approximate closely to the ideal antibacterial agent.

Despite this, absolute indications for their use are very few since the same effect can usually be achieved more rapidly with an antibiotic. Their principal use is for the treatment of urinary tract infection. Their applicability to the treatment of respiratory tract infection is more doubtful, and their value in alimentary tract infection has diminished owing to increasingly frequent resistance in enteropathogenic bacteria. The less soluble compounds remain useful in combination with neomycin for pre-operative suppression of the bowel flora. Some still regard sulphonamides as a useful adjunct in treating pneumococcal and *H. influenzae* meningitis, but their reliability as the sole treatment for meningococcal meningitis is threatened by the emergence of resistant strains. Among more exotic uses, sulphonamides appear currently to be the best treatment for nocardiosis, and, in combination with pyrimethamine, for toxoplasmosis, and perhaps for pyrimethamine-resistant malaria (p. 50).

It is a tenable position that except for a few special purposes, such as pre-operative suppression of the gut flora, sulphonamides should no longer be prescribed alone, but only in combination with trimethoprim, a drug which greatly enhances their effect. Its properties, and the wider indications which exist for this combined treatment, are described in the following chapter.

CHOICE OF A SULPHONAMIDE

There is no present need for the existence of so many different sulphonamides, and in our view there is no longer any need to attempt to balance their individual merits by a consideration of all the properties in which they differ. The following brief account only categorizes them and refers to some of the properties of those in commonest use.

Sulphonamides for General Use

Among the older compounds, sulphanilamide has been discarded because of its low activity, sulphacetamide for the same reason (except for use as eye drops) and sulphapyridine because of its toxicity. The following remain for consideration.

SULPHATHIAZOLE B.P.C. (2-sulphanilamido-thiazole) is highly potent, but peculiarly liable to cause side effects, and is now rarely prescribed alone.

SULPHADIAZINE B.P.C. (2-sulphanilamido-pyrimidine). This compound has the advantages of high potency, a rate of excretion such that adequate blood concentrations are easily maintained, and low protein binding, facilitating diffusion into the tissues and cerebrospinal fluid. Hence it is often regarded as the best choice for treating meningitis. Renal blockage has to be guarded against.

SULPHAMERAZINE (2-sulphanilamido-4-methylpyrimidine) is less potent than sulphadiazine, more highly protein-bound, more slowly excreted, and peculiarly liable to cause renal blockage. It is therefore unsuitable for administration alone in full doses.

SULPHADIMIDINE B.P. (2-sulphanilamido-4 : 6-methylpyrimidine; sulphamezathine, sulphamethazine). This compound is well absorbed, and excreted moderately slowly. Both the drug and its acetyl derivative are highly soluble, which renders the chance of renal blockage remote, and toxic effects of other kinds and sensitivity reactions are rare. These properties account for its high popularity in this country, but in others this does not obtain: in the United States, for instance, consumption is very small and diminishing (Zbinden, 1964). A good reason for this is its low potency: the concentrations required to inhibit many species according to our findings (Table II) are up to 8-fold higher than those of sulphadiazine, and according to Neipp (1964) some of these differences are much greater. Similar although less extreme differences have been observed in the curative doses for experimental infections. It also suffers by comparison with sulphadiazine in being acetylated to a greater degree and much more highly protein-bound (Fig. 2).

Sulphadimidine has evidently given satisfaction in clinical use, and it may seem unjustified to detract from its merits on largely theoretical grounds. It must nevertheless be pointed out that advantage can be taken of the higher potency of other compounds, and some of the risks of using them can be reduced by the use of one of the following combinations.

TRIPLE SULPHONAMIDES. The mixture originally advocated by Lehr contained 37 per cent of each of sulphadiazine and sulphathiazole and 26 per cent of sulphamerazine. Its main advantage is that each drug retains its individual solubility in the urine, and since the dose of each is small, so is the risk of renal blockage: indeed if adequate fluids and alkali are given it may well be negligible. Other advantages claimed are a reduced risk of sensitization reactions and the maintenance of a steadier blood level. Several modifications of the original " sulphatriad " are now in use.

Highly Soluble Compounds

The following are highly soluble, even in acid urine, in which they attain high concentrations, and have been largely used for treating urinary tract infections.

SULPHAFURAZOLE B.P. (3:4-dimethyl - 5 - sulphanilamido-isoxazole, sulfisoxazole, U.S.P., Gantrisin). According to our findings (Table III) this compound is highly active, and if given in sufficiently frequent doses to compensate for its rapid excretion, should serve for treating infections elsewhere as well as in the urinary tract.

SULPHAMETHIZOLE, B.P. (2-sulphanilamido-5-methyl-1:3:4-thiodiazole, Urolucosil, Thiosulphil).

SULPHACHLORPYRIDAZINE (3-sulphanilamido-6-chloropyridazine, Cosulid). This compound is credited with particularly high activity against *Esch. coli*. Table III confirms this, but the differences are small.

SULPHASOMIDINE B.P. (6-sulphanilamido-2:4-dimethylpyrimidine, sulphadimetine, Elkosin). This compound appears rather less active than sulphafurazole. It has also been used as a general purpose sulphonamide.

Compounds of Low Solubility

SUCCINYLSULPHATHIAZOLE B.P. (2(p-succinyl-sulphanilamido)-thiazole), sulfasuxidine, and Phthalylsulphathiazole B.P. (2(*p*-phthalyl-sulphanilamido)-thiazole, sulphathalidine) are very little absorbed and owe their activity to the slow liberation of sulphathiazole in the bowel. They may be given together with an antibiotic for pre-operative suppression of the bowel floral. (Sulphaguanidine B.P.C. is less suitable for this purpose because less potent and more absorbed.)

Long-Acting Compounds

These are further divisible into three categories according to their rate of excretion. " Medium "-long-acting, with half-lives such that two daily doses are given, include the following:

SULPHAMETHOXAZOLE (5-methyl-3-sulphanilamido-isoxazole, Gantanol) has a high potency (Table II) and is the compound with which trimethoprim is combined in the present commercial preparations of this drug.

SULPHASOMIZOLE (5-sulphanilamido-3-methyl-isothiazole, Bidizole). The only sulphonamide forming a sodium salt yielding a neutral solution, and thus suitable for intramuscular injection.

SULPHASYMAZINE (2-sulphanilamido-4, 6-diethyltriazine) has been used mainly for treating urinary tract infections: its rate of excretion can be accelerated 5-fold by alkalinizing the urine (Frisk & Hultman, 1966).

The best known long-acting compounds, of which only one daily dose need be given, are:

SULPHAMETHOXYPYRIDAZINE B.P. (3-sulphanilamido-6-methoxy-pyridazine, Lederkyn, Midicel).

SULPHADIMETHOXINE, B.P.C. (2 : 4-dimethoxy-6-sulphanilamido-1 : 3-diazine, Madribon).

SULPHAPHENAZOLE B.P.C. (3-sulphanilamido-2-phenylpyrazole, Orisulf).

SULPHAMETHOXYDIAZINE (2-sulphanilamido-5-methoxypyrimidine, Durenate).

Among these compounds sulphadimethoxine is the most highly protein-bound and sulphamethoxydiazine the least. Various merits have been claimed for each of them and some of these were discussed in previous editions of this book. According to our findings (Table II) none possesses any outstanding *in vitro* activity, and that of sulphaphenazole is distinctly inferior against all enterobacteria in contrast to the high activity against *Str. pyogenes*. No advantage is clearly discernible in their use except the convenience of a single daily dose, and against this has to be set the possible extra risk referred to on page 23.

Finally, much the longest acting compound is SULFADOXINE (formerly sulphormethoxine, 4-*p*-aminobenzenesulphonamido -5, 6-dimethoxypyrimidine, Fanasil) with which adequate blood levels can be maintained by giving 1 g. once a week. This compound has been commended for the prophylaxis of rheumatic fever and cerebrospinal fever, for the treatment of chronic bronchitis (Pines, 1967) and, rather surprisingly, in view of the low concentrations resulting from such slow excretion in the urine, for the single dose treatment of urinary tract infections (Grüneberg and Brumfitt, 1967). It also has an action in malaria (Laing, 1964). How liable this drug is to cause side effects seems still uncertain.

Sulphonamides for Special Uses

MARFANIL. This simple compound, *p*-aminomethylbenzene sulphonamide, now available as the hydrochloride under the name *sulfamylon,* has an interesting history. Synthesised in the U.S.A. where it was soon abandoned as being only feebly active, it was used by the Germans during the war, evidently with great success, as a local application to wounds for the prevention of gas gangrene. It has recently come into its own again as a local preparation for burns (page 315). It is active against *Ps. aeruginosa.* It rapidly diffuses through burned skin and is unusual in that it is not neutralised by *p*-aminobenzoic acid or tissue exudates.

SULPHASALAZINE. This compound of sulphapyridine and salicylic acid (*p*-(benzolsulphanyl-(amino-α-pyridine))-azo-salicylic acid, Salazopyrin, Azopyrin) is used almost exclusively for treating ulcerative colitis. The prolonged courses usually given are liable to cause side effects, including fever and rashes and blood dyscrasias. In a double blind trial, Baron *et al.* (1962) found sulphasalazine effective in acute attacks of ulcerative colitis, but side-effects are common. Truelove, Watkinson and Draper (1962) found corticosteroid therapy to be superior. In a controlled trial of sulphasalazine as maintenance therapy for ulcerative colitis, Misiewicz *et al.* (1965) found that the drug reduced the relapse rate.

PHARMACEUTICAL PREPARATIONS AND DOSAGE

PHTHALYL SULPHATHIAZOLE (Sulphathalidine, *Merck, Sharp and Dohme;* Thalazole, *May and Baker*)
Tablets, B.P., B.N.F.: 500 mg.; Mixture: 500 mg. per 5 ml. Dose: 5-10 g. daily in divided doses.

SUCCINYLSULPHATHIAZOLE (Sulfasuxidine, *Merck, Sharp and Dohme*)
Tablets, B.P., B.N.F.: 500 mg.; Mixture: 500 mg. per 5 ml. Dose: 10-20 g. daily in divided doses.

SULPHADIAZINE (Adiazine, *Fr.;* Microsulfon, *U.S.A.*)
Tablets, B.P., B.N.F.: 500 mg. Dose: Initial 3 g.; Subsequent: up to 4 g. daily in divided doses.

SULPHADIMETHOXINE (Madribon, *Roche*)
Tablets, B.P.: 500 mg.; U.S.N.F.: 250 and 500 mg.; Suspension, U.S.N.F.: 250 mg. per 5 ml. Dose: Initial: 1-2 g.; Subsequent: 500 mg. daily.

SULPHADIMIDINE (Sulphamethazine, *U.S.P.;* Sulphamezathine, and S-mez, *I.C.I.*)
Tablets, B.P., B.N.F.: 500 mg. Dose: *Systemic infections*: Initial: 3 g.; Subsequent: up to 6 g. daily in divided doses. *Urinary infections*: Initial: 2 g.; Subsequent: up to 4 g. daily in divided doses.

SULPHAFURAZOLE (Sulfisoxazole, *U.S.P.;* Gantrisin, *Roche*)
Tablets, B.P., B.N.F., U.S.P.: 500 mg. Dose: As for sulphadimidine. Sulphafurazole diethanolamine: Equiv. 2 g. sulphafurazole in 5 ml. Dose i/m: Not to exceed oral dose of sulphafurazole. Not more than 5 ml. one site.

SULPHAGUANIDINE
Tablets, B.P.C.: 500 mg. Dose: 10-20 g. daily in divided doses.

SULPHAMETHIZOLE (Urolucosil, *Warner;* Sulfurine, Thiolsulfil, Ultrasul, *U.S.A.*)
Tablets, B.P., B.N.F.: 100 mg.; U.S.N.F.: 250 mg. Suspension U.S.N.F.: 250 mg. per 5 ml. Dose: 100-200 mg. 4-6 hourly.

SULPHAMETHOXAZOLE (Gantanol, *Roche*)
Tablets, 500 mg. Syrup. 500 mg. per 5 ml. Dose: Initial: 2 g.; Subsequent: 1 g. 12 hourly. Not more than 3 g. per day.

SULPHAMETHOXYDIAZINE (Durenate, *F.B.A.* and Schering, *A.G.*)
Tablets, B.P.: 500 mg. Suspension 500 mg. per 5 ml. Dose: Initial: 1-2 g.; Subsequent: 500 mg. daily.

SULPHAMETHOXYPYRIDAZINE (Lederkyn, *Lederle;* Midicel, *Parke Davis*)
Tablets, 500 mg.; Suspension: 250 mg. per 5 ml. Dose: Initial: 1 g.; Subsequent: 500 mg. daily.

SULPHAPHENAZOLE (Orisulf, *Ciba*)
Tablets, B.P.C.: 500 mg. Suspension: 500 mg. per 5 ml. Dose: Initial: 1 g. 12 hourly for 2 days; Subsequent: 500 mg. 12 hourly.

SULPHASALAZINE (Salazopyrin, Asulfidine, *Pharmacia*)
Tablets, B.N.F.: 500 mg. Dose: 1 g. 4-6 hourly.

SULPHASOMIDINE (formerly Elkosin, *Ciba;* Aristamid, *Ger.*)
Tablets, B.P.: 500 mg. Dose: As for sulphadimidine.

SULPHASOMIZOLE (formerly Bidizole, *May and Baker;* Amidozol, *Fr.*)
Tablets, 500 mg. Dose: Initial: 1 g.; Subsequent: 500 mg. 12 hourly. Injection: Sodium sulphasomizole 1 g. in 3 ml. Dose i/m: Initial: 1-2 g. daily for 1-3 days; Subsequent: 1 g. daily; i/v: 1 g. in 250 ml. saline over 2-3 hours.

SULFADOXINE (Fanasil, *Roche*)
Tablets, 200, 500 mg. Injection: 1 g. in 4 ml. Dose: 1-2 g. as a single dose once weekly.

TRISULFAPYRIMIDINES (*equal parts sulphadiazine, sulphadimidine, sulpha-merazine;* numerous similar preparations)
Tablets, U.S.P.: 500 mg. Suspension, U.S.P.: 500 mg. per 5 ml. Dose: Initial: 4 g.; Subsequent: 1 g. 4 hourly.

REFERENCES

ANTON, A. H. (1960). *J. Pharmacol. exp. Ther.* **129**, 282.
ANTON, A. H. (1961). *J. Pharmacol. exp. Ther.* **134**, 291.
ANTON, A. H. (1968). *Clin. Pharmacol. Ther.* **9**, 561.
BARBER, M. & GARROD, L. P. (1963). *Antibiotic and Chemotherapy*, p. 26. Edinburgh: Livingstone.
BARON, J. H., CONNELL, A. M., LENNARD-JONES, J. E. & AVERY JONES, F. (1962). *Lancet* **1**, 1094.
BEVERIDGE, J., HARRIS, M., WISE, G. & STEVENS, L. (1964). *Lancet,* **2**, 593.
BØE, O. (1966). *Acta path. microbiol. scand.* **68**, 81.
BROWN, G. M., WEISMAN, R. A. & MOLNAR, D. A. (1961). *J. biol. Chem.* **236**, 2534.
BROWN, G. M. (1962). *J. biol. Chem.* **237**, 536.
CAHAL, D. A. (1965). In *Embryopathic Activity of Drugs,* ed. Robson, J. M., Sullivan, F. M. & Smith, R. L. London: Churchill.
CARON, G. A. & SARKANY, I. (1965). *Brit. J. Dermat.* **77**, 556.
CARROLL, O. M., BRYAN, P. A. & ROBINSON, R. J. (1966). *J. Amer. med. Ass.* **195**, 691.
DISCOMBE, G. (1952). *Brit. med. J.* **1**, 1270.
EVANS, D. A. P. & WHITE, T. A. (1964). *J. Lab. clin. Med.* **63**, 394.
FRISK, A. R. & HULTMAN, E. (1966). *Antimicrob. Agents & Chemother.* 1965, p. 672.
GRÜNEBERG, R. N. & BRUMFITT, W. (1967). *Brit. med. J.* **3**, 649.
HERMAN, L. G. (1959). *Antibiotic Ann.* (1958-9) p. 836.
HUTNER, S. H., NATHAN, H. A. & BAKER, H. (1959). *Vitamins and Hormones* **17**, 1.
LAING, A. B. G. (1964). *Brit. med. J.* **2**, 1439.
LUCEY, J. F. & DRISCOLL, T. J. (1961). In *Symposium on Kernicterus,* 1959. Toronto: Toronto University Press.
MADSEN, S. T., ØVSTHUS, Ø. & BØE, J. (1963). *Acta med. Scand.* **173**, 707.
MILLAR, J. W., SIESS, E. E., FELDMAN, H. A., SILVERMAN, C. & FRANK, P. (1963). *J. Amer. med. Ass.* **186**, 139.
MISIEWICZ, J. J., LENNARD-JONES, J. E., CONNELL, A. M., BARON, J. H. & AVERY JONES, F. (1965). *Lancet* **1**, 185.
MURDOCH, J. McC. (1965). *Practitioner* **194**, 26.
NEIPP, L. (1964). In *Experimental Chemotherapy,* vol. 2, p. 169, ed. Schnitzer, R. J. & Hawking, F. New York & London: Academic Press.
NEWBOULD, B. B. & KILPATRICK, R. (1960). *Lancet* **1**, 887.
O'DELL, G. B. (1959). *J. Paediat.* **55**, 268.
PAGET, G. E. & THORPE, E. (1964). *Brit. J. Pharmacol.* **23**, 305.
PATO, M. L. & BROWN, G. M. (1963). *Arch. Biochem. Biophys.* **103**, 443.
PINES, A. (1967). *Brit. med. J.* **3**, 202.
RICHMOND, M. H. (1966). *Symp. Soc. gen. Microbiol.* **16**, 301.
ROSE, G. A. & SPENCER, H. (1957). *Quart. J. Med.* **26**, 43.
RUSSELL, F. E. (1963). *J. clin Path.* **16**, 362.
SALVAGGIO, J. & GONZALEZ, F. (1959). *Ann. intern. Med.* **51**, 60.
SPARR, R. A. & PRITCHARD, J. A. (1958). *Obstet. Gynaec.* **12**, 131.
TRUELOVE, S. C., WATKINSON, G. & DRAPER, G. (1962). *Brit. med. J.* **2**, 1708.
WOODS, D. D. (1940). *Brit. J. exp. Path.* **21**, 74.
YOW, E. M. (1953). *Amer. Practit.* **4**, 521.
ZBINDEN, G. (1964). *Molecular Modification in Drug Design.* Advances in Chemistry Series No. 45, p. 25. Washington D.C.: American Chemical Society.

CHAPTER III

OTHER SYNTHETIC ANTIMICROBIAL AGENTS

SYNTHETIC agents active against mycobacteria are discussed in Chapter 25, those active against virus infections in Chapter 27, and those used principally or exclusively as topical applications in Chapter 18.

HEXAMINE

This agent, hexamethylenetetramine, was for many years the only drug capable of killing bacteria in the urine. It has no action *per se*, but in an acid medium is slowly decomposed with the liberation of formaldehyde. The odour of sweat is partly due to the action of skin bacteria and hexamine is included in some deodorant preparations where on contact with acid sweat it liberates formalin which inhibits bacterial activity. It is absorbed from the gut and mainly excreted unchanged in the urine. Because of the effect of acid, formalin will be liberated in the stomach unless the drug is given in enteric coated tablets. To ensure that this reaction shall be adequate in the urine the pH needs reducing to about 5·0. The treatment is therefore inapplicable to infection with any urea-splitting organism. All micro-organisms are susceptible to the action of formaldehyde, and hexamine may still have a place in treating infection by yeasts (*Candida* or *Torula*), which are completely resistant to antibiotics, and by otherwise resistant coliform bacilli. Some patients on the drug complain of frequent and burning micturition and it is still sometimes recommended that these side-effects be controlled by giving alkali—so guaranteeing an absence of any effect. Prolonged administration or high dosage may produce albuminuria, haematuria and bladder changes.

MANDELIC ACID and HEXAMINE MANDELATE

MANDELIC ACID. α-hydroxy-α-phenylacetic acid: white odourless crystals which turn yellow on exposure to light and should be protected. The therapeutic action of the ketogenic diet led to the identification by Rosenheim of mandelic acid as a drug which exerted an identical effect with much less trouble, expense and discomfort. Mandelic acid is excreted unchanged by the kidney, and is itself bactericidal: its action, like that of hexamine, is improved by reduction of the pH. All kinds of infections (again except that due to urea-splitting bacteria) are susceptible to it. It would undoubtedly be still a popular urinary antiseptic had not the introduction of the sulphonamides followed close on the heels of its discovery.

HEXAMINE MANDELATE. The two earlier drugs now seem rarely to be given alone: they have been ousted in popularity by this preparation, in which they are joined as a chemical compound. The pharmacological behaviour of this drug needs further elucidation (Garrod, 1959), but it can render the urine bactericidal, and certainly liberates formaldehyde. Since both of its components require an acid medium for activity, it should only be given when the urine is or can be rendered acid, and treatment should be controlled by daily pH estimations, if only by the use of multiple indicator papers. To give it to any patient whose urine remains alkaline is futile. The necessary pH 5 of the urine may only be achieved by giving acidifying agents such as ammonium chloride, or methionine which works by increasing the output of urinary sulphates. The large doses necessary may lead to central nervous disturbances, and gastro-intestinal upset is often such as to cause patients to abandon the treatment.

As with hexamine, excessive treatment may give rise to dysuria or haematuria, and occasional central nervous and gastrointestinal disturbances have been reported.

METRONIDAZOLE

1-(2-Hydroxyethyl)-2-methyl-5-nitroimidazole: an almost white crystalline powder, soluble 100 mg./ml. water; 5 mg./ml. alcohol; and 4 mg./ml. chloroform. Metronidazole is a potent trichomonacide, active in a concentration of about 2·5 μg./ml. It is inactive against candida and the majority of bacteria, but it is effective against Vincent's organisms, and has been shown to inhibit the Nicol's strain of *Tr. pallidum* in a concentration of 3·6-9·5 μg./ml. (Wilkinson *et al.*, 1967). It is absorbed by mouth, doses of 200 mg. producing serum levels of 2·5-13 μg./ ml. About 60 per cent is excreted in the urine (about 70 per cent in the unchanged form) giving levels of 50-390 μg./ml. It also appears in the saliva, peak levels up to 9·7 μg./ml. being found 3 hours after a 200 mg. dose on the third day of treatment (Stephen *et al.*, 1966).

Toxicity

Nausea, a metallic taste in the mouth, or furry tongue are fairly common. Rashes, central nervous symptoms, dysuria and dark urine have been occasionally reported. Leucopenia has been described but the changes are generally insignificant (Peterson *et al.*, 1967). Disulfiram-like flushing and hypotension are sufficiently common and severe in those taking alcohol while receiving metronidazole for the drug to have been used in the treatment of chronic alcoholism (Merry and Whitehead, 1968).

Clinical Use

The principal use of metronidazole is in the treatment of trichomoniasis in which it has generally been very successful. Re-treatment, intensive treatment or additional measures are required in some patients (p. 364). Metronidazole is as effective as penicillin in the treatment of Vincent's infection (p. 347). Its anti-spirochaetal effect has led to trials of its use in syphilis but it is considered inferior to penicillin. Its only importance in that connection is that it may lead to misdiagnosis since the serum of patients receiving the drug may immobilise treponemes in the T.P.I. test (Wilkinson *et al.*, 1967). Metronidazole has also been successfully used (in a dosage of 500 mg. daily for 5 days) in the treatment of giardiasis and (in a dosage of 800 mg. thrice daily) in the treatment of amoebiasis (Powel *et al.*, 1966).

NALIDIXIC ACID

1-Ethyl-7-methyl-4-oxo-1, 8-naphthyridine-3-carboxylic acid, was synthesized by Lesher *et al.* (1962). Its pale yellow crystals are slightly soluble in water and soluble in dilute alkali; solutions withstand autoclaving. It is active principally against Gram-negative organisms, the majority of which, with the exception of *Ps. aeruginosa,* are inhibited by 10 μg. per ml. or less. Gram-positive organisms are relatively resistant (Barlow, 1963).

Antibacterial Activity

The minimum inhibitory concentrations of nalidixic acid for common bacterial species are shown in Table IV. Nalidixic acid is bactericidal, although for some organisms concentrations substantially in excess of the M.I.C. are required. It is believed that nalidixic acid produces a lethal desynchronisation of bacterial metabolism by preventing the incorporation of precursors into DNA while permitting uninterrupted synthesis of RNA and protein (Cook *et al.,* 1966). Resistance is easily produced by serial passage of organisms in increasing concentrations of the drug and sometimes emerges during the treatment of patients (Atlas *et al.,* 1969).

TABLE IV

Sensitivity of Bacteria to Nalidixic Acid

	M.I.C. μg./ml.		M.I.C. μg./ml.
Staph. aureus	50	N. meningitidis	0·5-5
Str. pyogenes	500	H. influenzae	1-75
Str. pneumoniae	250	Brucella spp	7·5-10
Str. faecalis	500	Esch. coli	3·0-7·5
C. diphtheriae	500	Proteus spp	2·5-20
B. anthracis	75	Klebsiella spp	1·6-50
Clostridium spp	12·5-800	Salmonella spp	2·5-75
M. tuberculosis	250	Shigella spp	2·5-50
		Pseudomonas aeruginosa	4·0-500
		Bacteroides spp	200

Deitz, W. H., *et al.* (1964) Antimicrob. Agents Chemother.-1963, p. 584 Feldman, H. A. and Melnyk, C. *ibid*-1964, p. 440; Finegold, S. M. *et al., ibid*-1966, p. 189.

Absorption and Excretion

In serum, the drug is bound by protein with resultant decrease in antibacterial activity but the binding is readily reversed by dilution. The drug is readily absorbed from the gut and about 80 per cent of the dose is rapidly excreted in the urine, partly unchanged and partly as derivatives some of which are also antibacterially active. McChesney *et al.* (1964) found average peak plasma levels in normal subjects of about 25 μg./ml. following a dose of 1 g., the plasma half-life being about 1½ hours. About 4 per cent of 4 g. given over 12 hours appeared in the faeces. Excretion has been reported to be impaired in the premature infant but not in older children. Buchbinder *et al.* (1963) found no accumulation of the drug on a 6-hourly regimen of 1-2 g., the blood levels being <3·9-62·5 μg./ml.

The metabolites and their determination are discussed by McChesney *et al.* (1964) who found peak urine concentrations 3-5 hours after 500 mg. of 275 μg./ml. and 925 μg./ml. conjugated. The amount of free drug excreted was increased in alkaline urine.

Toxicity and side-effects

Nausea, rashes and C.N.S. disturbances, including seizures, have occurred in patients receiving the drug but these are usually transient and are not regarded as an indication for limiting the use of the drug. A two-week-old child developed haemolytic anaemia apparently as a result of the excretion of nalidixic acid in the breast milk of its treated mother (Belton and Jones, 1965). Studies in pregnant animals have not revealed any embryopathic effects and a number of pregnant patients have been treated without untoward effects. There is however no direct evidence that the drug may be safely given early in pregnancy. Caution is advised in giving the drug to patients with impaired renal, hepatic, or respiratory function.

Clinical Use

Nalidixic acid has been successfully used for the treatment of acute, chronic, and recurrent urinary tract infection, for the control of proteus infection by instillation into the bladder and for the prophylaxis of transurethral operations to cover the period of catheterization (Newman *et al.*, 1966; Conaghan and Ward-McQuaid, 1966).

NITROFURANS

Four nitrofuran compounds intended for different antibacterial uses are available : nifuratel (p. 432), nitrofurazone, applied locally, furazolidone, given for intestinal infections, and nitrofurantoin given for urinary infections. Some preparations available in the U.S.A. for local use contain nifuroxime (*anti*-2-hydroxyimino-methyl-5-nitrofuran). Many other nitrofurans have been synthesized. Some show superior antibacterial activity *in vitro* and some have had successful clinical trials, but none is at present commercially available. Furaltadone (Altafur) was at one time marketed as a broad-spectrum antibacterial agent for systemic use, but was subsequently withdrawn (Editorial, 1961).

Furazolidone

3 - (5 - Nitrofurfurylideneamino) - 2 - oxo - oxazolidine :   yellow odourless crystals almost insoluble in water and alcohol, slightly soluble in chloroform. Protect from light.

Furazolidone is bactericidal to a wide range of Gram-positive and negative organisms. In a dosage of 100 mg. 6-hourly (5 mg./kg./day for children) for 4-14 days, it has been successfully used for the treatment of a variety of bacterial gastrointestinal infections including salmonellosis and shigellosis. Similar treatment for 7 days is described as very effective in the eradication of *Giardia lamblia* infestation. Headache, nausea, diarrhoea, rashes and alcohol intolerance may occur.

Table V

Antibacterial Activity of Nitrofurans

	M.I.C. Nitrofurazone $\mu g./ml.$	M.I.C. Nitrofurantoin $\mu g./ml.$
Staph. aureus	10	4-30
Str. pyogenes	10	10
Str. viridans	25	8
Str. faecalis	25	4-125
N. gonorrhoeae	10	15
Esch. coli	10	0·4->250
Proteus spp	40	7·5->200
Klebsiella-Aerobacter spp	10-20	25->200
Salmonella spp	5-10	5-15
Shigella spp	5	5
Ps. aeruginosa	>200	>200

NITROFURANTOIN

1 - (5 - Nitrofurfurylideneamino) - hydantoin: yellow odourless crystals discoloured by alkalis and exposure to light from which it should be protected. Soluble: 50 μg./ml. alcohol; and 60 mg./ml. dimethylformamide. Its solubility in water increases markedly with pH: from 220 μg./ml. at pH 4·0 to 2·3 mg./ml. at pH 7·7.

Antibacterial Activity

Nitrofurantoin is active against many organisms responsible for urinary infection, particularly *Esch. coli. Ps. aeruginosa* and some *Klebsiella-Aerobacter* and *Proteus* strains are insensitive (Table V). The M.I.C. may greatly increase with increasing size of inoculum. It is bactericidal in concentrations not much above the M.I.C. but its activity may be reduced as much as 100-fold at pH 8 as compared with pH 5·5, and a bactericidal effect may only be obtained in an acid medium.

Resistant variants may be produced by passage in the presence of the drug and have been observed to emerge during the treatment of patients. There is no cross-resistance with other important antibacterial agents but nitrofurantoin antagonises *in vitro* the action of nalidixic acid and the two agents should not be prescribed together (p. 271).

A variety of biochemical abnormalities have been observed in organisms exposed to nitrofurantoin but its precise mode of action is unknown (Waterbury *et al.*, 1966).

Absorption and Excretion

Nitrofurantoin is well absorbed by mouth and rapidly excreted in the urine but very low levels appear in the plasma, apparently partly as the result of rapid tissue breakdown. Only about a third of the dose can be recovered from the urine. The peak plasma level appears 1-2 hours after an oral dose and has been found by many workers not to exceed 2·5 μg./ml. What little drug is present soon disappears, the plasma half-life being about 20 min. (Reckendorf *et al.*, 1963). Urine levels are usually in the range 15-46 μg./ml. and levels above the M.I.C. for the most sensitive organisms are detectable for about 6 hours.

Much higher levels are obtainable with intravenous infusion of sodium nitrofurantoin (not commercially available in this country) and some success has been claimed for this form of systemic therapy. Following conventional oral doses, the concentrations in milk and amniotic fluid are insignificant and the concentration in cord blood generally less than the maternal level (Perry and LeBlank, 1967). Since the maternal levels are so low there is little danger of foetal toxicity. Levels in prostatic fluid were only about $\frac{1}{4}$-$\frac{1}{2}$ the plasma level (Dunn and Stamey, 1967).

Nitrofurantoin is excreted by the kidney both in the glomerular filtrate and by tubular secretion. The drug is a weak acid and in alkaline urine about a third is reabsorbed by non-ionic back diffusion in the distal tubule. Calculations suggest that this could result in peri-tubular concentrations of the drug of the order of 12-48 μg/ml.—sufficient to exert a useful antibacterial effect (Shirmeister *et al.*, 1966). Direct assays of renal lymph (supposed to reflect the composition of renal interstitial fluid) have shown concentrations about twice those of the plasma. In azotaemic patients little appears in the urine and at the same time, there is some plasma accumulation of the drug and of potentially toxic metabolites resulting from its rapid breakdown. Nitrofurantoin is consequently contraindicated in renal failure (Sachs *et al.*, 1968).

Toxicity and side-effects

Nausea, vomiting and gastrointestinal upset may occur but are seldom severe enough to require withdrawal of treatment. Skin sensitization rarely occurs. There have been reports of anaphylaxis following nitrofurantoin, none fatal (Satter, 1966). Skin testing was unreliable. In some elderly patients a few days' therapy has been followed by dramatic onset of chills, cough and breathlessness resembling cardiac failure. Eosinophilia may be a striking feature of these. Peripheral neuropathy has developed in a number of patients sometimes following excessive treatment, but usually in those with impaired renal function. Onset may be sudden with increasing distal sensory disturbances, severe pain, depressed reflexes, and muscular wasting progressing to severe disablement. Heffelfinger and

Allen (1964) add a case of nitrofurantoin neurotoxity in a child. Treatment with 50 mg. 6 hourly was inadvertently continued for 94 days when the child was ataxic with numb extremities and wrist and foot drop. Recovery was complete 8 weeks after stopping treatment.

The neurotoxicity is evidently not simply an exaltation of the effects of uraemia since impaired nerve conduction can be demonstrated in normal subjects treated with conventional doses (Toole *et al.*, 1968). A possible role for folic acid deficiency in neuropathy has been considered since megaloblastic anaemia develops in occasional patients, perhaps as a toxic effect of the hydantoin moiety of nitrofurantoin. As with a number of other drugs, haemolytic episodes may occur in patients with G-6-PD deficiency (Pritchard *et al.*, 1965).

Clinical use

For practical purposes the use of nitrofurantoin is restricted to urinary tract infection (p. 370). Most success has been achieved with sensitive *Esch. coli* (Turck *et al.*, 1967). The low plasma levels achieved by the oral route make such treatment useless for systemic infection. Much higher and doubtless more toxic levels can be obtained by continuous intravenous infusion of sodium nitrofurantoin (not commercially available in this country) and some success has been claimed for such treatment of peritonitis and Gram-negative bacteraemia (Fadhli and Cross, 1965; Litvak and Melnick, 1966).

TRIMETHOPRIM

Trimethoprim, 2,4-diamino-(3,3,5-trimethoxybenzyl) pyrimidine was synthesized in the Burroughs Wellcome Laboratories, N.Y. (Hitchings and Bushby, 1961) and was released for general therapeutic use (as a mixture with sulphamethoxazole) in 1969. It is a weak base with a pKa of about 7·3 soluble to the extent of 44 μg./ml. water. The lactate is much more soluble: 50 mg./ml. water. It is active in concentrations achievable in the plasma against all the common pathogenic bacteria except mycobacteria and pseudomonas (Table VI). Its effect is predominantly bacteristatic.

TABLE VI

Sensitivity of bacteria to trimethoprim

	M.I.C. μg./ml.		M.I.C. μg./ml.
Staph. aureus	0·2–1	N. gonorrhoeae	8–128
Str. pyogenes	0·4–1	N. meningiditis	8
Str. pneumoniae	0·5–2	H. influenzae	0·12–1
Str. viridans	0·25	Bord. pertussis	3
Str. faecalis	0·25–0·5	Esch. coli	0·01–1
C. diphtheriae	0·4	K. pneumoniae	0·5–2
Cl. perfringens	50·0	Ent. aerogenes	1–3
M. tuberculosis	250	Proteus spp.	1–4
		Salmonella spp.	0·01–0·4
		Shigella spp.	0·4
		Ps. aeruginosa	100

Bushby, S. R. M. (1969) *Postgrad. med. J.* **45** (Suppl. Nov) 10; Waterworth, P. M. (1969) *ibid.*, p. 21; Williams *et al.* (1969) *ibid.*, p. 71.

Trimethoprim acts in the same sequential metabolic pathway as sulphonamide (a feature of great therapeutic importance) and is subject to the same difficulties of *in vitro* sensitivity testing due to the presence of inhibitors in the medium. The extent to which these difficulties can be overcome in practice by the use of suitable media containing lysed blood is discussed on page 462. Since trimethoprim is effective therapeutically, such inhibitors cannot be present in tissues in a form or concentration sufficient to interfere materially with the drug's action.

Mode of Action

All cells use forms of tetrahydrofolate as cofactors in the incorporation of 1-carbon fragments into the precursors of purines, thymidilate, serine and methionine. Amongst these essential reactions the synthesis of thymidilate has a special importance in that tetrahydrofolate is not only the carrier but the reductant of the 1-carbon fragment. As a result tetrahydrofolate is oxidized to dihydrofolate and must be regenerated by reduction—a process which is brought about through the agency of the enzyme dihydrofolate reductase. Inhibition of this enzyme is a general property of 2:4 diaminopyrimidines, but these compounds exhibit remarkable selectivity in that modification of the molecule can greatly increase the activity against the enzyme of one species while decreasing it against another (Hitchings, 1969).

Amongst therapeutically important examples of this class of agent, pyrimethamine inhibits mammalian and bacterial enzymes approximately equally but only in a concentration about 2000 times that needed to produce comparable inhibition of the plasmodial enzyme. In contrast, trimethoprim is extremely active against the bacterial enzyme, much less active against the plasmodial enzyme, and very feebly active against the mammalian enzyme which requires for comparable inhibition about 50,000 times the concentration which inhibits the bacterial enzyme, and 2000 times that which inhibits the plasmodial enzyme. Although its anti-plasmodial effect is plainly much less than its anti-bacterial effect, it is nevertheless sufficient to produce a useful degree of anti-malarial activity.

Differential affinity for the enzymes of different species is clearly of great importance in determining the selective toxicity of trimethoprim but there is an additional important difference in the way in which animals and parasites obtain their folate requirements. Bacteria and protozoa synthesize folic acid from para-aminobenzoic acid, while man and animals utilize preformed folic or folinic acid (leucovorin) from the diet. These two processes appear to be mutually exclusive: parasites which synthesize folic acid cannot absorb it preformed, and man and animals which absorb it preformed cannot synthesize it.

This difference has two important consequences. Firstly, any depressant effect of diaminopyrimidines on human folate metabolism may be overcome by feeding tetrahydrofolate supplements which the parasite cannot utilize (Whitman, 1969). Secondly, since sulphonamides inhibit the incorporation by parasites of p-aminobenzoic acid into dihydrofolate, sulphonamides and trimethoprim act sequentially in the same metabolic pathway. As a result, their combined action with sulphonamides is strongly synergic. There is about a 10-fold increase in activity when the agents are given together (Hitchings, 1961). Figure 3 shows the difference between parasite and human folic acid metabolism diagrammatically, and indicates the point at which sulphonamides and such folic acid antagonists as pyrimethamine and trimethoprim work.

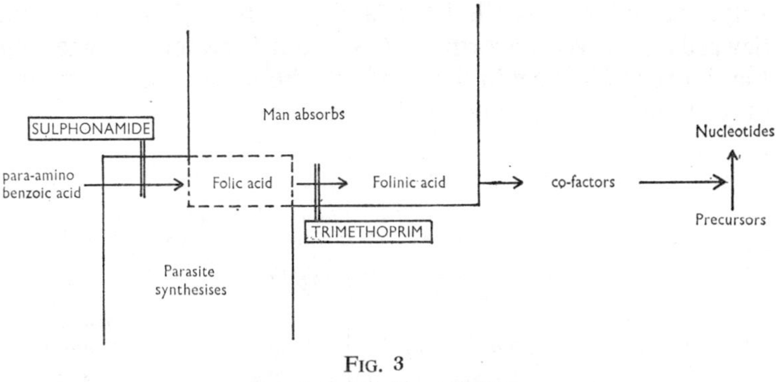

Fig. 3
Based on Hitchings (1961).

Synergy

The resulting increased activity of the two drugs when used together is readily demonstrated by any of the standard methods, and in chess-board titrations gives rise to a symmetrical isobologram (p. 272). This means that maximum potentiation occurs when the drugs are present in the ratio of their M.I.C.s. For example, an organism sensitive to 1 μg./ml. trimethoprim and 20 μg./ml. sulphonamide, will show maximum inhibition when exposed to a 1:20 mixture. This is the optimum ratio for many organisms, but for others proportionately more trimethoprim is required. Some (of which the neisseria are an important example) are more susceptible to sulphonamide than trimethoprim and the ratio must be reversed. An idea of the magnitude of increased susceptibility of various organisms to one drug in the presence of subinhibitory concentrations of the other is given in Table VII. In addition to lowering the concentration required to inhibit growth the mixture may be bactericidal, where either drug alone is bacteristatic.

Combinations of sulphonamides and folic acid antagonists can be further potentiated by the addition of purine antagonists (Hitchings, 1961: see Fig. 3). This approach led to the demonstration that *cyclo* guanil palmoate will protect man for months against challenge with *Plasmodium vivax* or *P. falciparum* (Elslager and Worth, 1965).

Polymyxin, which appears to damage membranous structures in bacteria (Merrick, 1965), acts synergically both with sulphonamides (Russell, 1963) and with trimethoprim (Noall, Sewards and Waterworth, 1962) against proteus, suggesting that it exerts its effect in the same metabolic sequence—presumably at the level of purine synthesis or beyond.

TABLE VII

Degree of potentiation of trimethoprim by sulphonamide

| | M.I.C. ($\mu g./ml.$) | | Mean Potentiation Factor* |
	Sulphafurazole	Trimethoprim	
Staph. aureus	4-8	0·12-0·5	5.4
Str. pyogenes	1-16	0·25-0·5	7
Str. pneumoniae	2-128	0·5-2	8·4
N. gonorrhoeae	0.5-8	32-64	25
H. influenzae	0.5-64	0·01-·0125	3·5
Esch. coli	4-32	0·12-0·5	5·7
Klebsiella spp.	8-64	0·5-1	4·6
Pr. mirabilis	4-16	0·5-2	26
Pr. vulgaris	4-16	0·5-2	10
Salmonella spp.	16-128	0·06-0·25	2·4
Shigella spp.	4-16	0·03-0·5	6·2

*Factor by which the M.I.C. of trimethoprim is reduced by presence of 9 parts of sulphafurazole (in the case of *N. gonorrhoeae*, 3 parts of sulphafurazole): Darrell *et al.* (1968) *J. clin. Path.*, **21**, 202.

Resistance

Organisms can be rendered resistant to trimethoprim *in vitro* by serial passage in increasing concentrations of the drug, enterobacteria becoming resistant to 500 $\mu g./ml.$ or more, after 12-35 passages (Bushby, 1969). Organisms capable of transferring resistance to other antibiotics have so far failed to transfer acquired resistance to trimethoprim (Bushby, 1969; Waterworth, 1969). Resistance has emerged in the course of treatment of patients infected with klebsiella and haemophilus. Such emergence of resistance so relatively early in the drug's therapeutic history must again be taken as a warning that it should not be used for infections which are almost certainly not of bacterial origin, for trivial infections which do not require antibacterial therapy, or for infections which can equally successfully and conveniently be treated with something else.

Synergy between the drugs is so marked that potentiation of trimethoprim by sulphonamide may be seen even in organisms which require such high concentrations of sulphonamide for inhibition that they would ordinarily be regarded as sulphonamide-resistant. Bushby (1969) found that of 194 strains resistant to 120 μg. or more sulphonamide/ml., 57 showed increased susceptibility to trimethoprim in the presence of 20 parts of sulphonamide. *Str. faecalis* which is generally regarded as solidly sulphonamide-resistant, also showed enhancement of trimethoprim inhibition in the presence of sulphonamide.

Absorption and Excretion

Trimethoprim is rapidly and near-completely absorbed from the gut, giving peak plasma levels of about 0·9-1·2 μg./ml. $1\frac{1}{2}$-$3\frac{1}{2}$ hours after a dose of 100 mg., and 2·2-3·2 μg./ml. after 250 mg. At these concentrations, 42-46 per cent of the drug is protein-bound. The plasma half-life is 6-12 hours (Schwartz and Ziegler, 1969). Excretion of the drug is almost wholly via the urine giving levels of 50-100 μg./ml. of which less than 8 per cent is in conjugated inactive forms. About 70 per cent of the drug is excreted in the first 24 hours, but detectable levels are present in the urine for 4-5 days during which time about 90 per cent of the dose can be recovered.

Sharpstone (1969) found the renal clearance of trimethoprim in the normal subject to be 19-148 ml./min., the wide variation being accounted for to a large extent by the influence of pH. Trimethoprim is a weak base and urinary excretion rises sharply with falling pH as the drug ionises and non-ionic back-diffusion in the tubules decreases. Trimethoprim clearance declines with renal function, but less rapidly than that of creatinine so that at the poorest function levels, trimethoprim clearance exceeds that of creatinine (supporting other evidence that the drug is partly excreted by active tubular secretion) and therapeutic concentrations of the drug are still found in the urine.

CHOICE OF MATCHING SULPHONAMIDE. In order to maintain in treated patients a ratio of trimethoprim to sulphonamide as close as possible to the synergic optimum, it was necessary to choose a sulphonamide with absorption and excretion characteristics as close as possible to those of trimethoprim. Sulpha-methoxazole was a particularly happy choice for this purpose since it combines pharmacokinetic behaviour closely similar to that of trimethoprim with high antibacterial activity (Table II).

The available preparations contain 5 times as much sulpha-methoxazole as trimethoprim and this produces a plasma level of sulphamethoxazole about 20-25 times the simultaneous level of trimethoprim, so achieving the optimum synergic ratio. Against *Neisseria* infections the optimum ratio is markedly different and it may be that for the treatment of infections with these organisms other formulations would be preferable (Garrod, 1969). Similarly, in renal failure differences in hand-ling of the two compounds may disturb the plasma ratio and dosage of the two components may need to be suitably adjusted if treatment of such patients is contemplated (Sharpstone, 1969).

Toxicity and Side Effects

Nausea, vomiting (occasionally severe enough to require withdrawal of treatment) and skin rashes have occurred in some patients. From now on, with the drug available only as a ready-made mixture with sulphamethoxazole, it will not be immediately plain which component is responsible for any re-actions which occur. The most serious forseeable toxic effect of trimethoprim is the induction of folate deficiency. The very low affinity of the drug for the mammalian enzyme and the possibility of by-passing any depressant effect by feeding folate supplements (which cannot be utilized by the parasite—p. 44) makes the likelihood of serious haematological disorder seem relatively remote.

Nevertheless it is plain that folate metabolism in man does not entirely escape the attentions of trimethoprim. In 10 sub-jects receiving the large dose of 1 g. per day, Whitman (1969) found bone marrow abnormalities in 8, and FiGlu excretion in 5. There was no evidence of abnormality in subjects re-ceiving 200 mg. per day, and O'Grady *et al.* (1969) found no evidence of folate deficiency in patients treated with small doses (see p. 381) for periods up to three years.

In the rat, doses greater than 200 mg/kg/day were teratogenic, but complete protection was afforded by leucovorin or dietary folate supplements. No abnormalities were produced in the rabbit (Udall, 1969). Williams *et al.* (1969) treated 120 patients with bacteriuria of pregnancy, half of whom were more than half way towards delivery, but 10 were less than 16 weeks pregnant, and in none of their infants was there any abnormality.

Clinical Use

The range of pathogens against which trimethoprim-sulphonamide combinations exert potent antibacterial effects opens up a wide field of potentially successful therapeutic exploration which has been reviewed by Garrod (1969).

There are records of highly successful treatment of septicaemia due to *Proteus* (Noall *et al.*, 1962; Cooper and Wald, 1964) and *Escherichia* (Darrell *et al.*, 1968) in which other treatment had completely failed. Success rates of 80-98 per cent are claimed in the treatment of gonorrhoea (Csonka, 1969; Schofield *et al.*, 1969) and the response of typhoid fever to the drug evidently compares favourably with that to chloramphenicol (Akinkugbe *et al.*, 1968; Pugsley *et al.*, 1969). The principal use of the drug so far, however, has been in the control of urinary and respiratory infections.

Treatment of urinary infection in hospitalised patients (Brumfitt *et al.*, 1969) and bacteriuria of pregnancy (Williams *et al.*, 1969) has produced cure rates (as judged by sterility of the urine one week after cessation of treatment) around 85 per cent. Encouraging results have also been obtained in the treatment of intractable infections of the urinary tract (Cox and Montgomery, 1969) and O'Grady *et al.* (1969) maintained ' sterile ' urine in 26/31 patients with long-standing urinary infections (many of whom had abnormalities of the urinary tract) for periods up to three years with a dosage which was progressively reduced until the majority of patients were receiving only one tablet twice a week (p. 381).

Disappointingly few agents of therapeutic value have emerged from the extensive attempts to synthesize bacterial antimetabolites which have now been pursued for many years. It is encouraging to see this important field of attempted genera-tion of new antimicrobial agents rewarded with so potent a substance as trimethoprim.

PYRIMETHAMINE

This agent, 2, 4-diamino-5-*p*-chlorophenyl-6-ethylpyrimidine, is principally used as a malaria suppressant, but has also been successfully given for the treatment of leishmaniasis and toxoplasmosis. In effective anti-parasitic doses the drug is more active than trimethoprim against mammalian dihydrofolate reductase and evidence of folate deficiency is more commonly seen during treatment. Its depressant effect on haemopoiesis disappears on withdrawing the drug and can be reversed during treatment by leucovorin.

Hurly (1959) showed that the minimum clearance dose of pyrimethamine for *Plasmodium falciparum* and *P. vivax* was reduced to about a tenth when sulphadiazine—which would not itself clear the parasites—was given simultaneously, and McGregor, Williams and Goodwin (1963) showed that the combination was effective against pyrimethamine-resistant malaria. It was while exploring the possibility that pyrimethamine-resistant *P. vivax* infection might respond to a combination of pyrimethamine and long-acting sulphonamide that Laing (1964) found that sulphadoxine, which gives therapeutic levels for a week following a single one gram dose, is by itself a potent schizonticide. Combinations of sulphonamide and pyrimethamine, shown to be superior to either drug alone in experimental toxoplasma infection, are at present the treatment of choice for human toxoplasmosis (Nolan and Rosen, 1968).

PHARMACEUTICAL PREPARATIONS AND DOSAGE

FURAZOLIDONE (' Furoxone ', *Smith, Kline and French*)
   Tablets B.P.C. 100 mg.; Suspension 100 mg./tablespoon (14 ml.). Dose: 400 mg. daily in divided doses.

HEXAMINE (' Methenamine ', *U.S.N.F.*)
   Tablets, B.P.C., U.S.N.F. 300 mg. and 500 mg. (should be dissolved in a large volume of water). Mixture, B.P.C. 650 mg. in 15 ml. Dose: 0.6-2 g. after meals.

HEXAMINE MANDELATE ('Methenamine mandelate', *U.S.P.;* 'Mandelamine' *Warner* and other proprietary names)
   Tablets 250 and 500 mg. Suspensions 250 and 500 mg. in 5 ml. Dose: 1 g. up to 4 times daily.

MANDELIC ACID usually given as *ammonium mandelate* (Mixture, *N.W.F.*
1 g./5 ml. Dose 15 ml. in water 3 times daily) or as *calcium mandelate*
(granules or suspension). Dose: 3 g. 4 times daily.

METRONIDAZOLE ('Flagyl', *May and Baker*)
Tablets B.P., B.N.F. 200 mg. Dose: 600 mg. daily in divided doses for
7 days.

NALIDIXIC ACID ('Negram', *Bayer Products*)
Tablets, B.N.F. 500 mg. Dose: 4 g. daily in divided doses.

NITROFURANTOIN ('Berkfurin', *Berk;* 'Furadantin', *Smith, Kline and French,*
'Furan', *Chelsea Drug and Chemical Co.*)
Tablets, B.P., B.N.F. 50 mg.; U.S.P. 50 mg. and 100 mg. Mixture, B.N.F.
25 mg. in 5 ml. Oral suspension, U.S.P. 0·5 per cent w/v. Dose: 50-150 mg.
6 hourly.

PYRIMETHAMINE ('Daraprim', *Burroughs Wellcome,* 'Malodice', *Specia*)
Tablets, B.P., U.S.P., B.N.F. 25 mg.; Elixir 6·25 mg./5 ml. Dose: (leishmaniasis and toxoplasmosis) 25-50 mg. daily.

TRIMETHOPRIM: Drapsules ('Bactrim', *Roche*) Tablets ('Septrin', *Burroughs
Wellcome*)
80 mg. trimethoprim + 400 mg. sulphamethoxazole; Paediatric tablets
20 mg. trimethoprim + 100 mg. sulphamethoxazole. Suspension 40 mg.
trimethoprim + 200 mg. sulphamethoxazole/5 ml. Adult dose: 1-2 tablets
(drapsules) twice daily.
Severe infections 2 tablets (drapsules) 3 times daily.

REFERENCES

AKINKUGBE, O. O., LEWIS, E. A., MONTEFIORE. D. & OKUBADEJO, O. A.
(1968). *Brit. med. J.* **3**, 721.
ATLAS, E., CLARK, H., SILVERBLATT, S. & TURCK, M. (1969) *Ann. intern. Med.,*
70, 713.
BARLOW, A. M. (1963). *Brit. med. J.* **2**, 1308.
BELTON, E. M. & JONES, R. V. (1965). *Lancet* **2**, 691.
BRUMFITT, W., FAIERS, M. C., PURSELL, R. E., REEVES, D. S. & TURNBULL,
A. R. (1969). *Postgrad. med. J.* **45** (Suppl. Nov.), 56.
BUCHBINDER, M., WEBB, J. C., ANDERSON LaV. & McCABE, W. R. (1963).
Antimicrob. Agents Chemother.—1962, p. 308.
BUSHBY, S. R. M. (1969). *Postgrad. med. J.,* **45** (Suppl, Nov.), 10.
CONAGHAN, J. P. and WARD-McQUAID, J. N. (1966). *Brit. J. Urol.* **38**, 199.
COOK, T. M., BROWN, K. G., BOYLE, J. V. & GOSS, W. A. (1966). *J. Bact.*
92, 1510.
COOPER, R. G. & WALD, M. (1964). *Med. J. Aust.* **2**, 93.
COX, C. E. & MONTGOMERY, W. G. (1969). *Postgrad. med. J.* **45** (Suppl.
Nov.), 65.
CSONKA, G. W. (1969). *Postgrad. Med. J.* **45** (Suppl. Nov.), 77.
DARRELL, J. H., GARROD, L. P. & WATERWORTH, P. M. (1968). *J. clin. Path.*
21, 202.
DUNN, B. L. & STAMEY, T. A. (1967). *J. Urol.* **97**, 505.
EDITORIAL (1961). *Brit. med. J.* **1**, 264.
ELSLAGER, E. F. & WORTH, D. F. (1965). *Nature (Lond.)* **206**, 630.
FADHLI, H. A. & CROSS, F. S. (1965). *Amer. J. Surg.* **109**, 160.
GARROD, L. P. (1959). *Roy. Coll. Physns. Edin.*, Publtn. No. 11.
GARROD, L. P. (1969). *Postgrad. med. J.* **45** (Suppl. Nov.), 52.
HEFFELFINGER, J. C. & ALLEN, R. J. (1964). *J. Pediat.* **65**, 611.
HITCHINGS, G. H. (1960-1961). *Trans. N.Y. Acad. Sci.* **23**, 700.
HITCHINGS, G. H. (1969). *Postgrad. med. J.* **45** (Suppl. Nov.), 7.
HITCHINGS, G. H. & BUSHBY, S. R. M. (1961). *Proc. 5th int. Cong. Biochem.*
(*Moscow*), *Sect.* **7**, p. 165. London. Pergamon.

HUGHES, D. T. D. (1969). *Postgrad. med. J.* **45** (Suppl. Nov.), 86.
HURLY, M. G. D. (1959). *Trans. roy. Soc. trop. Med. Hyg.* **53,** 412.
LAING, A. B. G. (1964). *Brit. med. J.* **2,** 1439.
LESHER, G. Y., FROELICH, E. J., GRUETT, M. D., BAILEY, J. H. & BRUNDAGE, R. P. (1962). *J. med. pharm. Chem.* **5,** 1063.
LITVAK, A. S. & MELNICK, I. (1966). *J. Urol.* **96,** 107.
McCHESNEY, E. W., FROELICH, E. J., LESHER, G. Y., CRAIN, A. V. R. & ROSI, D. (1964). *Toxicol. appl. Pharmacol.* **6,** 292.
McGREGOR, I. A., WILLIAMS, K. & GOODWIN, L. G. (1963). *Brit. med. J.* **2,** 728.
MERRICK, J. M. (1965). *J. Bact.* **90,** 965.
MERRY, J. & WHITEHEAD, A. (1968). *Brit. J. Psychiat.* **114,** 859.
NEWMAN, R. L., HOLT, R. J. & FRANKCOMBRE, C. H. (1966). *Arch. Dis. Child.* **41,** 389.
NOALL, E. W. P., SEWARDS, H. F. G. & WATERWORTH, P. M. (1962). *Brit. med. J.* **2,** 1101.
NOLAN, J. & ROSEN, E. S. (1968). *Brit. J. Ophthal.* **52,** 396.
O'GRADY, F., CHAMBERLAIN, D. A., STARK, J. E., CATTELL, W. R., SARDESON, J. M., FRY, I. K., SPIRO, F. I. & WATERS, A. H. (1969). *Postgrad. med. J.* **45** (Suppl. Nov.), 61.
PERRY, J. E. & LeBLANK, A. L. (1967). *Texas Rep. Biol. Med.* **25,** 265.
PETERSON, W. F., HANSEN, F. W., STAUCH, J. E. & RYDER, C. D. (1967). *Amer. J. Obstet. Gynec.* **97,** 472.
PINES, A., GREENFIELD, J. S. B., AAFAT, H. R., RAHMAN, M. & SIDDIQUI, A. M. (1969). *Postgrad. med. J.* **45** (Suppl. Nov.), 89.
POWELL, S. J., MacLEOD, I., WILMOT, A. J. & ELSDON-DEW, R. (1966). *Lancet* **2,** 1329.
PRITCHARD, J. A., SCOTT, D. E. & MASON, R. A. (1965). *J. Amer. med. Ass.* **194,** 457.
PUGSLEY, D. J., MWANJE, L.. PEARSON, C. & BLOWERS, R. (1969). *Postgrad. med. J.* **45** (Suppl. Nov.), 95.
RECKENDORF, H. K., CASTRINGIUS, R. G. & SPINGLER, H. K. (1963). *Antimicrob. Agents Chemother.*—1962, p. 531.
RUSSELL, F. E. (1963). *J. clin. Path.* **16,** 362.
SACHS, J., GEER, T., NOELL, P. & KUNIN, C. M. (1968). *New Engl. J. Med.* **278,** 1032.
SATTER, E. J. (1966). *J. Urol.* **96,** 86.
SCHIRMEISTER, J., STEFANI, F., WILLMANN, H. & HALLAUER, W. (1966). *Antimicrob. Agents Chemother.*—1965, p. 223.
SCHOFIELD, C. B. S., MASTERTON, G., MOFFET, M. & McGILL, M. I. (1969). *Postgrad. med. J.* **45** (Suppl. Nov.), 81.
SCHWARTZ, D. E. & ZIEGLER, W. H. (1969). *Postgrad. med. J.* **45** (Suppl. Nov.), 32.
SHARPSTONE, P. (1969). *Postgrad. med. J.* **45** (Suppl. Nov.), 38.
STEPHEN, K. W., McLATCHIE, M. F., MASON, D. K., NOBLE, H. W. & STEVENSON, D. M. (1966). *Brit. dent. J.* **121,** 313.
TOOLE, J. F., HAYES, D. M. & FELTS, J. H. (1968). *Arch. Neurol.* **18,** 680.
TURCK, M., RONALD, A. R. & PETERSDORF, R. G. (1967). *Antimicrob. Agents Chemother.*—1966, p. 446.
UDALL, V. (1969). *Postgrad. med. J.* **45** (Suppl. Nov.), 42.
WATERBURY, W. F., BOYDSTUN, J., CASTELLANI, A. G., FREEDMAN, R. & GAVIN, J. J. (1966). *Antimicrob. Agents Chemother.*—1965, p. 339.
WATERWORTH, P. M. (1969). *Postgrad. med. J.* **45** (Suppl. Nov.), 21.
WHITMAN, E. N. (1969). *Postgrad. med. J.* **45** (Suppl. Nov.), 46.
WILKINSON, A. E., RODIN, P., McFADZEAN, J. A. & SQUIRES, S. (1967). *Brit. J. vener. Dis.* **43,** 201.
WILLIAMS, J. D., BRUMFITT, W., CONDIE, A. P., REEVES, D. S. (1969). *Postgrad. med. J.* **45** (Suppl. Nov.), 71.

Chapter IV

PENICILLINS

1. NATURAL

Penicillin, the first of the antibiotics to come into general therapeutic use, is still in many ways the best. Indeed, some of its properties are unique, and it is nothing short of a miracle that so astonishing a substance should have been the first of its kind to be discovered. This is not to say that antibiotics were unknown before that time: many were discovered and used locally for therapeutic purposes much earlier, but this was the first which was suitable for systemic use in man.

The story of the discovery of penicillin by Fleming and of its isolation and systematic study by Florey, Chain and their colleagues in Oxford over ten years later, is now too well known to need re-telling. It took years of hard work to obtain penicillin in the pure state, and the unit of activity by which it had first to be measured, now known to represent 0·6 μg., has persisted to the present day, although all later penicillins are prescribed by weight.

BENZYL PENICILLIN

Physical and Chemical Properties

Penicillin can be prepared in quantity only by the original process of cultivating a mould forming it (a high-yielding mutant of a strain of *P. chrysogenum* is now used) in a suitable liquid medium. In the early stages of large-scale production it was found that four different penicillins were being formed, known as F, G, X and K. Of these G, or benzyl penicillin, had the most desirable properties, and its almost exclusive formation is ensured by adding the appropriate ' precursor ', phenylacetic acid, to the medium.

As formed, penicillin is an unstable acid, and in production it is converted to a salt, that of either potassium or sodium, which is more stable. The structure of benzyl penicillin is shown in the figure below. The potassium salt is what is commonly known as 'soluble' or 'crystalline' penicillin, both unsatisfactory terms, because they apply to any penicillin, but this salt is distinguishable from other forms of benzyl penicillin introduced later by its high degree of solubility in water and by its rapid absorption and excretion.

BENZYLPENICILLIN

a. Site of action of penicillinase

b. Site of action of amidase

STABILITY. Penicillin is stable in the dry state, but deteriorates slowly in solution, this process being accelerated by heat. Among many incompatible chemicals the most important is acid, since the action of gastric acid accounts for the loss of most of a dose of benzyl penicillin if it is swallowed. It is also destroyed by an enzyme, penicillinase, formed by various bacteria, including some staphylococci, various *Bacilli*, some species of *Proteus, Ps. aeruginosa,* other coliforms and the tubercle bacillus. Not all these penicillinases are the same. The resistance of staphylococci to penicillin in clinical practice is largely due to this factor: their intrinsic resistance may be comparatively low, but they appear to withstand high concentrations because in fact they destroy them. This can happen in the body, where further injury may be added to insult by interference with the action of the antibiotic on an accompanying sensitive species.

Anti-bacterial Activity

SPECIES SUSCEPTIBILITY. At one time bacteria were classed simply as sensitive or resistant to penicillin, but they exhibit degrees of sensitivity over an exceedingly wide range, and the fact that if necessary very large doses can be given enables infections by some moderately resistant species to be treated successfully. Table VIII states the concentrations usually required to inhibit the growth of the more sensitive organisms, which include almost all the Gram-positive pathogens and some of the Gram-negative. The least sensitive organisms listed among the latter are included because they can occur in the urine, where high concentrations of penicillin are easily attained.

ABNORMAL RESISTANCE. In some species naturally resistant strains are found: these include *Str. viridans*, resistant strains of which predominate in the mouth of patients undergoing penicillin treatment (Garrod and Waterworth, 1962) and *Staph. aureus*, in which resistance depends on penicillinase formation. Bacteria do not *acquire* resistance to penicillin, unless to a small extent during very prolonged treatment, and the sensitivity of most susceptible pathogens has remained unchanged despite years of extensive therapeutic use. An exception is the gonococcus, moderately resistant strains of which are now being encountered.

TYPE OF ANTI-BACTERIAL ACTION. In a nutrient medium (*i.e.* when bacterial growth can occur, but not otherwise) penicillin is bactericidal. About four hours is required to produce a high mortality, and this may proceed to extinction, or there may be a few survivors. This effect is best exerted by a concentration 5-10 times greater than the minimum inhibiting growth, and no increase above this level will accelerate it. Against many strains of two species, *Staph. aureus* and *Str. faecalis*, such an increase actually reduces the death rate, the so-called paradoxical zone phenomenon (Eagle, 1951). This behaviour of penicillin is unique, and no certain explanation for it is known, but one hypothesis is proposed by Eagle in his description of the phenomenon.

MODE OF ACTION. Recent work on the mode of action of penicillin explains why the antibiotic is only bactericidal to growing cells. The important work of Park and his colleagues has shown that certain nucleotides, all of which contain muramic acid, glutamic acid, alanine and lysine, accumulate within staphylococci growing in the presence of penicillin, and that similar nucleotides are components of the staphylococcal

3

TABLE VIII

Spectrum of Activity of Benzyl Penicillin

(Minimum inhibitory concentrations in μg./ml.)

	Gram-positive Organisms		Gram-negative Organisms	
Cocci	*Streptococcus pyogenes* (A)	0·006	*Neisseria gonorrhoeae*	0·003*
	Streptococcus pneumoniae	0·006	*Neisseria meningitidis*	0·012
	Streptococcus viridans	0·012*	*Neisseria catarrhalis*	0·012*
	Streptococcus faecalis	2		
	Staphylococcus aureus	0·012*		
	Staphylococcus albus	0·012*		
	Sarcina lutea	0·0015	*Haemophilus influenzae*	0·25 -1
Bacilli	*Bacillus anthracis*	0·01 -0·04	*Haemophilus pertussis*	0·5 -2
	Clostridium tetani	0·007-0·3	*Haemophilus ducreyi*	0·045-0·15
	Clostridium welchii	0·06 -0·25	*Bacteroides fragilis*	16*
	Clostridium oedematiens	0·007-0·015	*Bacteroides fusiformis*	0·06 -0·5
	Clostridium septicum	0·03	*Bacteroides melaninogenicum*	0·007-0·06
	Clostridium histolyticum	0·03	*Bacteroides necrophorus*	0·06 -0·12
	Corynebacterium diphtheriae	0·02 -0·6	*Escherichia coli*	20*
	Actinobacillus muris	0·06	*Klebsiella pneumoniae*	2-100
	Erysipelothrix rhusiopathiae	0·04 -0·08	*Proteus mirabilis*	8*
	Listeria monocytogenes	0·2 -0·6	*Salmonella* spp.	2-5
Fungi	*Actinomyces israeli*	0·02 -0·1	*Pasteurella septica*	0·5

* Denotes that some strains are more resistant.

Other sensitive species, the susceptibility of which cannot be measured in this way, are *T. pallidum* and other treponemata and a few of the larger viruses. *Leptospira* spp. are also sensitive to 0·05-0·5 μg./ml.

Resistant species not included in the Table are all organisms of the genera *Brucella, Mycobacterium, Pfeifferella, Pseudomonas, Vibrio, Proteus* (other than *P. mirabilis*). *Klebsiella aerogenes,* all fungi other than *A. israeli,* most viruses and all rickettsias.

The concentrations given for commoner species are the approximate mean of many estimations by various authors. Some of the less familiar are derived as follows: From the present writer's own observations *B. anthracis* (*Antibiot. and Chemother.* 1952, **2**, 689), *A. israeli* (*Brit. med. J.* 1952, **i**, 1263), *Bacteroides* (*Brit. med. J.* 1952, **ii**, 1529), *Clostridia* (*J. roy. Army med. Corps.* 1958, **104**, 209). For *C. diphtheriae* R. Cruickshank *et al.* (*Lancet* 1948, **ii**, 517), *E. rhusiopathiae* P. H. A. Sneath *et al.* (*Brit. med. J.* 1951, ii, 1063), *L. monocytogenes* I. A. Bakulov (Antibiotics 1959, **4**, 575), *H. pertussis* E. B. Wells *et al.* (*J. Pediat.* 1950, **36**, 752).

(This table also appears in a contribution by one of the authors (L. P. G.) to 'Experimental Chemotherapy ', cell wall. These observations have now been carried a stage further and it has been shown that, at least with staphylococci. penicillin acts by inhibiting the biosynthesis of cell wall mucopeptide, without interfering with protein synthesis (Mandelstam and Rogers, 1959). When growth takes place in the absence of a properly constituted cell wall, death of the cell

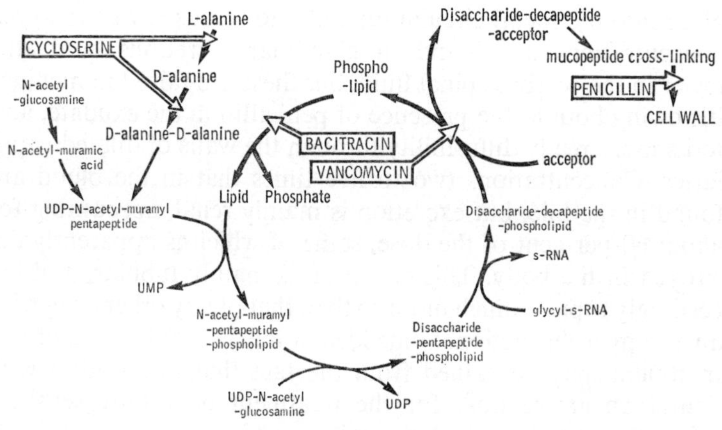

FIG. 4

Synthesis of bacterial cell wall showing sites of antibiotic inhibition. (Based on Matsuhashi *et al*, 1965. *Proc. nat. Acad. Sci. Wash. 54*, 587.)

occurs by lysis, but in the absence of growth osmotic sensitivity does not operate (Gale, 1960). Since the composition of cell walls differs this also explains the selective action of penicillin.

The cell wall is laid down as layers of a giant molecule, and its rigidity is due to a final process of cross-linking. It is with this process that penicillin interferes, as seen in Fig. 4, which also shows the points of action of other antibiotics on cell wall synthesis (Park, 1966).

The mode of action of methicillin has been shown to be similar (Rogers and Jeljaszewicz, 1961). The structural similarity between muramic acid and penicillins possessing anti-bacterial activity pointed out by Collins and Richmond (1962) may afford a rational approach to the development of new penicillins.

Pharmacology

The salts of benzyl penicillin are very freely diffusible: after intramuscular injection absorption occurs within a few minutes to produce a high concentration in the blood. Diffusion takes place into the foetal circulation and into serous cavities: lower concentrations are found in glandular secretions, and still lower in the cerebro-spinal fluid, but these are raised in meningitis owing both to the presence of penicillin in the exudate, and to its more ready diffusibility through the walls of dilated capillaries. Concentrations two to five times that in the blood are found in the bile, but excretion is mainly renal, accounting for about 60 per cent of the dose, some of which is apparently destroyed in the body. This excretion is mainly tubular, and exceedingly rapid—much more so than that of any other drug with an anti-microbic action. Some idea of the wasteful nature of this treatment may be gained from the fact that in an adult with anuria an ample dose for the treatment of a fully sensitive infection would be only 2,000 units.

The usual way of overcoming this difficulty is simply to give very large doses: the initially very high concentrations thus produced in the body are no bar to this because penicillin is virtually non-toxic. It is important to recognise that doubling the dose does not double the duration of effect. According to Eagle (1948) the doses required to maintain a blood level in excess of 0·16 unit per ml. for different periods are:

1 hour	20,000 units.
2 hours	50,000 ,,
3 ,,	140,000 ,,
4 ,,	235,000 ,,
6 ,,	600,000 ,,
8 ,,	1,400,000 ,,

These figures give a good idea of the dosage and intervals which must be observed if a *continuous effect* is considered necessary. It may not be: Eagle (1949) has also shown that it takes bacteria damaged but not killed by penicillin three to four hours to recover and resume growth. In some kinds of infection treatment which is intermittent to this degree may be satisfactory.

It has often been said that the blood level is not what matters, but that in the lesion: that penicillin diffuses into this when the blood level is high and persists there much longer. This is true of collections of exudate (Florey, Turton and Duthie, 1946), but not of inflammation in a vascular area without tissue destruction (Eagle, Fleischman and Levy, 1953), and it is to this category that most acute infections belong. It would certainly appear safer to administer doses calculated to maintain an effective concentration in the blood continuously, and by using forms of penicillin to be described later this is easily achieved.

One way of prolonging the action of each dose of penicillin is to administer another substance which interferes with tubular excretion. Probenecid (benemid) (Burnell and Kirby, 1951) serves this purpose well. It is used not so much for extending the intervals between doses as for maintaining higher blood levels between doses given at usual intervals when such levels are considered necessary, as in the treatment of endocarditis due to less sensitive streptococci.

Long-acting Forms of Benzyl Penicillin

The second possible way of prolonging the effect of a dose is to delay absorption. This was first achieved by suspending the calcium salt in a water-immiscible medium containing oil and beeswax. Much more satisfactory results have since been obtained with penicillin compounds of lesser solubility. The first of these was procaine penicillin, an equimolecular compound of penicillin and procaine, which is administered as a suspension of crystals which dissolve slowly at the site of injection. The ' peak ' blood level (which is not a peak but a plateau, and relatively low) is reached in about four hours, and the level falls slowly, being still detectable 24 hours after a moderate dose (Fig. 5).

Still less soluble and therefore longer-acting compounds are benethamine penicillin and benzathine penicillin, a single dose of which will provide a low concentration in the blood for four to five days and several weeks respectively. Various mixtures are available, some including the potassium salt for an immediate high level, and procaine penicillin and one of the least soluble compounds to sustain diminishing levels for a long period.

An orally administered form of benzathine penicillin (Penidural) converts the advantage of this compound when injected

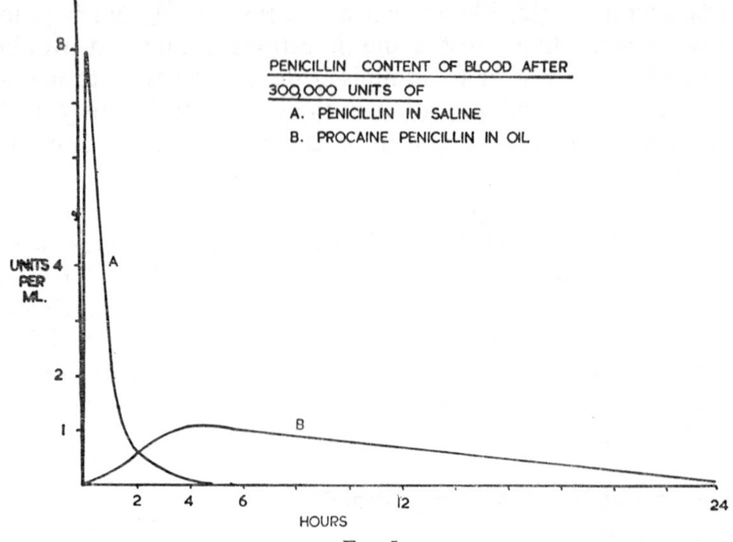

Fig. 5

Blood levels produced by the administration of penicillin in two different forms.

(Garrod (1950), reproduced by kind permission of the editor of the *British Medical Journal*.)

into a drawback, since, owing to its low solubility, little of a swallowed dose is absorbed. Henry, White and Meynell (1957) recovered only 6·7 per cent of an oral dose from the urine, in contrast to 30 per cent of an oral dose of phenoxymethyl penicillin, and over 70 per cent of a dose of either penicillin or procaine penicillin given intramuscularly. These tests were done in adults: benzathine penicillin appears to be better absorbed in children, but here account must be taken of the relatively large dose usually given in proportion to body weight. Even so the blood concentration most often found three hours after a dose of 300,000 units given to 101 children by Cathie and

MacFarlane (1953) was only 0·125 units per ml. In neonates a relatively still larger dose (150,000 units) of either benzathine or sodium penicillin produced higher and more sustained levels, with little to choose between the two treatments (Laurence and Alder, 1954). The only advantage of oral benzathine penicillin is palatability.

PHENOXYMETHYL PENICILLIN

The existence of several natural penicillins was recognised in early studies, and many more have been obtained by adding various derivatives of acetic acid to the fermentation medium as ‘ precursors ’. None of these is therapeutically important except phenoxymethyl penicillin, or penicillin V. which is obtained when phenoxyacetic acid is the precursor. This substance, originally described in 1948, but without its most important property having been detected, was re-discovered in Austria in 1953, and owes its value to acid stability: it is not destroyed in the stomach, and can therefore be given with confidence by mouth. Absorption is not in fact complete: the proportion of the dose recoverable from the urine is only 25 per cent (Heatley, 1956) but this was a great improvement on the absorption of benzyl penicillin, which is not only on the average much less, but unaccountably variable. Absorption is slower than that after injection, but excretion is equally rapid: hence a moderate dose needs repetition at intervals of four hours. Of different forms of penicillin V, the potassium salt is the best absorbed, the calcium salt next and the free acid least, that being their diminishing order of solubility: absorption is also better from a rapidly disintegrating tablet and after administration in the fasting state (Juncher and Raaschou, 1957).

It was for some time assumed that penicillin V has the same anti-bacterial activity as benzyl penicillin, but this is not so. It is rather *more* active against resistant staphylococci because more slowly destroyed by penicillinase, and slightly *less* active against streptococci, but much less active against Gram-negative species, including the gonococcus, *H. influenzae* and *Proteus* (Garrod, 1960a, b). These differences are exaggerated in the synthetic acid-resistant penicillins described later.

Penicillin V therefore affords a very convenient means of treating Gram-positive infections, but is not indicated for gonorrhoea or for Gram-negative infections involving the respiratory or urinary tract.

THERAPEUTIC APPLICATIONS

These are dealt with individually in the second part of this book, and need only be briefly reviewed here. In the first place, penicillin is almost wholly responsible for the fact that fatal haemolytic streptoccocal infection is now almost unheard of: in all serious forms of this infection, whether involving wounds, the air passages or the uterus, it is usually the treatment of choice. The pneumococcus is also invariably susceptible to it, and its efficacy can therefore be depended on in lobar pneumonia. In staphylococcal infections its value has been reduced by the increasing prevalence of resistant strains, but if the strain is sensitive natural penicillins are preferable to the synthetic.

Among its other principal uses may be mentioned the treatment of both syphilis and gonorrhoea, bacterial endocarditis and actinomycosis. Rarer indications for which it is highly effective are gas gangrene, anthrax and erysipeloid.

Dosage

Because both of the variety of its uses and of its lack of toxicity, the dosage of penicillin is remarkably elastic, certainly more so than that of any other drug. The factors determining the necessary dose are, first and foremost, the concentration required to inhibit the growth of the infecting organism, and the accessibility and gravity of the infection. If the inhibitory concentration is known or can be deduced, the aim should be to maintain one exceeding this, preferably several-fold, in the affected tissues. If these are intact and fully vascularized, the concentration in them will be much the same as that in the blood. If there are foci of suppuration or of necrosis, or fibrotic areas with a poor blood supply as in such a condition as actinomycosis, penetration is more difficult. A special indication for high dosage owing to inaccessibility is the attainment of an adequate concentration in the cerebro-spinal fluid in meningitis.

To translate these principles into practical terms, a fully sensitive infection in an area well supplied with blood should respond to 0·5 or even 0·25 g. of penicillin V given orally at intervals of four hours or to procaine penicillin given by injection in doses of 300,000 units (180 mg.) at intervals of 12 hours. Somewhat higher concentrations can be attained by increasing the dose of either of these preparations, but for maximum effects ' soluble ' (*i.e.* potassium) penicillin must be given either by intramuscular injection at intervals not exceeding six hours or by continuous intravenous infusion: the amount so administered may be anything from four to 20 million units daily or even more.

TOXICITY

Penicillin has no toxicity in the ordinary sense except when administered intrathecally: the dose by this route should never exceed 20,000 units, if indeed the route need be used at all, which is doubtful. It is almost impossible to poison a patient with penicillin if he has properly functioning kidneys, but if there is gross renal impairment the antibiotic may accumulate in the blood, in which the level should be estimated, the dose being reduced accordingly. Doses of 25 to 40 mega units of potassium penicillin daily given for presumed or known Gram-negative infections to 4 elderly patients, all with raised blood ureas, caused partial or complete loss of consciousness with myoclonic movements and sometimes generalized seizures (Bloomer, Barton & Maddock, 1967). From a study of 15 patients similarly treated (some with doses of up to 120 mega units daily) in whom the penicillin was assayed in the blood and cerebrospinal fluid, Smith, Lerner and Weinstein (1967) conclude that this ' neurotoxicity ' results only when a concentration of 10 units per ml. is exceeded in the c.s.f. These patients received either the Na or the K salt, the effects of which are not distinguished. An effect from the cation must be considered whenever large doses of a single salt are given, and it is now usually thought desirable in these circumstances to use a mixture of the Na and K salts. The disturbances which may follow massive doses of the Na salt are described by Brunner and Frick (1968).

The unique toxicity of penicillin for guinea-pigs, in which a single intramuscular dose is often fatal within a few days, seems finally to have been explained by the work of Farrar and Kent (1965). The two following effects in man may be classified as sensitivity reactions, but it is convenient to refer to them here.

NEPHRITIS. Very rarely patients receiving long courses of large doses of penicillin develop fever, eosinophilia, proteinuria and haematuria with a raised blood urea. Baldwin *et al.* (1968) describe 3 cases, in one of which persistence with the treatment ended in oliguria and death. The kidneys showed tubular necrosis and dense interstitial infiltration with mononuclears and eosinophiles.

HAEMOLYTIC ANAEMIA. This complication occurs only in patients who have been treated with penicillin before and again receive a prolonged course of large doses (commonly 20 mega units daily) usually for bacterial endocarditis. The haemolysis is due to the action of 1gG antibody on cells which have adsorbed the antibiotic. Rapid recovery ensues when administration is stopped. White *et al.* (1968) describe 2 cases and review the findings in 12 others.

SENSITIZATION REACTIONS

These present a more serious problem with penicillin than with any other antibiotic. Previous treatment is probably the usual cause of sensitization: various 'hidden contacts' (Siegel, 1959), such as consumption in milk, are possible causes; the idea that fungus infections may be responsible is less well founded. Reactions are of two kinds, the 'serum sickness' type, characterized by urticaria and fever; and immediate profound shock, which may be fatal within a few minutes. This condition, first recorded about 1952, has since been frequently described, some authors having knowledge of numerous cases (Cheng and Chiang, 1956; Rosenthal, 1958): penicillin is even described as having 'replaced foreign sera as the commonest cause of anaphylactic shock' (Kern and Wimberley, 1953). It usually follows a therapeutic injection, but has also been caused by oral administration, by local application, and by the injection of a minute dose as a test for sensitivity. The condition is one of profound vasomotor collapse, with an impalpable pulse, usually loss of consciousness, with or without facial or laryngeal oedema or a generalised rash.

Several authors (Hoigné and Schoch, 1959; Lewis, 1957; Tompsett, 1967) distinguish from this another kind of immediate reaction attributed to the accidental intravenous injection of a suspension of procaine penicillin, characterized by vertigo, disturbances of sensation (one of Tompsett's patients saw a green giraffe jump over her bed) and a sense of impending death: this can occur in individuals not sensitized to penicillin, as has sometimes been proved by giving a further dose without ill effects. Some other features, including tachycardia and cyanosis, may occur in either kind of reaction, and the two are not always easily distinguishable (Hoigné, 1962). Although sometimes regarded as manifestations of procaine poisoning, these reactions are undoubtedly due to blockage of pulmonary capillaries by the crystals, as demonstrated experimentally by Bell, Rannie and Wynne (1954). Bredt (1965) observed 7 cases after injections of Megacillin, a depot preparation containing no procaine, and prevented further cases by having the crystals in this milled to a smaller size.

Tests for sensitivity. Dermal tests, by the ' patch ', ' scratch ' or intradermal methods, are far from infallible, and seem better able to predict reactions of the serum sickness type than that of shock. Thus in a study in Taiwan (Idsöe and Wang, 1958), in which such tests were performed before therapeutic injection, the results were negative in each of five cases subsequently suffering from fatal shock and six having severe shock; they were positive only in a proportion of those later developing less severe shock or urticaria.

Further study of this problem has been pursued on three lines, and has produced an extensive recent literature which will not be fully reviewed here. One is the use of *penicilloyl-polylysine* for tests of sensitivity, based on the work of de Weck and Eisen (1961) and de Weck (1962). According to these authors, penicillin itself does not combine firmly enough with protein to produce an antigen: the actual haptene is penicillenic acid or a penicillenate or penicilloyl derivative of it. This substance is slowly formed from penicillin in solution. The result of a test with a solution of penicillin may thus depend on whether degradation products have formed in it. Penicillenic acid itself cannot be used for fear of producing sensitization, but the penicilloyl-polypeptide compound penicilloyl-polylysine is a suitable antigen and is said not to sensitize. (But Resnik and Shelley (1966) report shock following a repeat test with it.) The reliability claimed for this test by Parker *et al.* (1962) and in particular the claim that it gives no false negatives, have not always been confirmed by others. Rytel *et al.* (1963) in a study involving 1,022 patients given benzathine penicillin after a test, observed only 10 reactions, 7 being in negative test subjects, whereas about 70 others with a positive test did not react to the therapeutic dose. Smith, Johnson and Cluff (1966) tested 32 patients with penicilloyl-polylysine who had recently reacted to therapeutic penicillin: only 7 were positive, and these included neither of 2 patients whose reaction had been anaphylactic. Others (*e.g.* Finke *et al.*, 1965) have reported rather better results than these, but in no series have they been consistently correct.

Another method, the *basophil degranulation test* proposed by Shelley (1963) appears from a further study (Katz, *et al.*, 1964) to be a somewhat chancy procedure, and though others have used it in parallel with tests of different kinds, the results are unimpressive.

Impurities in penicillins as antigens. All work until very recently has been based on the belief that the sensitizing antigen is a combination of a penicillin derivative with body protein. The subject has now been much complicated by the discovery that a highly reactive pre-formed antigen may exist in penicillin itself (Batchelor *et al.*, 1967; Stewart, 1967). That found by these authors in 6-aminopenicillanic acid, and hence liable to be present in any semi-synthetic penicillin, is believed to be derived from the enzyme used in production, and that in benzyl penicillin from *P. chrysogenum* itself, each existing as a penicilloyl conjugate. It seems also that a reactive substance can be formed in a solution of pure benzyl penicillin by polymerization. Penicillin freed from the penicilloyl protein impurity (BRL 3000, " Purapen G ") produced no reaction in 11 sensitive volunteers who reacted to ordinary penicillin, but 9 reacted to both and 1 to the purified material only (Knudsen *et al.*, 1967). de Weck and Schneider (1969) contest the view that these impurities are responsible for reactions, at least to benzyl penicillin, on two grounds: that in animals they have found purified benzyl penicillin to retain its full immunogenicity, and that hydrolysed crude benzyl penicillin, which owing to the opening of the β-lactam ring cannot form penicilloyl conjugates, does not induce the formation of anti-penicilloyl antibodies.

ANTI-PENICILLIN ANTIBODIES. An agglutination test with penicillin-treated red cells is often positive, even in normal subjects or patients actually under treatment without ill effects. Positive results were obtained by Ascari & Gorman (1969) in 22·2 per cent of subjects with a history of reactions to penicillin and 37·8 per cent of treated syphilitics; Epp (1962) obtained them in over 50 per cent of all subjects and in a higher proportion of those with a history of a reaction. Levine *et al.* (1966) using an antigen prepared by coupling penicilloyl groups to red cells in a special suspending medium, obtained enormous titres, and demonstrated agglutinin in almost all of 76 ' consecutive ' patients, only one of whom had a history of a reaction to penicillin.

It seems that the method of preparing the cell suspension affects the frequency of positive results. These agglutinins can be either 1gM or 1gG, and the latter can function as ' blocking antibodies ', preventing the reaction between administered penicillin and the antibodies responsible for reactions.

These, the so-called ' skin-sensitizing ' antibodies, are certainly of two kinds, respectively responsible for urticarial and shock-like reactions. The former can be detected with penicilloyl-polylysine and the latter with benzyl penicillin itself, applied in a scratch test.

The expert application of these tests, if necessary employing different amounts of penicilloyl-polylysine, is recommended by de Weck and Schneider (1969) when penicillin treatment is strongly indicated in a supposedly sensitized patient, in a general review of this very complex subject, which should be consulted for further details. Apart from this only common sense precautions can be advocated, including regular inquiry about previous reactions whenever penicillin is to be given, extreme caution and preferably the substitution of other antibiotics in asthmatics and patients with other known sensitivities, and the immediate availability of adrenaline.

PHARMACEUTICAL PREPARATIONS

Benzyl penicillin (Na or K salt: 'crystalline' or 'soluble' penicillin. Vials containing 100,000 units and much more for solution for intramuscular injection. Dosage widely variable according to nature of condition treated: see text. Tablets containing 200,000 or 400,000 units or other amounts for oral administration. Also ointment, lozenges and other preparations.

Procaine benzyl penicillin. Available under numerous proprietary names as a suspension, usually containing 300,000 units per ml., or as a powdei for preparing such a suspension, for intramuscular injection. Some preparations (*e.g.* Fortified Procaine Penicillin Injection, B.P.) also contain benzylpenicillin. Dose 300,000 to 1,200,000 units; need usually be given only once daily.

Benzathine penicillin. Suspension usually containing 600,000 units per ml. for intramuscular injection: long interval dosage (one dose of 1,200,000 units monthly for rheumatic fever prophylaxis). Also available as tablets or suspension ('Penidural', Wyeth) for oral administration.

Phenoxymethyl penicillin (Penicillin V). Usually phenoxymethyl penicillin potassium ('Compocillin VK', Abbott; 'Crystapen V', Glaxo; 'Distaquaine V', Dista Products, and many others). Tablets containing 125 or 250 mg.: also as capsules and suspensions. Usual dose 250 mg. at 4- or 6-hourly intervals; this may be considerably exceeded, but gastric intolerance may result from larger doses.

REFERENCES

ASCARI, W. Q. & GORMAN, J. G. (1969). *Transfusion,* **9**, 35.
BALDWIN, D. S., LEVINE, B. B., McCLUSKEY, R. T. & GALLO, G. R. (1968). *New Engl. J. Med.* **279,** 1245.
BATCHELOR, F. R., DEWDNEY, J., FEINBERG, J. G. & WESTON, R. D. (1967). *Lancet* **2,** 1175.
BELL, R. C., RANNIE, I. & WYNNE, N. A. (1954). *Lancet,* **2**, 62.
BLOOMER, H. A., BARTON, L. J. & MADDOCK, R. K., Jr. (1967). *J. Amer. med. Ass.* **200**, 121.
BREDT, J. (1965). *Dtsch. med. Wschr.* **90,** 1602.
BRUNNER, F. P. & FRICK, P. G. (1968). *Brit. med. J.* **4,** 550.
BURNELL, J. M. & KIRBY, W. M. M. (1951). *J. clin. Invest.* **30,** 697.
CATHIE, I. A. B. & MacFARLANE, J. C. W. (1953). *Brit. med. J.* **1**, 805.
CHENG, C. L. & CHIANG, C-T. (1956). *Chinese med. J.* **74**, 513.
COLLINS, J. F. & RICHMOND, M. H. (1962). *Nature (Lond.)* **195, 142.**
EAGLE, H. (1948). *Ann. intern. Med.* **28,** 260.
EAGLE, H. (1949). *J. clin. Invest.* **28,** 832.
EAGLE, H. (1951). *J. Bact.* **62,** 663
EAGLE, H., FLEISCHMAN, R. & LEVI, MINA (1953). *J. Lab. clin. Med.* **41,** 122.
EPP, M. (1962). *Canad. J. pub. Hlth.* **53,** 79.
FARRAR, W. E. JR. & KENT, T. H. (1965). *Amer. J. Path.* **47,** 629.
FINKE, S. R., GRIECO, M. H., CONNELL, J. T., SMITH, M. C. & SHERMAN, W. B (1965). *Amer. J. Med.* **38,** 71.
FLOREY, M. E., TURTON, E. C. & DUTHIE, E. S. (1946). *Lancet* **2,** 405.
GALE, E. F. (1960). *Brit med. Bull.* **16,** 11.
GARROD, L. P. (1950). *Brit. med. J.* **2,** 453.
GARROD, L. P. (1960a). *Brit. med. J.* **1,** 527.
GARROD, L. P. (1960b). *Brit. med. J.* **2,** 1695.

GARROD, L. P. & WATERWORTH, PAMELA M. (1962). *Brit. Heart J.* **24**, 39.
HEATLEY, N. G. (1956). *Antibiot. Med.* **2**, 33.
HENRY, L., WHITE, G. & MEYNELL, M. J. (1957). *Brit. med. J.* **1**, 17.
HOIGNÉ, R. (1962). *Acta med. scand.* **171**, 201.
HOIGNÉ, R. & SCHOCH, K. (1959). *Schweiz. med. Wschr.* **89**, 1350.
IDSÖE, O. & WANG, K. Y. (1958). *Bull. Wrld Hlth Org.* **18**, 323.
JUNCHER, H. & RAASCHOU, F. (1957). *Antibiot. Med.* **4**, 497.
KATZ, H. I., GILL, K. A., BAXTER, D. L. & MOSCHELLA, S. L. (1964). *J. Amer. med. Ass.* **188**, 351.
KERN, R. A. & WIMBERLEY, N. A. JR. (1953). *Amer. J. med. Sci.* **226**, 357.
KNUDSEN, E. T., ROBINSON, O. P. W., CROYDON, E. A. P. & TEES, E. C. (1967). *Lancet* **2**, 1184.
LAURANCE, B. & ALDER, V. G. (1954). *Brit. med. J.* **2**, 1392.
LEVINE, B. B., FELLNER, M. J., LEVYTSKA, V., FRANKLIN, E. C. & ALISBERG, N. (1966). *J. Immunol.* **96**, 707, 719.
LEWIS, G. W. (1957). *Brit. med. J.* **1**, 1153.
MANDELSTAM, J. & ROGERS, H. J. (1959). *Biochem. J.* **72**, 654.
PARK, J. T. (1966). *Symp. Soc. gen. Microbiol.* **16**, 70.
PARKER, C. W., SHAPIRO, J., KERN, M. & EISEN, H. N. (1962). *J. exp. Med.* **115**, 821.
RESNIK, S. S. & SHELLEY, W. B. (1966). *J. Amer. Med. Ass.* **196**, 740.
ROGERS, H. J. & JELJASZEWICZ, J. (1961). *Biochem. J.* **81**, 576.
ROSENTHAL, A. (1958). *J. Amer. med. Ass.* **167**, 1118.
RYTEL, M. W., KLION, F. M., ARLANDER, T. R. & MILLER, L. F. (1963). *J. Amer. med. Ass.* **186**, 894.
SHELLEY, W. B. (1963). *J. Amer. Med. Ass.* **184**, 171.
SIEGEL, B. B. (1959). *Bull. Wrld. Hlth. Org.* **21**, 703.
SMITH, H., LERNER, P. I. & WEINSTEIN, L. (1967). *Arch. intern. Med.* **120**, 47.
SMITH, J. W., JOHNSON, J. E. III & CLUFF, L. E. (1966). *New Engl. J. Med.* **274**, 998.
STEWART, G. T. (1967). *Lancet* **2**, 1177.
TOMPSETT, R. (1967). *Arch. intern. Med.* **120**, 565.
WECK, A. L. DE (1962). *Schweiz. med. Wschr.* **92**, 1155.
WECK, A. L. DE & SCHNEIDER, C. H. (1969). *Minnesota Med.* **52**, 137.
WECK, A. L. DE & EISEN, H. N. (1960). *J. exp. Med.* **112**, 1227.
WHITE, J. M., BROWN, D. L., HEPNER, G. W. & WORLLEDGE, S. M. (1968). *Brit. med. J.* **3**, 26.

CHAPTER V

PENICILLINS

2. SEMI-SYNTHETIC PENICILLINS AND CEPHALOSPORINS

THE existence of the penicillin ' nucleus ', 6-aminopenicillanic acid, in *Penicillium chrysogenum* fermentations was first detected by discrepancies between the results of chemical and microbiological assays, and more was found to be formed in the absence of added precursor (Batchelor *et al.*, 1959). The second discovery made at this time was that this substance

6−amino−penicillanic acid   7−amino−cephalosporanic acid

could also be prepared in quantity from benzyl or phenoxymethyl penicillin by the action of an enzyme derived from other micro-organisms: the effect of this amidase is to separate the side chain (for site of action see p. 54). The amidase acting on benzyl penicillin is obtainable from numerous enterobacteria (*Escherichia, Klebsiella,* etc.) and that attacking phenoxymethyl penicillin is derived from moulds (*e.g. Streptomyces lavendulae* (Batchelor *et al.*, 1961).

Until this discovery different penicillins could only be obtained by adding precursors to the medium, among which only derivatives of acetic acid were effective. The availability of the nucleus itself enabled side chains in a great variety to be attached by a semi-synthetic process. In the Beecham Research Laboratories, where these discoveries were made, over 2,000 new penicillins have been prepared by this process, and those which have come into therapeutic use possess one or more of

70

TABLE IX

CLINICALLY USEFUL PENICILLINS

Side Chain	Approved Name and Full Chemical Name	Trade Names	Important Properties
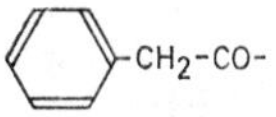 $-CH_2-CO-$ (benzene ring)	**Benzyl penicillin** 6-phenylacetamido penicillanic acid		
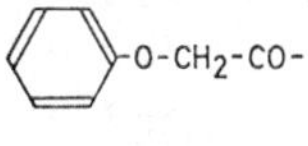 $-O-CH_2-CO-$ (benzene ring)	**Phenoxymethyl penicillin** Penicillin V 6-phenoxyacetamido penicillanic acid		Acid-resistant
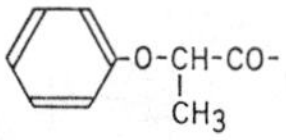 $-O-CH-CO-$ with CH_3 (benzene ring)	**Phenethicillin** DL-6-(α-phenoxypropionamido) penicillanic acid	Broxil	Acid-resistant
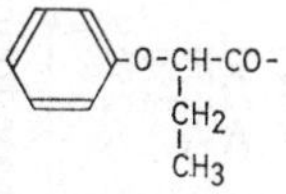 $-O-CH-CO-$ with CH_2-CH_3 (benzene ring)	**Propicillin** DL-6-(α-phenoxy-n-butyramido) penicillanic acid	Brocillin Ultrapen	Acid-resistant
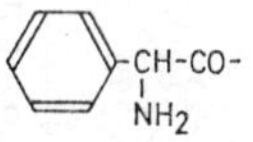 $-CH-CO-$ with NH_2 (benzene ring)	**Ampicillin** 6-(D(-)-α-aminophenylacetamido) penicillanic acid	Penbritin	Active against Gram-negative bacilli Acid-resistant
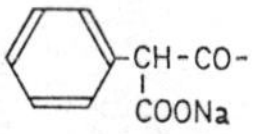 $-CH-CO-$ with $COONa$ (benzene ring)	**Carbenicillin** Disodium α-carboxy-benzyl-penicillin	Pyopen	Active against Gram-negative bacilli
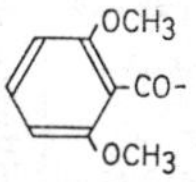 OCH_3 ... $-CO-$ ... OCH_3 (benzene ring)	**Methicillin** 6-(2,6 dimethoxybenzamido) penicillanic acid	Celbenin	Penicillinase-resistant
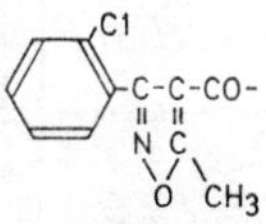 Cl ... $-C-C-CO-$ ring with N, C, O, CH_3 (benzene ring)	**Cloxacillin** 6-(5-Methyl-3-orthochlorophenyl-isoxazole-4-carboxyamido) penicillanic acid	Orbenin	Penicillinase-resistant Acid-resistant

the following advantages: (1) resistance to acid, (2) resistance to penicillinase, (3) broader spectrum. The names, structures, and important properties of those in established use in Great Britain are stated in Table IX.

ACID-RESISTANT PENICILLINS (PHENOXYPENICILLINS)

The property of acid resistance, permitting a reliable effect from oral administration, was not new, since it already existed

TABLE X

Sensitivity of Bacteria to the Penicillins

Usual Minimum Concentration (μg.ml.) causing Complete Bacteristasis with a Moderate Inoculum

	Benzyl Penicillin	Phenoxy-methyl Penicillin	Phenethi-cillin	Propicillin	Phenbeni-cillin	Ampicillin	Methi-cillin	Cloxa-cillin
1. Highly Sensitive Species								
Staph. aureus*	0·03	0·03	0·03	0·06	0·125	0·06	2	0·125
Str. pyogenes	0·015	0·015	0·03	0·03	0·03	0·03	0·125	0·06
Str. pneumoniae	0·015	0·015	0·06	0·03	0·015	0·06	0·25	0·25
B. anthracis	0·008	0·015	0·06		0·06	0·06	0·125	0·5
Cl. welchii	0·06							
N. gonorrhoeae	0·015	0·03	0·125	0·125	0·125	0·125	0·06	0·5
N. meningitidis	0·03	0·125	1		0·125	0·06	0·25	0·5
N. catarrhalis	0·03	0·125			0·125	0·015	0·25	1
2. Less Sensitive Species								
Str. faecalis	2	4	4		4	2	32	32
H. influenzae	1	4	4		4	0·25	2	16
Salmonella spp.	8	128	>250		128	2	>250	250
Salm. typhi	4	64	250		64	1	>250	250
Shigella spp.	16	64			64	4	>250	128
Esch. coli	64	128	>250		64	8	>250	250
Proteus mirabilis*	32	128	>250		250	4	250	250
Proteus mirabilis†	>250	>250	>250	>250	>250	>250	>250	>250
Proteus vulgaris	>250	>250	>250	>250	>250	64	>250	>250
Proteus rettgeri	4 - >250	>250	>250	>250	>250	2 - >250	>250	>250
Proteus morgani	>250	>250	>250	>250	>250	128 - >256	>250	>250
Klebsiella aerogenes	>250	>250	>250	>250	>250	16 - >250	>250	>250

* Non-penicillinase-forming.   † Penicillinase-forming.

in phenoxymethyl penicillin (p. 61). Despite this property, only about 25 per cent of the dose is absorbed, and better absorption is the main advantage of the semi-synthetic penicillins in this class, phenethicillin (Knudsen and Rolinson, 1959), propicillin (Williamson, Morrison and Stevens, 1961), and phenbenicillin (Rollo, Somers and Burley, 1962). Details of their anti-bacterial activity are given in Table X. Like phenoxymethyl penicillin they are almost as active as benzyl penicillin against sensitive Gram-positive bacteria, but they share and in some instances exaggerate the deficiencies of phenoxymethyl penicillin in dealing with various Gram-negative species. Their clinical application should be restricted accordingly.

The therapeutic efficacy of these penicillins is the product of three factors, anti-bacterial activity, efficiency of absorption, and extent of protein binding in the blood. The last two tend to cancel one another: thus phenbenicillin, although attaining much the highest *total* blood levels, is also by far the most highly protein-bound, with the result that the level of *free* antibiotic is the lowest among these four compounds. The only adequate study taking all these factors into account is that of Bond, Lightbown, Barber and Waterworth (1963) who assayed not only total but free antibiotic in the blood of volunteers at intervals after a dose, as well as studying the anti-bacterial activity of the four compounds *in vitro* in the presence and absence of serum. Their conclusion as to the order of merit for treating staphylococcal and streptococcal infections are expressed in Table XI. Phenbenicillin is no longer available.

A sufficient dose of any of these drugs given at 4-hour intervals should serve any ordinary suitable purpose. If any of them is to be used for a serious and unusual purpose, notably for bacterial endocarditis, its suitability should be verified by an accurate test of the sensitivity of the organism *to the penicillin which it is proposed to use*. It cannot be assumed that the result will be the same as that to be obtained with benzylpenicillin.

PENICILLINASE-RESISTANT PENICILLINS

Of far greater practical importance than the discovery of the acid-resistant penicillins was the discovery that changes in the side-chain of penicillin can protect the central β-lactam ring from the action of penicillinase without removing anti-bacterial activity. Several such penicillins are now available for clinical use. They comprise a single compound, methicillin, which is acid-labile and has therefore to be injected, and a group, the isoxazolyl penicillins, which are also acid-stable and can hence be given orally.

TABLE XI

Comparison of Four Phenoxypenicillins on the Basis of the Ratio of Total or Free Blood Level to the Appropriate Minimum Inhibitory Concentration

Ratio	Total Blood Level				Free Blood Level			
	M.I.C. in Serum				M.I.C. in Broth			
Organism	*Staph. aureus*		*Str. pyogenes*		*Staph. aureus*		*Str. pyogenes*	
Time	1 hr.	2 hrs.	1 hr.	2 hrs.	1 hr.	2 hrs.	1 hr.	2 hrs
Phenoxymethyl-penicillin	9·0	3·48	37·5	14·5	6·0	3·7	24·0	14·7
Phenethicillin	13·4	8·0	13·4	8·0	10·7	7·3	21·3	14·6
Propicillin	4·7	2·87	14·2	8·6	2·3	1·8	9·3	7·3
Phenbenicillin	2·74	2·4	5·48	4·1	0·56	0·44	4·7	3·7

Methicillin

CHEMISTRY. Methicillin is 2:6 dimethyloxybenzyl penicillin (Table IX) and is supplied as the sodium salt. It is readily soluble in water, but solutions are very unstable. Neutral solutions lose 50 per cent of their activity in five days at room temperature and 20 per cent when stored at 5°C. Acid solutions are much more unstable and at pH 2·0 half the activity is lost in 20 minutes at room temperature (Rolinson *et al.*, 1960).

ANTI-BACTERIAL ACTIVITY. Methicillin is highly resistant to staphylococcal penicillinase, although less so to the penicillinase of many other species (Rolinson *et al.*, 1960). It is, therefore, equally active against penicillin-sensitive and penicillinase-producing strains of *Staph. aureus*. On the other hand, its activity is much less than that of benzyl penicillin against most other penicillin-sensitive species (Table X).

Methicillin, like benzyl penicillin, is actively bactericidal in optimum concentrations, but, at least against staphylococci, may be less so in higher concentrations. Its activity against other species is inferior to that of benzyl penicillin, and there is no indication for its use except a severe penicillin-resistant staphylococcal infection.

RESISTANCE IN STAPHYLOCOCCI. Strains of *Staph. aureus* resistant to methicillin, thought at first not to exist and then to be exceedingly rare, are now being encountered more frequently: the percentage resistant among many thousands of strains tested at the Central Public Health Laboratory rose from 0·06 in 1960 to 0·97 in 1964 (Dyke, Jevons and Parker, 1966) and to 4·11 per cent in 1969 (Parker and Hewitt, 1970). Much higher frequencies of resistance in strains isolated from infections in hospitals have been reported from France (Chabbert *et al.*, 1965), Switzerland (Benner and Kayser, 1968; Kayser and Hollinger, 1968) and Denmark (Siboni and Poulsen, 1968). It is now clear that such infections may not respond to treatment with methicillin alone, and the strains concerned are usually resistant to many other antibiotics. An appropriate treatment for serious infections of this nature may be a combination of methicillin or cephalothin with kanamycin, which exerts a synergic bactericidal effect (Bulger, 1967).

Although these strains form large amounts of penicillinase, they do not destroy methicillin, as has been asserted: their resistance is intrinsic. Only a small minority of the cells in these cultures appears resistant (Sutherland and Rolinson, 1964a)—except on a medium containing an excess of electrolytes, such as 5 per cent NaCl (Barber, 1964)—with the result that a diffusion test of sensitivity with a light inoculum may give a misleading result. Methods for detecting methicillin resistance are discussed in Chapter XXVIII.

Resistance to methicillin is much commoner in *Staph. albus*: Kjellander and Finland (1963) found 10 per cent of clinical isolates resistant. They formed penicillinase, but also possessed intrinsic resistance.

PHARMACOLOGY. Methicillin is not acid-resistant and has, therefore, to be administered by intramuscular (or intravenous) injection. Like benzyl penicillin it is rapidly excreted and injections must, therefore, be frequent. The usual regime is 1 g. every four hours for the first 24 hours and every six hours thereafter but much larger doses can and may have to be given, and their effect can be reinforced with probenecid. Only about 40 per cent of the drug in the blood is protein-bound, an important fact in assessing its relative merits.

Toxicity. Methicillin has in general the same low toxicity as benzyl penicillin, but has apparently caused bone marrow depression, mainly affecting leucocytes, in a few patients (McElfreh and Huang, 1962: Levitt *et al.*, 1964). Nephritis has also been described (Brauninger and Remington, 1968) and its occurrence has been advanced in the United States as a reason for preferring isoxazolyl penicillins to methicillin. Condemnation because of this very rare complication seems unjustifiable when it is remembered that benzyl penicillin can have the same effect: among patients with penicillin nephritis described by Baldwin, Levine and McCluskey (1968), 3 had been treated with methicillin, 3 with benzyl penicillin, and one with both (see p. 64). Patients sensitized to benzyl penicillin will usually, although not always, react to methicillin.

Isoxazolyl Penicillins

These compounds combine resistance to penicillinase with resistance to acid. The series of 3:5-disubstituted 4-isoxazolyl penicillins was originally described by Doyle *et al.* (1961), and among them cloxacillin was first brought into use in this country and oxacillin in the United States. Their sodium salts are readily soluble in water and neutral solutions are stable at room temperature for 24 hours. They also show a similar degree of resistance to acid to that of phenoxymethyl penicillin.

Cloxacillin is 3-chlorophenyl-5-methyl-4 isoxazolyl penicillin. The usual inhibitory concentration for all staphylococci is about 0·12-0·25 μg. per ml.: *i.e.* cloxacillin has fully eight times the *in vitro* activity of methicillin, although still considerably less than that of benzyl penicillin against sensitive strains. It is slightly less resistant than methicillin to staphylococcal penicillinase, with the result that a 2-4 fold higher concentration may be required to inhibit a large inoculum. Activity is diminished even more by protein: in 95 per cent serum this reduction is 8-fold (Barber and Waterworth, 1964). The susceptibility of all other species is less than that to benzyl penicillin (Table X), but that of *Str. pyogenes* is noteworthy, since cloxacillin—or oxacillin (Simon and Sakai, 1963)—will eliminate a streptococcal infection complicated by the presence of penicillinase-forming staphylococci when benzyl penicillin has failed because of local inactivation.

Cloxacillin and methicillin exhibit cross-resistance: the position with regard to staphylococci is thus the same for both antibiotics.

PHARMACOLOGY. Cloxacillin should be administered before meals, since food interferes with absorption. Even so this is incomplete: higher blood levels are produced by intramuscular injection, when 30 per cent of the dose is excreted in the urine, compared with 20 per cent after an oral dose (Kislak, Eickhoff and Finland, 1965). About 10 per cent of an oral dose is excreted in the bile ((Nayler *et al.*, 1962). It is clear from excretion studies that much of the drug is unaccounted for, evidently owing to inactivation in the body.

The usual dose recommended is 500 mg. orally or 250 mg. intramuscularly at 6-hour intervals: this can be increased if necessary and reinforced with probenecid. Absorption is better than that of oxacillin: differences of up to 2-fold in favour of cloxacillin have been reported in the blood levels attained (Report, 1962; Turck, Ronald and Petersdorf, 1965). The degree of protein binding is very high, as would be expected from the effect of serum on activity *in vitro*. Toxicity is low, and no special effects have been reported.

OXACILLIN. This compound, 3-methyl-5-phenyl-4-isoxazolyl penicillin, has been extensively used and studied in the United States while similar studies of cloxacillin have been pursued in this country. As would be expected from the fact that only a single chlorine atom distinguishes them, their properties are closely similar and call for no separate description. As already stated, oxacillin is less well absorbed and this difficulty has been overcome in some clinical studies by intramuscular injection for the early stages of severe infections. Its activity against penicillinase-forming staphylococci is also slightly less, and these differences have led some American authors (Sidell *et al.*, 1964) to compare it unfavourably with cloxacillin. It also seems that oxacillin may be more rapidly destroyed in the body (Gravenkemper *et al.*, 1965): in patients with ' end-stage kidney disease ' having regular renal dialysis, the oxacillin level in the blood fell to *nil* in eight hours after a 1 g. dose (Bulger *et al.*, 1964).

DICLOXACILLIN. This more recently introduced compound, which is 3(2,6-dichlorphenyl)-5-methyl-4-isoxazolyl penicillin, furnished as the sodium monohydrate, has interesting properties, well described in comparison with those of cloxacillin and oxacillin by Gravenkemper *et al.* (1965). Its inhibitory concentration for both sensitive and resistant staphylococci is somewhat lower than that of the other two compounds, and it is also highly active against streptococci and pneumococci. The concentrations attained in the blood exceed those of cloxacillin by 2-fold, just as those of cloxacillin exceed those of oxacillin to the same degree, and these concentrations are better sustained. This difference is due not only to better absorption, but to slower excretion: Rosenblatt *et al.* (1968) found the renal clearances of oxacillin, cloxacillin and dicloxacillin to be 226·8, 162·2 and 113·7 ml./min. respectively. These authors and Naumann and Kempf (1965) have also shown that >70 per cent of a dose of dicloxacillin is excreted in the urine, the figures for both other compounds being lower (oxacillin 55·5 and cloxacillin 62, according to Rosenblatt *et al.*, 1968). The main defect of dicloxacillin is its very high degree of protein binding: according to these authors the percentages bound are oxacillin 94-96, cloxacillin 93-95 and dicloxacillin 95-97.

FLUCLOXACILLIN. This new compound, now undergoing clinical trial, is 3-(2-chloro-6-fluorophenyl)-5-methyl-4-isoxazolyl penicillin. Its anti-bacterial activity is almost identical with that of cloxacillin, but it is much better absorbed after oral administration, the blood levels attained being about double those produced by the same dose of cloxacillin at all times up to 4 hours. Protein binding has been determined as 94·7 per cent, in a test showing oxacillin 93·1 and dicloxacillin as 96·9 per cent. The usual dose proposed, which may be exceeded if necessary, is 250 mg. either orally or intramuscularly at intervals of 4-6 hours (Sutherland *et al.*, 1970).

Other Penicillinase-Resistant Penicillins

The properties of the following three compounds, so far as they are ascertainable by *in vitro* experiment, are well described and compared by Barber and Waterworth (1964).

DIPHENICILLIN (ANCILLIN). This is 2-biphenylyl penicillin, the properties of which are similar to those of oxacillin, including spectrum, resistance to penicillinase, and high protein binding, but with the difference that it is less acid-stable and hence less well absorbed (Gourevitch *et al.*, 1962). Sabath, Klein and Finland (1963) confirmed and extended these findings, including incomplete and variable absorption, and in their therapeutic study Klein, Sabath, Steinhauer and Finland (1963) gave the antibiotic parenterally to most of their patients. The results compared unfavourably with those obtained with methicillin in a previous series of severe staphylococcal infections.

NAFCILLIN is 6-(2-ethoxy-1-naphthamido) penicillanic acid. Its anti-bacterial activity was studied by Lane (1964) and by Klein and Finland (1963) who also studied absorption, which was irregular and incomplete, although no specific reason for this is adduced. Hence in an extensive clinical trial in severe staphylococcal infections Eickhoff, Kislak and Finland (1965a) used mainly the parenteral route in a dose of usually 6 but up to 18 g. daily, sometimes with probenecid. Results compared favourably with those obtained with methicillin, oxacillin, etc. According to Kind *et al.* (1970) the relatively low blood levels attained by nafcillin are due, not to defective absorption, but to inactivation in the liver.

QUINACILLIN is 3-carboxy-2-quinoxalinyl penicillin, furnished as the disodium salt. The original description by Richards, Housley and Spooner (1963) contains most of what is known about it. Staphylococci are the only organisms highly sensitive to it, even streptococci being considerably less so than to other similar penicillins. It is highly resistant to staphylococcal penicillinase and not highly protein-bound, but although resistant to acid, is so poorly absorbed by the oral route that parenteral injection is advisable. Emphasis has been laid on the fact that it is an exceptionally poor inducer of penicillinase (Smith, Hamilton-Miller and Knox, 1964), which may have some therapeutic advantage. Methicillin-resistant strains are highly and uniformly resistant to quinacillin (Barber and Waterworth, 1964). Clinical results are lacking.

General Therapeutic Efficacy

All these penicillinase-resistant penicillins have been used mainly for treating severe staphylococcal infections. These are notoriously varied in nature, and many occur in patients with a still greater variety of predisposing conditions, some of these being of the gravest nature in themselves. Hence all extensive clinical studies embrace a mixture of patients with pneumonia, septicaemia, wound infections, etc., with sometimes a few of endocarditis or meningitis, many occurring as a complication of malignant disease, or serious cardiac, hepatic or renal lesions, often in elderly subjects. Such miscellaneous clinical material does not lend itself to an assessment of the relative value of antibiotics which are themselves closely related, and no attempt at such an analysis will be made here.

The main choice lies between methicillin, which has much the lowest intrinsic anti-staphylococcal activity, but of which 60 per cent in the blood is free, and one of the isoxazolyl or other acid-resistant compounds, with higher anti-bacterial activity, but of which perhaps only 5 per cent is free. These contrasting properties are largely self-cancelling, and the probability is that adequate doses of almost any of these penicillins will achieve very similar effects. The possibilities of reducing protein binding by displacement with other drugs which have been explored by Kunin (1966) do not seem hopeful. Initial treatment of a severe staphylococcal infection should always be with one of these penicillins unless or until the strain has been shown to be sensitive to benzylpenicillin.

BROAD SPECTRUM PENICILLINS

Adicillin

This is the name now given to cephalosporin N, one of three distinct antibiotics formed by the Sardinian *Cephalosporium* referred to in the succeeding section. It is identical with synnematin B, an antibiotic isolated by Gottshal *et al.* in 1951 from a mould of the *Tilachlidium* genus. It is a penicillin with a side-chain derived from D-α-aminoadipic acid, which, although much less active than benzyl penicillin against Gram-positive cocci, is rather more so against various Gram-negative species, including *Salm. typhi*. Although it gave promising results in the treatment of typhoid fever (Benavides *et al.*, 1955) it has never been manufactured in quantity: this is understood to be due to difficulties in purification.

Ampicillin

This semi-synthetic compound, α-aminobenzyl penicillin, was first described by Rolinson and Stevens (1961). It is administered orally as the free acid, which unlike most other penicillins is soluble only to the extent of about 10 per cent in water.

ANTI-BACTERIAL ACTIVITY. Ampicillin is slightly less active than benzyl penicillin against most Gram-positive bacteria, but slightly more so against *Str. faecalis*. It is destroyed by staphylococcal penicillinase, and is therefore not indicated for resistant staphylococcal infections. *Listeria monocytogenes* is highly sensitive (Seeliger, Laymann and Finger, 1967) and several recent papers (Weingartner and Ortel, 1967; MacNair, White and Graham, 1968; Seeliger and Matheis, 1969) commend ampicillin for the treatment of listeriosis.

The outstanding property of ampicillin is an activity four to eight times greater than that of benzyl penicillin against various Gram-negative bacilli (Table X), including *H. influenzae*, *Salmonella* and *Shigella* spp., non-penicillinase-forming *Proteus mirabilis*, and most strains of *Esch. coli* (Sutherland and Rolinson, 1964b; Anderson *et al.*, 1964). *Kl. pneumoniae* may be sensitive, but *Kl. aerogenes*, penicillinase-forming *Proteus*, and *Pseudomonas* spp. are resistant, as are other coliform bacilli forming a penicillinase. *Kl. aerogenes* possesses a high degree of intrinsic resistance, apart from its capacity to destroy ampicillin enzymically (Hamilton-Miller, 1965). The effect of ampicillin, like that of benzyl penicillin, is bactericidal.

PHARMACOLOGY. Ampicillin is resistant to acid, and is well absorbed when administered orally, but not completely*: 30

---

* An ester of ampicillin has now been described, pivaloyloxymethyl-D-α-aminobenzyl penicillinate, which is much better absorbed than ampicillin itself (v. Daehne *et al.*, 1970)

per cent of an oral dose is recoverable from the urine, but 60-70 per cent of an intramuscular (Naumann, 1965), for which reason the parenteral route may be preferred for maximal effect. This can also be enhanced with probenecid. When different oral doses are compared, plotting the dose against the blood concentration gives a straight line (Knudsen, Rolinson and Stevens, 1961): *i.e.* the same proportion of a large dose is absorbed as of a small, whereas the larger the dose of a tetracycline, the less the proportion absorbed. The peak concentration is reached in about 2 hours, and the subsequent fall is gradual, a detectable amount persisting for 6 hours after a moderate dose (250 mg.).

Although excretion is mainly renal, fairly high concentrations are attained in the bile. The report by Brown and Acred (1961) of a level in the bile of dogs 300 times that in the blood, does not seem to represent conditions in the human biliary tract, since Ayliffe and Davies (1965) found a mean difference of only 9-fold (extremes 3- 48-fold) in a series of patients. There were wide variations in the content among patients with normal biliary tracts: in those with obstructive lesions it was very low or nil. These observations have been confirmed and extended by Mortimer, Mackie and Haynes (1969). Blecher *et al.* (1966) have shown that ampicillin accumulates and persists in the amniotic fluid, evidently in consequence of renal excretion by the foetus: in most specimens the level exceeded 2·5 μg. per ml. after 3 maternal doses of 500 mg.

Ampicillin can also be administered intramuscularly or intravenously, the sodium salt, which behaves identically (Eickhoff, Kislak and Finland, 1965b) being more suitable by the latter route. High concentrations are attained in the cerebrospinal fluid in patients with purulent meningitis when 150-200 mg. per kg. are given intravenously daily (Naumann, 1965) although ampicillin, like benzyl penicillin, traverses the normal blood-brain barrier in very small amounts. Impairment of renal function reduces the rate of excretion, and the dose can be reduced accordingly: renal dialysis will reduce the blood level (Höffler, Stegemann and Scheler, 1966).

Toxic Effects. Ampicillin appears to be as free from toxicity as benzyl penicillin. Apart from occasional gastric intolerance, the only significant side effects seen have been rashes, which are decidedly commoner than with other penicillins. A large-scale survey by Shapiro *et al.* (1969) showed that 9·5 per cent of patients treated with ampicillin developed rashes and only 4·5 per cent of those given other penicillins. The route of administration was not a factor, but the effect of dosage was not analysed: it may be significant that a series of patients of whom 20 per cent had rashes were given 6 g. daily (Sleet, Sangster and Murdoch, 1964). Both because the rash is sometimes erythematous and not urticarial and because its onset may be delayed, it seems likely that a mechanism differing from true sensitization to penicillin may sometimes be responsible. A rash almost invariably results when ampicillin is given to a patient with glandular fever.

CLINICAL APPLICATIONS. Early reports dealt largely with the treatment of urinary tract infections. Ampicillin is unquestionably the best penicillin for this purpose when the organism is sensitive: it is not only more active than benzyl penicillin (although the same species are moderately sensitive to this) but has the great practical advantage of oral administrability. The phenoxy penicillins, although also administrable by mouth, are insufficiently active against Gram-negative species.

The high hopes originally entertained of efficacy in enteric fever have not altogether been fulfilled. This and other important uses are discussed in the later chapters on the treatment of alimentary tract and respiratory tract infections and meningitis.

Hetacillin

This derivative of 6-aminopenicillanic acid ('Versapen', Bristol) was said to be a new chemical entity, 'the first penicinate': It is described as 6-(2,2-dimethyl-5-oxo-4-phenyl-1-imidazolidinyl)-3,3-dimethyl-7-oxo-4-thia-1-azabicyclo (3.2.0) heptane-2-carboxylic acid (Hardcastle *et al.*, 1966). Its range and degree of antibacterial activity are said in earlier papers to be very similar to those of ampicillin. According to Bunn, Milicich and Lunn (1965) and Tuano *et al.* (1966) it is more slowly excreted than ampicillin, each dose therefore having a more prolonged effect. It is acknowledged that hetacillin undergoes hydrolysis with the formation of ampicillin, both *in vitro* and in the body, but the first descriptions of this change do not specify its rate or extent. According to the recent observations of Sutherland and Robinson (1967) this hydrolysis is rapid and complete, both *in vitro* and in the blood: these authors even suggest that hetacillin may itself have no anti-bacterial activity, but this cannot be determined since the formation of ampicillin begins immediately on solution. The *in vitro* activities of hetacillin and ampicillin against 15 species of bacteria were identical, as would be expected. Comparative studies of absorption showed lower initial blood levels from hetacillin, and only such prolongation of effect in some experiments as would be accounted for by the time required for conversion to ampicillin. It seems from these findings that hetacillin is only another form in which to administer ampicillin and possesses no advantages over it.

Carbenicillin

This compound, numbered 2064 in the Beecham Research Laboratories series, is disodium α-carboxybenzyl penicillin (Knudsen, Rolinson and Sutherland, 1967). It is distinguished from all other penicillins by its degree of activity against *Ps. aeruginosa,* most strains of which are inhibited *in vitro* by 25 or 50 μg./ml. (Table XII). It is also active against all species of *Proteus* and some other enterobacteria, but inferior to benzyl penicillin against Gram-positive species. Its action is bactericidal.

It must be administered by injection and gives a peak level at 1 hour with some persistence to 6 hours (about 25 and 4 μg./ml. respectively after a dose of 1 g.). Probenecid enhances these levels and excretion is renal. Usual dosage is 1 g. at 4-hour intervals, but larger doses, if necessary by intravenous drip, are safe. The results of treating 74 patients are reported by Brumfitt, Percival and Leigh (1967), including 54 with urinary tract infections and 14 with Gram-negative bacteriaemia. Among the latter only 2 out of 7 with *Ps. aeruginosa* infection responded, but all of those with *Esch. coli* or *Proteus* infections: success was also less frequent in *Ps. aeruginosa* urinary infections. Jones and Lowbury (1967) obtained encouraging results in *Ps. aeruginosa* infection of experimental burns, with some verification in the clinical field.

Massive dosage was highly successful in the hands of Van Rooyen *et al.* (1967) in treating this infection in a series of very extensive burns, but the impression is gaining ground that whenever a systemic effect is necessary it may be unwise to rely on carbenicillin alone. Several authors, among whose observations those of Sonne and Jawetz (1969) are perhaps the most convincing, have demonstrated synergy between carbenicillin and gentamicin, and it is now a common practice to administer both. In our own experience this combination was effective even in a case of *Pseudomonas* endocarditis, although in a patient whose greatly impaired renal function enabled very high carbenicillin blood levels to be maintained. Cooper, Rice and Penfold (1969) used this combination successfully in four very severe *Ps. aeruginosa* infections in children, two having septicaemia and two including one of these leukaemia.

TABLE XII

Minimum Inhibitory Concentrations of Carbenicillin (µg./ml.)

Escherichia coli	5
*Proteus mirabilis**	2·5
„ *morganii*	5
„ *rettgeri*	2·5
„ *vulgaris*	5
Pseudomonas aeruginosa	50
Klebsiella aerogenes	250
*Staphylococcus aureus**	0·5
Streptococcus pyogenes	0·25
„ *pneumoniae*	0·5
„ *faecalis*	25

* non-penicillinase-forming
(From Knudsen, Rolinson & Sutherland, 1967.)

An added reason for using this combination is that during treatment with carbenicillin alone *Ps. aeruginosa* may become resistant. Such strains were recovered from 17 patients by Darrell and Waterworth (1969), 5 of whom had been treated with carbenicillin and 10 with other penicillins. Lowbury *et al.* (1969) report the appearance and rapid predominance of highly resistant strains in the Burns Unit at Birmingham.

The possible usefulness of carbenicillin in *Proteus* infections should not be forgotten. *P. mirabilis*, if penicillinase-forming, is resistant, as it is to ampicillin, but the other three species which are resistant to ampicillin and in general also to the cephalosporin antibiotics, are sensitive, and for infections of the urinary tract or elsewhere caused by these less common species carbenicillin may be the antibiotic of choice. The sensitivities of these organisms to four antibiotics are stated in simplified form in Table XIII.

TABLE XIII

Antibiotic Sensitivities of Proteus Species

	Ampicillin	*Carbeni-cillin*	*Cephalori-dine*	*Kanamycin*
P. mirabilis	+	+	+	+
„ (penicillinase-forming)	0	0	+	+
P. morganii	0	+	0	+
P. rettgeri	0	+	0	+
P. vulgaris	0	+	0	+

+ = sensitive
0 = resistant

CEPHALOSPORINS

This group of antibiotics, the early studies of which at Oxford are described by Florey (1955) and then later by Abraham (1962) is formed by a species of *Cephalosporium* cultivated from the sea near a sewage outfall off Sardinia by Brotzu, who used the crude products of its growth with some success for treating typhoid fever and brucellosis. When the culture was examined at Oxford it was found to produce three quite distinct antibiotics, cephalosporin N, a penicillin (adicillin: p. 80), cephalosporin P, an antibiotic of steroid structure similar to fucidin (p. 206) and cephalosporin C.

Cephalosporin C

The existence of this substance among the products of the mould was not even detected for several years, and the yield was at first so small that great difficulty was experienced in obtaining enough for essential laboratory tests. It has the same side chain as cephalosporin N, attached to a nucleus now known as 7-aminocephalosporanic acid (p. 70). The degree of antibacterial activity of cephalosporin C is only moderate, but the property which attracted most attention, at that time unique among antibiotics of this general structure, was a high degree of resistance to staphylococcal penicillinase: moreover it competitively inhibited the action of penicillinase on benzyl penicillin (Abraham and Newton, 1956). It was shown to be therapeutically active in mice and to have a very low toxicity.

Thanks to the prophetic foresight of its discoverers, determined and prolonged attempts were made to obtain an adequate yield, and when this had been achieved, chemical manipulations, similar to those being applied at the same time to the penicillin nucleus, were undertaken to improve its performance. The substitution of other side chains greatly enhanced antibacterial activity and three valuable derivatives so produced are now in therapeutic use. These are cephalothin, the first to come into use, cephaloridine and cephalexin.

Cephalothin

This derivative is 7-(thiophene-2-acetamido)-cephalosporanic acid, supplied as the sodium salt. The range of its anti-bacterial activity, and that of cephaloridine, may be seen from Table XIV,

TABLE XIV

Minimum Inhibitory Concentrations (μg. per ml.)

	Cephalothin	*Cephaloridine*
Staph. pyogenes pen. sens.	0·25	0·12
,, pen. res.	0·25-0·5	0·12-0·25
Strep. pyogenes	0·06	0·007
,, *pneumoniae*	0·06-0·12	0·015-0·03
faecalis	32	8-16
N. gonorrhoeae	0·25-0·5	4
N. meningitidis	0·12-0·5	0·5-1
H. influenzae	2-8	4-16
Esch. coli	2-8	2-4
Salm. typhi	0·5-2	2
Sh. flexneri	1-2	1-2
Pr. mirabilis	4-8	8
Kl. edwardsii	1-4	1-4
Kl. aerogenes	2-32	2-8
Ent. aerogenes	128-256	128-256

(Condensed from Barber and Waterworth, 1964)

4

condensed from the findings of Barber and Waterworth (1964) in whose paper cephaloridine is referred to as Ceph 87/4. All staphylococci, whether penicillinase-forming or not, and streptococci (except *S. faecalis*) are highly sensitive. *Neisseria* spp. are sensitive and *H. influenzae* less so. Among enterobacteria *Esch. coli, Salmonella* and *Shigella* spp. are inhibited by concentrations not exceeding 8 μg per ml., as is *Proteus mirabilis,* whether penicillinase-forming or not. This is a point of distinction from ampicillin, which is destroyed by the penicillinase of this species. The three other species of *Proteus* (not in the Table) are variable but in general resistant. *Kl. edwardsii (pneumoniae)* is sensitive, as to a rather lesser degree is *Kl. aerogenes,* but *Enterobacter aerogenes* is much more resistant. This difference is evidently that referred to by Benner *et al.* (1965b) employing different nomenclature. They distinguish the species by motility, and contrast *Aerobacter,* which is motile, and highly resistant to cephalothin and cephaloridine, but sensitive to various other drugs including tetracycline, chloramphenicol, streptomycin and sulphonamides, with the non-motile *Klebsiella* which is frequently resistant to these other drugs, but consistently sensitive to the cephalosporins. *Pseudomonas* spp. are all highly resistant.

Serum somewhat reduces the activity of cephalothin, but the inoculum effect with penicillinase-producing staphylococci is small. On the other hand methicillin-resistant staphylococci are also more resistant to cephatholin, and here the inoculum effect is large.

The cephalosporin antibiotics, like penicillins, are bactericidal, and like them, they inhibit the synthesis of staphylococcal cell walls (Abraham, 1959).

PHARMACOLOGY. Absorption after oral administration is quite inadequate, and administration is by intramuscular injection; adequate blood levels can be maintained by giving 1 g. at intervals of 4-6 hours. Excretion is mainly renal, and tubular. According to Kunin and Atuk (1966) cephalothin loses activity in the body, its half-life in " severely oliguric " patients being comparatively short whereas that of cephaloridine is much prolonged. Perkins, Smith and Saslaw (1969) found much less difference in their behaviour: both are removed by peritoneal dialysis. Penetration into the cerebrospinal fluid is poor (Vianna and Kaye, 1967; Lerner, 1969). Unlike cephalothin, cephaloridine is excreted via the glomeruli.

CLINICAL APPLICATIONS. Patients sensitized to penicillin do not react to cephalosporins: hence they may be indicated on this account for a variety of infections susceptible to both, and several clinical studies report successful use for pneumococcal and Group A streptococcal infections (Turck *et al.*, 1965; Perkins and Saslaw, 1966). The second important property of cephalothin is its activity against penicillin-resistant staphylococci, and many patients with severe staphylococcal infections including pneumonia, septicaemia and endocarditis have been treated with a high proportion of successes (Walters, Romansky and Johnson, 1963; Merrill *et al.*, 1966). Doses of up to 12 g. daily have been used. Superinfections with *Pseudomonas* or resistant *Klebsiella* are liable to occur and may be fatal. The third principal use is for Gram-negative infections, mainly of the urinary tract, caused by sensitive enterobacteria: it is noteworthy in this connection that cephalothin has a rather broader spectrum than ampicillin.

SIDE EFFECTS. Injections may be painful, and rashes are sometimes produced: thus cephalothin, although without effect on a penicillin-sensitive patient, may itself sensitize. It is claimed that cephalothin does not cause the renal damage which may be produced by cephaloridine, and although there are at least two cases in the literature in which it seems that this may have occurred, it can be accepted that the relative degree of risk is much smaller.

Cephaloridine

This derivative, resulting from the addition of not one but two side chains to the nucleus, is described chemically as 7-[(2-thienyl) acetamido]-3-(1-pyridylmethyl)-3-cephem-4-carboxylic acid betaine. It was made available at the end of 1964, its properties being described by Muggleton, O'Callaghan and Stevens (1964). These authors give particulars of its *in vitro* activity and the results of therapeutic tests in mice in which its CD_{50} was shown to be lower than that of four other appropriate antibiotics for infections by *Staph. aureus, Esch. coli* and *Pr. mirabilis*. After an intramuscular dose of 500 mg. in man the blood content was >12 μg. per ml. at 1 hour and still nearly 2 μg. per ml. at 6 and 8 hours. About 80 per cent of the dose was excreted in the urine.

This paper was accompanied by an account of clinical results (Murdoch *et al.*, 1964) in 6 cases of septicaemia, 4 of pneumococcal meningitis, for which intrathecal injections were also given, and 24 of pyelonephritis. Among later clinical reports are those of Apicella, Perkins and Saslaw (1966a) on 92 patients with a variety of infections and by the same authors (1966b) on the treatment of endocarditis.

The properties of cephaloridine and the indications for its use are very similar to those of cephalothin, and it seems necessary only to point out the differences between them. Cephaloridine has three advantages: rather greater activity against some bacteria, better stability in the body, and indifference to protein effect. Another is that injections are less painful than those of cephalothin. It also attains better concentrations than cephalothin in the cerebrospinal fluid in the presence of meningitis: Oppenheimer, Beaty and Petersdorf (1969) in an experimental study found peak c.s.f. levels as percentages of those in the blood to be for cephaloridine 10·9, cephalothin 5·6 and methicillin 2·9.

On the other hand it has one serious disadvantage which was not at first appreciated. The large inoculum effect in tests with penicillinase-forming staphylococci first noted by Barber and Waterworth (1964) and found to be still larger by Kislak, Steinhauer and Finland (1966), suggests that cephaloridine is more susceptible than had been supposed to the action of penicillinase. Ridley and Phillips (1965) have shown that when a heavy inoculum is used, the minimum inhibitory concentration of cephaloridine for different strains of staphylococci varies widely, those possessing multiple antibiotic resistance and particularly those resistant to methicillin being inhibited only by much higher concentrations than those at first reported. Benner *et al.* (1965a) have also shown that some strains destroy cephaloridine rapidly, but not cephalothin, and suggest that the latter is preferable for treating infections due to such organisms. Burgess and Evans (1966) report the failure of cephaloridine to control a staphylococcal endocarditis, blood cultures remaining positive despite the demonstrated presence of high concentrations of the antibiotic in the same specimens of blood.

It must be concluded that cephaloridine cannot always be relied on for treating one of the principal infections for which it was first recommended. It is in fact doubtful whether any single antibiotic can regularly be depended on to control staphylococcal endocarditis: a combination with another antibiotic which has been shown to be totally bactericidal *in vitro* may be necessary (Chap. XVI).

SIDE EFFECTS. Rashes due to sensitization may occur as with cephalothin. A much more serious possible effect is that on the kidney. That large doses of cephaloridine cause necrosis of the proximal convoluted tubules has been amply demonstrated in animals. There is a wide variation in species susceptibility, a single dose of only 90 mg./kg. producing this change in the rabbit, the doses required in the monkey, guinea-pig and mouse being 300, 400 and 3100 mg./kg. (Atkinson *et al.*, 1966). In the mouse and hen the effect can be prevented by giving probenecid (Child and Dodds, 1967). It is well recognized that only moderate doses may cause the appearance of large numbers of hyaline casts in the urine. Larger doses—8 g. daily or more—have unquestionably sometimes caused increasing proteinuria with a raised blood urea, going on in some cases to oliguria and renal failure, the lesion responsible being a tubular necrosis. We ourselves know of several patients in whom in retrospect it seems that this must have occurred, although the reason for it was unsuspected at the time. In severely ill patients renal failure is not uncommon and may be produced in other ways, but careful observers with extensive experience of the use of this drug have satisfied themselves that it has sometimes been responsible for renal damage. Kaplan, Reisberg and Weinstein (1968) observed it in 4 out of 7 patients given 12 g. daily, and Steigbigel *et al.* (1968) attributed renal failure in 2 out of 7 patients in whom it occurred out of a total of 122 treated directly to cephaloridine. In one case in each of these series it was fatal. Two further cases reported by Galbraith (1967) had not received such large doses. It seems advisable that at least the possibility of this effect should be more widely recognized.

ORAL CEPHALOSPORINS

Neither cephalothin nor cephaloridine is absorbed from the alimentary tract in sufficient amount to exert a therapeutic effect, and much effort has evidently been devoted to finding a derivative which is. Two are now being studied, and one is already commercially available.

Cephaloglycin

This derivative, which is 7-(D-α-aminophenyl acetamido)-cephalosporanic acid, was first described by Wick and Boniece (1965) five years ago. It is absorbed from the alimentary tract only to a limited extent: Kunin and Brandt (1968) could detect none in the blood after a 500 mg. dose, and Applestein *et al.* (1968) observed a peak level of 1·5 μg./ml. after a dose of 1 g. Fairly high concentrations are found in the urine, and some success has been obtained in treating urinary tract infections (Ronald and Turck, 1967). Perkins, Glantz and Saslaw (1969) used it not only for this purpose but even for treating pneumonia, the pneumococcus being a highly sensitive organism. Despite some success they conclude that cephaloglycin should be reserved for the continuation of successful treatment begun with an injectable cephalosporin. Cephaloglycin is unstable in an alkaline medium, and it is suggested that sensitivity tests by a dilution method in broth should be read after 12 hours. In view of this instability it is difficult to trace the fate of this substance in the body, but it is clear that not more than about 10 per cent of a dose is excreted in the urine.

Cephalexin

Cephalexin, which is 7-(D-α-amino-α-phenylacetamido)-3-methyl-3-cephem-4-carboxylic acid, has like cephaloglycin a closely similar anti-bacterial spectrum to that of cephalothin, but with a somewhat lower degree of activity against most species (Thornhill *et al.*, 1969). Unlike cephaloglycin it is stable, and very well absorbed: mean 1-hour blood levels after doses of 250, 500 and 1,000 mg. were 6·8, 17·6 and 25 μg./ml., falling to 0·6, 1·5 and 3·1 μg./ml. at 4 hours. Urinary recovery in 6 hours was from 85 to 96 per cent of the dose given

(Perkins, Carlisle and Saslaw, 1968). Similar findings are reported by Braun *et al.* (1968). In experimental streptococcal infection in monkeys oral cephalexin had an efficacy equal to that of cephalothin but inferior to that of cephaloridine, each of these being of course administered by injection (Saslaw and Carlisle, 1969). Cephalexin has now been fairly extensively used, mainly for urinary tract and respiratory infections (Symposium, 1970) but it is still difficult to assess its merits, apart from that of convenience of administration, in comparison with those of the injectable cephalosporins.

Bacterial Resistance to the Cephalosporins

It is important to recognize that staphylococci resistant to methicillin are also abnormally resistant to both cephalothin and cephaloridine. How effective the latter are in the treatment of infections caused by such strains cannot yet be judged. These fortunately exceptional organisms are thus not fully susceptible to any of this general group of antibiotics. Appropriate sensitivity tests for assessing the behaviour of individual strains are discussed in Chapter XXVIII.

The natural resistance of some Gram-negative species is in part intrinsic, and in part dependent on enzymic destruction of the antibiotic. The distribution of 'cephalosporinase' the enzyme responsible, as described by Fleming, Goldner and Glass (1963), corresponds to that of resistance among enterobacteria. Although also a β-lactamase, this enzyme has little action on benzyl penicillin. Hamilton-Miller, Smith and Knox (1965) determined the action of cell-free extracts of various Gram-negative species on benzyl penicillin, ampicillin and cephaloridine, and observed several patterns of activity, some extracts destroying ampicillin more rapidly than cephaloridine or vice versa. Jack and Richmond (1970) classify β-lactamases from Gram-negative bacteria in eight distinct types on the basis both of their patterns of relative activity and of other characters.

PHARMACEUTICAL PREPARATIONS

PHENETHICILLIN POTASSIUM ('Broxil', Beecham). Tablets of 125 or 250 mg., and syrup. Dosage of this and the two following as for phenoxymethyl penicillin.

PROPICILLIN POTASSIUM ('Brocillin', Beecham; 'Ultrapen', Pfizer). Tablets of 125 or 250 mg., and syrup.

METHICILLIN (Sodium methicillin, 'Celbenin', Beecham). Vials of 1 g. for solution for intramuscular injection: the solution should be freshly prepared (particularly unstable if the distilled water is acid from dissolved CO_2). Usual adult dose 1 g. at 4-hour intervals, but this may be increased if necessary to a total of 12 or 18 g. daily.

CLOXACILLIN (Sodium cloxacillin, 'Orbenin', Beecham). Capsules of 250 mg. (oral) and vials containing 250 mg. for solution in 1·5 ml. water for intramuscular injection. Usual adult oral dose 500 mg. at 6-hour intervals, administered *before* meals: admixture with food in bulk greatly reduces absorption. Half this dose intramuscularly produces similar blood levels, but larger amounts, up to 8 g. daily, have been given by this route for severe infections.

FLUCLOXACILLIN ('Floxapen', Beecham). Capsules of 250 mg. Usual dose 250 mg. at 6-hour intervals.

OXACILLIN (Sodium Oxacillin, 'Prostaphlin', Bristol Laboratories). Preparations and dosage as for cloxacillin.

AMPICILLIN ('Penbritin', Beecham). Capsules of 250 and 500 mg.; vials of 100, 250 and 500 mg. for solution for intramuscular injection; also tablets and syrup. Adult dose from 250 mg. orally at 6-hour intervals to a total of up to 6 g. daily given at the same intervals intramuscularly.

CARBENICILLIN ('Pyopen', Beecham). Vials of 1 g. and 5 g. for solution for intramuscular or intravenous injection. Dosage: urinary tract infections 1-2 g. 6-hourly. Systemic infections 2 g. 6-hourly. (*Pseudomonas* 20-30 g. intravenously daily).

CEPHALORIDINE ('Ceporin', Glaxo). Vials of 250, 500 and 1,000 mg. for solution for intramuscular injection. Dose 250 mg. or more (up to 1·5 g.) at 6-hour intervals.

CEPHALOTHIN ('Keflin', Lilly). Preparations and doses as for cephaloridine.

CEPHALEXIN ('Ceporex', Glaxo, 'Keflex', Lilly). Tablets 250 mg. and syrup: dosage 250 mg. or more 6-hourly up to 4 g. daily.

REFERENCES

ABRAHAM, E. P. (1959). *Endeavour* **18,** 212.

ABRAHAM, E. P. (1962). *Pharmacol. Rev.* **14,** 473.

ABRAHAM, E. P., & NEWTON, G. G. F. (1956). *Biochem. J.* **63,** 628.

ANDERSON, K. N., KENNEDY, R. P., PLORDE, J. J., SHULMAN, J. A. & PETERSDORF, R. G. (1964). *J. Amer. med. Ass.* **187,** 555.

APICELLA, M. A., PERKINS, R. L. & SASLAW, S. (1966a). *Amer. J. med. Sci.* **251,** 266.

APICELLA, M. A., PERKINS, R. L. & SASLAW, S. (1966b). *New Engl. J. Med.* **274,** 1002.

APPLESTEIN, J. M., CROSBY, E. B., JOHNSON, W. D. & KAYE, D. (1968). *Appl. Microbiol.* **16,** 1006.

ATKINSON, R. M., CURRIE, J. P., DAVIS, B., PRATT, D. A. H., SHARPE, H. M. & TOMICH, E. G. (1966). *Toxicol. appl. Pharmacol.* **8,** 398.

AYLIFFE, G. A. J. & DAVIES, A. (1965). *Brit. J. Pharmacol.* **24,** 189.

BALDWIN, D. S., LEVINE, B. B., McCLUSKEY, R. T. & GALLO, G. R. (1968). *New Engl. J. Med.* **279,** 1245.

BARBER, M. (1964). *J. gen. Microbiol.* **35,** 183.

BARBER, M. & WATERWORTH, P. M. (1964). *Brit. med. J.* **2,** 344.

BATCHELOR, F. R., CHAIN, E. B., RICHARDS, M. & ROLINSON, G. N. (1961). *Proc. roy. Soc. B.* **154,** 522.

BATCHELOR, F. R., DOYLE, F. P., NAYLER, J. H. C. & ROLINSON, G. N. (1959). *Nature (Lond.)* **183,** 257.

BENAVIDES, V. L., OLSON, B. H., VARELGA, G. & HOLT, S. H. (1955). *J. Amer. med. Ass.* **157**, 989.
BENNER, E. J., BENNET, J. V., BRODIE, J. L. & KIRBY, W. M. M. (1965a). *J. Bact.* **90**, 1599.
BENNER, E. J. & KAYSER, F. H. (1968). *Lancet* **2**, 741.
BENNER, E. J., MICKLEWAIT, J. S., BRODIE, J. L. & KIRBY, W. M. M. (1965b). *Proc. Soc. exp. Biol. (N.Y.)* **119**, 536.
BLECHER, T. E., EDGAR, W. M., MELVILLE, H. A. H. & PEEL, K. R. (1966). *Brit. med. J.* **1**, 137.
BOND, J. M., LIGHTBOWN, J. W., BARBER, M. & WATERWORTH, P. M. (1963). *Brit. med. J.* **2**, 956.
BRAUN, P., TILLOTSON, J. R., WILCOX, C. & FINLAND, M. (1968). *Appl. Microbiol.* **16**, 1684.
BRAUNINGER, G. E. & REMINGTON, J. S. (1968). *J. Amer. med. Ass.* **203**, 103.
BROWN, D. M. & ACRED, P. (1961). *Brit. med. J.* **2**, 197.
BRUMFITT, W., PERCIVAL, A. & LEIGH, D. A. (1967). *Lancet* **1**, 1289.
BULGER, R. J. (1967). *Lancet* **1**, 17.
BULGER, R. J., LINDHOLM, D. D., MURRAY, J. S. & KIRBY, W. M. M. (1964). *J. Amer. med. Ass.* **187**, 319.
BUNN, P. A., MILICICH, C. & LUNN, J. S. (1966). *Antimicrob. Agents & Chemother.* 1965: p. 947.
BURGESS, H. A. & EVANS, R. J. (1966). *Brit. med. J.* **2**, 1244.
CHABBERT, Y. A., BAUDENS, J. G., ACAR, J. F. & GERBAUD, G. R. (1965). *Rev. franc. clin. biol.* **10**, 495.
CHILD, K. J. & DODDS, M. G. (1967). *Brit. J. Pharmacol.*, **30**, 354.
COOPER, R. G., RICE, J. C. & PENFOLD, J. L. (1969). *Med. J. Aust.* **1**, 517.
v.DAEHNE, W., FREDERIKSEN, E., GUNDERSEN, E., LUND, F., MORCH, P., PETERSEN, H. J., ROHOLT, K., TYBRING, L. & GODTFREDSEN, W. O. (1970). *J. med. Chem.* **13**, 607.
DARRELL, J. H. & WATERWORTH, P. M. (1969). *Brit. med. J.* **3**, 141.
DOYLE, F. P., LONG, A. A. W., NAYLER, J. H. C. & STOVE, E. R. (1961). *Nature (Lond.)* **192**, 1183.
DYKE, K. G. H., JEVONS, M. P. & PARKER, M. T. (1966). *Lancet* **1**, 835.
EICKHOFF, T. C., KISLAK, J. W. & FINLAND, M. (1965a). *New Engl. J. Med.* **272**, 699.
EICKHOFF, T. C., KISLAK, J. W. & FINLAND, M. (1965b). *Amer. J. med. Sci.* **249**, 163.
FLEMING, P. C., GOLDNER, M. & GLASS, D. G. (1963). *Lancet* **1**, 1399.
FLOREY, H. W. (1955). *Ann. intern. Med.* **43**, 480.
GALBRAITH, H. J. B. (1967). *Brit. J. clin. Pract.* **21**, 331.
GOTTSHALL, R. Y., ROBERTS, J. M., PORTWOOD, L. M. & JENNINGS, J. C. (1951). *Proc. Soc. exp. Biol. (N.Y.)* **76**, 307.
GOUREVITCH, A., HOLDREGE, C. T., HUNT, G. A., MINOR, W. F., FLANNIGAN, C. C., CHENEY, L. C. & LEIN, J. (1962). *Antibiotic and Chemother.* **12**, 318.
GRAVENKEMPER, C. F., BENNETT, J. V., BRODIE, J. L. & KIRBY, W. M. M. (1965). *Arch. intern Med.* **116**, 340.
HAMILTON-MILLER, J. M. T. (1965). *J. gen. Microbiol.* **41**, 175.
HAMILTON-MILLER, J. M. T., SMITH, J. T. & KNOX, R. (1965). *Nature (Lond.)* **208**, 235.
HARDCASTLE, G. A. JR., JOHNSON, D. A., PANETTA, C. A., SCOTT, A. I. & SUTHERLAND, S. A. (1966). *J. organic Chem.* **31**, 897.
HÖFFLER, D., STEGEMANN, I. & SCHELER, F. (1966). *Dtsch. med. Wschr.* **91**, 206.
JACK, G. W. & RICHMOND, M. H. (1970). *J. gen. Microbiol.* **61**, 43.
JONES, R. J. & LOWBURY, E. J. L. (1967). *Brit. med. J.* **3**, 79.
KAPLAN, K., REISBERG, B. & WEINSTEIN, L. (1968). *Arch. intern. Med.* **121**, 17.
KAYSER, F. H. & HOLLINGER, A. (1968). *Dtsch. med. Wschr.* **93**, 1933.

KIND, A. C., TUPASI, T. E., STANDIFORD, H. C. & KIRBY, W. M. M. (1970). *Arch intern Med.* **125,** 685.

KISLAK, J. W., EICKHOFF, T. C. & FINLAND, M. (1965). *Amer. J. med. Sci.* **249,** 636.

KISLAK, J. W., STEINHAUER, B. W. & FINLAND, M. (1966). *Amer. J. med. Sci.* **251,** 433.

KJELLANDER, J. O. & FINLAND, M. (1963). *Proc. Soc. exp. Biol.* (*N.Y.*) **113,** 1031.

KLEIN, J. O. & FINLAND, M. (1963). *Amer. J. med. Sci.* **246,** 10.

KLEIN, J. O., SABATH, L. D., STEINHAUER, B. W. & FINLAND, M. (1963). *Amer. J. med. Sci.* **246,** 385.

KNUDSEN, E. T. & ROLINSON, G. N.(1959). *Lancet* **2,** 1105.

KNUDSEN, E. T., ROLINSON, G. N. & STEVENS, S. (1961). *Brit. med. J.* **2,** 198.

KNUDSEN, E. T., ROLINSON, G. N. & SUTHERLAND, R. (1967). *Brit. med. J.* **3,** 75.

KUNIN, C. M. (1966). *Clin. Pharmacol. Ther.* **7,** 166.

KUNIN, C. M. & ATUK, N. (1966). *New Engl. J. Med.* **274,** 654.

KUNIN, C. M. & BRANDT, D. (1968). *Amer. J. med. Sci.* **255,** 196.

LANE, W. R. (1964). *Med. J. Aust.* **2,** 499.

LERNER, P. I. (1969). *Amer. J. med. Sci.* **257,** 125.

LEVITT, B. H., GOTTLIEB, A. J., ROSENBERG, I. R. & KLEIN, J. J. (1964). *Clin. Pharmacol. Ther.* **5,** 301.

LOWBURY, E. J. L., KIDSON, A., LILLY, H. A., AYLIFFE, G. A. J. & JONES, R. J. (1969). *Lancet* **2,** 448.

McELFRESH, A. E. & HUANG, N. N. (1962). *New Engl. J. Med.* **266,** 246.

MacNAIR, D. R., WHITE, J. E. & GRAHAM, J. M. (1968). *Lancet* **1,** 16.

MERRILL, S. L., DAVIS, A., SMOLENS, B. & FINEGOLD, S. M. (1966). *Ann. intern. Med.* **64,** 1.

MORTIMER, P. R., MACKIE, D. B. & HAYNES, S. (1969). *Brit. med. J.* **3,** 88.

MUGGLETON, P. W., O'CALLAGHAN, C. H. & STEVENS, W. K. (1964). *Brit. med. J.* **2,** 1234.

MURDOCH, J. McC., SPIERS, C. F., GEDDES, A. M. & WALLACE, E. T. (1964). *Brit. med. J.* **2,** 1238.

NAUMANN, P. (1965). *Dtsch. med. Wschr.* **90,** 1085.

NAUMANN, P. & KEMPF, B. (1965). *Arzneimittel Forsch.* **15,** 139.

NAYLER, J. H. C., LONG, A. A. W., BROWN, D. M., ACRED, P., ROLINSON, G. N., BATCHELOR, F. R., STEVENS, S. & SUTHERLAND, R. (1962). *Nature* (*Lond.*) **195,** 1264.

OPPENHEIMER, S., BEATY, H. N. & PETERSDORF, R. G. (1969). *J. Lab. clin. Med.* **73,** 535.

PARKER, M. T. & HEWITT, J. H. (1970). *Lancet* **1,** 800.

PERKINS, R. L., CARLISLE, H. N. & SASLAW, S. (1968). *Amer. J. med. Sci.* **256,** 122.

PERKINS, R. L., GLONTZ, G. E. & SASLAW, S. (1969). *Clin. Pharmacol. Ther.* **10,** 244.

PERKINS, R. L. & SASLAW, S. (1966). *Ann. intern. Med.* **64,** 13.

PERKINS, R. L., SMITH, E. J. & SASLAW, S. (1969). *Amer. J. med. Sci.* **257,** 116.

REPORT FROM SIX HOSPITALS (1962). *Lancet* **2,** 634.

RICHARDS, H. C., HOUSLEY, J. R. & SPOONER, D. F. (1963). *Nature* (*Lond.*) **199,** 354.

RIDLEY, M. & PHILLIPS, I. (1965). *Nature* (*Lond.*) **208,** 1076.

ROLINSON, G. N. & STEVENS, S. (1961). *Brit. med. J.* **2,** 191.

ROLINSON, G. N., STEVENS, S., BATCHELOR, F. R., WOOD, J. C. & CHAIN, E. B. (1960). *Lancet* **2,** 564.

ROLLO, I. M., SOMERS, G. F. & BURLEY, D. M. (1962). *Brit. med. J.* **i,** 76.

RONALD, A. R. & TURCK, M. (1967). *Antimicrob. Agents & Chemother.* —1966, p. 83.

ROSENBLATT, J. E., KIND, A. C., BRODIE, J. L. & KIRBY, W. M. M. (1968). *Arch. intern. Med.* **121**, 345.

SABATH, L. D., KLEIN, J. O. & FINLAND, M. (1963). *Amer. J. med. Sci.* **246**, 129.

SASLAW, S. & CARLISLE, H. N. (1969). *Amer. J. med. Sci.* **257**, 395.

SEELIGER, H. P. R., LAYMANN, V. & FINGER, H. (1967). *Dtsch. med. Wschr.* **92**, 1095.

SEELIGER, H. & MATHEIS, H. (1969). *Dtsch. med. Wschr.* **94**, 853.

SHAPIRO, S., SLONE, D., SISKIND, V., LEWIS, G. P. & JICK, H. (1969). *Lancet* **2**, 969.

SIBONI, K. & POULSEN, E. D. (1968). *Dan. med. Bull.* **15**, 161.

SIDELL, S., BULGER, R. J., BRODIE, J. L. & KIRBY, W. M. M. (1964). *Clin. Pharmacol. Therap.* **5**, 26.

SIMON, H. J. & SAKAI, W. (1963). *Pediatrics* **31**, 463.

SLEET, R. A., SANGSTER, G. & MURDOCH, J. McC. (1964). *Brit. med. J.* **1**. 148.

SMITH, J. T., HAMILTON-MILLER, J. M. T. & KNOX, R. (1964). *Nature (Lond.)* **203**, 1148.

SONNE, M. & JAWETZ, E. (1969). *Appl. Microbiol.* **17**, 893.

STEIGBIGEL, N. H., KISLAK, J. W., TILLES, J. G. & FINLAND, M. (1968.) *Arch. intern. Med.* **121**, 24.

SUTHERLAND, R., CROYDON, E. A. P. & ROLINSON, G. N. (1970). *Brit. med. J.* **4**, 455.

SUTHERLAND, R. & ROBINSON, O. P. W. (1967).*Brit. med. J.* **2**, 804.

SUTHERLAND, R. & ROLINSON, G. N. (1964a). *J. Bact.* **87**, 887.

SUTHERLAND, R. & ROLINSON, G. N. (1964b). *J. clin. Path.* **17**, 461.

SYMPOSIUM (1970). *Postgrad. med J.* **47**, Suppl. Oct.

THORNHILL, T. S., LEVISON, M. E., JOHNSON, W. W. & KAYE, D. (1969). *Appl. Microbiol.* **17**, 457.

TUANO, S. B., JOHNSON, L. D., BRODIE, J. L. & KIRBY, W. M. M. (1966). *New Engl. J. Med.* **275**, 635.

TURCK, M., ANDERSON, K. N., SMITH, R. H., WALLACE, J. F. & PETERSDORF, R. G. (1965). *Ann. intern. Med.* **63**, 199.

TURCK, M., RONALD, A. & PETERSDORF, R. G. (1965). *J. Amer. med. Ass.* **192**, 961.

VAN ROOYEN, C. E., ROSS, J. F., BETHUNE, G. W. & MACDONALD, A. C. (1967). *Canad. med. Ass. J.* **97**, 1227.

VIANNA, N. J. & KAYE, D. (1967). *Amer. J. med. Sci.* **254**, 216.

WALTERS, E. W., ROMANSKY, M. J. & JOHNSON, A. C. (1963). *Antimicrobial Agents and Chemotherapy—1962*, 706.

WEINGARTNER, L. & ORTEL, S. (1967). *Dtsch. med. Wschr.* **92**, 1098.

WICK, W. E. & BONIECE, W. S. (1965). *Appl. Microbiol.* **13**, 248

WILLIAMSON, G. M., MORRISON. J. K. & STEVENS. K. J. (1961). *Lancet* **1**, 847.

CHAPTER VI

AMINOGLYCOSIDES

1. STREPTOMYCIN

UNLIKE penicillin, streptomycin was discovered as the result of a deliberate search for antibiotics. Starting in 1939, Waksman and his colleagues examined a large series of micro-organisms, particularly soil bacteria, for activity against Gram-negative bacilli. The first antibiotic of any value resulting from this investigation was streptothricin, which was isolated in 1942 by Waksman and Woodruff from a strain of *Streptomyces lavendulae,* but was subsequently found to be too toxic for clinical use. In 1944, after more than ten thousand micro-organisms had been examined, Schatz, Bugie and Waksman recorded the isolation of streptomycin from a strain of *Streptomyces griseus,* found in a diagnostic culture from a chicken's throat.

Different strains of *Streptomyces griseus* vary very much in antibiotic production. Some strains appear to produce no antibiotics, others produce streptomycin; and yet others produce grisein or the antifungal agent, candicidin. The species was first isolated by Krainsky in Russia in 1914 and soon after by Waksman and Curtis (1916). When this original strain was tested in 1946 it produced no antibiotics, but after irradiation, a streptomycin-producing variant was obtained (Waksman and Lechevalier, 1953).

CHEMICAL PROPERTIES

Streptomycin is readily soluble in water and is a strong base. Many organic and inorganic salts have been prepared, of which the sulphate is the most important preparation, and is the only one listed in the British Pharmacopoeia, since it causes the least pain and irritation at the site of injection.

Streptomycin sulphate is a white almost colourless substance with a slightly bitter taste. It is very soluble in water and

almost insoluble in alcohol. Watery solutions are acid, those
containing 250 mg./ml. having a pH as low as 4·5. Solutions
are stable for long periods at a pH between 3 and 7 and a
temperature below 28° C.; solutions kept in the cold retain their
potency for at least a year.

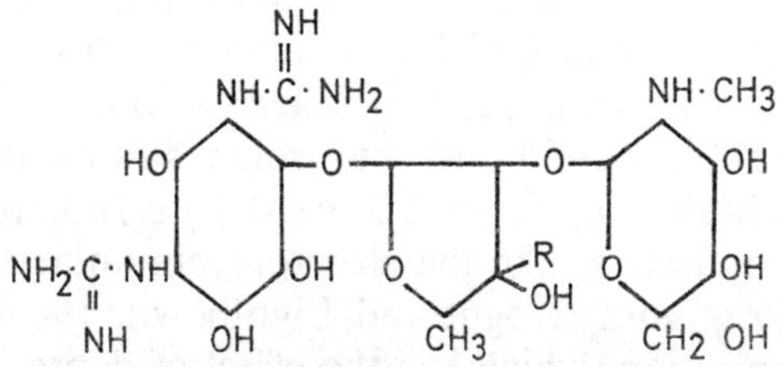

FIG. 6
Structure of Streptomycin (R=CHO) and Dihydrostreptomycin
(R=CH₂OH).

ANTI-BACTERIAL ACTIVITY

Streptomycin is a bactericidal antibiotic particularly active
against *Mycobacteria,* Gram-negative bacilli and some strains
of staphylococci. Streptococci and pneumococci are relatively
resistant, and anaerobic sporing bacilli and fungi almost completely insensitive (Table XV).

TABLE XV

Sensitivity of Bacteria to Streptomycin

Usual minimum inhibitory concentration (μg./ml.) with a moderate
inoculum.
N.B. The results given below are those obtained with sensitive strains,
which have not previously been in contact with streptomycin.
Resistant variants are common with all species.

Gram-negative Bacteria		Gram-positive Bacteria	
Esch. coli	2 - 4	Staph. aureus	2
Kl. aerogenes	2	Str. pyogenes	32
Kl. pneumoniae	1	Str. pneumoniae	64
Proteus spp.	4 - >256	Str. faecalis	64 - >256
Ps. aeruginosa	16 - 64	Clostridium spp.	> 128
Salm. typhi	8 - 16		
Salm. paratyphi	4 - 8		
Salm. spp.	4 - 16	Myco. tuberculosis	0·5
Sh. sonnei	2 - 4		
Sh. flexneri	2 - 8		
N. gonorrhoeae	4		

The anti-bacterial activity of streptomycin is greatest in a slightly alkaline medium (pH 7·8) and is considerably reduced in media with a pH of 6·0 or less. Streptomycin is so sensitive to the effect of pH that the natural acidity of a solution of streptomycin sulphate may be sufficient to depress its anti-bacterial activity. Krauss *et al.* (1968) found that 20 μg./ml. streptomycin sulphate (pH 7·1) inhibited a strain of pneumo-cocci, while 50 μg./ml. (pH 6·8) failed to do so. It is less active under anaerobic conditions, but some strains of anaerobic cocci are inhibited by from 2·0 to 10·0 μg./ml. It seems that anaerobic conditions, like the streptomycin antagonist isolated from *Ps. aeruginosa* (Kogut and Lightbown, 1963), act by in-hibiting respiration, which has the effect of depressing strepto-mycin uptake. Anaerobiosis also limits the stimulation of RNA synthesis which precedes the death of sensitive strains exposed to streptomycin (Stern *et al.*, 1966).

Mode of Action

Garrod (1948) drew attention to the bactericidal action of streptomycin in concentrations which can be attained in the blood-stream. Thus a population of 95 million staphylococci per ml. was completely extinguished in eight hours by 20 μg. streptomycin per ml.; 50 and 200 μg./ml. extinguished it in four and two hours respectively and 2,000 μg./ml. produced a 99·8 per cent mortality in 10 minutes. Thus, unlike penicillin, which has a quite low optimum concentration for bactericidal effect, above which no enhancement is obtainable, strepto-mycin behaves like an ordinary germicide, the velocity of its bactericidal action increasing progressively with rise in con-centration.

The bactericidal effect of concentrations readily attainable in the body is also exerted against *Myco. tuberculosis*. This would account for the therapeutic efficiency of treatment with a single daily dose which does not maintain a consistently bacteristatic concentration in the blood stream. Streptomycin is more actively bactericidal to rapidly multiplying than to resting cells, but unlike penicillin is capable, under certain circumstances, of killing bacteria which are not multiplying (Eagle and Saz, 1955).

Streptomycin is rapidly taken up by bacteria with the result that the negative surface charge falls and the cells tend to agglutinate. There is an associated rapid loss of potassium from the cell, but it seems unlikely that this permeability change, which is transient, plays an important part in the lethal effect of streptomycin.

Protein Synthesis

It was early established that streptomycin, like tetracycline and chloramphenicol, interferes with bacterial protein synthesis but the means by which this is evidently brought about is one of the most fascinating anti-bacterial effects yet uncovered. On the DNA template the cell assembles three kinds of RNA: transfer-RNA (t-RNA), ribosomal-RNA (r-RNA) and messenger-RNA (m-RNA). Ribosomal-RNA is utilized, with protein, in the construction of ribosomes—small bodies, lying free in the cytoplasm or attached to the cytoplasmic membrane, which are concerned with protein synthesis. Messenger-RNA takes from DNA to the ribosomes the code which fixes the order in which amino acids are assembled into protein.

Amino acids are activated by combination with ATP and the activated amino acid is transported to the ribosomes by a t-RNA specific to that type of amino acid. On the ribosome the amino acids are united in the order specified by the m-RNA, and the t-RNA is released to transport more amino acid. This sequence of events is summarized in Fig. 7 where the sites of action of chloramphenicol, tetracycline, erythromycin and streptomycin are shown. The growing peptide chain is attached to one of two sites on the ribosome by the most recently added amino acid which is also located on the m-RNA by its t-RNA carrier. The amino acid to be next added (determined by correspondence between its t-RNA and the m-RNA codon) is attached to the second site on the ribosome (Fig. 7, A). The growing peptide is now transferred enzymically to the attached amino acid (Fig. 7, B). When transfer has occurred, the peptide chain is moved back to the first site, the t-RNA which attached the chain is released, and the messenger moved along in relation to the ribosome (a process called ' translocation ') so that the next codon is opposite the amino acid attachment site. The next amino acid is then attached (Fig. 7, C) and the whole cycle repeated.

After binding to the surface, streptomycin enters the cell and becomes attached to the ribosome. It has no effect on m-RNA or its binding by the ribosome but appears to exert its effect on the ribosome itself (Leon and Brock, 1967). The linkage of amino acids continues but the effect on the ribosome is such that the information supplied by the attached messenger-RNA is mis-read and the wrong amino acid is incorporated into the growing peptide chain (Fig. 7, D).

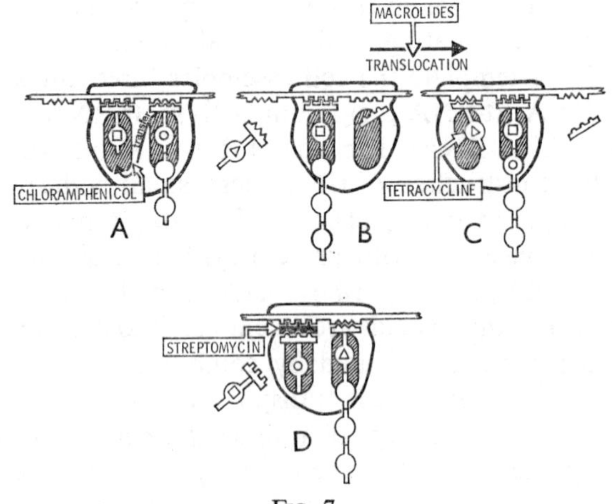

FIG. 7

Protein synthesis: (A) The growing peptide chain is transferred to the amino acid which has recently attached to the ribosome. The t-RNA which attached the peptide is released and the m-RNA moves in relation to the ribosome (B→C) bringing the next codon in apposition to the amino acid site. The amino acid specified by the codon and carried by its specific t-RNA, attaches to the ribosome (C); the peptide chain is transferred to it and the whole cycle is repeated.

The degree of infidelity introduced into protein replication by this process is very small. Major deletions of amino acid sequences do not occur and it appears that the lesion involves misplacement of a single amino acid. Estimations of the numbers of streptomycin molecules required to inhibit protein synthesis strongly suggest that the specific biochemical lesion is brought about by attachment of a single streptomycin molecule to one of the nucleotides of the coding triplet. This very discrete lesion is sufficient for the continuation of the peptide sequence to fail, or for protein to be manufactured which is unable to fulfil its enzymic or structural function. The effect of streptomycin on cell growth is relatively slow and it is probable that considerable accumulation of faulty protein occurs before cell function ceases. Streptomycin produces a number of later effects on the cell, such as permeability changes and impairment of respiration, which might result from imperfections in the protein molecules concerned in those functions or might be independent effects of the drug. Either way it is probable that it is these effects, rather than the protein derangement itself which are directly responsible for cell death.

Acquired Resistance

Nearly all species of bacteria, including the tubercle bacillus, are capable of yielding variants showing a gross increase in resistance to streptomycin after only a few passages in the presence of the antibiotic *in vitro* or within a few days (for the tubercle bacillus a few weeks) of the beginning of streptomycin treatment. It was soon realised that this rapid emergence of streptomycin-resistant cultures was due to the fact that any large population of bacteria was liable to contain a few cells resistant to 1,000 μg. per ml. streptomycin which were readily selected by the antibiotic. Streptomycin-resistant strains sometimes have a reduced growth-rate and may be of decreased virulence, but many, at any rate, appear to be as virulent as streptomycin-sensitive strains.

Resistance appears to arise from several discrete mechanisms. In *Esch. coli* and *Str. pneumoniae* it appears to result from ribosomal alterations due to a specific ribosomal protein which is coded for at the streptomycin resistance locus (Leboy *et al.*, 1964). It appears possible that while high level resistance results from reduced ribosomal susceptibility to streptomycin, low level resistance is due to decreased uptake of the antibiotic (Gundersen, 1967). R-factor mediated resistance (p. 254) is different in that it results from inactivation of streptomycin by a specific enzyme (Yamada *et al.*, 1968).

It is not infrequent to find strains of meningococci, *Staph. aureus, Esch. coli, Ps. aeruginosa, Proteus* and *Myco. tuberculosis* which are actually favoured by the presence of the antibiotic or completely dependent on it. Spotts and Stanier (1961) proposed that the conditions of streptomycin sensitivity, resistance and dependence are due to alternate states of a single ribosomal protein. Ribosomes from sensitive bacteria are sensitive to the action of streptomycin, and ribosomes from resistant bacteria resistant. In certain conditions, ribosomes from streptomycin-dependent bacteria require streptomycin to function (Likover and Kurland, 1967). The results of streptomycin deprivation of streptomycin-dependent cells are those which would be expected if streptomycin were required by the cell to reverse an ambiguity of protein synthesis introduced by mutation. A good deal of evidence derived from study of various agents and conditions which will induce and reverse ambiguity of protein synthesis strongly support the view that streptomycin acts in this way in dependent bacteria (Brock, 1966). The antigenicity and virulence of streptomycin-dependent variants of *Salm. typhi* is unchanged (Reitman, 1967).

Cross Resistance

There is complete cross resistance between streptomycin and dihydrostreptomycin, and partial cross resistance between streptomycin and neomycin, kanamycin and paromomycin. This is usually one way: strains that have developed resistance to neomycin and kanamycin nearly always show a significant increase in resistance to streptomycin (Table XIX, p. 120) while streptomycin-resistant bacteria are frequently still sensitive to neomycin and kanamycin (Brock, 1964). These cross-resistances probably arise from differences in the ribosomal sites of action of the antibiotics (Tanaka *et al.*, 1964).

PHARMACOLOGY

Absorption

Streptomycin is not absorbed in any quantity from the intestinal tract. Its activity in the gut is retained and it is excreted unchanged in the faeces. It may, therefore, be used orally for its action on bacteria in the lumen of the intestine.

INTRAMUSCULAR INJECTION. For systemic treatment streptomycin is usually administered by this route. Injections are liable to be painful. The levels obtained are shown in Table XVI. In patients treated for tuberculosis, Line *et al.* (1970) found considerable variation in the same patient on repeat testing, the peak levels following a dose of 0·75 g. sometimes differing by as much as 50 μg./ml.

TABLE XVI

Plasma Levels of Streptomycin

	Dose	Peak Plasma Level		Plasma Half-life Hours
		Hour	μg./ml.	
Adult	0·5G		16-42	2·4-2·7
	1·0G	$\frac{1}{2}$-1$\frac{1}{2}$	25-50	
Adult over 40 yrs	0·75G		26-58	up to 9·0
Premature Infant	10 mg. per kg.	2	17-42	7·0

Adcock, J. D. & Hettig, R. A. (1946). *Arch. intern. Med.* **77,** 179.
Buggs, C. W., *et al.* (1946). *J. clin. Invest.* **25,** 94.
Axline, S. G. & Simon, H. J. (1965). *Antimicrob. Agents Chemother.* 1964, p. 135.
Line, D. H. *et al.* (1970).

In premature infants the ability to excrete streptomycin is impaired (Table XVI) and therapeutic levels (10 μg./ml. or more) are still present 4-5 hours after 5 mg./kg. (half the adult dose). As renal function declines with age too, so in patients over the age of 40 streptomycin tends to persist longer in the blood (Table XVI) and in older adults excretion is commonly incomplete at 24 hours (Line *et al.*, 1970).

INTRATHECAL ADMINISTRATION. Since streptomycin does not readily reach the cerebro-spinal fluid after systemic administration, intrathecal injections may be necessary in the treatment of meningitis, unless a second drug, which passes into the cerebro-spinal fluid, is being used at the same time. A daily dose of 100 mg. in 10 ml. of normal saline produces levels of 750-2,000 μg./ml. after 1-3 hours and detectable concentrations after 24 hours. Such intrathecal injections may produce meningeal irritation demonstrated by a marked increase in the number of polymorphonuclear cells in the C.S.F.

Distribution and Excretion

TISSUES. Streptomycin diffuses fairly rapidly into most body tissues. It is distributed as if it were present in extracellular fluid only, and does not readily penetrate into cells. Little or no streptomycin can be demonstrated inside macrophages in the presence of therapeutic blood levels, even when the cells are actively phagocytic (Bonventre *et al.*, 1967). Appreciable concentrations of streptomycin have been found in most organs of the body, in postmortem studies, with the notable exception of the brain. A case has been recorded in which the brain tissue contained no detectable streptomycin, although a concentration of 15·8 μg. per ml. was present in the cerebrospinal fluid.

SEROUS CAVITIES AND ABSCESSES. In ascites, streptomycin appears in the peritoneal fluid within a short time of an intramuscular injection in concentrations about one-quarter to one-half those present in the blood. Diffusion into pleural fluid appears to be rather slower, but after repeated injections higher concentrations are reached, so that streptomycin levels in pleural fluid may be equal to those in the blood.

Streptomycin does not penetrate into thick-walled abscesses but significant amounts are usually present in tuberculous cavities.

PASSAGE THROUGH PLACENTA. Streptomycin has been shown to pass through the placenta to give levels in cord blood similar to those in maternal blood.

URINE. Streptomycin is rapidly excreted in the urine, when the kidneys are normal, but the amount excreted in 24 hours differs very much in different individuals. Excretion is by glomerular filtration and is unaffected by agents which block tubular secretion. The renal clearance is 30-70 ml./min. and between 30 and 90 per cent of the dose is usually excreted in the first 24 hours, some being destroyed or retained in the body. The concentrations of streptomycin in the urine are often very high: urinary levels of 300-400 μg. per ml. after doses of 0·5 g. and 1,000 μg. per ml. or more after doses of 1 g. are not uncommon. In oliguria, the plasma half life is prolonged to 50-100 hours and dosage must be reduced if toxic levels are to be avoided. Adequate levels can usually be obtained if following a normal dose, half the usual dosage is given at 3-4 day intervals (Kunin, 1967).

BILE. Small amounts of streptomycin, probably less than one per cent, are excreted in the bile and levels of from 3 to 12·5 μg./ml. have been recorded.

FAECES. Large amounts of streptomycin appear in the faeces after oral administration, since the antibiotic is neither absorbed nor inactivated in the intestine. The effect is cumulative and a concentration of 9 mg. per g. faeces has been recorded after 1 g. streptomycin daily for six days.

TOXICITY AND SIDE-EFFECTS

Pain and irritation at the site of injection of streptomycin are common, but are probably less severe with the sulphate than with the hydrochloride. The pain can be relieved by giving the antibiotic in association with procaine.

Many patients experience unpleasant symptoms within a few hours of an intramuscular injection of streptomycin, such as paraesthesiae in and round the mouth, vertigo and ataxia, headaches and lassitude and ' muzziness in the head '. These are often trivial, but in ambulant patients in whom blood levels are appreciably higher than in those at rest, they are sometimes sufficient to render the patient unable to work.

Varpela (1964) offers some evidence that foetal abnormalities may be more common in pregnant patients receiving streptomycin, isoniazid and P.A.S. for tuberculosis, but the situation is complicated and the correlation is not easy to sustain.

Effects on Eighth Nerve

The most serious toxic effect of streptomycin is vestibular disturbance. In early clinical trials of streptomycin in tuberculosis the drug was given in a daily dose of 2 g. and in the first American series the incidence of vertigo was 96 per cent, and in the first British report it was 66 per cent. If the daily dose was only 1 g. the incidence of vertigo was greatly reduced and with half this dose rarely occurred earlier than the forty-fifth day of treatment. Animal experiments confirm that the principal toxic effect of streptomycin is on the sensory epithelia of the labyrinth. Cats treated with a single dose of 400 mg. per kg. became ataxic and remained so for more than 24 hours (Wersall and Hawkins, 1962). Those treated with a daily dose of 100-200 mg. per kg. became incoordinated after 16-19 days and with continuation of treatment lost their righting reflexes and eventually had difficulty in standing. Some recovery occurred after cessation of treatment but they were still unable to jump without falling and some showed the circling movement characteristic of chronic vestibular damage. Severe degenerative changes were found in the vestibular hair cells and supporting cells, and the thicker vesiculated nerve fibres and the nerve chalices disappeared.

The vestibular end-organs are essential to the development of the typical symptoms of motion sickness, and even partial impairment of vestibular function will afford some protection. This has led to the treatment of patients suffering from Meniere's disease with just enough streptomycin to produce unsteadiness. On prolonged follow-up, there was no recurrence and none had developed deafness (Graybiel *et al.*, 1967).

Nevertheless there is no doubt that both in man and animals, damage to hearing can occur. Robinson and Cambon (1964) described two cases of congenital hearing loss in children born to mothers treated with streptomycin in pregnancy, and amongst 17 children whose mothers had received the drug, Conway and Birt (1965) found abnormalities in the caloric test in 6 and in the audiogram in 4. In all 8 monkeys treated with streptomycin, Igarashi *et al.* (1966) found pathological changes in the organ of Corti in addition to vestibular damage.

There is a good deal of evidence that the incidence of vestibular disturbance is related to total dosage and also to excessive blood levels maintained for shorter periods. Two other factors are important: the age of the patient and the state of renal function. In the patient over 40 the risk of damage is higher and when it does occur compensation is less good than in younger patients. In the cases reported by Erlanson and Lundgren (1964) two thirds of the patients had received a total dose of only 4-10 g. over 5-14 days, but in some the daily dose was high, and two thirds had impaired renal function. Line *et al.* (1970) studied 27 patients treated with 0·75 g. streptomycin daily for tuberculosis, 8 of whom became dizzy within 6 weeks of starting treatment. There was no significant relation between incidence of dizziness and peak streptomycin level, but a highly significant relation with the 24 hour level. Serum levels exceeding 3 μg./ml. at 24 hours were found in 5 out of 8 dizzy patients but only 2 out of 18 unaffected patients, and both of these had had their dosage reduced when it was found that their renal function was impaired.

While there is no doubt of the importance of excessive dosage, there is also considerable individual variation in susceptibility to the drug. In their studies in monkeys, Igarashi *et al.* (1966) found damage to the cristae which varied from very slight to very severe and which bore no relation to the amount of drug given. Prazic *et al.* (1964), who emphasize the possibility of damage to hearing after only a few doses of streptomycin, describe a family of 7 in which 4 sisters all became deaf after receiving 5-30 g. streptomycin. The hearing of the remaining members of the family was normal and there was no history of familial deafness. It may be that such familial susceptibility to streptomycin was implicated in the case of a mother treated in pregnancy and her child both of whose audiograms were abnormal (Conway and Birt, 1965).

The possibility of toxic effects needs taking into account, therefore, not only in connection with a long course given for tuberculosis, but when streptomycin is prescribed for shorter periods for other purposes. Among 22 patients with eighth nerve damage, affecting vestibular function in 21 and hearing in three, seen by Cawthorne and Ranger (1957), only four had been treated for tuberculosis: none had received more than 20 g., and 12 had had only 10 g. or less. Some of their diagnoses imply renal insufficiency, and most of them were middle aged or elderly. In some cases the antibiotic had been given only as 'cover' for what should have been a clean operation. It is quite unjustifiable to use streptomycin for such a purpose in anyone in whom there is any possibility of impaired renal function, including that which naturally accompanies the advance of age. When such impairment exists, either the dose should be carefully regulated by the results of blood assays, or alternative treatment should be adopted. It is evident from the work of Line *et al.* (1970) that if the 24 hour serum level exceeds 3 μg./ml., the dosage should be reduced.

All recent authors are agreed that there is no foundation for the claim that streptomycin pantothenate is less ototoxic than other preparations (Erlanson and Lundgren, 1964; Igarashi, 1966). The comparative incidence of toxicity encountered by Willemot *et al.* (1962) was:

TABLE XVII

Relative Ototoxicity of Streptomycin Preparations

	Average dose g.	*Number of patients*	*Ototoxic %*
Streptomycin	105	91	12
Streptomycin pantothenate	106	104	11·5
Streptomycin plus dihydro-streptomycin	79	100	22·7
Dihydrostreptomycin pantothenate	67	47	44·7

Hypersensitivity

Skin rashes and drug-fever occur in about 5 per cent of treated patients. They are usually trivial and respond to antihistamine treatment so that in most cases streptomycin therapy can be continued, although this should be done with caution, since occasionally severe and even fatal exfoliative dermatitis may develop.

Skin sensitization is also common in nurses and dispensers who handle streptomycin and may lead to severe dermatitis, sometimes associated with periorbital swelling and conjunctivitis. This can be avoided by care in the giving of injections, the use of cartridge syringes and the wearing of gloves and masks.

Desensitization of those who handle streptomycin is usually possible, but may take several months and quite severe reactions may occur even with the minute doses used. Cover with antihistamines or corticosteroids, together with the use of repeated minute doses, instead of steadily increasing ones, may help to reduce the reactions but will not necessarily eliminate them.

Patients showing hypersensitivity during therapy are generally much more readily desensitized. Reactions most frequently develop between 4 and 6 weeks, but may appear after the first dose or after 6 months' treatment. Desensitization may be achieved by giving 20 mg. prednisolone daily plus 10 daily increments from 10-100 mg. streptomycin followed by 10 daily increments from 0·1-1·0 g. (Hutfield, 1965).

Lal and Ferguson (1963) gave increasing doses of streptomycin every six hours. By the ninth day, the whole dose was tolerated in a single injection and the patients were able to continue treatment without reaction.

Neuromuscular Blockade

Several antibiotics have attracted attention because of their capacity to produce neuromuscular blockade (pp. 124 and 192). According to Hokkanen (1964) streptomycin and its relatives function as membrane stabilizers in the same way as curare, reducing the sensitivity of the post-junctional end-plate membrane to the depolarizing effect of acetyl-choline. To give some idea of the potency of these compounds, Lullmann and Reuter (1960) have estimated that if D-tubocurarine has a blocking value of 1,000, that of polymyxin B is 5, neomycin 2·5, streptomycin 0·7, dihydrostreptomycin 0·6, and kanamycin 0·5. Their effect is, therefore, relatively feeble and it is rare for streptomycin to show any neuromuscular blocking effects in those whose neuromuscular mechanisms are normal. However, as Hokkanen points out, antibiotics are customarily given in much larger amounts than curare and it is relatively common to see blocking effects in patients who are also receiving muscle relaxants or anaesthetics or in those suffering from myasthenia gravis (Toivakka and Hokkanen, 1965).

Other Toxic Effects

Agranulocytosis and aplastic anaemia have occasionally been recorded.

CLINICAL APPLICATION

The most important use of streptomycin is in the treatment of tuberculosis. On account of the danger of streptomycin-resistant tubercle bacilli emerging during treatment it should be given in combination with one of the other anti-tuberculous drugs (Chap. XXIII).

Apart from this streptomycin is the most effective antibiotic for the treatment of plague and tularaemia and sometimes, also, for infections due to *Ps. aeruginosa* and *Proteus* and other coliform bacilli. In the treatment of infections with coliform bacilli, particularly of the urinary tract, large doses should be given for a short period, and combined therapy should be considered, since unless the infection is sterilized within a day or two of the onset of treatment drug-resistant strains are almost certain to appear.

Streptomycin is a good drug to give in combination with penicillin, since both are bactericidal antibiotics (Chap. XVI) and this combination is often useful in the treatment of bacterial endocarditis. Streptomycin in combination with tetracycline is considered by some to be the most effective antibiotic treatment for brucellosis.

Since streptomycin is not absorbed from the intestinal tract, oral administration may be used for its effect on the intestinal flora. It is disappointing in the treatment of intestinal infections, but may be of value for depressing the normal bowel flora prior to abdominal surgery. For this purpose it is best given in association with another antibiotic.

Dihydrostreptomycin

Dihydrostreptomycin (Fig. 6) was first produced by catalytic reduction of streptomycin and has since been isolated from cultures of *Streptomyces humidus* in Japan (Imamura *et al.,* 1956).

Its solubility, stability, antibacterial activity, distribution and excretion are similar to those of streptomycin.

TOXICITY. It was introduced with the claim that its ' chronic neurotoxicity ' is less than that of streptomycin. Unfortunately, although less liable to cause vestibular disturbance, it is much more liable to cause deafness (Table XVII). Moreover this usually develops after the course of treatment is over, an interval of two months being common and six not unheard ot. There is thus no possibility of minimizing damage by stopping treatment at its first sign. Marcus *et al.* (1963) examined 35 deaf children who had received medication as premature infants and found that 29 had had dihydrostreptomycin in excess of the standard dose. The deafness is often complete and almost always permanent. It is therefore not surprising that dihydrostreptomycin has now been omitted from the B.P.

Because the carbonyl group through which streptomycin binds to protein is hydrogenated in dihydrostreptomycin, it is not antigenic and does not cause sensitization (Cronin, 1965). Commercial preparations of dihydrostreptomycin are contaminated with streptomycin—from which they are produced—and this is probably responsible for reports of skin sensitivity to dihydrostreptomycin in man.

CLINICAL APPLICATION. On the principle that it has no countervailing advantages over streptomycin, and deafness is worse than vertigo and ataxia, dihydrostreptomycin should probably never be prescribed at all.

PHARMACEUTICAL PREPARATIONS AND DOSAGE

STREPTOMYCIN SULPHATE (Streptolin, *Glaxo;* Streptoquaine, *Dista*)

INJECTION: B.P., B.N.F., equiv. 330 mg. in 1 ml.; U.S.P., equiv. 1 g. in 2 ml. and 2·5 ml.; equiv. 5 g. in 10 ml. and 12·5 ml. Dose: i.m.: 0·5-1·0 g. daily; intrathecal: 100 mg.

REFERENCES

BONVENTRE, P. F., HAYES, R. & IMHOFF, J. (1967). *J. Bact.* **93**, 445.
BROCK, T. D. (1964). *Fed. Proc.* **23**, 965.
BROCK, T. D. (1966). *Symp. Soc. gen. Microbiol.* **16**, 131.
CAWTHORNE, T. & RANGER, D. (1957). *Brit. med. J.* **1**, 1444.
CHIOSA, L. & MANOLESCU, A. (1965) *Arch. int. Pharmacodyn.* **156**, 161.
CONWAY, N. & BIRT, B. D. (1965). *Brit. med. J.* **2**, 260.
CRONIN, A. E. (1965). *Aust. J. Dermat.* **8**, 78.
EAGLE, H. & SAZ, A. K. (1955). *Ann. Rev. Microbiol.* **9**, 173.
ERLANSON, P. & LUNDGREN, A. (1964). *Acta med. scand.* **176**, 147.
GARROD, L. P. (1948). *Brit. med. J.* **1**, 382.
GRAYBIEL, A., SCHUKNECHT, H. F., FREGLY, A. R., MILLER, E. F. & MCLEOD.
    M. E. (1967). *Arch. Otolaryng.* **85**, 156.
GUNDERSEN, W. B. (1967). *Acta path. microbiol. scand.* **69**, 214.
HOKKANEN, E. (1964). *Acta neurol. scand.* **40**, 346.
HUTFIELD, D. C. (1965). *Brit. J. vener. dis.* **41**, 210.
IGARASHI, M., MCLEOD, M. E. & GRAYBIEL, A. (1966). *Acta Oto-laryng.*
    Suppl. **214**, 1.

IMAMURA, A., HORI, M., NAKAZAWA, K., SHIBATA, M., TATSUOKA, S. & MIYAKE, A. (1956). *Proc. imp. Acad. (Japan)* **32,** 648.
KOGUT, M. & LIGHTBOWN, J. W. (1963). *Biochem. J.* **89,** 18p.
KRAINSKY, A. (1914). *Zbl. Bakt. 2. Abt.* **41,** 649.
KRAUSS, M. R., KING, J. C. & COX, R. P. (1968). *J. Bact.* **95,** 2413.
KUNIN, C. M. (1967). *Ann. intern. Med.* **67,** 151.
LAL, S. & FERGUSON, A. D. (1963). *Tubercle (Edin.)* **44,** 360.
LEBOY, P. S., COX, E. C. & FLAKS, J. G. (1964). *Proc. nat. Acad. Sci., Wash.* **52,** 1367.
LEON, S. A. & BROCK, T. D. (1967). *J. molec. Biol.* **24,** 391.
LIKOVER, T. E. & KURLAND, C. G. (1967). *J. molec. Biol.* **25,** 497.
LINE, D. H., POOLE, G. W. & WATERWORTH, P. M. (1970). *Tubercle (Lond.)* **51,** 76.
LÜLLMAN, H. & REUTER, H. (1960). *Antibiot. et Chemother. (Basel)* **1,** 375.
MARCUS, R. E., SMALL, H. & EMANUEL, B. (1963). *Arch. Oto-laryng.* **77,** 198.
PRAZIC, M., SALAJ, B. & SUBOTIC, R. (1964). *J. Laryngol.* **78,** 1037.
REITMAN, M. (1967). *J. infect. Dis.* **117,** 101.
ROBINSON, G. C. & CAMBON, K. G. (1964). *New Engl. J. Med.* **271,** 949.
SCHATZ, A., BUGIE, E. & WAKSMAN, S. A. (1944). *Proc. Soc. exp. Biol. (N.Y.)* **55,** 66.
SPOTTS, C. R. & STANIER, R. Y. (1961). *Nature (Lond.)* **192,** 633.
STERN, J. L., BARNER, H. D. & COHEN, S. S. (1966). *J. molec. Biol.* **17,** 188.
TANAKA, N., SASHIKATA, K., NISHIMURA, T. & UMEZAWA, H. (1964). *Biochem. biophys. Res. Commun.* **16,** 216.
TOIVAKKA, E. & HOKKANEN, E. (1965). *Acta neurol. Scand.* **41,** Suppl. **13,** 275.
VARPELA, E. (1964). *Acta tuberc. scand.* **45,** 53.
WAKSMAN, S. A. & CURTIS, R. E. (1916). *Soil Sci.* **1,** 99.
WAKSMAN, S. A. & LECHEVALIER, H. (1953). *Guide to the Classification and Identification of the Actinomycetes and their Antibiotics.* Baltimore: The Williams and Wilkins Co.
WAKSMAN, S. A. & WOODRUFF, H. B. (1942). *Proc. Soc. exp. Biol. (N.Y.)* **49,** 207.
WERSALL, J. & HAWKINS, J. E. (1962). *Acta oto-laryng.* **54,** 1.
WILLEMOT, J. P., PANNIER, R., VAN DE CALSEYDE, P. & VYNCKIER, H. (1962) *Acta tuberc. belg.* **53,** 128.
YAMADA, T., TIPPER, D. & DAVIES, J. (1968). *Nature (Lond.)* **219,** 288.

CHAPTER VII

AMINOGLYCOSIDES

2. THE NEOMYCIN GROUP

THIS group of antibiotics, to be included with streptomycin in the general term aminoglycosides, shares the following properties:

1. A wide range of bactericidal activity, including both Gram-positive and Gram-negative species and *Mycobacteria*.

2. Slow acquisition of bacterial resistance, in contrast to single-step behaviour in relation to streptomycin.

3. A high degree of mutual cross-resistance.

4. Pharmacological behaviour like that of streptomycin: *i.e.*, little absorption from the alimentary tract, and fairly slow renal excretion in unchanged form after intramuscular injection, affording therapeutic blood levels for 6-8 hours.

5. A strong tendency to damage the auditory branch of the eighth nerve, with some possibility also of damage to the kidney. These risks are such that two of the group are not usually administered parenterally at all.

The first to be discovered, neomycin, was originally hailed as a second line of defence in treating tuberculosis, but deafness so often resulted that this treatment fell into disrepute. Since then various other ways of using neomycin have been devised, involving either direct local application or oral administration, which entail little or no risk of toxic effects.

Three closely similar antibiotics which have since been described are framycetin, kanamycin and paromomycin, and some of their properties can be described together. Gentamicin, which is another aminoglycoside, will be described separately, since it differs distinctly in several properties from the others.

DISCOVERY

NEOMYCIN, or more accurately the neomycin complex, was first isolated by Waksman and Lechevalier in 1949 from a strain of *Streptomyces fradiae*. The crude material has been shown to contain two chemically similar, biologically active components, which have been named neomycin B and C (Dutcher *et al.*, 1951). Neomycin A, the first homogeneous compound with biological activity to be isolated from crude concentrations, was subsequently discovered to be a degradation product.

FRAMYCETIN. In 1947 Decaris noticed a pink mould growing on a damp patch on the wall of his home in Paris. He cultivated the mould and identified it as a strain of *Streptomyces lavendulae* and found that culture filtrates were bactericidal for many species of Gram-positive and Gram-negative bacteria. These findings were not published until 1953 (Decaris, 1953). Further extraction and purification of the antibiotic were carried out in the research laboratories of Roussel.

KANAMYCIN was isolated in 1957 by a group of workers in Japan from a strain of *Streptomyces kanamyceticus* (Umezawa *et al.*, 1957). Crude preparations have been shown to contain two active components, referred to as kanamycin and kanamycin B.

PAROMOMYCIN was isolated from a strain of *Streptomyces rimosus* from the soil of Colombia in 1959 (Coffey *et al.*, 1959).

CHEMICAL PROPERTIES

Neomycin B and C

Both of these antibiotics consist of two paired components. A deaminohexose (neosamine B or C) linked to D-ribose forms one component, and this is linked to neamine, which consists of a diaminohexose and 2-deoxystreptamine (Rinehart, Woo and Argoudelis, 1958; Abraham and Newton, 1960). Commercial preparations of neomycin contain a mixture of neomycin B and C.

Framycetin

According to Rinehart *et al.* (1960) framycetin is identical with neomycin B, but this is disputed by the manufacturers.

Framycetin differs in any case from neomycin, since the latter is a mixture of B and C.

Kanamycin

Kanamycin has the empirical formula $C_{18}H_{36}N_4O_{11}$. Like streptomycin it consists of three components linked glycosidically. The components are: 6-amino-6-deoxy-D-glucose, 3-amino-3-deoxy-D-glucose and 2-deoxystreptamine (Cron *et al.*, 1958).

Paromomycin

Paromomycin consists of two components, glucosamine (paromamine) and a disaccharide paromobiosamine, joined to an inositol derivative (Haskell, French and Bartz, 1959).

The following are identical with paromomycin (Schillings and Schaffner, 1962) and will therefore not be further described: aminosidine (marketed in Italy as Gabbromycina), catenulin and hydroxymycin.

All these antibiotics are thus bases, of which the sulphates are usually employed in therapeutics. These are white crystalline powders freely soluble in water: solutions are very stable.

ANTI-BACTERIAL ACTIVITY

The whole of this group shows the same 'spectrum' of activity. Among Gram-positive organisms, staphylococci are highly sensitive and streptococci much less so. All the principal enterobacteria are sensitive except *Ps. aeruginosa*, which is relatively resistant to the whole group with the single exception of gentamicin. *Myco. tuberculosis* is also sensitive, but only two members of the group (streptomycin and to a much less extent kanamycin) are used in the treatment of tuberculosis. Table XVIII, giving the results of tests on numerous recent isolates of common bacteria, shows the degree of susceptibility of different species and such differences as there are between the activities of different members of the group.

The effect exerted is rapidly bactericidal like that of streptomycin, and activity is greater on the alkaline side of neutrality. but the degree of pH effect differs. The -fold differences in activity (against *Staph. aureus*) between media of pH 5·5 and 8·5 found by Garrod (1959) were for streptomycin 512, neomycin 64, framycetin 32, kanamycin 16 and paromomycin 8.

TABLE XVIII

Mean Minimum Inhibitory Concentrations (µg. per ml.) of Aminoglycoside Antibiotics*

	No. of Strains	Strepto-mycin	Neomycin	Kanamycin	Framycetin	Paromo-mycin	Genta-micin
Staph. aureus	29	2	0·5	1	0·5	1	0·125
Str. faecalis	32	64	64	32	64	64	8
Esch. coli	22	8	8	4	8	8	1
Klebsiella spp.	20	4	2	2	2	2	1
Aerobacter spp.	10	4	2	2	2	2	0·5
P. mirabilis	6	8	8	4	8	8	2
P. vulgaris	6	4	4	4	4	4	1
P. morgani	10	8	8	4	8	4	1
P. rettgeri	7	4	8	2	8	4	1
Ps. aeruginosa	31	32	32	128	32	512	4
Salmonella spp.	14	16	2	2	2	2	1
Shigella spp.	17	8	8	4	8	8	2

* Tests mainly of recent isolates at Hammersmith Hospital by plate dilution method with 2-fold differences. Means are of $\log_2$ of M.I.C. to the nearest $\log_2$. In the series tested strains showing a clearly abnormal degree of resistance (sometimes following treatment with the antibiotic) were omitted from these calculations.

An exceptional property claimed only for paromomycin is an effect on *E. histolytica,* which is inhibited *in vitro* by a concentration of from 2 to 10 μg. per ml. It was also effective in the treatment of intestinal amoebiasis of rats and dogs when administered orally, and was active against amoebic hepatitis in hamsters when given subcutaneously (Thompson *et al.,* 1959).

Acquired Resistance

Bacteria become resistant to members of this group slowly, although some change may be seen during the treatment of an individual patient. Frequent and long-continued use for a particular purpose certainly seems liable eventually to generate resistance in the pathogen at which it is aimed. The treatment of nasal staphylococcus carriers has had this effect (Harrison, Beavon and Griffin, 1959; Quie, Collin and Cardle, 1960), and in some hospitals resistance in staphylococci is now not uncommon. The use of Polybactrin spray (neomycin-bacitracin-polymyxin) may well have contributed largely to this: a majority of the numerous strains resistant to neomycin and kanamycin examined by Barber and Waterworth (1966) were also resistant to bacitracin. An epidemic of infection by a resistant strain in a Burns Unit where neomycin was being used locally and kanamycin systemically is described by Lowbury *et al.* (1964): this was a single organism described as 'an atypical 83A', and colonized burns in a majority of patients treated with these antibiotics, but was found in few patients not so treated, and disappeared when their use was given up. This is by no means the only instance in which the administration of an antibiotic has apparently favoured colonization or infection by staphylococci resistant to it: other examples are described by Knight and Holzer (1954) and Simon (1963).

Among enterobacteria, strains of *Esch. coli* from infants, and of this and other organisms from patients with urinary tract infections, treated with kanamycin, are now not uncommonly resistant. Resistance has also been seen in enterobacteria from the faeces of patients treated orally: we ourselves have found resistant strains of *Proteus* in patients given neomycin for pre-operative bowel preparation. The time may come, if liberal oral use for this and other purposes continues, when this group, and kanamycin in particular, can no longer be relied on for treating *Proteus* infections.

Cross-resistance

Most naturally occurring resistant strains, and all those trained to resistance *in vitro,* are almost equally resistant to all four members of this group (Kunin *et al.,* 1958; Andrieu *et al.,* 1959). On the other hand we have seen strains of enterobacteria which have become resistant, particularly after oral treatment, only to the antibiotic used and not to other members of this group. There is a less close relationship with streptomycin, which tends to be one-way: *i.e.* training to resistance to any of the neomycin group produces a substantial increase in resistance to streptomycin, but when streptomycin resistance is induced, the increase in resistance to the neomycin group is much less. Naturally occurring resistance is even less closely related, or not at all, in that streptomycin-resistant bacteria may be fully sensitive to neomycin.

TABLE XIX

Cross Resistance among Antibiotics of the Neomycin Group
Index of Increase in Resistance to*

Antibiotic to which habituated	Streptomycin	Neomycin	Framycetin	Kanamycin	Paromomycin
Streptomycin	10	5	4	5	5
Neomycin	6	8	8	8	8
Framycetin	6	8	8	9	10
Kanamycin	6	9	9	10	9
Paromomycin	6	8	8	8	9

* *e.g.* $8 =$ Increased 2^8-fold (*i.e.* 256-fold).

A typical example of the results of training may be seen in Table XIX. A 1,024-fold increase in resistance to streptomycin resulted in no more than a 32-fold increase in resistance to the other four antibiotics, but training to each of these raised streptomycin resistance to a relatively greater degree, as well as producing approximately the same level of resistance in all four.

PHARMACOLOGY

Oral Administration

None of the antibiotics described in this chapter is absorbed in any quantity from the alimentary canal. Like streptomycin, they retain their activity in the gut and, after oral administration, are excreted unchanged in the faeces. Small quantities are absorbed and if large doses are given orally for long periods, as in the treatment of hepatic coma, toxic concentrations may occur (see below).

Parenteral Administration

Kanamycin administered by intramuscular injection behaves similarly to streptomycin with regard to blood levels, distribution and excretion (Cronk and Naumann, 1959; Berger *et al.*, 1959; Boger and Gavin, 1960).

After a single intramuscular dose of 0·5 g. peak blood levels occur in about one hour and are of the order 10-20 μg./ml.; thereafter they decrease exponentially with time. Excretion is mainly via the kidneys, and takes place by glomerular filtration; a small amount is also excreted in the bile. *Neomycin* behaves in the same way as kanamycin, but the latter has now almost entirely replaced it for purposes requiring intramuscular injection.

Framycetin and *paromomycin* are not administered parenterally.

TOXICITY

All this group are ototoxic and are also liable to cause renal damage. It is presumably for this reason that parenteral administration of framycetin and paromomycin has never been recommended, although Teik and Siew (1964) treated 7 severe staphylococcal infections with intramuscular aminosidine (paromomycin) without causing deafness, possibly because the total dose given never exceeded 15 g. Neomycin is also liable to produce deafness, but this tendency is decidedly less in kanamycin, which is hence the only antibiotic in this group to be recommended for systemic use. An interesting contrast is afforded by two cases of enterococcal endocarditis described by Garrod and Waterworth (1962) for whom the usual combination of penicillin and streptomycin was unsuitable owing to very high bacterial resistance to the latter. Neomycin was substituted in one and kanamycin in the other, each given in a dose of 1 g. daily for six weeks. The patients were of approximately the same age, and both recovered, but whereas the neomycin caused total deafness, the hearing of the patient given kanamycin was unaffected.

Nevertheless kanamycin can also cause deafness if either the daily or the total dose given is excessive (Winfield *et al.*, 1958), or after the normal daily dose of 1 g. if there is any impairment of renal function (Lecca *et al.*, 1959). Some of the seven patients so afflicted in the series of Erlanson and Lundgren (1964) had a total dose of less than 10 g., and all but one of them had reduced renal function, two being anuric. Renal insufficiency is unfortunately common in the intractable urinary infections for which this antibiotic is indicated, and the utmost care is necessary both in assessing renal efficiency and controlling dosage accordingly, verifying that it is not excessive by blood assays. Atuk, Mosca and Kunin (1964) treated 10 uraemic patients in this way without toxic effects. A scheme for prolonging the interval between doses in accordance with the serum creatinine level is proposed by Sørenen *et al.* (1967).

Oral administration is relatively innocuous except for two possibilities. In surgical patients it carries a remote risk—considerably less than that of administering a tetracycline, and only if a staphylococcus resistant to this group is in the environment—of producing staphylococcal enterocolitis. Secondly, when neomycin is given in large doses for long periods to patients with hepatic failure, and if their kidneys are unequal to excreting the small amounts absorbed, it may accumulate in the blood and occasionally cause deafness (Last and Sherlock, 1960).

CLINICAL APPLICATION

Neomycin

It should be understood that for many of the purposes here described, other members of this group are alternatives.

Topical Application. Neomycin is a valuable agent for the local treatment of superficial infections with staphylococci and many Gram-negative bacilli. To avoid the development of resistant strains it is best used in combination with another agent, such as bacitracin, chlorhexidine or, for infection due to *Ps. aeruginosa,* polymyxin. Neomycin in combination with chlorhexidine or bacitracin is also useful in the treatment of staphylococcal nasal carriers. The recent appearance of neomycin-resistant strains has reduced the value of this proceeding.

Prolonged application to skin lesions of either neomycin or framycetin may cause sensitization, usually to both antibiotics (Kirton and Munro-Ashman, 1965).

Oral Administration. This has three distinct objects, one being the treatment of an acute intestinal infection. There is no dispute about the efficacy of neomycin or kanamycin in infantile gastro-enteritis due to pathogenic *Esch. coli* (Rogers *et al.,* 1956), although the emergence of resistant strains of the organism now threatens this. It is not so clear that benefit can be expected in *Salmonella* or *Shigella* infections, and results as regards elimination of the subsequent carrier state have been disappointing. The supposedly synergic combination of neomycin with ampicillin also failed in this task in the hands of Pettersson, Klemola and Wager (1964).

Neomycin is also useful as an intestinal antiseptic prior to abdominal surgery, for which purpose it may be administered with sulphathalidine or bacitracin (p. 356). Finally oral neomycin has been recommended for prolonged suppression of the intestinal flora in hepatic failure (Dawson, McLaren and Sherlock, 1957). In connection with any long-continued administration, it should be recognized that atrophic changes in the intestinal mucosa may result, with malabsorption of fats and carbohydrates (Jacobson and Faloon, 1961). According to Cheng and White (1962) there is also interference with the absorption of phenoxymethyl penicillin.

Inhalation. Neomycin aerosol is strongly commended by some authors for the treatment of bronchial infections, particularly bronchiectasis. The antibiotic is absorbed from the lung, and if this treatment is overdone, deafness may result.

INTRAPERITONEAL APPLICATION. Neomycin has been introduced into the peritoneal cavity at operation for the prevention or treatment of peritonitis, sometimes in what appear to be excessive amounts (2-3 g. or even more): respiratory depression or apnoea may result. Craig *et al* (1966) review reports of this effect and describe experiments in dogs showing that neomycin potentiates the action of muscle relaxants.

INTRAVESICAL APPLICATION. Neomycin solution may be introduced into the urinary bladder after cystoscopy etc. to kill any bacteria accidentally introduced. Thornton, Lytton and Andriole (1966) commend irrigation with a solution containing 40 mg. neomycin and 20 mg. polymyxin B per l. for preventing the establishment of infection during catheter drainage prolonged up to 10 days.

Framycetin

This antibiotic is used like neomycin for treating skin infections and nasal carriers of staphylococci.

According to Louwette and Lambrechts (1958) it is also as effective as neomycin in infantile *Esch. coli* enteritis.

Framycetin has also been recommended for suppression of the intestinal flora prior to operation (Shidlovsky, Marmell and Prigot, 1956). It was compared for this purpose by Stratford and Dixson (1964) with a larger dose of neomycin and found nevertheless to be superior to it: *Esch. coli, Str. faecalis* and even *Cl. welchii* totally disappeared from the faeces of 10 out of 12 patients given framycetin, but from only 8 out of 17 of those given neomycin. Results in the treatment of post-operative infection were also better in a small series.

In France framycetin is sometimes injected intrathecally as part of the treatment of acute meningitis.

Kanamycin

The uses which kanamycin shares with others of this group are the treatment of infantile gastro-enteritis and the suppression of the bowel flora, whether pre-operatively or in patients with hepatic disease.

Like neomycin it has been introduced into the peritoneal cavity, but with a more limited object and in more reasonable amounts. Cohn, Cotlar and Richard (1963) treated 360 patients, most with established peritonitis, by local instillation (1 g. in 50 ml. for an adult) with what are claimed to be excellent results: the treatment is specially commended for young children with peritonitis complicating appendicitis.

PARENTERAL ADMINISTRATION. This is the only antibiotic of the group which it now seems advisable to administer by repeated intramuscular injection. The necessity to limit the dose in accordance with renal function has already been stated, and it may be added that the length of the course should also be limited, if possible to 7-10 days. With these provisos, kanamycin may be the drug of choice for infections due to coliform organisms, particularly *Proteus* spp., resistant to other antibiotics. With the arrival of methicillin it is doubtful whether kanamycin has a place in the treatment of staphylococcal infections. Murdoch, Geddes and Syme (1962) recorded complete cure in 50 of 55 patients treated with kanamycin sulphate for infections with coliform bacilli, including five with septicaemia.

Kanamycin is also a recognized second line drug for the treatment of tuberculosis.

Paromomycin

Clinical reports on the use of this antibiotic refer mainly to oral administration. Good results in various forms of enteritis are claimed by Mössner (1962). A convincing account of effects in acute infantile enteritis by Kahn, Stein and Wayburne (1963) is referred to in Chapter XXI. According to Weinstein, Samet and Meade (1961) paromomycin is superior to neomycin in suppressing the bowel flora, but they made no direct comparison of the two, and their bacterial counts in faeces before administering paromomycin (up to 10^{18} aerobes per g.) are impossibly high.

The main difference between paromomycin and other aminoglycosides is its activity against *E. histolytica*. Excellent results were reported with paromomycin in an extensive study involving treatment of 432 patients with amoebic dysentery in 12 different countries in Asia, Africa and the Americas (Courtney *et al.*, 1960).

GENTAMICIN

This antibiotic is produced by a strain of *Micromonospora purpurea* and has two closely similar components. The available preparation is the sulphate. Its distinguishing characters are greater antibacterial activity combined with greater toxicity than those of related antibiotics.

ANTIBACTERIAL ACTIVITY (see Table XVIII). According to Weinstein *et al.* (1964) the inhibitory concentration of gentamicin is lower than that of neomycin or kanamycin for all enterobacteria tested, including species of *Aerobacter, Escherichia, Klebsiella* and *Salmonella. Proteus* spp. are also sensitive, but *P. vulgaris* least so. The most significant activity is against *Ps. aeruginosa,* shown by these authors to be 5-10 times greater than that of neomycin or kanamycin. This is fully confirmed by Barber and Waterworth (1966), who examined 25 recently isolated strains and found them decidedly more sensitive to gentamicin than to either kanamycin or streptomycin.

The actual M.I.C. of gentamicin for sensitive strains of *Ps. aeruginosa* found by different workers varies considerably. The probable explanation for this has been proposed by Garrod and Waterworth (1969) who found that the result of any such test can vary as much as 32-fold with the magnesium content of the medium: Mg, which is essential for the growth of this species and enhances its pigment production, also with increasing concentration reduces its apparent sensitivity to this antibiotic. Since this is a factor very difficult to control, the test is better conducted by direct comparison with another strain of the same organism having a known normal sensitivity.

Activity against streptococci is only moderate, although again claimed to exceed that of neomycin or kanamycin. The only Gram-positive species of therapeutic interest is *Staph. aureus,* in connection with which the findings of Barber and Waterworth (1966) are both extensive and decisive. They tested 102 strains with normal sensitivity to kanamycin (M.I.C. most often 1 μg. per ml.) and found gentamicin four times more active (M.I.C. of majority 0·25 μg. per ml.). They also tested 57 strains resistant to both kanamycin and neomycin (the majority also to bacitracin) and found that with two minor exceptions their sensitivity to gentamicin was normal. Naturally acquired resistance to neomycin and kanamycin may therefore be unaccompanied by resistance to gentamicin. It was shown by these authors in training experiments that a considerable degree of crossing results when resistance is artificially produced.

The action of gentamicin is bactericidal, and influenced in the usual way by *p*H, but to different degrees according to bacterial species (Rubenis, Kozij and Jackson, 1964); these authors also showed that high concentrations of NaCl greatly depress its activity.

PHARMACOLOGY AND DOSAGE. Like the rest of this group gentamicin is almost unabsorbed from the alimentary tract, and is administered by intramuscular injection. Absorption, distribution and excretion also do not apparently differ: the peak concentration in the blood is reached in about one hour, and an effective concentration persists for six to eight hours according to the dose (Black *et al.*, 1964). Excretion is mainly renal, over 80 per cent being recoverable from the urine.

The dose originally recommended was 0·5 mg. per kg. (i.e. about 40 mg. for an adult of average weight) at 8-hour intervals. This may suffice for some purposes, but as shown by Darrell and Waterworth (1967) the blood concentration produced by this does not for long exceed the M.I.C. for *Ps. aeruginosa*, and if a systemic effect is required it must clearly be increased. These authors also report that three strains of *Ps. aeruginosa* isolated after unsuccessful treatment on this low scale of dosage had become more resistant. It is now usually considered that a dose of 80 mg. three times a day is safe if renal function is normal.

CLINICAL APPLICATIONS. Gentamicin has been used largely for the treatment of urinary tract infections caused by *Ps. aeruginosa* and otherwise resistant organisms, results of which are reported by Bulger, Sidell and Kirby (1963), Klein, Eickhoff and Finland (1964), Brayton and Louria (1964) and Jao and Jackson (1964). Although only a moderate proportion of such treatments have been fully successful, this is to be explained by the choice of patients, many of whom had underlying conditions precluding any permanent cure. Among more immediately serious infections, *Pseudomonas* or other coliform pneumonia is referred to in some of these reports, and examples of bacteriaemia showing some response. *Pseudomonas aeruginosa* meningitis was successfully treated in an infant (Klein *et al.*, 1964), and a septicaemia due to the same organism was overcome by larger doses than usual at the cost of total loss of labyrinthine function (Jao and Jackson, 1964). Some of the patients treated for *Ps. aeruginosa* infection of burns both locally and parenterally had also positive blood cultures and responded well to the combined treatment.

The dilemma posed by a systemic infection, for which an adequate dose entails a serious risk of toxic effect, is probably best resolved by combination with another antibiotic. In *Ps. aeruginosa* infections this should be carbenicillin, with which gentamicin has been shown to act synergically. The use of this combination is discussed on page 85. Another combination strongly commended by Martin *et al.* (1969) for other forms of ' gram-negative rod bacteriaemia ' is gentamicin + cephaloridine. This paper was a contribution to a symposium, the report of which should be consulted for information about other clinical applications of gentamicin.

Various forms of local application have been successful, the effect evidently being mainly or wholly on the highly sensitive staphylococcus. A 0·1 per cent cream has been used for burns, bedsores, various forms of dermatitis and for the nasal staphylococcus carrier state. Oral administration for pre-operative suppression of the bowel flora is said to be successful with much smaller doses than those of neomycin used for this purpose, and would have, at least at present, the advantage of presenting no risk of enterocolitis due to a neomycin-resistant staphylococcus.

Toxic Effects. The only known toxic effect, apart from the suspicion of an occasional effect on the kidney, is on the vestibular branch of the eighth nerve: slight effects on the auditory branch have also been observed. This is a very real risk, particularly in patients with any impairment of renal function. In the series of 57 patients reported on by Jao and Jackson (1964), five suffered various degrees of loss of labyrinthine function. Four of these had raised blood ureas; the fifth was the *Pseudomonas* septicaemia already referred to, for whom larger doses than usual were considered necessary. Subsequent experience shows that labyrinthine damage occurs only if the blood level exceeds 10 μg./ml. This can be prevented by lengthening the interval between doses of 80 mg. from 8 hours to as long as 48 hours in accordance with the degree of impairment of renal function (Gingell and Waterworth, 1968). During such treatment it should be verified by blood assays that the expected levels are not being exceeded.

PHARMACEUTICAL PREPARATIONS

NEOMYCIN SULPHATE ('Mycifradin', *Upjohn;* 'Neomycin', *Glaxo;* 'Nivemycin', *Boots*). Supplied as tablets containing 500 mg. for oral administration: usual dose 4-6 g. daily, and in vials of 500 mg. sterile powder for parenteral administration, the dose not normally exceeding 1 g. daily: also in numerous creams, powders, etc. for local application, often combined with other antibacterial substances. In future, doses are to be stated in units. The minimum acceptable potency of a preparation is 650 units per mg.

KANAMYCIN SULPHATE ('Kannasyn', *Bayer;* 'Kantrex', *Bristol Laboratories,.* Available for parenteral administration in vials containing 1·43 g. (= 1 g. kanamycin base) (Kannasyn), or in vials of a stable aqueous solution containing 500 mg. in 2 ml. or 1 g. in 3 ml. (Kantrex Injection). Usual dose 1 g. daily. Also in capsules or suspension for oral administration: usual dose up to 2 g. daily for intestinal infections and up to 6 g. daily for a short period for pre-operative bowel preparation.

FRAMYCETIN SULPHATE ('Soframycin', *Roussel*). Tablets of 250 mg. for oral administration: dosage as for kanamycin. Also as ointment, nasal spray solution, etc.

PAROMOMYCIN SULPHATE ('Humatin', *Parke Davis*). Capsules of 250 mg. and syrup for oral administration: dosage similar to the foregoing.

GENTAMICIN SULPHATE ('Garamycin', *Schering Corporation;* 'Genticin', *British Schering;* 'Cidomycin', *Roussel*). Genticin and Cidomycin are supplied for intramuscular injection in vials containing a solution of 80 mg. of the base in 2 ml. with certain excipients.

REFERENCES

ABRAHAM, E. P. & NEWTON, G. G. F. (1960). *Brit. med. Bull.* **16,** 3.
ANDRIEU, G., MONNIER, J. & BOURSE, R. (1959). *Pr. méd.* **67.** 718.
ATUK, N. O., MOSCA, A. & KUNIN, C. (1964). *Ann. intern. Med.* **60,** 28.
BARBER, M. & WATERWORTH, P. M. (1966). *Brit. med. J.* **1,** 203.
BERGER, S. H., BERGSTROM, W. H. & WEHRLE, P. F. (1959). *Antibiot. Ann.* 1958-59, p. 684.
BLACK, J., CALESNICK, B., WILLIAMS, D. & WEINSTEIN, M. J. (1964). *Antimicrob. Agents and Chemother.*—1963, p. 138.
BOGER, W. P. & GAVIN, J. J. (1960). *Antibiot. Ann.* 1959-60. p. 393.
BRAYTON, R. G. & LOURIA, D. B. (1964). *Arch. intern. Med.* **114,** 205.
BULGER, R. J., SIDELL, S. & KIRBY, W. M. M. (1963). *Ann. intern. Med.* **59,** 593.
CHENG, S. H. & WHITE, A. (1962). *New Engl. J. Med.* **267,** 1296.
COFFEY, G. L., ANDERSON, L. E., FISHER, M. W., GALBRAITH, M. M., HILLEGAS, A. B., KOHBERGER, D. L., THOMPSON, P. E., WESTON, K. S. & EHRLICH, J. (1959). *Antibiot. and Chemother.* **9,** 730.

COHN, I., COTLAR, A. M. & RICHARD, L. (1963). *Amer. Surg.* **29,** 756.
COURTNEY, K. O., THOMPSON, P. E., HODGKINSON, R. & FITZSIMMONS, J. R. (1960). *Antibiot. Ann.* 1959-60, p. 304.
CRAIG, H. V., GUILLET, G. G., WALKER, J. A. & ARTZ, C. P. (1966). *Amer. Surg.* **32,** 27.
CRON, M. J., FARDIG, O. B., JOHNSON, D. L., WHITEHEAD, D. F., HOOPER, J. R. & LEMIEUX, R. U. (1958). *J. Amer. chem. Soc.* **80,** 4115.
CRONK, G. A. & NAUMANN, D. E. (1959). *J. Lab. clin. Med.* **53,** 888.
DARRELL, J. H. & WATERWORTH, P. M. (1967). *Brit. med. J.* **2,** 535.
DAWSON, A. M., MCLAREN, J. & SHERLOCK, S. (1957). *Lancet* **2,** 1263.
DECARIS, L. J. (1953). *Ann. Pharmacol. franç.* **2,** 44.
DUTCHER, J. D., HOSANSKY, N., DONIN, M. N. & WINTERSTEINER, O. (1951). *J. Amer. chem. Soc.* **73,** 1384.
ERLANSON, P. & LUNDGREN, A. (1964). *Acta med. scand.* **176,** 147.
GARROD, L. P. (1959). *Royal College of Physicians of Edinburgh,* Publication No. 11.
GARROD, L. P. & WATERWORTH, P. M. (1962). *J. clin. Path.* **15,** 328.
GARROD, L. P. & WATERWORTH, P. M. (1969). *J. clin. Path.* **22,** 534.
GINGELL, J. C. & WATERWORTH, P. M. (1968). *Brit. med. J.* **2,** 19.
HARRISON, K. J., BEAVON, J. & GRIFFIN, E. (1959). *Lancet* **1,** 908.
HASKELL, T. H., FRENCH, J. C. & BARTZ, Q. R. (1959). *J. Amer. chem. Soc.* **81,** 3480, 3481, 3482.
JACOBSON, E. D. & FALOON, W. W. (1961). *J. Amer. med. Ass.* **175,** 187.
JAO, R. L. & JACKSON, G. G. (1964). *J. Amer. med Ass.* **189,** 817.
KAHN, E., STEIN, H. & WAYBURNE, S. (1963). *Lancet* **2,** 703.
KIRTON, V. & MUNRO-ASHMAN, D. (1965). *Lancet* **1,** 138.
KLEIN, J. O., EICKHOFF, T. C. & FINLAND, M. (1964). *Amer. J. med. Sci.* **248,** 528.
KNIGHT, V. & HOLZER, A. R. (1954). *J. clin. Invest.* **33,** 1190.
KUNIN, C. M., WILCOX, C., NAJARIAN, A. & FINLAND, M. (1958). *Proc. Soc. exp. Biol. (N.Y.)* **99,** 312.
LAST, P. M. & SHERLOCK, S. (1960). *New Engl. J. Med.* **262,** 385.
LECCA, G. G., TERRY, J., MAGGIOLO, L. & MORALES, A. (1959). *J. Amer. med. Ass.* **170,** 2064.
LOUWETTE, R. & LAMBRECHTS, A. (1958). *Brit. med. J.* **1,** 868.
LOWBURY, E. J. L., BABB, J. R., BROWN, V. I. & COLLINS, B. J. (1964). *J. Hyg. (Lond.)* **62,** 221.
MARTIN, C. M., CUOMO, A. J., GERAGHTY, M. J., ZAGER, J. R. & MANDES, T. C. (1969). *J. infect. Dis.,* **119,** 506.
MÖSSNER, G. (1962). *Dtsch. med. Wschr.* **87,** 185.
MURDOCH, J. McC., GEDDES, A. M. & SYME, J. (1962). *Lancet* **1,** 457.
PETTERSSON, T., KLEMOLA, E. & WAGER, O. (1964). *Acta med. scand.* **175,** 185.
QUIE, P. G., COLLIN, M. & CARDLE, J. B. (1960). *Lancet* **2,** 124.
RINEHART, K. L. JR., WOO, P. W. K. & ARGOUDELIS, A. D. (1958). *J. Amer. chem. Soc.* **80,** 6461.
RINEHART, K. L. JR., ARGOUDELIS, A. D., GOSS, W. A., SOHLER, A. & SCHAFFNER, C. P. (1960). *J. Amer. chem. Soc.* **82,** 3938.
ROGERS, K. B., BENSON, R. P., FOSTER, W. P., JONES, L. E., BUTLER, E. B. & WILLIAMS, T. C. (1956). *Lancet* **2,** 599.
RUBENIS, M., KOZIJ, V. M. & JACKSON, G. G. (1964). *Antimicrob. Agents and Chemother.*—1963, p. 153.
SCHILLINGS, R. T. & SCHAFFNER, C. P. (1962). *Antimicrob. Agents and Chemother.*—1961, p. 274.
SHIDLOVSKY, B. A., MARMELL, M. & PRIGOT, A. (1956). *Antibiot. Ann.* 1955-6, p. 118.
SIMON, H. J. (1963). *Proc. Soc. exp. Biol. (N.Y.)* **113,** 518.
SØRENEN, A. W. S., SZABO, L., PEDERSEN, A. & SCHARFF, A. (1967). *Postgrad. med. J.,* 1967 Suppl. 'The Clinical Aspects of Kanamycin', p. 37.
STRATFORD, B. C. & DIXSON, S. (1964). *Med. J. Aust.* **1,** 74.

TEIK, K. O. & SIEW, L. G. (1964). *Med. J. Malaya* **19**, 8.
THOMPSON, P. E., BAYLES, A., HERBST, S. F., OLSZEWSKI, B. & MEISEN-HELDER, J. E. (1959). *Antibiot. and Chemother.* **9**, 618.
THORNTON, G. F., LYTTON, B. & ANDRIOLE, V. T. (1966). *J. Amer. med. Ass.* **195**, 179.
UMEZAWA, H., UEDA, M., MAEDA, K., YAGISHITA, K., KONDÖ, S., OKAMI, Y., UTAHARA, R., ÖSATO, Y., NITTA, K. & TAKEUCHI, T. (1957). *J. Antibiot.* *(Tokyo). Series A.* **10**, 181.
WAKSMAN, S. A. & LECHEVALIER, H. A. (1949). *Science* **109**, 305.
WAKSMAN, S. A., KATZ, E. & LECHAVALIER, H. A. (1950). *J. Lab. clin. Med.* **36**, 93.
WEINSTEIN, M. J., LUEDEMANN, G. M., ODEN, E. M. & WAGMAN, G. H. (1964). *Antimicrob. Agents and Chemother.*—1963, p. 1.
WEINSTEIN, L., SAMET, C. A. & MEADE, R. H. (1961). *J. Amer. med. Ass.* **178**, 891.
WINFIELD, M., CRISP, G. O., MAXWELL, M. H. & KLEEMAN, C. R. (1958). *Ann. N.Y. Acad. Sci.* **76**, 140.

CHAPTER VIII

CHLORAMPHENICOL

CHLOROMYCETIN, or chloramphenicol as it is now named, was the first broad spectrum antibiotic to be discovered. It was isolated independently by Burkholder from an actinomycete from the soil of Venezuela (Ehrlich *et al.*, 1947) and by Carter, Gottlieb and Anderson (1948) from a similar organism found in a sample of soil from a compost heap in Illinois. In 1948 the two groups of workers in collaboration isolated the antibiotic in crystalline form. Within a year its structural formula was established and a substance identical with the natural product was synthesized and given the name chloramphenicol, which has now been accepted as the official name for the antibiotic. A method of synthesizing chloramphenicol from *p*-nitroacetphenone has proved practicable on a large scale, and alone among clinically important antibiotics chloramphenicol is manufactured synthetically. Early work leading to the synthesis of chloramphenicol is reviewed by Brock (1961).

CHLORAMPHENICOL

Chemical Properties

Chloramphenicol consists of yellowish-white crystals with an intensely bitter taste. Its solubility is about 2·5 mg./ml. water and about 400 mg./ml. alcohol. Aqueous solutions have a *p*H of about 5·5 and are extremely stable. They keep indefinitely at ordinary room temperature if protected from light, and will withstand boiling. Some hydrolysis occurs on autoclaving.

Relation of Structure to Function

There are four isomers of chloramphenicol, all of which have been synthesized. The other three have 1 per cent or less

132

Table XX

Sensitivity of Bacteria to Chloramphenicol

	M.I.C. µg./ml.		M.I.C. µg./ml.
C. diphtheriae	0·5-3·0	*H. influenzae*	0·2-0·5
Str. pneumoniae	1·0-4·0	*Pasteurella* spp.	0·2-10
Actino. israeli	1·0-4·0	*H. pertussis*	0·2-12·5
Clostridium spp.	1·5->500	*N. meningitidis*	0·5-1·5
Str. pyogenes	2·0-4·0	*N. gonorrhoeae*	0·5-1·5
B. anthracis	2·5-5·0	*Kl. pneumoniae*	0·5-2·0
Str. faecalis	4·0-12	*Salmonella* spp.	0·5-10
Staph. aureus	4·0-12	*Kl. aerogenes*	0·5-30
Myco. tuberculosis	12-25	*Brucella* spp.	0·8-2·5
		Esch. coli	0·8-8·0
		Bacteroides spp.	1·0-8·0
		Salm. typhi.	2·0-4·0
		Sh. sonnei.	2·5-6·0
		Proteus spp.	2·5-64
		Ps. aeruginosa	50-125

McLean, I. W. *et al.* (1949). *J. clin. Invest.* **28**, 953.
Chen, C. H. *et al.* (1949). *South. med. J.* **42**, 986.
Garrod, L. P. (1952). *Antibiot. Chemother.* **2**, 689.
Garrod, L. P. (1952). *Brit. med. J.* **1**, 1263.
Garrod, L. P. (1955). *Brit. med. J.* **2**, 1529.
Welch, H. *et al.* (1952). *Antibiot. Chemother.* **2**, 693.

of the activity of the natural antibiotic. Many structurally related compounds have been synthesized, but so far none with greater activity than natural chloramphenicol. The structure of the side chain is critical to antibacterial activity but contrary to the original view the precise nature of the aromatic ring is of little importance (von Strandtmann *et al.*, 1967).

Antimicrobial Activity

Chloramphenicol is active against a wide range of Gram-positive and Gram-negative bacteria (Table XX). Its most novel property at the time of its discovery was a high degree of activity against all species of rickettsia. Agents of the psittacosis-lymphogranuloma group are also susceptible. Chloramphenicol is much less active than penicillin or tetracycline against Gram-positive cocci. Penicillin inhibits some organisms at a concentration of 0·01 unit per ml. or less; very few organisms are sensitive to less than 1 µg. per ml. of chloramphenicol. Nevertheless, *Salm. typhi, H. influenzae* and *H. pertussis* are more susceptible to chloramphenicol than to almost any other antibiotic, a fact to be remembered in considering indications for clinical use. Chloramphenicol is strictly bacteristatic against almost all bacterial species including salmonella, brucella, escherichia, streptococci and staphylococci. Its purely bacteristatic effect on *Salm. typhi* is shown in Figure 8. In the highest concentrations of chloramphenicol the viable count remains stationary, and there is no decline in the number of living organisms as there would be with a bactericidal agent.

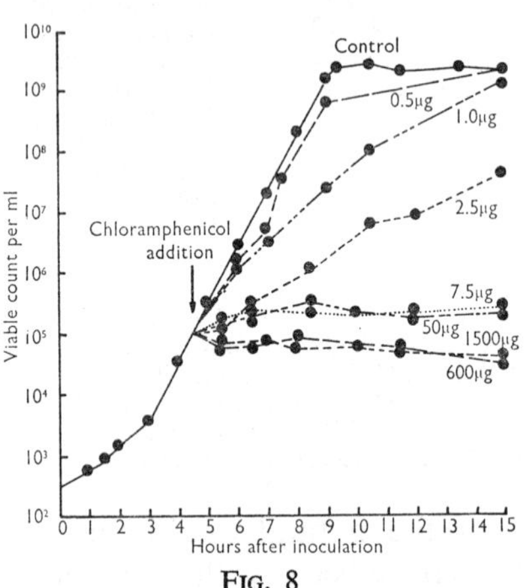

FIG. 8

The purely bacteristatic effect of chloramphenicol. Growth is slowed or halted but there is no significant decline in the number of viable organisms. (From Brock, 1964.)

Activity *in vivo*

The same bacteristatic effect is seen *in vivo*. Mice infected with *Salm. typhimurium* can be protected by chloramphenicol but when treatment is stopped, death occurs from multiplication of the original—and still chloramphenicol-sensitive—strain. This emphasizes the major role which must be played by the host during the period of growth suppression if the organism is to be eliminated. The incapacity of the mouse to destroy the organism even when its growth is suppressed is shown by the behaviour of salmonella in mouse cells. *Salm. typhi* grows rapidly within the cells and although it can be inhibited within a few minutes by exposure to chloramphenicol, the organism remains viable for long periods and will regrow on removal from exposure to the drug (Showacre *et al.*, 1961). Similar reappearance of the organism when chloramphenicol is withdrawn is seen in the treatment of human typhoid carriers (Woodward and Smadel, 1964).

Mode of Action

Chloramphenicol has no effect on oxidative phosphorylation, permeability, or the synthesis of DNA or bacterial cell wall; but at concentrations corresponding with those which inhibit bacterial growth it is a potent inhibitor of protein synthesis. It now appears that this is brought about by inhibition of the enzymic transfer of the growing peptide chain to the newly attached amino acid (p. 101).

Acquired Resistance

Resistant strains of various bacterial species have been isolated by serial passage in increasing concentrations of chloramphenicol. The resistant strains are mutants and resistance can arise at a number of different genetic loci on the bacterial chromosome (Reeve and Suttie, 1968). As the concentration of chloramphenicol is increased, mutants resistant at more than one locus emerge, and as each new locus is affected, resistance increases in a step-wise fashion. Resistant mutants commonly grow less rapidly than the sensitive parent strain and show antigenic and morphological changes including loss of flagella. The biochemical basis of this resistance has not so far been elucidated.

The chloramphenicol molecule can be attacked at a number of different points by bacteria and the degradation products have no antibacterial activity. Naturally occurring chloramphenicol-resistant *Staph. aureus* evidently owe their resistance to inactivation of the agent by an inducible acetylase (Shaw and Brodsky, 1968). Such resistance can be spontaneously lost, or ' cured ' by acridines, suggesting a plasmid location for the responsible gene (p. 253). An analogous situation exists in *Escherichia* where the capacity to acetylate chloramphenicol accounts for the resistance of many clinical isolates. In this species too the location of the gene controlling synthesis of the enzyme is extrachromosomal, and it may be transferred in conjugation accounting for R-factor mediated resistance (p. 255).

Chloramphenicol resistance in *Pseudomonas aeruginosa* is apparently not dependent on enzymic destruction of the drug, and the situation in resistant strains of *Proteus, Klebsiella* and *Aerobacter* is variable (Okamoto *et al.,* 1967; Sompolinsky *et al.,* 1968).

Dependent strains which will not grow, or grow very poorly, in the absence of chloramphenicol have also been described.

Cross Resistance

There is cross resistance between chloramphenicol and tetracyclines in *Esch. coli* but not in other species. Low-order cross resistance between chloramphenicol and erythromycin has also been described (Barber, Csillag and Medway, 1958).

Practical Applications

Resistance in wild strains has emerged slowly but has been seen in a variety of species, including *Salm. typhi* (Agarwal, 1962). Coliform bacilli readily acquire resistance and those causing urinary infections are not uncommonly resistant. Resistance is uncommon in staphylococci, at least in this country, but the proportion of resistant strains of all species increases with the use of chloramphenicol. For example, Koch (1960) reported that chloramphenicol consumption in her hospital fell to low levels in 1952 when blood dyscrasia was reported but

TABLE XXI

Percentages of Strains Resistant to Chloramphenicol

	Escherichia	Proteus	Pseudo-monas	Staph. aureus	Str.faecalis
1953	12	22	59	2	4
1958	53	47	99	34	40

From Koch, M. L. (1960).

increased after 1955 with increasing use of the drug as organisms became resistant to other agents. The increased proportion of resistant organisms between 1953 and 1958 is shown in Table XXI. There was a direct correlation between the use of the drug and the emergence of resistant strains. The much greater increase in the proportion of resistant Gram-positive cocci is attributed to the fact that in 1953 a substantial proportion of the Gram-negative bacilli were already resistant—a reflection of the greater ease with which resistance is acquired by these organisms.

PHARMACOLOGY

Absorption and Distribution

The usual route of administration is oral, and the peak blood levels obtained are shown in Table XXII. The dissolution and absorption of poorly soluble compounds like chloramphenicol depends to an important extent on particle size. Direct comparisons show that preparations containing large particles may give blood levels only $\frac{1}{4}$-$\frac{1}{2}$ those arising from

TABLE **XXII**

Serum Levels of Chloramphenicol after Oral Adminstration in Patients of Different Ages

Age	Dose mg./kg.	Peak		Half-life Hours
		Hour	μg./ml.	
Adult	7(0·5 g.)	2-3	8-13	2-5
	30(2 g.)		15-25	
1-2 days	50	6-12	30-40	24-28

Glazko *et al.* (1968) *Clin. Pharmacol. Therap.* **9**, 472.
Weiss *et al.* (1960) *New Engl. J. Med.*, **262**, 787.

small particles (Glazko *et al.*, 1968). Reducing or increasing the dose has a proportionate effect on the level attained. This falls comparatively slowly, and since there is some cumulative effect, a level of 4-6 μg. per ml. can be maintained by giving 0·5 g. at six-hour intervals, or a correspondingly higher one by raising the dose.

Children can neither swallow the capsules given to adults nor tolerate the exceedingly bitter taste of the free drug. The alternative for them is a suspension of chloramphenicol palmitate, a tasteless compound which is itself inert, but is hydrolyzed in the gut, liberating chloramphenicol.

Very young infants are deficient in the ability to form glucuronides and their glomerular and tubular excretion capabilities are low. The rate of disappearance of chloramphenicol from the blood is consequently greatly prolonged (Table XXII) and in the new-born the dose and frequency of administration must be reduced (p. 143) if toxic quantities of the drug are not to accumulate.

PARENTERAL ADMINISTRATION. Simple suspensions of finely ground chloramphenicol are available which are suitable only for intramuscular injection. Chloramphenicol sodium succinate, on the other hand, which is freely soluble, and undergoes hydrolysis in the tissues with the liberation of chloramphenicol, can be injected in a small volume intramuscularly, intravenously or subcutaneously.

The levels of the drug after administration by these routes differ little from those following the same dose by the oral route. The peak level is of course attained immediately after intravenous injection. In contrast to this, the absorption of an intramuscularly injected suspension appears to be slower (peak at 4-5 hours) than that from the bowel, detectable blood levels persisting longer (half-life 4-6 hours).

Excretion

About 60 per cent of the chloramphenicol in the blood is bound to protein. Studies of organ distribution have shown the diminishing order of concentration to be kidney, liver, lung, heart, spleen, muscle and brain. Free diffusion occurs into serous effusions, and into the foetal circulation. Penetration into all parts of the eye has also been demonstrated. Perhaps most important of all, the concentrations attained in the cerebro-spinal fluid are higher than those of any other antibiotic: they amount to 30-50 per cent of those in the blood even in the absence of meningitis. Glandular secretions also contain some of the antibiotic: its presence in the saliva occasions a bitter taste and accounts for changes in the oral flora.

Before excretion, most of the chloramphenicol in the body is inactivated either by conjugation with glucuronic acid or by reduction to inactive aryl amines, and the main site of these processes is the liver. Excretion is mainly renal: 90 per cent of the dose can be detected in the urine by chemical methods, but only about 10 per cent of this amount is unaltered antibiotic. Chloramphenicol itself is excreted by the glomeruli, but excretion of its inactive derivatives is also by active tubular secretion. Excretion diminishes linearly with renal function. At a creatinine clearance of less than 20 ml./min., maximum concentrations of 10-20 μg./ml. of urine are found in contrast to 150-200 μg./ml. in the normal. Despite this, blood levels of active chloramphenicol are only marginally elevated but micro-biologically inactive metabolites accumulate. This may explain the poor results found in some (especially elderly) patients (Lindberg *et al.*, 1966).

About 3 per cent of the administered dose is excreted in the bile but only about 1 per cent appears in the faeces and that mostly in inactive forms. The idea that high concentrations of chloramphenicol can be demonstrated in the bile appears to have come from studies in the rat, in which, in contrast to man, the bile is a principal route of excretion.

Side Effects and Toxicity

Chloramphenicol passed the usual toxicity tests in animals, and had been in world-wide use for several years before it was recognized as a potentially highly dangerous bone marrow depressant. More years passed before it was observed to be the cause of the ' grey syndrome ' in infants, another usually fatal condition. It thus has the unenviable distinction of exerting lethal toxic effects of two different kinds. Other effects are of only minor importance.

ALIMENTARY TRACT. Soreness of the mouth is fairly common if a course of treatment exceeds one week. It is attributable to depression of the normal flora by the antibiotic in the saliva and consequent overgrowth of *Candida albicans*. Mild cases show little change, but in the more severe there is a frank stomatitis: it is possible that vitamin B deficiency or even a direct action of the antibiotic on the epithelium, which in the tongue shows atrophic changes, may also play some part. Nausea, vomiting and diarrhoea, although they may occur, are much less common and less severe than those capable of being caused by tetracyclines.

Marrow Aplasia. A few isolated reports of granulo-cytopenia and aplastic anaemia following chloramphenicol therapy appearing about 1950 attracted little attention. The storm burst in 1952, when a succession of papers described such effects, not merely in single cases but in series. The immediate alarm sharply restricted the use of the drug, but soothing propaganda has since restored this to a high level, despite further warnings (Dameshek, 1960).

Simple granulocytopenia is uncommon: the usual effect is a total aplasia of the marrow. The first signs are purpura and pallor, and a blood count reveals a deficiency of all blood cells including platelets. Most patients die despite repeated transfusions. Survival is most likely in those with early onset of dyscrasia in which few cell types are depressed (Best, 1967). A few patients survive with protracted aplasia and in them myeloblastic leukaemia may ultimately supervene (Brauer and Dameshek, 1967). In over 400 cases reviewed by Best (1967) manifestations appeared *during* treatment in only 22 per cent. In 10 per cent there was an interval between the cessation of treatment and onset of dyscrasia of 130 days or more. Cause and effect may thus never be connected.

The frequency of marrow aplasia in treated patients is unknown. Several estimates have been made but are all suspect because of difficulty in establishing the size of the population at risk. The value of such overall figures is also doubtful because some physicians have given very large doses or treated thou-sands of patients (Lietman *et al.*, 1964; Woodward and Smadel, 1964) without encountering haematological abnormali-ties, while others have seen several cases of aplastic anaemia over a limited period. One of us saw three cases, two of them fatal, among an estimated number of 1,200 patients treated with chloramphenicol at St. Bartholomew's Hospital up to 1952. Apparently the profession is divided into those who, perhaps having seen chloramphenicol cause marrow aplasia, fear this effect and rarely use the drug, and a larger number who ignore this possibility because it seems too remote and prescribe chloramphenicol freely.

It has several times been suggested (though there is no direct evidence for this) that the toxic agent is not chloramphenicol itself but some metabolite, and that marked differences in the incidence of aplasia may be explained by some genetic pre-disposition. This idea is attractive, but as Best (1967) points out, difficult to reconcile with the extreme rarity of aplasia in more than one member of a family. Further light has been shed on the problem by the finding that characteristic haematolo-gical abnormalities regularly follow the administration of chloramphenicol although, fortunately, these have not so far been seen to progress to aplastic anaemia. The abnormalities are vacuolization of the pro-erythroblasts, reticulocytopenia, thrombocytopenia, and a raised serum iron level. Associated sideroblastosis and a fall in the white cell count also some-times occur. Contrary to the initial supposition that chloram-phenicol owes its marrow suppressive action to its nitro group, these changes occur when analogues of chloramphenicol are given in which the nitro group has been substituted (Suhrland and Weisberger, 1962).

The same changes develop more readily in severely ill patients (Gussoff and Lee, 1966) especially where renal or hepatic disease interferes with excretion or conjugation.

Although this has been disputed, there seems no doubt that repeated blood counts can be a safeguard: significant changes, of which a diminished reticulocyte count is the earliest, can be detected at a stage at which the process is reversible. There is overall a good deal of evidence that toxicity is more common in patients receiving high doses or prolonged treat-ment. This relationship is well shown in Figure 9 taken from the study of McCurdy (1963). Equally well shown, however, is the development of toxicity in a small number of patients whose total exposure to the drug was low. If these haematological changes are related to aplasia—and the occasional pancyto-penia which develops suggests that they are—it is evident that some patients are at grave risk from even the smallest doses.

Chloramphenicol is a phenylalanine analogue, and diverse observations link chloramphenicol with phenylalanine meta-bolism. Chloramphenicol inhibits the intestinal uptake of phenylalanine, and the morphological abnormalities induced in red cells by the antibiotic resemble those seen in phenylala-nine deficiency. There is at present, however, no undisputed evidence to support the unifying hypothesis that chloramphenicol toxicity in some way operates through phenylalanine metabolism (Weksler *et al.*, 1968).

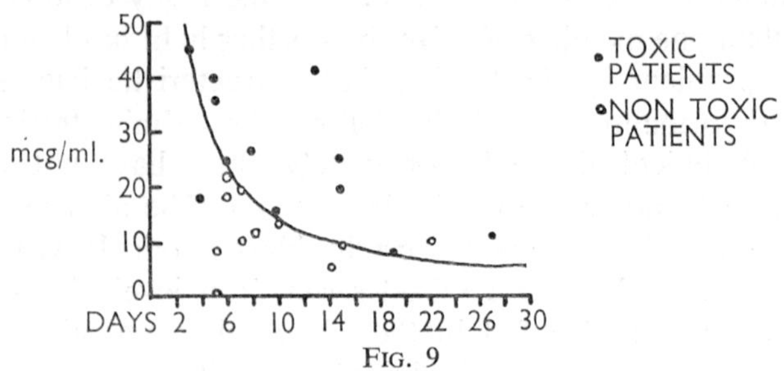

Fig. 9

Relationship between plasma concentration of chloramphenicol 2-3 hours after a dose, and duration of therapy in patients with bone marrow suppression compared with those without marrow effect. (McCurdy, 1963.)

Looked at from the other side—that is to say not how many patients given chloramphenicol developed aplasia, but how many patients with aplasia had previously received chloramphenicol—the evidence against chloramphenicol is very strong. By the end of 1963 the Registry of Blood Dyscrasias of the American Medical Association had collected 674 cases of drug-induced marrow aplasia (Erslev, 1964). Chloramphenicol was implicated in 299 of these and had been the sole drug administered in 151—more cases than all the rest of the listed drugs put together. Its nearest rivals as the sole implicated drug (which incidentally included sulphonamides) were each associated with 18 cases. Despite the publicity given to the relationship between aplasia and chloramphenicol over the years, Sharp (1963), reporting 40 cases of marrow aplasia associated with chloramphenicol collected by the Association of Clinical Pathologists in this country, again commented that the drug had frequently been given for trivial reasons and in extravagant doses.

THE ' GREY SYNDROME ' IN INFANTS. The practice of giving large doses of chloramphenicol by injection to new-born infants prophylactically seems to have arisen about 1957. Indications mentioned by various authors were prematurity, premature rupture of the membranes, and among post-natal factors such conditions as lethargy and abdominal distension. It is remarkable that in none of these reports was there the slightest evidence that this treatment served any useful purpose. The infants remained well for two or three days, when vomiting, refusal to suck and abdominal distension were succeeded by flaccidity, an ashen colour and hypothermia (the ' grey syndrome '), this circulatory collapse being followed by death within a few hours. In what was described as an ' outbreak ' of neonatal deaths among full term infants in Los Angeles, the condition was at first thought to be some obscure infection, and the dose of chloramphenicol was actually increased in an endeavour to overcome it: nine infants died from this cause in only two months.

The doses given were from 100 to 160 mg./kg. daily by intramuscular injection and in infants so treated blood levels climb to as high as 170 μg. per ml. This results from the deficient capacity of the infant to conjugate and excrete chloramphenicol (Weiss *et al.*, 1960). It is accordingly recommended that the daily dose in the full term and premature infant should be limited to 50 and 25 mg. per kg. respectively. A consideration of the wider question of the utility of this antibiotic in these circumstances seems overdue.

OPTIC NEURITIS. A number of cases have been described of optic neuritis in children with cystic fibrosis of the pancreas, receiving prolonged chloramphenicol treatment for pulmonary infection. Partial restoration of sight has followed stopping the drug and treatment with large doses of B complex vitamins (Cocke *et al.*, 1966). While insisting on the value of chloramphenicol in the management of cystic fibrosis, Lietman *et al.* (1964) emphasize the need to pay special attention to the visual acuity.

Clinical Applications

There is great diversity of opinion on this subject, depending on the degree of importance to be attached to the possibility of toxic effects. We believe that this possibility should not be disregarded, and the following principles, which have frequently been enunciated, should therefore be not only assented to but observed.

1. Chloramphenicol should never be prescribed for minor infections. There have been many tragic fatalities following its use for trivial conditions such as respiratory catarrh.

2. It is currently still the drug of choice in typhoid fever and other severe salmonella infections. Some authorities take the view that these are the *only* indications. *H. influenzae* meningitis or pneumonia might be considered another, but it seems that ampicillin is an effective alternative. Pertussis may be an indication in severe cases at an early age and if treatment can be begun early enough. It should be prescribed for other serious infections only when these are resistant, or much less sensitive, to other antibiotics.

3. Both the daily dose (usually not exceeding 2 g.) and the duration of the course (*e.g.* 10 days) should be limited. Prolonged treatment is almost certainly more dangerous, and repeated courses are reputed to be, although no one has formulated any precise rules to meet this: presumably a recent history of a course of treatment should be considered a contra-indication to another.

4. During treatment a reticulocyte count should be performed at intervals not exceeding two days: if a fall is observed a full blood examination will decide whether the drug should be stopped. Suhrland and Weisberger (1962, 1963) believe increase in the serum iron above 80 μg. per 100 ml. to be a sensitive index of toxicity.

Chloramphenicol has a very similar antibacterial spectrum to the tetracyclines which are often antibacterially more active and, although not free from toxicity, are innocent of the production of fatal aplastic anaemia. It is therefore pertinent to consider in what circumstances chloramphenicol is to be preferred. Brock (1964) has assembled extensive direct comparisons of the efficacy of chloramphenicol and tetracyclines in a number of experimental infections. As he comments, there must be reservations about the transfer of these findings to man but they are sufficiently in accord with human therapeutic experience, where that is available, to form a useful guide. Part of his summary of these experiments is reported in Table XXIII.

It appears that in the treatment of the majority of experimental infections chloramphenicol fails to show any special advantages. Nevertheless, many clinicians, guided by their own experience, believe it to be a most valuable drug, preferring it in many situations to agents which on other evidence might be expected to be superior. There is no doubt that chloramphenicol can be, and frequently has been, life saving in the treatment of severe infections. It is also unique amongst readily available antibiotics in producing a condition which is commonly irreversible and fatal. The onus is on anyone who prescribes it to show that he has excellent reasons for doing so.

TABLE XXIII

Comparative Survey of the in vivo *Activity of Chloramphenicol and Chlortetracycline in Various Experimental Infections*

Infecting Organism	Chloramphenicol	Chlortetracycline
Brucella	Ineffective; may potentiate infection	Effective
V. cholerae	Effective in large doses	Effective in lower doses
H. pertussis	Effective	More effective
C. diphtheriae	Completely ineffective	Moderately effective
T. pallidum	Weakly effective	Moderately effective
L. canicola	Completely ineffective	Effective
Lymphogranuloma venereum	Effective	More effective
Psittacosis	Delays multiplication	Eradicates

From Brock (1964).

PHARMACEUTICAL PREPARATIONS AND DOSAGE

CHLORAMPHENICOL (Alficetyn, *Allen and Hanburys;* Chloromycetin, *Parke Davis;* Kemicetine, *Carlo Erba;* numerous other proprietary names).

Capsules, B.P., B.N.F.: 250 mg. U.S.P., 50, 100, 250 mg. Injections: Suspension, U.S.N.F.: 1 and 2 g.; Chloramphenicol sodium succinate, U.S.P.: equiv. 1 g. Mixture, B.N.F., U.S.P.: Chloramphenicol palmitate, equiv. 125 mg. per 4 ml. Dose: 1·5-3 g. daily in divided doses. Children 25-50 mg. per kg. per day in divided doses. Premature infant: not more than 25 mg. per kg. per day.

REFERENCES

AGARWAL, S. C. (1962). *Bull. Wld Hlth Org.* **27,** 331.
BARBER, M., CSILLAG, A. & MEDWAY, A. J. (1958). *Brit. med J.* **2,** 1377.
BEST, W. R. (1967). *J. Amer. med. Ass.* **201,** 181.
BRAUER, M. J. & DAMESHEK, W. (1967). *New Engl. J. Med.* **277,** 1003.
BROCK, T. D. (1961). *Bact. Rev.* **25,** 32.
BROCK, T. D. (1964). In *Experimental Chemotherapy,* vol. 3, p. 119, ed. Schnitzer, R. J. & Hawking, F. New York: Academic Press.
CARTER, H. E., GOTTLIEB, D. & ANDERSON, H. W. (1948). *Science* **107,** 113.
COCKE, J. G., BROWN, R. E. & GEPPERT, L. J. (1966). *J. Pediat.* **68,** 27.
DAMESHEK, W. (1960). *J. Amer. med. Ass.* **174,** 1853.
EHRLICH, J., BARTZ, Q. R., SMITH, R. M., JOSLYN, D. A. & BURKHOLDER, P. R. (1947). *Science* **106,** 417.
ERSLEV, A. J. (1964). *J. Amer. med. Ass.* **188,** 531.
GLAZKO, A. J., KINKEL, A. W., ALEGNANI, W. C. & HOLMES, E. L. (1968). *Clin. Pharmacol. Therap.* **9,** 472.
GUSSOFF, B. D. & LEE, S. L. (1966). *Amer. J. med. Sci.* **251,** 8.
KOCH, M. L. (1960). *Antibiot. and Chemother.* **10,** 364.
LIETMAN, P. S., DI SANT' AGNESE, P. A. & WONG, V. (1964). *J. Amer. med. Ass.* **189,** 924.
LINDBERG. A. A., son NILSSON, L. H., BUCHT, H. & KALLINGS, L. O. (1966). *Brit. med. J.* **2,** 724.
McCURDY, P. R. (1963). *Blood* **21,** 363.
OKAMOTO, S., SUZUKI, Y., MISE, K. & NAKAYA, R. (1967). *J. Bact.* **94,** 1616.
REEVE, E. C. R. & SUTTIE, D. R. (1968). *Genet. Res.* **11,** 97.
SHARP, A. A. (1963). *Brit. med. J.* **1,** 735.
SHAW, W. V. & BRODSKY, R. F. (1968). *J. Bact.* **95,** 28.
SHOWACRE, J. L., HOPPS, H. E., DuBUY, H. G. & SMADEL, J. E. (1961). *J. Immunol.* **87,** 153.
SOMPOLINSKY, D., ZIEGLER-SCHLOMOWITZ, R. & HERCZOG, D. (1968). *Canad. J. Microbiol.* **14,** 891.
SUHRLAND, L. G. & WEISBERGER, A. S. (1962). *Amer. J. med. Sc.* **244,** 16.
VON STRANDTMANN, M., BOBOWSKI, G. & SHAVEL, J. Jr. (1967). *J. med. Chem.* **10,** 888.
WEISS, C. F., GLAZKO, A. J. & WESTON, J. K. (1960). *New Engl. J. Med.* **262,** 787.
WEKSLER, M. E., BOURKE, E. & SCHREINER, G. E. (1968). *Clin. Pharmacol. Therap.* **9,** 647.
WOODWARD, T. E. & SMADEL, J. E. (1964). *Ann. intern. Med.* **60,** 144.

CHAPTER IX

TETRACYCLINES

IN 1948, when aureomycin, the first of the tetracyclines, was discovered, the only other antibiotics in general use were penicillin and streptomycin. Each of these had a limited range of activity, and each had to be given by injection. Aureomycin differed from them in having a wide range of activity, including most organisms susceptible to either and some to neither of them, and a second advantage, shared with chloramphenicol, which was discovered at about the same time, of being administrable by the mouth.

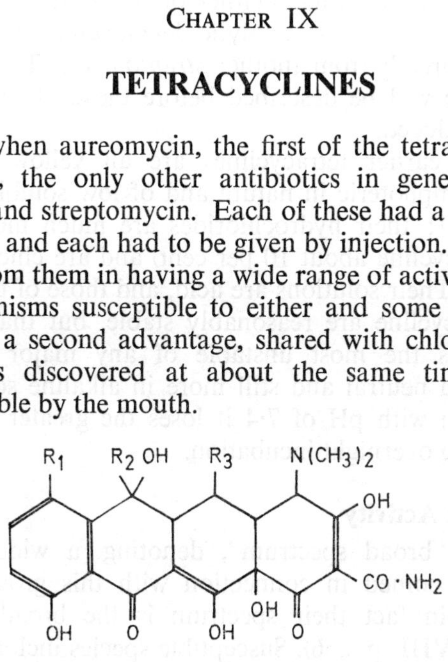

	R_1	R_2	R_3
Tetracycline	H	CH_3	H
Chlortetracycline	Cl	CH_3	H
Oxytetracycline	H	CH_3	OH
Demethylchlortetracycline	Cl	H	H

FIG. 10

Structure of tetracyclines.

The tetracyclines are a family of closely related antibiotics, to which additions are still being made after over 20 years. The first, aureomycin, was so called from the golden yellow colour of the colony of *Streptomyces aureofaciens*, the organism forming it. Two years later (1950) 'Terramycin' derived from *Streptomyces rimosus*, was introduced, and within a further two years their structure was ascertained (Fig. 10), which differs only in the presence of a Cl atom in one and an OH group in the other. The names chlortetracycline and oxytetracycline were then proposed for them, and in 1953 tetracycline was introduced, which has neither of these attachments: this can be obtained either by catalytic dehalogenation of chlortetracycline or directly from another *Streptomyces*. The properties of these three will be described before those of several more recently introduced.

The three earlier tetracyclines are all yellow crystalline substances, amphoteric in nature and of low solubility (about 0·05 per cent): their hydrochlorides are much more soluble (that of tetracycline about 10 per cent) and are chiefly used in therapeutics. Their solutions are acid, and those of tetracycline and oxytetracycline are reasonably stable, but that of chlortetracycline is the most unstable of any major antibiotic, particularly in neutral and still more in alkaline solution: in nutrient broth with pH of 7·4 it loses the greater part of its activity during overnight incubation.

Anti-microbic Activity

The term 'broad spectrum', denoting a wide range of activity, was coined in connection with this group of antibiotics, and in fact their spectrum is the broadest known (Table XXXVIII, p. 266). Susceptible species include not only those, mainly Gram-positive, which are also sensitive to penicillin, but many Gram-negative species which are not, and in addition rickettsias and *chlamydia* (p. 447). Like penicillin the tetracyclines are active against *T. pallidum* and other treponemata: unlike it, they also have some action on the tubercle bacillus. The only large group of fully resistant pathogenic organisms are the fungi (not including that of actinomycosis, which is highly sensitive). The possible indications for administering tetracyclines, to be considered later, are therefore very numerous.

INDIVIDUAL DIFFERENCES IN ACTIVITY. These are only of the order of two-fold, and may therefore not be of much consequence. Chlortetracycline, provided that the test is read after about 18 hours (further incubation alters the results, owing to its instability) can be shown to be the most active against all the pathogenic Gram-positive cocci, particularly staphylococci and pneumococci. Oxytetracycline is the most active against *Ps. aeruginosa* and tetracycline against *Proteus,* although the inhibitory concentrations for these species are considerably higher. There are no consistent differences among numerous other susceptible species.

ACQUIRED RESISTANCE. The acquisition of resistance to tetracyclines is a slow process, and is not often observed during the treatment of an individual patient, Nevertheless resistant strains of various coliform bacilli and of staphylococci have gradually become fairly common; indeed, tetracycline resistance has come to be regarded as the hall-mark of a virulent and troublesome staphylococcus. Resistance in haemolytic streptococci, first observed as long ago as 1952 in the special environment of a Burns Unit where tetracyclines had been extensively used (Lowbury and Hurst, 1956), has since been reported in strains isolated from the throat: Kuharic *et al.* (1960) found 20 per cent of strains in Seattle resistant, and Mitchell and Baber (1965) 32 per cent of a large number isolated in Bristol from throat swabs and other sources. The frequency of resistance in South-west Essex (Robertson, 1968) has remained steady at about the same level for several years, and varies with the site of origin, being highest in strains from infections of the ear, wounds and skin. Anyone who formerly regarded tetracyclines as suitable for treating acute sore throats and other possibly streptococcal infections should be warned.

Even more discouraging, since it comprises much the largest field of present use of tetracyclines, is the appearance of resistance in pneumococci. Earlier reports of this, reviewed in the last edition of this book, refer to small numbers of patients or to isolated outbreaks of infection due to a single serological type in elderly chronic bronchitics in institutions. It was not to be expected that such strains would indefinitely remain rarities, and the recent studies of Percival, Armstrong and Turner (1969) show that at least in Liverpool they have not. The frequency of resistance in strains from in-patients at the Royal Infirmary rose from 6 per cent in 1967 to 23 per cent in 1968, and at least half of these infections were judged to have been acquired outside hospital. Among patients attending general practitioners and chest clinics the corresponding figures were

7 and 12 per cent. The degree of resistance (M.I.C. of the order of 50 μg./ml.) is such as to preclude any possibility of successful treatment. No such steep increase in resistance has been observed in *H. influenzae,* although strains with some diminution in sensitivity have been seen.

Another organism now showing resistance is *Cl. welchii.* Johnstone and Cockcroft (1968) of Vancouver report that tetracycline given to a road casualty 'known to be allergic to penicillin' failed to prevent gas gangrene, and his arm had to be amputated. The strain of *Cl. welchii* responsible was tetracycline-resistant, as were 11 out of 102 further strains from human sources subsequently tested. Another objection to the emergency use of tetracycline for this purpose is that shock delays its absorption (Owen-Smith, 1969).

An organism resistant to one tetracycline is equally or almost equally resistant to any other.

MODE OF ACTION. Antibiotics are classified as bactericidal and bacteristatic, and the tetracyclines decidedly belong in the second category. There may be no such thing as pure bacteristasis, and there is some evidence that high concentrations of tetracyclines cause a steeper fall in the viable count than low ones, but the process is very gradual, with numerous survivors after as long as 24 hours. It is now known that tetracyclines belong to the group of antibiotics acting by interference with protein synthesis, the stage affected being probably the formation of peptide linkages. Resistance may be due to decreased permeability to the antibiotic.

Pharmacology

Although it is possible to prepare solutions suitable for intravenous or even intramuscular injection, the usual route of administration is oral, in capsules containing the hydrochloride.

ABSORPTION. This takes place from all levels of the alimentary tract from the stomach onwards (Gray *et al.,* 1953) but is never complete, and the larger the dose the lower is the proportion of it absorbed. Both because defective absorption militates against effective treatment and because the principal side effects are due to retention of the antibiotic in the bowel, much attention has been devoted to this problem, which has eluded complete solution so far as the earlier tetracyclines are concerned. Two factors appear to be involved. One is simply solubility: the hydrochlorides are reasonably soluble in water, giving a highly acid solution, but in a neutral or alkaline medium they tend to be precipitated, or (as when liberated in the intestine) not to dissolve. Secondly, tetracyclines combine with divalent metals, of which calcium is likely to be present in the largest amount. This was not appreciated for some years, and it is interesting in retrospect that calcium phosphate was actually used as a filler in capsules (Dearborn *et al.*, 1957) long after it had been shown that aluminium hydroxide, which must act in a similar way, interferes with absorption (Waisbren and Hueckel, 1950): this substance had been added to chlortetracycline to allay the gastric disturbance sometimes produced.

When the general significance of this reaction was grasped studies were made of the effect of appropriate additions to the contents of tetracycline capsules on the blood levels attained, and it was shown that calcium phosphate reduced absorption, whereas citric acid or sodium metaphosphate, which combine with calcium and thus render it unavailable for combination with the antibiotic, increased it substantially (Welch *et al.*, 1957; Sweeney *et al.*, 1957). Phosphate is now commonly included in the capsule to enhance absorption either as an addition or in combination with the antibiotic as a tetracycline phosphate complex, but it must not be supposed that this solves the problem: a variable and sometimes large proportion of the dose remains unabsorbed.

DISTRIBUTION. The blood level curve is a plateau, having a slow rise and a still slower fall. Factors contributing to this persistence are (1) continued absorption, (2) biliary excretion and reabsorption, (3) protein binding, the extent of which has been determined as 47, 20 and 24 per cent for chlor- and oxytetracycline and tetracycline respectively (Kunin, Dornbush and Finland, 1959). Tetracycline attains the highest level and chlortetracycline the lowest, but the differences are not large: maxima on ordinary doses (*e.g.* 250 mg. six-hourly) are of the

6

order of 2-4 μg./ml. with a small cumulative increase. Tetra-cyclines behave much like penicillin in their diffusion into serous cavities, the foetal circulation and glandular secretions. They enter the cerebro-spinal fluid somewhat more freely, concentrations of tetracycline found there being about 10 per cent of those in the blood: those of chlor- and oxytetracycline are somewhat lower (Wood and Kipnis, 1954). A unique feature of their behaviour is deposition in bone in areas where bone is being laid down: here they remain detectable for long periods. Similar deposition in teeth is referred to in the next section.

EXCRETION. Tetracyclines are freely excreted in both bile and urine. In the former the concentrations attained are 10-20 times those in the blood: much of the antibiotic so excreted must be re-absorbed. Urinary excretion accounts for rather over 20 per cent of an oral dose and 50 per cent of an intravenous: the difference between these figures is explained by incomplete absorption from the bowel, and the balance unaccounted for even after injection denotes degradation in the body. Variable but often very large amounts ($>$1,000 μg./g.) are found in the faeces when administration is oral.

PARENTERAL ADMINISTRATION. Suitable solutions can be administered by slow intravenous infusion, a usual dose being 0·5 g. twice daily. Advantages of this route are the immediate effect and the certainty of attaining an adequate blood level, the factor of variable absorption from the alimentary tract being eliminated. The level is also well maintained, doubtless owing largely to biliary excretion and reabsorption.

Side Effects

At the time when the first edition of this book was in preparation, alimentary tract superinfections were almost the only side-effects recognized from the use of these drugs. It is indeed strange that in 1963, after many years of world-wide use, a series of new accusations should have been levelled against them. The climate of suspicion engendered by the thalidomide disaster had some responsibility for this.

Several of these accusations have little foundation. The authors who alleged teratogenicity on the basis of a single infant with finger deformities have since reported that ' in 3 or 4 instances the administration to the mother of penicillin in early pregnancy had been followed by the birth of a malformed baby ' and proceeded to suggest that all antibiotics should be avoided in pregnant women (Carter and Wilson, 1963). Renal damage evidenced by proteinuria, glycosuria and amino-aciduria has been caused by improperly stored capsules of tetracycline (Frimpter *et al.*, 1963): it is now known that this is due to a toxic epimer, epianhydrotetracycline, which is only formed in the presence of not only moisture but an acid. This was citric acid included in the capsule to promote absorption: this formulation has naturally been abandoned, and hence this toxic effect has not been and will not be seen again. It is also doubtful whether alleged effects on skeletal development have an adequate basis. This is certainly not to be found in experiments in echinoderm larvae and chick embryos referred to by Cohlan, Bevelander and Tiamsic (1963), but these authors also observed a diminution in the rate of growth of the fibula in premature infants given the excessive dose of 100 mg. per kg. tetracycline daily for 9-12 days. A lesser effect was produced by a smaller dose, but stopping the treatment was usually followed immediately by accelerated growth. There is no evidence of any permanent effect, and a bony deformity so produced has yet to be seen.

A minor and unexplained side effect described by Fields (1961) in two out of an unstated number of infants treated with tetracycline is bulging of the anterior fontanelle: it disappeared when treatment was stopped.

Two other effects require more serious consideration.

STAINING OF TEETH. Tetracyclines are deposited in teeth during the early stages of calcification, just as they are in calcifying bone. This may occur *in utero* if the mother is treated after the fifth month, when calcification of the deciduous teeth begins (Kline, Blattner and Lunin, 1964) or be produced by treatment of the child after birth. For the effect to be visible as yellow staining a certain total dose must be exceeded: the relationship between dosage and effect was well studied by Wallman and Hilton (1962). Different tetracyclines produce different degrees and shades of pigmentation (Owen, 1963) and varying degrees of hypoplasia may accompany it. The main objection to this change is cosmetic, and this applies particularly to the second dentition: it is thus important to remember when the permanent teeth begin to be formed, and it would also be useful to know for how long after this pigmentation can still be produced. The permanent incisors begin to be formed six months after birth, the canines and premolars after two years, and the molars after three to four years (Witkop and Wolf, 1963). There seems to have been no thorough study of the relationship between age at the time of tetracycline treatment and dental staining, but an effect on the anterior teeth seems likely to be small after the third year. Tetracycline treatment is therefore to be avoided in early childhood except for imperative indications or unless a short course will suffice.

Liver Damage. It has been known since the work of Lepper *et al.* (1951) that tetracyclines given in excessive doses parenterally as well as orally can damage the liver. Little more was heard of this effect until Schulz *et al.* (1963) reported the deaths of six women treated for pyelitis during pregnancy with large intravenous doses of tetracycline. They had exhibited jaundice, fever, azotaemia, electrolyte disturbances, and in some cases haemorrhage from the alimentary tract. The main lesion found at post portem was diffuse fine droplet fatty degeneration of the liver. Excessive dosage—from 3·5 to 6 g. daily—was evidently the main factor in this disaster. Whalley, Adams and Combes (1964) describe five similar cases with only one death, in four of which ' 1-2 g. ' was given intravenously daily, and the fifth, only mildly affected and without jaundice, received only 1 g. orally daily. These authors performed tetracycline blood assays, and found levels up to 40-60 μg. per ml. during treatment, and substantial amounts in blood collected up to two weeks later. Kunelis, Peters and Edmondson (1965) described 16 cases of ' fatty liver of pregnancy ' in 12 of which tetracycline had been given intravenously or intramuscularly, usually in doses of 2 g. or more daily, for pyelonephritis. The remaining four had had no tetracycline, and Ober and LeCompte (1955) earlier described an apparently identical condition as idiopathic: indeed it may well be of the same nature as the ' acute yellow atrophy ' of late pregnancy described long before by Sheehan

(1940). Dowling and Lepper (1964) review other reported cases, including one unassociated with pregnancy but evidently resulting from excessive dosage.

A total daily dose of tetracycline by the intravenous route of 1 g. is adequate for most purposes, and should rarely be exceeded. Whether pyelonephritis, for which the treatment has usually been given in pregnancy, plays an important part by delaying elimination of the antibiotic has not been actually determined. The alternative possibility is that the liver itself is specially liable to damage in pregnancy: Kunelis *et al.* (1965) make the specific suggestion that it may be more sensitive to agents which depress protein anabolism. That tetracycline interferes to some extent with protein synthesis in the human body as well as in the bacterial cell seems evident from observations such as those of Shils (1963), who draws attention to the consequences which may result from this when renal function is impaired: these include increased urinary loss of nitrogen with a rising blood urea, acidosis, anorexia, nausea and vomiting and loss of weight. Some of these patients die with uncontrollable electrolyte disturbances and recognition of the seriousness of their condition may be delayed because the urinary output is commonly normal or increased (Lew and French, 1966). Tetracyclines should evidently not be given to patients with impaired renal function or, in the interests of both mother and foetus, in late pregnancy.

It remains to consider side-effects involving the alimentary tract, which have been recognized as a drawback to the use of this group of antibiotics from early days.

GASTRO-INTESTINAL DISTURBANCES. Nausea and vomiting are presumably due to a direct irritant effect of the drug on the gastric mucosa. Possibly diarrhoea can also be so caused, but this and other effects are more often the result of superinfection, *i.e.* the replacement of the suppressed normal flora by antibiotic-resistant organisms. It is here that the broad spectrum effect operates to the patient's disadvantage: most of the flora of the mouth, and even of the more complex flora of the lower bowel, including lactobacilli and clostridia as well as streptococci and the normal coliforms, are sensitive, and their suppression leaves a vacuum liable to be filled by less well-disposed inhabitants. These are of three kinds.

1. *Candida albicans* can produce effects at three levels: in the mouth its proliferation can cause anything from simple soreness to frank and extensive thrush, which may spread to the pharynx and even the bronchi; in the bowel it can be manifested by diarrhoea, and at the other end of the alimentary tract it commonly causes pruritus ani.

2. *Proteus* and *Pseudomonas* species resistant to tetracyclines may become predominant in the bowel and diarrhoea is common.

3. *Staphylococcus aureus* causes the most serious super-infection: the responsible strain is always resistant to tetracycline and often to other antibiotics. This dangerous condition, first described as a complication of treatment with oxytetracycline (Jackson *et al.*, 1951), can in fact be produced by any tetracycline, even one given by the intravenous route (Lundsgaard-Hansen *et al.*, 1960), when its direct action on the bowel must result from biliary excretion; it has also often been caused by treatment with penicillin and streptomycin together, and less often by other antibiotics. The epidemic at the Radcliffe Infirmary, Oxford, embracing 31 cases with 14 deaths (Cook *et al.*, 1957) suggests that cross-infection with an endemic strain is the usual source of the infection. The condition is seen almost exclusively in surgical patients post-operatively, and the operation most commonly followed by it (14 of the Oxford series) is gastrectomy. The emptiness of the bowel in such patients is probably an important factor. The lesion is a superficial necrosis of large areas of small intestinal mucosa, and the clinical manifestations are a profuse watery diarrhoea, with stools swarming with staphylococci, leading to dehydration and circulatory collapse. Treatment includes stopping the offending antibiotic, administering another to which the staphylococcus is or is likely to be sensitive (methicillin or perhaps vancomycin: see p. 354) and fluid replacement. Detection at an early stage by staining films of faeces from all patients with post-operative diarrhoea may enable the development of the full syndrome to be prevented.

There is some evidence that gastro-intestinal disturbances are less often caused by tetracycline than by chlor- and oxytetracycline: indeed, the fact that it is better tolerated was a leading claim made for tetracycline when it was introduced. It should be remembered in this connection that the doses of chlortetracycline originally given were larger than those of tetracycline usually given today.

Vitamin B supplements are usually said to be advisable for patients given these antibiotics for more than a few days, although this is disputed, but it is doubtful whether vitamin deficiency is the usual basis of any of these side effects.

NEWER TETRACYCLINES

Several new tetracyclines have been introduced recently. They possess the same general properties as the foregoing, and only those in which they differ need be described.

Demethylchlortetracycline

This substance, of which a general account is given by Finland and Garrod (1960) is formed by a mutant strain of *Streptomyces aureofaciens,* and is chlortetracycline without the methyl group in the R_1 position (p. 147). It is astonishing that subtracting this one attachment should have such profound effects. One of these is to confer a high degree of stability, in contrast to the remarkable instability of chlortetracycline. Anti-bacterial activity exceeds that of tetracycline against most species by a factor of about two. Absorption is better than that of tetracycline, and excretion is considerably slower, the rate of renal clearance being 43 per cent of that of tetracycline. This may be due, at least in part, to a higher degree of protein binding than that of the older tetracyclines. The result of these differences in behaviour is that a smaller dose will give at least an equal blood level for a longer time, and indeed the usual daily dose is four 150 mg. capsules when that of tetracycline would be four of 250 mg. It is believed that larger doses than this of demethylchlortetracycline are more liable than those of other tetracyclines to cause gastro-intestinal disturbance, although statistical proof of this is unavailable on a convincing scale.

These findings with regard to absorption and excretion have been confirmed by several groups of workers, but in consequence of one conflicting report (Roberts *et al.,* 1961) a further cross-over test on an impressive scale was carried out, which not only confirmed that the average blood levels produced by 300 mg. demethylchlortetracycline given twice a day equal those produced by 250 mg. tetracycline given four times a day, but showed further that if the former is given in doses of 150 mg. four times a day the levels produced are substantially higher (Sweeney, Dornbush and Hardy, 1962).

Demethylchlortetracycline has the minor drawback of causing photo-sensitization: patients taking it should avoid prolonged exposure to sunlight.

Rolitetracycline

This tetracycline compound (pyrrolidinomethyl tetracycline), known as Reverin in Germany, the country of its origin, unlike any of the foregoing is highly soluble in water (>1 g./ml.), giving a neutral solution. It is thus easily administered intravenously in full doses, and by this means exceptionally high blood and tissue levels can be attained (Otte, 1960; Knothe and Mahler, 1959). There are enthusiastic reports of its clinical use, mainly from the Continent. Its toxicity somewhat exceeds that of tetracycline, and there would appear to be some possibility of the kind of liver damage observed when chlortetracycline was given in large doses parenterally. Although administered only by injection, its use in surgical cases can result in staphylococcal enterocolitis: six cases with two deaths are reported by authors from Berne (Lundsgaard-Hansen *et al.*, 1960).

Lymecycline

This compound (tetracycline-L-methylenelysine), produced in Italy and known as Tetralysal, is formed by a reaction between tetracycline, formaldehyde and L-lysine (Cassano *et al.*, 1961). Like the foregoing it is highly soluble (1 g. in 0·4 ml.), and is said to be particularly well absorbed when given orally, permitting lower dosage and reducing (or according to some statements eliminating) alimentary tract side effects. It can also be administered by intramuscular or intravenous injection. Its *in vitro* activity is stated as identical with that of tetracycline.

Most of the publications on this product are Italian, and those dealing with absorption and excretion include none reporting estimations in the faeces: these should afford the best evidence of good absorption, particularly in subjects shown to be poor absorbers of tetracycline. The finding of de Carneri and Manfredi (1962) that doubling the dose increases the blood level by 82 per cent is suggestive: an increase so nearly corresponding to the increase in the dose is not to be expected with other tetracyclines. In this country Whitby and Black (1964) obtained conflicting results: lymecycline gave higher blood levels than tetracycline in volunteers, but lower ones in treated patients. The 24-hour urinary excretions of tetracycline and lymecycline in volunteers were 21 and 28 per cent of the dose respectively: this figure for lymecycline is less than half that reported in some Italian studies. In their clinical study these authors observed no difference in the frequency of side effects: diarrhoea, sore mouth, etc. occurred in 13 out of 58 patients given lymecycline and in 10 out of 44 given tetracycline. The dose of lymecycline given was smaller, as in the study of Pines *et al.* (1964) who observed side-effects in 13 out of 66 patients with chronic bronchitis treated with lymecycline and 23 out of 69 given tetracycline: an apparent fallacy in these results has been pointed out by Stratford (1965). In view of these conflicting and equivocal findings, final judgment on the merits of this form of tetracycline must be suspended.

Clomocycline

('Megaclor'), described as N-methylolchlortetracycline, is another Italian product for which similar advantages are claimed. It has a solubility in water of over 1:1 over a wide range of *p*H, and because of this is said to be much better absorbed than less soluble tetracyclines. Its instability is claimed to be an advantage as accountable for minimal deposition in bone (Tubaro, 1964). There is less published evidence about this product than about lymecycline, and some of the same questions call for an independent and authoritative answer in connection with both. It is supplied in capsules containing 170 mg. of which one four times a day is said usually to be an adequate dose.

Methacycline

It is claimed for this compound (6-methylene oxytetracycline: Rondomycin) that its anti-bacterial activity *in vitro* somewhat exceeds that of demethylchlortetracycline, that this difference in its favour is greater *in vivo* (mouse infections) and that it is better absorbed (English *et al.*, 1962). Remington and Finland (1962), on the other hand, found the blood levels produced by methacycline and demethylchlortetracycline to be very similar, except that the latter diminished more slowly. There was little difference between the two in activity against the organisms used for assay. No notable information about this drug has become available possibly because its manufacturers have concentrated more attention on the newer derivative, doxycycline.

Doxycycline

This compound, which is a α-6-deoxytetracycline, is described by English (1966) as possessing similar *in vitro* activity to that of methacycline and demethylchlortetracycline, and similar therapeutic activity against streptococcal, staphylococcal and *P. multocida* infections in mice when administered subcutaneously: on the other hand the curative dose by oral administration was less, a difference attributed to better absorption. From a further study (English, 1967) using different methods it was calculated that the percentage of an oral dose of doxycycline absorbed exceeded that of several other tetracyclines (including methacycline) by a factor of over 3. The observations of Rosenblatt *et al.* (1967) suggest a different or additional explanation: they found that doses of 100 mg. doxycycline and 300 mg. demethylchlortetracycline gave similar blood levels, but showed that this was due, not to better absorption (about the same proportion of the dose of each being excreted in the urine), but to slower excretion, the renal clearances of the two drugs being respectively 15·95 and 36·49 ml. per min.

An advantage of this drug is that owing to its slow excretion only one daily dose need be given. According to Fabre *et al.* (1967) an initial dose of 200 mg. followed by 100 mg. daily serves to maintain a blood level of between 1·5 and 3 μg./ml. Favourable clinical results are reported by Rennau and Schmiedel (1968) in infections of the lungs and bronchi and of the urinary and biliary tracts.

Minocycline

This derivative was first described by Redin (1967). It is 7-dimethylamino-6-demethyl-6-deoxytetracycline. It appears to be exceptionally well absorbed after oral administration, about one quarter of the dose of demethylchlortetracycline being required to produce the same blood level. Therapeutic activity in mice exceeded that of tetracycline, often by a wide margin, in 9 out of 10 infections studied. It was also much more active than either tetracycline or PAS in *Myco. tuberculosis* infection. Its most interesting property is its activity both *in vitro* and *in vivo* against staphylococci resistant to tetracycline: effective doses against mouse infections by 12 such strains varied from 0·3 to 14 mg. per kg., whereas tetracycline was ineffective at 1 g. per kg. We have had the opportunity of examining this compound and found that its *in vitro* activity greatly exceeds that of tetracycline against tetracycline-resistant strains, not only of staphylococci, but of *Str. pyogenes, Str. faecalis,* and *Esch. coli.* This difference does not extend to resistant pneumococci or to any other enterobacteria (*Proteus, Pseudomonas, Klebsiella, Salmonella* or *Shigella*). An explanation of why minocycline retains activity against tetracycline-resistant strains of some species but not of others would be of great interest.

In a later *in vitro* study Fedorko, Katz and Allnoch (1968) emphasize the activity of minocycline against strains of staphylococci resistant to other tetracyclines. This is also confirmed by Steigbigel, Reed and Finland (1968) in one of the largest series of determinations of M.I.C. ever published. It embraces 7 tetracyclines and 421 strains of 21 varieties of bacteria. From a vast mass of data they calculate an order of merit based on the percentage of total strains inhibited by each tetracycline either in a lower concentration than by any other or in one not bettered by any other. These percentages, with the organisms most sensitive to each tetracycline are minocycline 67 (staphylococci and streptococci), doxycycline 38 (enterococci), methacycline 32 (*H. influenzae*), chlortetracycline and demethylchlortetracycline each 20 and tetracycline and oxytetracycline each 4. Some clinical results with minocycline are reported by Frisk and Tunevall (1969).

CLINICAL APPLICATIONS

Thanks to their exceptionally broad spectrum, tetracyclines are indicated for a greater variety of infections than any other antibiotic. This fact encourages their choice, particularly by the general practitioner, when a bacteriological diagnosis is unavailable.

Much of their prescription in this country is for infections of the respiratory tract. It used to be said that all organisms capable of causing pneumonia were susceptible, but as resistant strains of pneumococci have become more prevalent this ceases to be true of the most important of them. It holds good for most Gram-negative infection, for psittacosis and infections with *Rickettsia burneti* and *Myocoplasma pneumoniae*. Resistance in haemolytic streptococci is now common, and the prescription of tetracyclines for acute throat infections is therefore inadvisable. Much the largest consumption is in the treatment of chronic bronchitis, for which the efficacy of tetracyclines is exceeded only by that of chloramphenicol, the long term administration of which is dangerous, and possibly by trimethoprim.

Brucellosis is an absolute indication. Other uses which may be indicated are for urinary tract infections and infections of the skin. Tetracyclines also afford an alternative to penicillin and for the treatment of actinomycosis, anthrax and syphilis. Other possible or definite indications are for cholera, granuloma venereum, lymphogranuloma inguinale, leptospirosis, relapsing fever, trachoma, tularaemia and typhus.

Tetracyclines are also valuable in mixed infections, notably peritonitis, for which one of them is certainly the most effective single antibiotic, and probably also better than mixtures of others. On the other hand prophylactic administration to surgical patients should be avoided if possible. A general contra-indication to the use of tetracyclines is any condition in which a bactericidal effect is essential: thus they have no place in the treatment of bacterial endocarditis.

PHARMACEUTICAL PREPARATIONS

TETRACYCLINE HYDROCHLORIDE ('Achromycin', *Lederle;* 'Tetracyn', *Pfizer,* and other names).
    Capsules and Tablets B.P., B.N.F. 200 mg., Proprietary 50 mg., U.S.P. 50, 100 and 250 mg., Elixir B.N.F. 125 mg./5 ml., Oral Suspension 250 mg./5

ml., Injection B.P., B.N.F. (i.m.) 200, 400 mg. Proprietary and U.S.P. 100, 250 and 500 mg. Usual adult dose 250 mg. 4 times a day, which may be doubled for severe infections. Dose by intramuscular or intravenous routes should rarely exceed 1 g. daily.

CHLORTETRACYCLINE HYDROCHLORIDE ('Aureomycin ', *Lederle*).
Capsules B.P. 250 mg., Proprietary 50 mg., U.S.N.F. 50, 100 and 250 mg., Injection B.P., B.N.F., U.S.N.F. 100, 250, 500 mg. Dosage: See Tetracycline hydrochloride.

OXYTETRACYCLINE HYDROCHLORIDE ('Terramycin', *Pfizer;* 'Imperacin' *I.C.I.*).
Capsules and Tablets B.N.F. 250 mg., U.S.N.F. 50, 100 and 250 mg. Syrup 125 mg./5 ml., Oral Suspension 250 mg./5 ml. Injection B.P., B.N.F., U.S.N.F. 100, 250 and 500 mg., Proprietary 50 mg. (in 2 ml.). Dosage: see Tetracycline hydrochloride.

DEMETHYLCHLORTETRACYCLINE HYDROCHLORIDE('Ledermycin', 'Declomycin' *Lederle*).
Capsules B.P., B.N.F. 150 mg., U.S.N.F. 75 and 150 mg., Tablets 300 mg., Syrup, B.N.F., U.S.N.F. 75 mg./5 ml., Oral Suspension U.S.N.F. 15 mg./ ml.: usual dose 150 mg. 4 times a day, but may be increased. No parenteral preparation. Also ointment and syrup.

ROLITETRACYCLINE (' Reverin ', *Hoechst,* Synetrin, Velocycline *U.S.A.*).
Available as vials of the pure substance for solution for intramuscular or (preferably) intravenous injection. Usual dose 250 mg. twice daily.

LYMECYCLINE (' Tetralysal ', *Carlo Erba*).
Capsules containing equivalent of 150 mg. tetracycline base. Injection (i.m.) 100 mg. Usual dose one capsule 4 times a day.

METHACYCLINE HYDROCHLORIDE (' Rondomycin ', *Pfizer*).
Capsules of 150 mg. Syrup 75 mg./5 ml.: usual dose one capsule 4 times a day.

CLOMOCYCLINE (' Megaclor', *Pharmax*).
Capsules of 170 mg. Syrup 85 mg./5ml.: usual dose one capsule 4 times a day.

DOXYCYCLINE (' Vibramycin ', *Pfizer*).
Capsules 100 mg.: dosage 100 to 200 mg. once a day.

REFERENCES

CARTER, M. P. & WILSON, F. (1963).*Lancet* 1, 1267.
CASSANO, A., FILICE, A., COSTA, C. & TRIMARCO, C. (1961). *Rif. med.* 75, 1383.
COHLAN, S. Q., BEVELANDER, G. & TIAMSIC, T. (1963). *Amer. J. Dis. Child.* 105, 453.
COOK, J., ELLIOTT, C., ELLIOT-SMITH, A., FRISBY, B. R. & GARDNER, A. M. N. (1957). *Brit. med. J.* 1, 542.
DEARBORN, E. H., LITCHFIELD, J. T. JR., EISNER, H. J., CORBETT, J. J. & DUNNETT, C. W. (1957). *Antibiot. Med.* 4, 627.
DE CARNERI, I. & MANFREDI, N. (1962). *Arzneimittal-Forsch.* 12, 1174.
DOWLING, H. F. & LEPPER, M. H. (1964). *J. Amer. med. Ass.* 188, 307.
ENGLISH, A. R. (1966). *Proc. Soc. exp. Biol. (N.Y.)* 122, 1107.
ENGLISH, A. R. (1967). *Proc. Soc. exp. Biol. Med.* 126, 487.
ENGLISH, A. R., MCBRIDE, T. J. & RIGGIO, R. (1962). *Antimicrob. Agents and Chemotherapy*—1961, p. 462. Detroit.
FABRE, J., PITTON, J. S., VIRIEUX, C., LAURENCET, F. L., BERNHARDT, J. P. & GODEL, J. C. (1967). *Schweiz. med. Wschr.* 97, 915.

FEDORKO, J., KATZ, S. & ALLNOCH, H. (1968). *Amer. J. med. Sci.* **255**, 252.

FIELDS, J. P. (1961). *J. Pediat.* **58**, 74.

FINLAND, M., & GARROD, L. P. (1960). *Brit. med. J.* **2**, 959.

FRIMPTER, G. W., TIMPANELLI, A. E., EISENMENGER, W. J., STEIN, H. S. & EHRLICH, L. I. (1963). *J. Amer. med. Ass.* **184**, 111.

FRISK, A. R. & TUNEVALL, G. (1969). *Antimicrob. Agents Chemother.*, 1968, p. 335.

GRAY, W. D., HILL, R. T., WINNE, R. & CUNNINGHAM, R. W. (1953). *J. Pharmacol. exp. Ther.* **109**, 223.

JACKSON, G. G., HAIGHT, T. H., KASS, E. H., WOMACK, C. R., GOCKE, T. M. & FINLAND, M. (1951). *Ann. intern. Med.* **35**, 1175.

JOHNSTONE, F. R. C. & COCKCROFT, W. H. (1968). *Lancet* **1**, 660.

KLINE, A. H., BLATTNER, R. J. & LUNIN, M. (1964). *J. Amer. med. Ass.* **188**, 178.

KNOTHE, H. & MAHLER, J. (1959). *Dtsch. med. Wschr.* **84**, 1687.

KUHARIC, H. A., ROBERTS, C. E. JR., & KIRBY, W. M. M. (1960). *J. Amer. med. Ass.* **174**, 1779.

KUNELIS, C. T., PETERS, J. L. & EDMONDSON, H. A. (1965). *Amer. J. Med.* **38**, 359.

KUNIN, C. M., DORNBUSH, A. C. & FINLAND, M. (1959). *J. clin. Invest.* **38**, 1950.

LEPPER, M. H., WOLFE, C. K., ZIMMERMAN, H. J., CALDWELL, E. R. JR., SPIES, H. W. & DOWLING, H. F. (1951). *Arch. intern. Med.* **88**, 271.

LEW, H. T. & FRENCH, S. W. (1966). *Arch. intern. Med.* **118**, 123.

LOWBURY, E. J. L. & HURST, L. (1956). *J. clin. Path.* **9**, 59.

LUNDSGAARD-HANSEN, P., SENN, A., ROOS, B. & WALLER, U. (1960). *J. Amer. med. Ass.* **173**, 1008.

MITCHELL, R. G. & BABER, K. G. (1965). *Lancet* **1**, 25.

OBER, W. B. & LeCOMPTE, P. M. (1955). *Amer. J. Med.* **19**, 743.

OTTE, H. J. (1960). *Zbl. Bakt.* 1, Abt. Orig. **180**, 569.

OWEN, L. N. (1963). *Arch. oral Biol.* **8**, 715.

OWEN-SMITH, M. S. (1969). *J. roy. Army med. Corps* **115**, 23.

PERCIVAL, A., ARMSTRONG, E. C. & TURNER, G. C. (1969). *Lancet* **1**, 998.

PINES, A., PLUCINSKI, K., GREENFIELD, J. S. B. & MITCHELL, R. C. (1964). *Brit. med. J.* **2**, 1495.

REDIN, G. A. (1967). *Antimicrob. Agents and Chemother.*—1966, p. 371.

REMINGTON, J. S. & FINLAND, M. (1962). *Clin. Pharmacol. & Therap.* **3**, 284.

RENNAU, H. & SCHMIEDEL, A. (1968). *Münch. med. Wschr.* **110**, 1136.

ROBERTS, C. E. JR., PERRY, D. M., KUHARIC, H. A. & KIRBY, W. M. M. (1961). *Arch. intern. Med.* **107**, 204.

ROBERTSON, M. H. (1968). *Brit. med. J.* **3**, 349.

ROSENBLATT, J. E., BARRETT, J. E., BRODIE, J. L. & KIRBY, W. M. M. (1967). *Antimicrob. Agents and Chemother.*—1966, p. 134.

SCHULZ, J. C., ADAMSON, J. S., WORKMAN, W. W. & NORMAN, T. D. (1963). *New Engl. J. Med.* **269**, 999.

SHEEHAN, H. L. (1940). *J. Obstet. Gynaec. Brit. Emp.* **47**, 49.

SHILS, M. E. (1963). *Ann. intern. Med.* **58**, 389.

STEIGBIGEL, N. H., REED, C. W. & FINLAND, M. (1968). *Amer. J. med. Sci.* **255**, 179.

STRATFORD, B. C. (1965). *Brit. med. J.* **1**, 922.

SWEENEY, W. M., HARDY, S. M., DORNBUSH, A. C. & RUEGSEGGER, J. M. (1957). *Antibiot. Med.* **4**, 642.

SWEENEY, W. M., DORNBUSH, A. C., & HARDY, S. M. (1962). *Amer. J. med. Sci.* **243**, 296.

TUBARO, E. (1964). *Brit. J. Pharmacol.* **23**, 445.

WAISBREN, B. A. & HUECKEL, J. S. (1950). *Proc. Soc. exp. Biol.* (*N.Y.*) **73**, 73.

WALLMAN, I. S. & HILTON, H. B. (1962). *Lancet* **1**, 827.

WELCH, H., LEWIS, C. N., STAFFA, A. W. & WRIGHT, W. W. (1957). *Antibiot. Med.* **4,** 215.
WHALLEY, P. J., ADAMS, R. H. & COMBES, B. (1964). *J. Amer. med. Ass.* **189,** 357.
WHITBY, J. L. & BLACK, H. J. (1964). *Brit. med. J.* **2,** 1491.
WITKOP, C. J. & WOLF, R. O. (1963). *J. Amer. med. Ass.* **185,** 1008.
WOOD, W. S. & KIPNIS, G. P. (1953). *Antibiot. Ann.* 1953-54, p. 98.

CHAPTER X

MACROLIDES

THIS is a group of closely similar antibiotics, the more widely used of which were discovered in 1952-4. They all consist of a macrocyclic lactone ring—to which they owe the generic name macrolide—and to which sugars are attached. The chemical inter-relationships of the macrolides are reviewed by Celmer (1966). All have a similar antibacterial spectrum which closely resembles that of penicillin. Erythromycin, the first to be discovered, has the highest activity, at least *in vitro,* and has been used more extensively and studied more thoroughly than either oleandomycin or spiramycin, which rank next in importance and are commercially available. About 35 antibiotics with the basic macrolide structure have now been described.

ERYTHROMYCIN

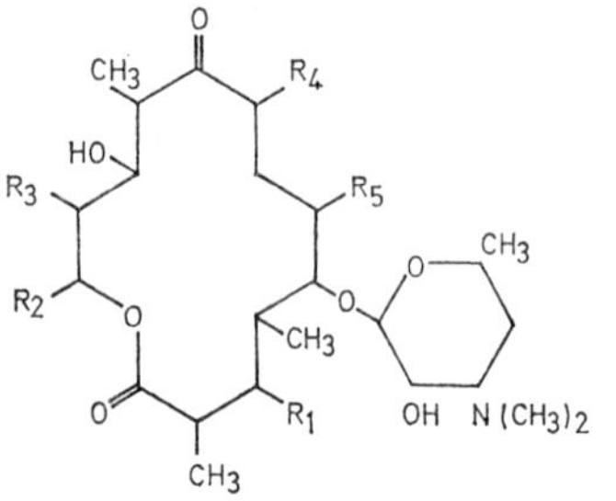

	Erythromycin A	Oleandomycin
R_1	L – cladinose	L – oleandrose
R_2	$CH_2 \cdot CH_3$	CH_3
R_3	$<^{CH_3}_{OH}$	CH_3
R_4	CH_3	$<^{CH_2}_{O}$
R_5	$<^{CH_3}_{OH}$	CH_3

FIG. 11
Structure of macrolides.

This antibiotic was obtained in 1952 in the Lilly Research Laboratories, Indianapolis, from a strain of *Streptomyces erythreus* derived from soil from the Philippines. Its structure is shown in Fig. 11. There are three erythromycins, of which B and C possess lesser activity. Erythromycin is a faintly yellow crystalline weak base, soluble only to the extent of about 0·1

166

per cent in water, but readily so in ethanol and other organic solvents. Neutral solutions are stable for many weeks at 5°C, but at room temperature there is some loss after a few days: at a pH below 5 loss of activity is rapid.

Esters of erythromycin can be prepared which possess a pharmacological advantage to be referred to later.

Anti-bacterial Activity

The sensitivity of pathogenic bacteria to erythromycin is shown in Table XXIV. Among the factors often affecting bacteristatic activity, inoculum size has only a small effect except

TABLE XXIV

Sensitivity of Bacteria to Erythromycin

Usual minimum concentration (μg./ml.) causing complete bacteristasis with a moderate inoculum.

Gram-positive Bacteria		Gram-negative Bacteria	
Str. pneumoniae	0·01 - 0·2	N. gonorrhoeae	0·04 - 0·4
Str. haemolyticus		N. meningitidis	0·2 - 1·6
Group A	0·02 - 0·2	H. influenzae	0·4 - 3·1
B	0·04 - 0·4	H. pertussis	0.2
C	0·04 - 0·8	Brucella abortus	10
Str. viridans	0·02 - 3·1	Brucella melitensis	0·3
Str. faecalis	0·6 - 3·1	Esch. coli	8 - 300
Staph. aureus	0·01 - 1·6	Shigella spp.	100 - 200
Staph. albus	0·2 - 3·1	Salmonella spp.	100 - 200
C. diphtheriae	0·2 - 3·1	Kl. aerogenes	>100
Cl. tetani	0·2 - 0·6	Kl. pneumoniae	>100
Cl. welchii	0·1 - 0·2	Proteus spp.	>100
Mycobacterium spp.	0·4 - 6·25	Ps. aeruginosa	>100

Haight and Finland (1952). *Proc. Soc. exp. Biol. (N.Y.)* **81**, 175.
Heilman *et al.* (1952). *Proc. Mayo Clin.* **27**, 285.
Lowbury and Hurst (1959). *J. clin. Path.* **12**, 163.
Powell *et al.* (1953). *Antibiot. Chemother.* **3**, 165.

at extremes of the possible range. The addition of up to 50 per cent of serum has little effect, but pH is an important factor, activity increasing with increase in pH up to 8·5.

Noteworthy features of the spectrum are uniformly high activity against pneumococci and haemolytic streptococci of group A. *Staph. aureus* is rather less sensitive and where erythromycin has been extensively used highly resistant strains have readily emerged. The more vulnerable Gram-negative genera *Neisseria* and *Haemophilus* are also sensitive, and the hardier enterobacteria generally resistant although some strains of *Escherichia* are inhibited (and killed) by as little as 8 μg./ml. Erythromycin also exerts anti-rickettsial (*R. prowazeki*) activity in the embryonated egg, and an action inferior to that of chlortetracycline on the *Chlamydia* of lymphogranuloma venereum.

Although the action of erythromycin is predominantly bacteristatic in low concentrations, somewhat higher ones are distinctly if slowly bactericidal, there being few survivors after 24 hours' exposure. The behaviour of the antibiotic in some tests of combined action (for example, Fig. 3B in Garrod and Waterworth, 1962) is also proof of such an effect. A peculiar feature of the action of erythromycin in combination is its synergic effect with penicillin, only on strains of staphylococci resistant to both (Herrell, Balows and Becker, 1960). This exceptional effect, the only parallel to which is in the combined action of penicillin and fucidin on staphylococci forming small amounts of penicillinase, has a peculiar mechanism (p. 208) which has been neatly elucidated by Waterworth (1963).

Mode of Action

Erythromycin inhibits bacterial growth through competing with amino acid for ribosomal binding sites (Mao and Wiegand, 1968). The mechanisms of action of chloramphenicol and lincomycin (as well as other macrolides and forocidins—Vazques, 1967) are closely similar, but Cundliffe and McQuillen (1967) suggest that chloramphenicol interrupts the transfer reaction, while erythromycin interrupts translocation (p. 101). The resistance of many Gram-negative bacteria to the drug probably resides in a barrier effect of the cell wall since high concentrations of erythromycin accumulate inside Gram-positive but not Gram-negative bacilli (Mao and Putterman, 1968) and Taubeneck (1962) found that a stable L form (which has no cell wall) of *Proteus mirabilis* was more than a thousand times more sensitive to erythromycin than its parent strain.

Acquired Bacterial Resistance

It was soon apparent that staphylococci and many other species can readily develop resistance to erythromycin *in vitro*, strains of *Staph. aureus,* enterococcus and *Str. pneumoniae* developing 500-fold increases in resistance after 3-12 subcultures in the antibiotic, and strains of *Str. pyogenes* and *Str. viridans* showing 20-fold increases in resistance after 20 passages.

Increased resistance is not often observed to develop during successful short term treatment, but during more prolonged treatment of infections more difficult to eradicate, such as endocarditis, it is common. Where such resistant staphylococci emerge, they may spread rapidly in a hospital where the use of erythromycin is extensive. Reports have begun to appear of resistant strains of pneumococci (Cooper *et al.,* 1968) and of haemolytic streptococci which spread to several contacts (Sanders *et al.,* 1968). Such reports are likely to be dismissed as curiosities of no therapeutic importance, but the appearance of resistance in such highly susceptible species to so relatively little used an agent highlights the extent to which current therapeutic practice is encouraging the emergence of resistant organisms.

Characteristics of Resistant Strains

Resistance to this group of antibiotics is not associated with drug destruction and no drug-inactivating enzyme or other type of antagonist has been demonstrated. The resistant mutants are capable of growing in an increased concentration of the unchanged antibiotic. The resistance is only moderately stable and resistant variants often consist of a mixed population, the individual cells of which have a wide variation in sensitivity to erythromycin. Erythromycin-resistant mutants of *Staph. aureus* are frequently deficient in other properties. Thus they often give rise to small colonies with relatively little pigment production on the usual nutrient media and may produce little or no coagulase. These changes are more frequent after passage in erythromycin *in vitro* but may also be seen when erythromycin resistance occurs *in vivo*. Biological deficiencies of this sort, together with the instability of the resistance in some cases, probably account for the fact that erythromycin in moderate doses is sometimes effective in the treatment of experimental infection with erythromycin-resistant staphylococci.

Cross-resistance

There is a curious difference in the extent of cross resistance between organisms passaged in increasing concentrations of macrolides and those isolated from patients. When staphylococci are passaged separately in erythromycin, spiramycin, oleandomycin and carbomycin resistance to all four antibiotics develops to the same extent and at approximately the same rate. Complete cross resistance with all four was also shown by staphylococci passaged in leucomycin (Waterworth, 1960).

As shown by Garrod (1957), however, erythromycin-resistant staphylococci isolated from patients are not necessarily resistant to spiramycin and oleandomycin. He studied 45 erythromycin-resistant strains of *Staph. aureus* isolated from patients in hospital in various parts of England and found that 15 were resistant to erythromycin, spiramycin and oleandomycin, whereas 30 were resistant to erythromycin only. Similarly, amongst the erythromycin-resistant strains from a number of hospitals in America, English and Fink (1961) found 80 per cent to be oleandomycin-sensitive. Organisms also occur which are resistant to oleandomycin, but sensitive to erythromycin.

Garrod (1957) showed that the strains showing the dissociated type of resistance consisted of cells the majority of which were sensitive to erythromycin, but growth on a medium containing the antibiotic produced a uniformly and highly resistant population. A unique feature of the behaviour of such organisms is that in the presence of erythromycin they are also resistant to oleandomycin or spiramycin, although in its absence they are fully sensitive. This extraordinary behaviour (Fig. 12) is undoubtedly the basis of the ' antagonism ' between erythromycin and spiramycin described by Chabbert (1956). A culture illustrating it in another way is shown in Figure 13. It has been explained by Weaver and Pattee (1964) who showed that erythromycin is the specific inducer of an enzyme the possession of which confers resistance to erythromycin and other macrolides. In the absence of erythromycin, this enzyme is lost and the population again becomes sensitive. An apparently identical situation occurs with lincomycin (Barber and Waterworth, 1964): erythromycin-resistant staphylococci sensitive to lincomycin in the absence of erythromycin

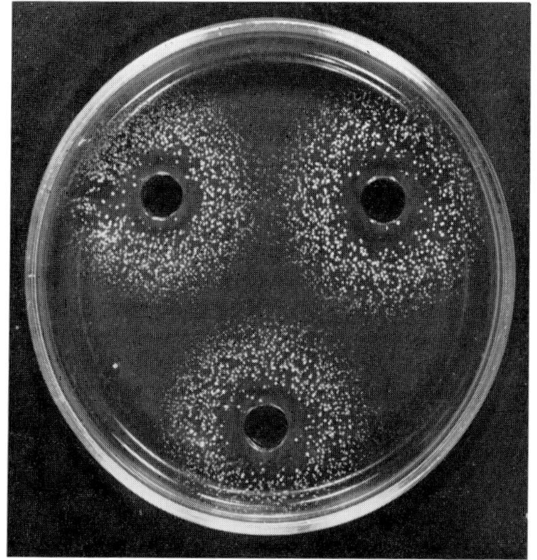

Nutrient agar plate containing 1 µg. oleandomycin per ml., surface-inoculated with a strain of staphylococcus having the dissociated type of erythromycin resistance, with three cups containing erythromycin solutions of 100 (*top right*), 50 (*below*), and 25 (*top left*) µg./ml. Growth of all but very few colonies is inhibited within a few millimetres of the cups: in a zone surrounding this the erythromycin permits growth despite the presence of oleandomycin. Elsewhere oleandomycin inhibits it.

(Garrod (1957) reproduced by kind permission of the Editor of the *British Medical Journal*.)

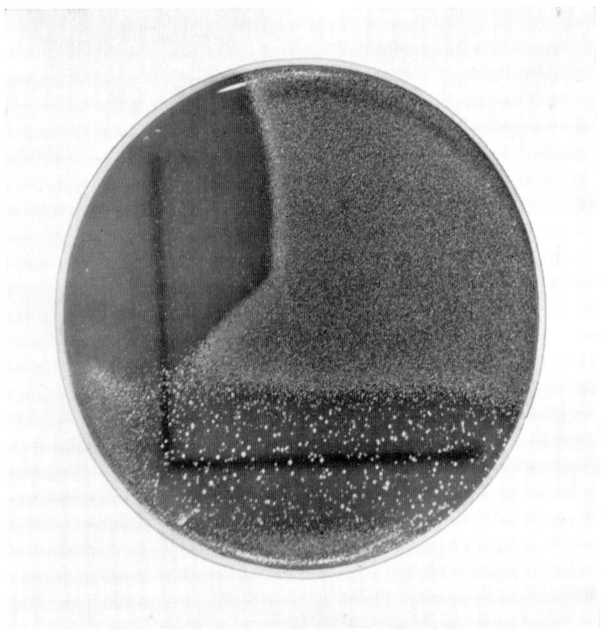

FIG. 13

Blood agar plate into which antibiotics have diffused from paper strips previously applied in positions denoted by lines. Vertical line=spiramycin (strip dipped in 1,000 μg./ml. solution); horizontal=erythromycin (250 μg./ml.). Surface-inoculated after removal of strips with a staphylococcus of the dissociated resistant type. Spiramycin acting alone is strongly inhibitory: where erythromycin encroaches on its area this action is totally abolished. Erythromycin inhibits the majority of the population, which includes only a small proportion of highly resistant cells: this action is not affected by the additional presence of spiramycin.

may be resistant in its presence. This adds further to the great similarity between the macrolides and lincomycin despite its very different chemical structure (p. 212).

Cross-resistance of a lower order has also been demonstrated between erythromycin and chloramphenicol (Barber, Csillag and Medway, 1958).

PHARMACOLOGY

Absorption

The acid lability of erythromycin base necessitates administration in a form giving protection from gastric acid. Gelatin capsules were not wholly satisfactory and better, although delayed, absorption is ensured by enteric-coated tablets. Even so, absorption is evidently not complete, although there is some cumulative effect, the blood level usually rising to 1-2 μg./ml. two to four hours after each dose when the six-hourly administration of 250 mg. capsules has continued for two or three days. There is some individual variation, adequate levels not being attained at all in a few subjects. An alternative is to give capsules of erythromycin stearate, which is so formulated as to be resistant to gastric acid, and broken down in the intestine liberating the base.

Much better absorption follows the administration of the propionyl ester of erythromycin. The propionyl ester is now prepared in the form of its lauryl sulphate, which possesses the two advantages of tastelessness and resistance to gastric acid. This compound, officially named erythromycin estolate (B.P.C., 1963) gives higher blood levels than the propionyl ester. That it is not without countervailing disadvantages will be made clear in a later section. The serum levels obtained after single doses of various preparations are given in Table XXV.

PARENTERAL INJECTION. The glucoheptonate and lactobionate of erythromycin are suitable for intravenous injection and are useful for attaining an immediate effect and higher blood levels (Table XXV). Intramuscular injection is also possible but causes pain, and the dose should not exceed 100 mg. The lactobionate has also been used for local instillation in infections of the pleural cavity and for inhalation, a 100 mg. dose by this route producing therapeutic levels both in the bronchial secretion and in the blood for four hours (Lopez-Belio *et al.*, 1957).

Distribution

Erythromycin is at first uniformly distributed throughout the organs and tends to be retained longer in the liver and spleen

TABLE XXV

Erythromycin Serum Levels in Man

Preparation	Dose mg.	Route	Peak Hrs.	Peak µg./ml.	Half life hrs.
Base	250 500 1,000	oral	3-4 2-4 4	0·25-0·5 0·9-1·4 1·3-1·5	2-4
Stearate fasting	250 500	oral	2 2-4	1·3 0·4-1·8	
after food	500		2-4	0·1-0·4	2-4
Propionate fasting	500		2-4	0·4-1·9	3-5
after food	500	oral	4	0·3-0·5	3-4
Estolate fasting	250 500	oral	2-4 1-2	0·9-2·4 1·4-5·0	2-4
after food	500		2-4	1·8-5·2	
Gluconate diethylcarbamate lactobionate glucoheptonate	500 500 300	I/M I/V I/V	½-1 0 0	2·7-5·0 11·5-30·0 20·0-80·0	1-1·5 1-2

Davis, D. S. & Romansky, M. J. (1955). *Antibiot. Ann.* 1954-5, p. 286.
Griffith, R. S. (1955). *Antibiot. Ann.* 1954-5, p. 269.
Griffith, R. S. & Black, H. R. (1962). *Antibiot. Chemother.* **12**, 398.
Griffith, R. S. & Black, H. R. (1964). *Amer. J. med. Sci.* **247**, 69.
Hirsch, H. A. & Finland, M. (1959). *Amer. J. med. Sci.* **237**, 693.
Lopez-Belio, M. & Takimura, Y. (1955). *Antibiot. Ann.* 1954-5, p. 295.
Reichelderfer, T. E. *et al.* (1960). *Antibiot. Ann.* 1959-60, p. 899.

than in the blood (Table XXVI). In a comparison of the persistence of various macrolides in the tissues of monkeys, Eidus *et al.* (1962) found that spiramycin (p. 176) had by far the longest life but that erythromycin was next in order. Only very low levels are attained in the cerebro-spinal fluid. Furgiuele (1964) found good penetration into the aqueous humour after oral erythromycin. Levels of 0·1 μg. per ml. occurred when the serum level was 0·36 μg. per ml. There was no demonstrable penetration into the vitreous.

Excretion

Erythromycin is excreted both in the urine and in the bile but only a fraction of the dose can be accounted for in this way. Subjects receiving 1 g. a day of propionyl erythromycin gave concentrations in the urine of 13-46 μg. per ml. With similar doses of erythromycin base, only about 8-20 mg. could be recovered from the urine in 24 hours, the concentrations being about 11-24 μg. per ml. (Griffith, 1959). Studies in the dog suggest that what little is excreted in the glomerular filtrate is partially re-absorbed by the tubules.

Fairly high concentrations are found in the bile in man but nothing like the high concentrations found in the rat. Peak concentrations of 10 μg. per ml. in subjects receiving the propionyl ester; 64 μg. per ml. in those receiving the base were reported by Hammond and Griffith (1961). The bile-serum concentration ratio in man was only about 4 for the propionyl ester, and 30 for the base whereas the corresponding values for the rat were about 20 times as much (Lee *et al.*, 1959). It is possible that the smaller excretion of the propionyl ester into the bile accounts in part for its better maintained serum levels. Even so, only about 1·5 per cent of the dose of the base (0·2 per cent of the ester) appears in the bile in the first eight hours.

With so little recoverable from the urine and bile, the greater part of the drug must be broken down in the body. Mao and Tardrew (1965) have shown that an enzyme capable of demethylating erythromycin is widely distributed in rabbit tissues, the greatest activity being found in the liver. The importance of non-renal mechanisms of elimination in man is shown by the finding of Kunin and Finland (1959) that the serum half-life of erythromycin is only increased about four-fold in the anuric patient while the half-life of penicillin is increased about 20-fold.

Toxicity and Side Effects

No toxic effects of any consequence have ever been recorded from the administration of erythromycin base. This unfortunately cannot be said of erythromycin estolate: according to Robinson (1961) about 12 per cent of patients given either this drug or a similar ester of oleandomycin for more than 14 days develop signs of liver damage. These consist of upper abdominal pain, fever, hepatic enlargement, a raised serum bilirubin, with or without actual jaundice, and eosinophilia. The condition may mimic viral hepatitis, cholecystitis or pancreatitis. The report by Kohlstaedt (1961) suggests a much lower incidence. From 15 million doses administered, 33 cases of jaundice had been reported. In a series of more than 11,000 patients, including 300 receiving prophylactic treatment for a year or more, no jaundice occurred. Whatever the incidence may be, it is astonishing that such reactions were not recognized earlier, and these revelations contributed to the atmosphere of suspicion about unsuspected toxic drug effects which developed about this time. Kuder (1960) had shortly before reviewed the side effects in over 20,000 patients treated with the propionyl ester or the estolate without commenting on jaundice. Yet Ticktin and Robinson (1963) have since claimed that evidence of hepatic abnormality is demonstrable in over a third of those receiving the estolate.

In contrast, Grönroos *et al.* (1967) found no clinical and scarcely any biochemical evidence of hepatic derangement amongst 37 patients treated with 250 mg. erythromycin estolate four times daily for 10 days.

Nevertheless, ample well documented cases of clinical jaundice have now been reported. There have been no deaths and on stopping the drug recovery has been complete (McKenzie and Doyle, 1966). Once patients have recovered, recurrence of symptoms can be produced by giving the estolate but not by giving the base or stearate (Brown, 1963). This together with the relative frequency of the reaction after second courses of the drug, peripheral eosinophilia and other evidence of sensitivity, and the histological appearances (Popper *et al.*, 1965) suggest that the reaction results from a mixture of intrahepatic cholestasis of hypersensitive origin and liver cell necrosis. As Ticktin and Robinson (1963) point out, the development of abnormal liver function in more than a third of those treated with the estolate (or with the related triacetyl oleandomycin) strongly suggests a direct hepatotoxic effect in addition to any sensitivity which may be responsible for more severe manifestations in susceptible individuals.

Erythromycin in any form may cause gastro-intestinal disturbances. Kuder (1960) found gastro-intestinal symptoms in 5·7 per cent of patients treated with the propionate and 2 per cent of those treated with the estolate. Nausea and vomiting were more common with the propionate and diarrhoea with the estolate. He and Kohlstaedt (1961) agreed that possible allergic effects occurred in about 0·5 per cent of patients.

In view of the apparently similar modes of action of erythromycin and chloramphenicol it is interesting that the macrolides have not been described as giving rise to aplasia. Erythromycin, tetracycline and chloramphenicol all depress haemoglobin synthesis by bone marrow cultures, but while chloramphenicol slightly impairs iron uptake by erythroblasts and greatly impairs iron incorporation into haem, erythromycin and tetracycline depress iron uptake but have no effect on its haem incorporation. Moreover, the cells appear to be considerably less sensitive to erythromycin and tetracycline than to chloramphenicol (Vas *et al.*, 1964).

It would be wrong to give the impression, by reviewing the side effects which have been reported, that erythromycin is a toxic substance. Leaving aside the special problem of the hepatotoxicity of the estolate, there is no doubt that erythromycin is one of the most innocuous antibiotics in current use.

OLEANDOMYCIN

This antibiotic was isolated in 1954 in the laboratories of Charles Pfizer & Co. from a strain of *Streptomyces antibioticus*. Its *in vitro* activity is less than that of erythromycin but greater than that of spiramycin: the factor by which that of erythromycin exceeds it was found to be two to four for *Staph. aureus* and about 10 for *Str. pyogenes*. Like erythromycin it is incompletely absorbed, and an ester, triacetyloleandomycin, gives improved blood levels, but this, like erythromycin estolate, can cause liver damage. Gilbert (1962) found abnormal liver function tests in 50 per cent of patients given triacetyloleando-mycin for more than 10 days and 5 per cent developed jaundice.

Oleandomycin has been extensively used as a 1:2 mixture with tetracycline (Sigmamycin) a combination for which synergic properties were claimed by English *et al.* (1956). Garrod (1957) could not confirm this, even with one of these authors' own strains of staphylococcus, and Jones and Finland (1957) also dispute the utility of this combination on the basis of assays of the anti-bacterial activity of the serum of subjects to whom tetracycline was given alone and in combination with oleandomycin, erythromycin or spiramycin.

SPIRAMYCIN

Spiramycin (Rovamycin) was obtained in 1954 in the Rhone-Poulenc Research Laboratories from a strain of *Streptomyces ambofaciens* derived from a sample of soil collected near Paris (Pinnert-Sindico *et al.*, 1955). This organism forms three closely related antibiotics, of which spiramycin A is used therapeutically.

Spiramycin has a substantially lower *in vitro* activity than erythromycin: 16-32-fold against *Staph. aureus,* 8-16-fold against *Str. pyogenes,* and 4-8-fold against *Str. pneumoniae.*

If spiramycin had no other property tending to compensate for its lesser anti-bacterial activity, the clinical results claimed for it would be difficult to understand. It seems that this property may be exceptional persistence in the tissues. Macfar-lane *et al.* (1968) who successfully used the drug for the preven-tion of post-prostatectomy staphylococcal sepsis, found levels 12 hours after a dose of 1 g. in man of 0·25 μg./ml. in serum, 5·3 μg./ml. in bone, 6·9 μg./ml. in pus, and 4 hours after the dose, 10·6 μg./ml. in saliva. As with erythromycin, high levels were found in the prostate (27 μg./ml.) after repeated dosage. It is evident from comparative studies of different macrolides (Eidus *et al.,* 1962; Sutherland, 1962) that at a time when the spiramycin content of the blood has fallen to a low level, high concentrations persist in the organs, whereas the organ content of erythromycin, oleandomycin or carbomycin declines much more rapidly (Table XXVI).

It must be accepted that this behaviour helps to account for such therapeutic success as spiramycin has achieved: whether it fully compensates for so considerable a deficiency in anti-bacterial activity is doubtful. It should be remembered that these organ assays were done after single large doses: the organ content during continual administration at intervals of four or six hours is not likely to differ so much.

TABLE XXVI

Concentrations of Antibiotic in Organs (µg./g.) and Blood (µg./ml.) of Mice 6 and 24 hrs. after Single Oral Dose of 500 mg. per kg.

	Spiramycin		*Erythromycin*		*Oleandomycin*		*Carbomycin*	
	6 hrs.	*24 hrs.*	*6 hrs.*	*24 hrs.*	*6 hrs.*	*24 hrs.*	*6 hrs.*	*24 hrs.*
Spleen	122	164	80	6	114	4	97	22
Kidney	107	108	5	<1	5	<1	7	<1
Lung	87	103	43	<1	42	<1	18	>1
Heart	56	46	2·5	2	22	3	6	<3
Liver	150	32	37	<1	170	<1	3	<1
Blood	11.2	3·9	16	5	8·6	1.8	16	7·2

Benazet and Dubost (1959). *Antibiot. Ann.* 1958-9, p. 211.

CARBOMYCIN

Carbomycin (Magnamycin) was discovered in the laboratories of Chas. Pfizer & Co. as a product of *Streptomyces halstedii* (Tanner *et al.*, 1952). Its anti-bacterial activity is inferior to that of erythromycin, and it is very poorly and ir-regularly absorbed from the alimentary tract. Finland *et al.* (1953) came to the conclusion that it ' cannot be recommended as a useful antibiotic in bacterial infections '.

CLINICAL APPLICATIONS

When erythromycin was introduced it was acclaimed as a new barrier to the onslaught of the staphylococci, some of which were already resistant to all its predecessors. Restrictions on its use were advised in order to preserve its value for this purpose as long as possible. Since that time our resources have multiplied remarkably and one of the newer agents will almost always be preferred for a resistant staphylococcal infection.

This still leaves a large field of usefulness in pneumococcal and streptococcal infections, for which erythromycin is at least a natural second choice in patients sensitive to penicillin. Figure 14 shows that erythromycin is the most active agent *in vitro* against *Str. pneumoniae.* There is ample evidence of its efficacy in the treatment of pneumococcal and streptococcal infection (Limson, 1961). For streptococcal infection Breese *et al.* (1966) found penicillin G, triacetyl oleandomycin and erythromycin estolate to be equally effective and Moffet *et al.* (1964)

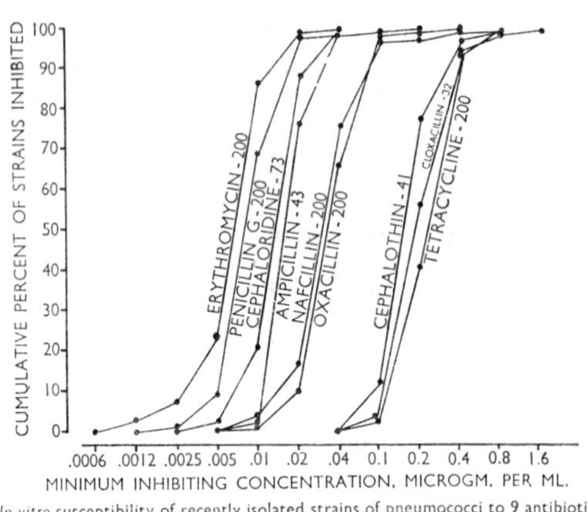

In vitro susceptibility of recently isolated strains of pneumococci to 9 antibiotics

FIG. 14

Redrawn from Kislak *et al.* (1965). *Amer. J. med. Sci.* 250, 261.

found that patients treated with erythromycin estolate were less liable to relapse than those treated with phenoxymethyl penicillin. Otitis media due to *Haemophilus influenzae* was found to respond satisfactorily to erythromycin estolate (Sell and Sanders, 1964). It should, therefore, be well suited to the treatment of mixed bronchial infections with *Str. pneumoniae* and *H. influenzae.* Erythromycin appears to be as effective as penicillin in the treatment of diphtheria and some authors regard it as the drug of choice in the treatment of carriers. The advisability of using it in severe infections depends in part on the ultimate view taken of the hepatic toxicity of erythromycin estolate since the absorption of other forms is sometimes inadequate. Some authors have found that despite the higher serum levels achieved by erythromycin estolate, the clinical response is no better than to the stearate or succinate (Billow *et al.,* 1964). If this is confirmed there will be no valid reason for using the potentially more toxic estolate. Since it appears to take 10 days or more to produce liver changes and these are reversible, our own feeling at present is that if erythromycin must be given by mouth for severe infection—and perfectly satisfactory parenteral preparations are available—the estolate should be used unless the patient is known to have been treated with it before. It should not be given for more than 10 days. Above all, those using the drug should be alert to the significance of any indication of hepatic derangement.

Erythromycin is certainly a useful antibiotic to have available when it seems desirable to ring the changes in dealing with endemic staphylococcal infection. There is much to be said for combining it with another antibiotic in order to discourage acquired bacterial resistance.

The merits of the other macrolides are more difficult to assess. Spiramycin, owing to its peculiar tissue distribution, is the most interesting although intrinsically the least active. It has been used in the treatment of ocular toxoplasmosis, but is inferior to pyrimethamine (Nolan and Rosen, 1968). Spiramycin inhibits the growth of some experimental tumours, but the claim that it might be useful in the treatment of skin cancer has not been substantiated (Klein *et al.*, 1965). Oleandomycin is intermediate in activity with no known special advantage, and in its best absorbed form is hepatotoxic. It is doubtful whether any of the remaining macrolides has any place in current therapeutics.

PHARMACEUTICAL PREPARATIONS AND DOSAGE

ERYTHROMYCIN (Erythrocin, *Abbott* (stearate); Ilotycin, *Lilly* (base). Numerous other proprietary names and preparations of various salts). Tablets 100 mg.; B.P., B.N.F.: (base) 250 mg.; B.P. (Stearate) equiv. 250 mg.; U.S.P. (base or various salts or esters): equiv. 100 and 200 mg. Mixture, B.N.F.. equiv. 80 mg. per 4 ml.; Oral suspension, U.S.P.: equiv. 200 mg. per 5 ml. Injection, U.S.P. (Gluceptate, lactobionate, ethylsuccinate, etc.) 250 mg.; 500 mg. and 1 g. Dose: 1-2 g. daily in divided doses.

ERYTHROMYCIN ESTOLATE (Propionyl erythromycin lauryl sulphate; Ilosone, *Lilly*).
Capsules: Equiv. 125 and 250 mg. erythromycin base; Suspension: equiv. 125 mg. erythromycin base per 5 ml. Dose: 1-2 g. daily in divided doses for not more than 10 days.

SPIRAMYCIN (Rovamycin, *May & Baker*).
Tablets and capsules of 250 mg., and syrup. Usual dose 0·5-1 g. 4 times daily.

OLEANDOMYCIN (Oleandomycin phosphate).
Capsules containing equivalent of 250 mg. of base: sterile powder for solution for intramuscular injection. Usual oral dose 250-500 mg. 4 times daily.

REFERENCES

BARBER, M., CSILLAG, A. & MEDWAY, A. J. (1958). *Brit. med. J.* **2**, 1377.
BARBER, M. & WATERWORTH, P. M. (1964). *Brit. med. J.* **2**, 603.
BILLOW, B. W., THOMPSON, E. A., STERN, A. & FLORIO, A. (1964). *Curr. ther. Res.* **6**, 381.
BREESE, B. B., DISNEY, F. A. & TAPLEY, W. B. (1966). *Amer. J. Dis. Child.* **111**, 128.
BROWN, A. R. (1963). *Brit. med. J.* **2**, 913.
CELMER, W. D. (1966). *Antimicrob. Agents Chemother.* 1965, p. 144.
CHABBERT, Y. (1956). *Ann. Inst. Pasteur* **90**, 787.
COOPER, R. G., RISCHBIETH, H. G. & VESEY, B. (1968). *Med. J. Aust.* **1**, 1131.
CUNDLIFFE, E. & McQUILLEN, K. (1967). *J. molec. Biol.* **30**, 137.
EIDUS, L., MANIAR, A. C. & FURESZ, J. (1962). *Chemotherapia, Basel* **4**, 398.
ENGLISH, A. R. & FINK, F. C. (1961). *Antibiot. Chemother.* **11**, 648.
ENGLISH, A. R., McBRIDE, T. J., VAN HALSEMA, G. & CARLOZZI, M. (1956). *Antibiot. Chemother.* **6**, 511.
FINLAND, M., PURCELL, E. M., WRIGHT, S. S. & LOVE, B. D. (1953). *New Engl. J. Med.* **249**, 310.
FURGIUELE, F. P. (1964). *Amer. J. Ophthal.* **58**, 443.
GARROD, L. P. (1957). *Brit. med. J.* **2**, 57.
GARROD, L. P. & WATERWORTH, P. M. (1962). *J. Clin. Path.* **15**, 328.
GILBERT, F. I. (1962). *J. Amer. med. Ass.* **182**, 1048.
GRIFFITH, R. S. (1959). *Antibiot. Ann.* 1958-9, p. 364.
GRÖNROOS, J. A., SAARIMAA, H. A. & KALLIOMÄKI, J. L. (1967). *Curr. therap. Res.* **9**, 589.
HAMMOND, J. B. & GRIFFITH, R. S. (1961). *Clin. Pharmacol. Therap.* **2**, 308.
HERRELL, W. E., BALOWS, A. & BECKER, J. (1960). *Antibiot. Med.* **7**, 637.
JONES, W. F. & FINLAND, M. (1957). *New Engl. J. Med.* **257**, 481.
KLEIN, E., STOLL, H. L., MILGROM, H., CASE, R. W., TRAENKLE, H. L., GRAHAM, S., LAOR, Y. & HELM, F. (1965). *J. invest. Derm.* **44**, 351.
KOHLSTAEDT, K. G. (1961). *J. Amer. med. Ass.* **178**, 89.
KUDER, H. V. (1960). *Clin. Pharmacol. Ther.* **1**, 604.
KUNIN, C. M. & FINLAND, M. (1959). *J. clin. Invest.* **38**, 1509.
LEE, C.-C., ANDERSON, R. C., HENDERSON, F. G., WORTH, H. M. & HARRIS, P. N. (1959). *Antibiot. Ann.* 1958-9, p. 354.
LIMSON, B. M. (1961). *Antibiot. Chemother.* **11**, 630.
LOPEZ-BELIO, M., TAKIMURA, Y., FORNATTO, E. J. & HOLINGER, P. H. (1957). *Antibiot. Ann.* 1956-7, p. 152.
MACFARLANE, J. A., MITCHELL, A. A. B., WALSH, J. M. & ROBERTSON, J. J. (1968). *Lancet* **1**, 1.
MAO, J. C-H. & PUTTERMAN, M. (1968). *J. Bact.* **95**, 1111.
MAO, J. C-H. & TARDREW, P. L. (1965). *Biochem. Pharmacol.* **14**, 1049.
MAO, J. C-H. & WIEGAND, R. G. (1968). *Biochem. Biophys. Acta* **157**, 404.
McKENZIE, I. & DOYLE, A. (1966). *Med. J. Aust.* **1**, 349.
MOFFET, H. L., CRAMBLETT, H. G., BLACK, J. P., SHULENBERGER, H., SMITH, A. & WILLIAMS, A. Y. (1964). *Antimicrob. Agents Chemother.*—1963, 759.
NOLAN, J. & ROSEN, E. S. (1968). *Brit. J. Ophthal.* **52**, 396.
PINNERT-SINDICO, S., NINET, L., PREUD'HOMME, J. & COSAR, C. (1955). *Antibiot. Ann.* 1954-5, p. 724.
POPPER, H., RUBIN, E., GARDIOL, D., SCHAFFNER, F. & PARONETTO, F. (1965). *Arch. intern. Med.* **115**, 128.
ROBINSON, M. M. (1961). *J. Amer. med. Ass.* **178**, 89.
SANDERS, E., FOSTER, M. T. & SCOTT, D. (1968). *New. Engl. J. Med.* **278**, 538.
SELL, S. H. W. & SANDERS, R. S. (1964). *Antimicrobial. Agents Chemother.*—1963, 756.
SUTHERLAND, R. (1962). *Brit. J. Pharmacol.* **19**, 99.
TANNER, F. W. JR., ENGLISH, A. R., LEES, T. M. & ROUTIEN, J. B. (1952). *Antibiot. Chemother.* **2**, 441.

TAUBENECK, U. (1962). *Nature (Lond.)* **196,** 195.
TICKTIN, H. E. & ROBINSON, M. M. (1963). *Ann. N.Y. Acad. Sci.* **104,** 1080.
VAS, M. R., BAIN, B. & LOWENSTEIN, L. (1964). *Nature (Lond.)* **204,** 1100.
VAZQUEZ, D. (1967). *Life Sci.* **6,** 845.
WATERWORTH, P. M. (1960). *Antibiot. and Chemother.* **10,** 101.
WATERWORTH, P. M. 1963). *Clin. Med., Winnetka.* **70,** 941.
WEAVER, J. R. & PATTEE, P. A. (1964). *J. Bact.* **88,** 574.

CHAPTER XI

PEPTIDES

THE peptide antibiotics form a large group of which very few have found any therapeutic application. They are composed of peptide-linked amino acids which commonly include both D- and L-forms and some unusual compounds. Perlman and Bodanszky (1966) list the amino acid composition of 18 families of antibiotic peptides and 37 others. Characteristic non-amino acid moieties, like the long chain fatty acids of the polymyxins (p. 188), also occur. Ring formation is common. The peptides bind to bacterial membranes and it is suggested that the cyclic molecules, or aggregates of them, may form false pores through which the flux of ions which accompanies their antibacterial effect occurs (Mueller and Rudin, 1967).

Antibiotic peptides are commonly produced in families of closely related compounds which sometimes differ only in one amino acid residue. The separation of these close relatives may be so difficult that there is doubt about the homogeneity of some of the compounds and hence doubt about the number of members of the family. There are also strong resemblances between some of the members of different families. This kind of inter-relationship is illustrated in Figure 15, which shows that the tyrocidines not only closely resemble one another but that half the tyrocidine molecule is made up of the amino acid sequence of gramicidin S.

The majority of the peptide antibiotics are more active against Gram-positive organisms, but the compounds which are of greatest therapeutic importance, the polymyxins, are more active against Gram-negative organisms. This has suggested that there is a connection between antibacterial range and the number of basic groups in the molecule (Table XXVII). Most peptide antibiotics are powerful bactericidal agents, but their clinical use is limited by their high toxicity, particularly to the kidneys.

It is of interest that almost all peptide antibiotics have been isolated from the genus *Bacillus,* and that no other type of antibiotic has emerged from this genus. Those that have found a place in clinical medicine are gramicidin, bacitracin, isolated in the United States in 1945, the polymyxins, discovered independently in Britain and America in 1947 and

TABLE XXVII

Antibiotic	Number of basic groups	Active against Gram-positive or Gram-negative organisms
Polymyxin	6	—
Colistin	5	—
Circulin	5	—
Gramicidin	2	+ and —
Bacitracin	2	+
Tyrocidine	1	+
Staphylomycin	0	+
Capreomycin	4	+ and — and *Myco. tuberculosis*

Herr, E. B. Jr., (1963). *Antimicrob. Agents Chemother.* 1962, p. 201.

capreomycin which is active against mycobacteria and has been found moderately effective in the treatment of human tuberculosis (Schwartz, 1967).

None of the antibiotic peptides isolated from other species of bacteria has found a place in clinical medicine.

GRAMICIDIN

This was the first in the field and came from the pioneer work of Dubos (1939) which preceded the extraction and purification of penicillin. It is produced by an aerobic sporing bacillus, *B brevis,* originally isolated from soil. Crude extracts of cultures of this bacillus yielded an alcohol-soluble bactericidal substance, tyrothricin, from which two antibiotics, gramicidin and tyrocidine, were separated (Dubos and Hotchkiss, 1941). There are at least four gramicidins in the substance isolated by Dubos (Ramachandran, 1963) and a further compound designated gramicidin S (Soviet), the structure of which is indicated in Figure 15, was obtained from a strain of *Bacillus brevis* by Gause and Brazhnikova (1944).

7

Anti-bacterial Activity

Gramicidin is active against most species of aerobic and anaerobic Gram-positive bacteria, including mycobacteria. Pneumococci and haemolytic streptococci are the most sensitive and aerobic sporing bacilli the least. Staphylococci also

Tyrocidine	R_1	R_2
A	L-Phe	D-Phe
B	L-Try	D-Phe
C	L-Try	D-Try

GRAMICIDIN S

$$\left[\begin{array}{l} \text{L-Val} - \text{L-Orn} - \text{L-Leu} - \text{D-Phe} - \text{L-Pro} \\ \text{L-Pro} - \text{D-Phe} - \text{L-Leu} - \text{L-Orn} - \text{L-Val} \end{array} \right]$$

TYROCIDINES

$$\left[\begin{array}{l} \text{L-Val} - \text{L-Orn} - \text{L-Leu} - \text{D-Phe} - \text{L-Pro} \\ \text{L-Tyr} - \text{L-Glu-NH}_2 - \text{L-Asp-NH}_2 - R_1 - R_2 \end{array} \right]$$

Fig. 15

Structure of gramicidin S and tyrocidines (Ruttenberg *et al.*, 1965).

tend to be relatively resistant: *Str. viridans* and *Str. faecalis* give intermediate results. With all species there is considerable strain variation. *N. gonorrhoeae* and *N. meningitidis* are sensitive to high concentrations. Gram-negative bacilli are completely insensitive probably due to the presence of surface phospholipids which inhibit the action of gramicidin.

Tyrothricin, which contains only 15 to 20 per cent gramicidin, is about as active against pneumococcal infection in mice as gramicidin itself, although the other component of tyrothricin, tyrocidine, is inactive *in vivo*. It has been suggested therefore, that there is a synergic action between tyrocidine and gramicidin, a situation reminiscent of the more recently discovered peptolides (p. 187).

Toxicity and Use

Gramicidin is highly toxic by intravenous injection and gives rise to extensive liver and kidney damage. It is also toxic to erythrocytes and inhibits growth in tissue cultures.

Therapeutically, gramicidin is of historical interest only. It should never be given systemically and has no special properties to justify its inclusion in mixtures for local application (p. 303).

BACITRACIN

Bacitracin was the outcome of a study of the bacterial flora of contaminated civilian wounds in the Presbyterian Hospital, Columbia University (Johnson, Anker and Meleney, 1945). It was observed that following direct plating of material from the injured tissue, bacteria sometimes appeared on blood agar plates that were not subsequently recovered from broth cultures made at the same time from the same material. This occurred most frequently when the broth cultures contained a large number of aerobic Gram-positive sporing bacilli. The cell-free filtrate of one such bacillus was found to have strong antibiotic activity. Further extraction and purification led to the isolation of a group of closely related polypeptide antibiotics, designated bacitracin A, B and C after Tracy, the patient from whom the bacillus was originally isolated.

Anti-bacterial Activity

Bacitracin is highly active against many species of Gram-positive bacteria and the pathogenic *Neisseriae*. Although strains of *Staph. aureus* are usually sensitive, they are rather less so than most other Gram-positive bacteria. Haemolytic streptococci of Lancefield's Group A are so much more sensitive than streptococci of other groups (Table XXVIII) that bacitracin sensitivity can be used as a screening test for the identification of Group A streptococci. Discs (containing 0·05 unit) suitable for this purpose are commercially available (Streamer *et al.*, 1962).

MODE OF ACTION. Bacitracin has been known for a long time to inhibit bacterial cell wall synthesis causing cell wall precursors to accumulate. It now appears that bacitracin interferes with the final dephosphorylation in cycling the phospholipid carrier which transfers mucopeptide to the growing cell-wall skeleton (Fig. 4, p. 57: Siewert and Strominger, 1967). As with other peptide antibiotics, bacitracin binds to the cell membrane increasing the efflux of ions. It thus differs from penicillin and cycloserine in affecting cell-wall synthesis at the level of the cell membrane and consequently, unlike those agents, is active against protoplasts.

TABLE XXVIII

Bacitracin	Streptococci, Lancefield Group:				
	A	B	C	G	Not A, C, G
Sensitive	2345	2	12	5	22
Resistant	22	5	279	40	505

Maxted, W. R. (1953). *J. clin. Path.* **6,** 224.

Toxicity

The bacitracins are not absorbed by the oral route. All are nephrotoxic when given parenterally, bacitracin C apparently being the most toxic and bacitracin B the least.

Patients treated with the antibiotic can develop proteinuria associated with acute depression of renal tubular function which persists for weeks.

Administration and Clinical Application

Being a bactericidal agent, bacitracin has occasionally been used in the treatment of difficult cases of endocarditis—usually in combination with other agents. With the steady accumulation of less toxic bactericidal antibiotics it now has little or no place in therapy and preparations for systemic use are no longer ordinarily available. It is still included in some preparations for local application (p. 303) and has been successfully used (in combination with kanamycin) for peritoneal irrigation in patients with gastrointestinal perforation (Noon *et al.*, 1967). Absorption may occur from such use or from local applications to ulcerated areas and resulting anaphylaxis has been described (Comaish and Cunliffe, 1967).

PEPTOLIDES

The antibiotics of this group also consist of cyclically linked amino acids (Schröder and Lübke, 1963). They are particularly active against streptococci and staphylococci. Amongst the better studied are ostreogrycin (Garrod and Waterworth, 1956), staphylomycin (Van Dijk *et al.*, 1957), streptogramin (Vazquez, 1962), mikamycin (Yamaguchi and Tanaka, 1964), and pristinamicin (Barber and Waterworth, 1964). They each consist of several components, pairs of which commonly act synergically. Some components of the differently named agents appear to be identical (Bodanszky and Ondetti, 1964).

Organisms trained to resistance by serial passage show cross-resistance with the macrolides which they resemble in being inhibitors of protein synthesis. The peptolides are, however, more actively bactericidal. Some have been used in the treatment of staphylococcal septicaemia with ' spectacular ' results. Despite this success and their high order of bactericidal activity *in vitro,* they have not been made commercially available in this country and there is no reason at present to believe that they are likely to supplant the better known anti-staphylococcal agents. On the other hand, pristinamycin (Pyostacine, *Rhone Poulenc*) is marketed in France and there is now an extensive literature, mainly French, on its clinical use. It has been employed almost exclusively in infections by staphylococci, most strains of which are inhibited by less than 1 μg./ml. Administration is oral, 2-3 g. being given daily in divided doses.

POLYMYXINS

The polymyxins are a group of basic polypeptide antibiotics derived from a spore-bearing soil bacillus and with a selective action against Gram-negative bacilli. They were first isolated in 1947 independently in one laboratory in Britain (Ainsworth, Brown and Brownlee, 1947) and two in the United States (Stansly, Shepherd and White, 1947; Benedict and Langlykke, 1947). The British investigators called the antibiotic ' aerosporin ' since they identified the bacillus as *B. aerosporus*. The American investigators identified the bacillus as *B. polymyxa* and called the antibiotic polymyxin. Comparative studies in the two laboratories proved the identity of the two bacilli and the name polymyxin was accepted (Symposium, 1949).

Chemical Properties

Five chemically distinct polymyxins have been identified and are designated A, B, C, D, and E. Their structures are given by Vogler and Studer (1966). Polymyxin A is the antibiotic originally named aerosporin and polymyxin D is the polymyxin isolated by Stansly, Shepherd and White in 1947. Some consist of more than one component. For example, polymyxin B is composed of polymyxins B1 and B2 which are separated with difficulty. Colistin, an antibiotic isolated by Koyama *et al.* (1950) in Japan has been shown to consist of two components, colistin A and B, identical with polymyxin E1 and E2 (Suzuki *et al.*, 1964). All five polymyxins are basic polypeptides and contain the fatty acid D-6-methyloctan-1-oic acid and the amino acids L-$\alpha\gamma$-diaminobutyric acid and L-threonine.

The structures of polymyxin B1, B2 and colistin A (polymyxin E1) are shown in Figure 16.

$$\text{L-DAB-NH}_2 - \text{R}_1 - \text{L-Leu} - \text{L-DAB-NH}_2$$
$$\text{L-DAB} - \text{L-Thr} - \text{L-DAB-NH}_2$$
$$\text{L-DAB-NH}_2 - \text{L-Thr} - \text{L-DAB-NH}_2 - \text{R}_2$$

	R_1	R_2
Polymixin B₁	D-Phe	6-methyl-octanoyl
Polymixin B₂	D-Phe	6-methyl-heptanoyl
Polymixin E₁ Colistin A	D-Leu	6-methyl-octanoyl

FIG. 16

Structure of polymyxins.

Leu=leucine; Thr=threonine; Phe=phenylalanine; DAB=di-amino-butyric acid.

Suzuki, T. *et al.* (1963). *J. Biochem.* (*Japan*) **54,** 173, 412, 555.
Suzuki, T. *et al.* (1964). *J. Biochem.* (*Japan*) **56,** 335.
Wilkinson, S. & Lowe, L. A. (1964). *Nature* (*Lond.*) **204,** 993.

The polymyxins commercially available are polymyxin B, under the name polymyxin, and polymyxin E, under the name colistin. Since pure preparations are not obtainable the activity and dosage of polymyxin is usually referred to in units. 1 mg. of pure polymyxin B base is equivalent to 10,000 units.

1 mg. of colistin base approximates to 30,000 units. Both preparations are supplied as the sulphate or the sulpho-methyl derivative (p. 193).

Anti-bacterial Activity

All the polymyxins have a similar anti-bacterial spectrum, although there are slight quantitative differences in their activity *in vitro*. Several investigators have shown that polymyxin and colistin have a very closely similar anti-bacterial activity (Fekety, Norman and Cluff, 1962; Eickhoff and Finland, 1965). Nearly all species of Gram-negative bacilli are highly sensitive to polymyxin and on a weight for weight basis

TABLE XXIX

Sensitivity of Bacteria to Polymyxins
M.I.C. μg. per ml.

	Colistin sulphate	Sulphomethyl-Colistin	Polymyxin B sulphate
Staph. aureus	(11) 75-300	(11) >100	(1·2) 50-200
Str. pyogenes	33	33	10->80
Str. faecalis	>100	>100	>100
Str. viridans	33->100	33->100	33->100
C. diphtheriae	—	—	10
Myco. tuberculosis	—	—	>80
N. meningitidis	4-33	>33	>100
H. influenzae	0·4-0·8	—	0·02
Br. abortus	>100	>100	>100
A. aerogenes	0·02-33 (>100)	0·4->100	0·02-11 (>100)
Kl. pneumoniae	0·01-1·2	0·01-3·7 (>100)	0·02-0·4
Esch. coli	0·01-25 (>100)	0·04->100	0·02-11 (>100)
Proteus spp.	>100	>100	>100
Ps. aeruginosa	0·14-10 (50)	1·2-33	0·02-3·7 (50)
Salmonella spp.	0·01-0·8 (4)	0·04-0·4 (4)	0·02-0·4 (1·2)
Shigella spp.	0·01-0·8 (3)	0·1-0·14 (16)	0·01-0·75

The minimum inhibitory concentrations reported for occasional exceptionally sensitive or resistant strains are shown in brackets.

Graber, C. O. *et al.* (1960). *Antibiot. Ann.* 1959-60, p. 77.
Ross, S. *et al.* (1960). *Ibid.*, p. 89.
Schwartz, B. S. *et al.* (1960). *Ibid.*, p. 41.
Wright, W. W. & Welch, H. (1960). *Ibid.*, p. 61.
Courtieu, A. L. *et al.* (1961). *Ann. Inst. Pasteur. Suppl.* **4**, 14.
Postic, B. & Finland, M. (1961). *Amer. J. med. Sci.* **242**, 551.
Fekety, F. R. *et al.* (1962). *Ann. intern. Med.* **57**, 214.
Taylor, G. & Allison, H. (1962). *Brit. med. J.* **2**, 161.

are usually more sensitive to polymyxin than to any other antibiotic. Notable exceptions are bacteria of the *Proteus* group, all of which are highly resistant. The pathogenic Gram-negative cocci, *N. gonorrhoeae* and *N. meningitidis,* and all species of Gram-positive bacteria and fungi are also resistant.

Fekety, Norman and Cluff (1962) compared the bacteristatic and bactericidal activity of polymyxin, colistin, streptomycin, kanamycin, chloramphenicol and tetracycline against 85 strains of *Esch. coli,* 70 of *Klebsiella,* 95 of *Ps. aeruginosa* and 22 of paracolon bacilli. They found that polymyxin and colistin were almost identical in activity and were as good as, or better than, any of the other antibiotics against 94 per cent of *Esch. coli,* 86 per cent of *Klebsiella,* 93 per cent of *Ps. aeruginosa* and 50 per cent of paracolon bacilli.

Polymyxin is also highly active against most strains of *Shigella* and *Salmonella* and *H. influenzae.* It is more active than any other antibiotic, including chloramphenicol, against most strains of *H. pertussis.* The sensitivity of common organisms is shown in Table XXIX. Classical *Vibrio cholerae* and the El Tor vibrio are sufficiently different in sensitivity to polymyxin for this to be used to distinguish them. As judged by disc or well methods, the classical vibrio is sensitive, while the El tor vibrio, apart from few exceptional strains, is resistant (Roy *et al.,* 1965). Because of its wide activity against Gram-negative organisms, polymyxin has been used in a number of selective media (see for example Davis and Davis, 1965).

INHIBITION BY SERUM. When mixed with large amounts of serum the polymyxins lose about 50 per cent of their activity *in vitro.*

Mode of Action

Cytological and other studies suggest that the disruptive effects of polymyxins on the bacterial cell are secondary to damage to the plasma membrane (Kaye and Chapman, 1963), the cyclic structure and size of the molecule being important in producing this effect (Sebek, 1967). Such damage might be expected to affect the permeability of the cell and there is considerable evidence that this occurs. Kawamata and Nakajima (1966) have shown that sub-inhibitory doses of colistin will make *Esch. coli* susceptible to erythromycin and penicillin presumably by facilitating their penetration into the cell. Other examples of synergic activity which have been put to therapeutic use are the combinations of polymyxin with sulphonamide and trimethoprim (p. 45).

ACQUIRED RESISTANCE. Bacteria do not readily develop resistance to polymyxin *in vitro*. Resistant strains of *Ps. aeruginosa* and other coliform bacilli have been obtained by passage *in vitro*, and with these strains there is complete cross-resistance between polymyxin and colistin (Hirsch *et al.*, 1960). Differences in resistance amongst related organisms, for example, *V. cholerae* and *V. el tor* (p. 190) evidently reside not in the cell-membranes, which are equally susceptible, but in penetrability to the drug of the cell-walls (Biswas and Mukergee, 1967).

Absorption, Distribution and Excretion

None of the polymyxins is absorbed from the alimentary tract and even after parenteral administration blood levels of active antibiotic are usually low (Table XXX), probably because, as mentioned above, polymyxin loses 50 per cent of its

TABLE XXX

Serum Levels of Various Polymyxin Derivatives in Man after a Dose (I.M.) Equivalent to 60 mg. Polymyxin B Sulphate

	Peak	
	Hr.	*μg. per ml.*
Polymyxin B Sulphate	1	1·46
Sulphomethyl polymyxin B		1·98
Sulphomethyl polymyxin E	2	1·58

From Barnett, Bushby and Wilkinson (1964).

activity in the presence of serum. Somewhat higher levels are obtained by repeated administration, but levels obtained in different individuals are very variable. The levels tend to be higher in children.

Although polymyxin is excreted mainly by the kidneys there is a considerable lag in urinary excretion. With a daily dose of 3 mg./kg. polymyxin B or E sulphate, only about 0·1 per cent of the dose is recovered in the first 12 hours, but concentrations varying from 40 to 400 μg./ml. can be found from 24 hours onwards.

Toxicity

All the polymyxins are nephrotoxic and cause damage to the epithelium lining the convoluted tubules, with resultant proteinuria. The polymyxins have achieved a reputation for renal toxicity in clinical practice, however, which is largely undeserved. There is no doubt that polymyxins A, C, and D are too nephrotoxic for use and that polymyxin B and E (colistin) can produce renal damage (Elwood *et al.*, 1966). Nevertheless, a number of investigators have shown that by proper control of dosage even patients with pre-existing renal failure can be safely treated. Tallgren *et al.* (1965) concluded that patients with different kidney diseases show different susceptibilities to the toxic effects of polymyxin. That the therapeutic efficiency of polymyxin in these circumstances can outweigh its nephrotoxicity is demonstrated by the improvement in renal function which occurs as infection is controlled (Atuk *et al.*, 1964).

Pain and tissue injury can occur at the site of injection and neurological symptoms such as paraesthesiae with typical numbness and tingling around the mouth, dizziness and weakness all occur but are usually mild.

Pharmacological Activities

In addition to their antibacterial activities the polymyxins have two pharmacological effects of some interest. They liberate histamine and 5HT (Levy, 1967) and they exert curariform effects on striped muscle and other effects on smooth muscle (Ramos *et al.*, 1963). The effect of polymyxin on human mast cells is shown by the altered pattern of excretion of mast cell products during treatment with polymyxin (Asboe-Hansen and Clausen, 1964).

Kubikowski and Szreniawski (1963) have reviewed the mechanisms of neuromuscular blockade by antibiotics. Several cases of apnoea have been reported following polymyxin therapy, some with other pareses. This effect has not been described in patients with normal renal function (Lindesmith *et al.*, 1968) and presumably results from the high plasma levels which may develop (100 μg./ml. in one patient). It is possible that the cationic polymyxins, which owe their antibacterial effect to interaction with the lipid-rich anionic bacterial cell membrane, exert a similar effect on the lipid-rich synaptic membranes so interfering with conduction (Naiman and Martin, 1967). Perkins (1964) has suggested that this effect should be particularly considered when polymyxin treatment is contemplated in patients with debilitating diseases, hypoxia or impaired renal function or already receiving muscular relaxants, corticosteroids or sedatives (p. 111).

SULPHOMETHYL POLYMYXINS

By treatment with formalin and sodium bisulphite, some or all of the 5 amino-groups of the polymyxins can be replaced by sulpho-methyl groups. Sulphomethyl derivatives of both polymyxin B and of colistin (polymyxin E) are commercially available. The substituted compounds differ considerably in their properties from the parent antibiotics. They are relatively painless on injection, less toxic, less active antibacterially (Table XXIX), and more rapidly excreted by the kidney.

There has been some argument about the basis of these differences. The situation is complicated by the fact that the derivatives consist of undefined mixtures of the mono-, di-, tri-, tetra- and penta-substituted compounds—all of which might theoretically have different properties—and by the fact that the more substituted compounds readily dissociate in solution. The experimental toxicity of the sulphomethyl-colistin commercially available in America (Coly Mycin) is so different from that available in this country (Colomycin) that the two compounds probably differ considerably in their degree of sulphomethylation.

Barnett, Bushby and Wilkinson (1964) showed that solutions of the compounds increase progressively in antibacterial activity on incubation until activity approaching that of the parent polymyxin is obtained. They argued from this and other evidence that the sulphomethyl derivatives are relatively non-toxic, inactive compounds which owe their effect to the liberation of the parent polymyxin. Beveridge and Martin (1967) confirmed that the sulphomethyl derivatives rapidly dissociate into more active compounds but found that the parent polymyxin was liberated only if the compounds were boiled. They conclude that the less substituted compounds must possess intrinsic antibacterial activity.

The liberation of more active compounds on incubation considerably complicates the determination of minimum inhibitory concentrations, since the results are compounded of the activities of substances liberated during incubation of the cultures. Similar problems occur in attempting to measure the level of the compounds in biological fluids by microbiological methods. The minimum inhibitory concentrations for common organisms of polymyxin B sulphate, colistin sulphate and sulphomethyl colistin are shown in Table XXIX. In a direct comparison of the antibacterial activity of colistin and polymyxin sulphates with their sulphomethyl derivatives, Eickhoff and Finland (1965) found the sulphates to be about eight times more active. The results obtained by various authors for the serum concentrations of sulphomethyl colistin are shown in Table XXX and Table XXXI.

In the mouse, the compounds differ considerably in their toxicity but the more toxic the compound, the more effective it is therapeutically. Nord and Hoeprich (1964) showed that polymyxin B was more toxic to white mice than colistin; that the sulphomethyl derivatives were considerably less toxic, and that the activity of the compounds against *Ps. aeruginosa* was in the same order as their toxicity. For a given antibacterial effect, an equally toxic dose of each of the compounds would have to be given. O'Grady and Pennington (1967) showed that the same was true of the sulphomethyl derivatives in the treatment of an experimental pseudomonas infection in the mouse. The LD_{50} for sulphomethyl colistin was almost three times that for sulphomethyl polymyxin B, but almost three times the dose of sulphomethyl colistin had to be given to achieve the same therapeutic result.

In the dog, Vinnicombe and Stamey (1969) found a larger differential in the toxicity of the compounds as measured by depression of renal function. An intravenous dose of 5 mg./kg.

polymyxin B sulphate, which produced average serum and urine levels of 30 and 60 μg./ml. depressed the G.F.R. and renal plasma flow by about 60 per cent. The same dose of

TABLE XXXI

Serum Levels of Sulpho-methyl Colistin in Man.

Dose i/m	Patients	Peak		Half life hrs.
		Hr.	µg. per ml.	
2 mg./kg.		2-3	6-15	6-12
4 mg./kg.	Adult	3-5	17-25	6-10
5 mg./kg.		4	25	5
2·5 mg./kg.	Children	1	5	2-3

Forni, P. V. & Guidetti, E. (1956). *Minerva Med.* **2**, *Suppl.* **77**, 823.
Ross, S. *et al.* (1960). *Antibiot. Ann.* 1959-60, p. 89.
Wright, W. W. & Welch, H. (1960). *Antibiot. Ann.* 1959-60, p. 61.
Colley, E. W. & Frankel, H. L. (1963). *Brit. med. J.* **2**, 790.

sulphomethyl polymyxin B produced average serum and urine levels of 14·5 and 165 μg./ml. and depressed renal function by 20-25 per cent. In contrast, 40 mg./kg. of sulphomethyl colistin, which produced much higher serum and urine levels of 57 and 1,020 μg./ml., had no depressant effect on renal function. When sulphomethyl polymyxin B was given in a dose (25 mg./kg.) which produced about the same urine levels (999 μg./ml.) but higher serum levels (143 μg./ml.), both the G.F.R. and renal plasma flow were reduced by more than 80 per cent.

In both the mouse and the dog, therefore, the toxicity of the compounds increases in the order: sulphomethyl colistin, sulphomethyl polymyxin B, polymyxin B sulphate. The antibacterial activity of the compounds *in vivo* has not been compared in the dog and it is not known, therefore, whether their therapeutic activity parallels their toxicity as it does in the mouse. If the dog is a better guide than the mouse to renal toxicity in man, then sulphomethyl colistin appears on this evidence to be much the safest compound.

Because the derivatives are more rapidly excreted by the kidneys, their half-life is shorter than that of the parent compounds. Serum levels are not augmented by probenecid and extra-renal mechanisms probably take part in excretion (Baines and Rifkind, 1964). There is disagreement about the effect of peritoneal dialysis on the plasma half-life, but it is in any case not great. Described differences in the effect of haemodialysis may well depend on the membrane used. Curtis and Eastwood (1968) who review the findings of various workers suggest a dose of 2-3 mg./kg. every three days for patients in severe renal failure. There does not seem to be excessive retention of sulphomethyl colistin in the new-born (Lawson and Hewstone, 1964).

Following a dose of 150 mg. sulphomethyl colistin intravenously, none could be detected in the amniotic fluid three hours later. Very low plasma levels (about 0·45 μg./ml.) were found in both mothers and infants born 6-20 hours later. A dose of 30-40 mg. injected into the amniotic fluid of patients not in labour was still present 18 hours later (MacAuley and Charles, 1967).

Relative painlessness on intramuscular injection and low toxicity have caused sulphomethyl polymyxins to be generally used in recent years where systemic polymyxin therapy is indicated. Barnett, Bushby and Wilkinson (1964) have questioned the rationale of this on the ground that if the toxicity and antibacterial activity of the derivatives are due to the liberation of free polymyxin, therapy could be more accurately controlled by giving polymyxin sulphate intravenously. In addition, as the sulphomethyl derivatives are more rapidly excreted, tissue levels are likely to be lower than with polymyxin sulphate. As long as there is argument about the mode of action and pharmacology of these compounds, many will still no doubt prefer to give the sulphomethyl derivatives by the more convenient intramuscular route. For oral and local application, the more active polymyxin sulphate should be used.

CLINICAL APPLICATION

Before the advent of gentamicin (p. 126) and carbenicillin (p. 84), polymyxin B or E was unchallenged as the drug of choice for the treatment of infections due to *Ps. aeruginosa* and also in infections with some other coliform bacilli, but the poor blood levels obtainable with polymyxin must be taken into consideration.

URINARY INFECTION. Success has been claimed particularly in the treatment of pseudomonas urinary infection (Rodger *et al.*, 1965; Brumfitt *et al.*, 1966). There has naturally been concern about treating urinary tract infection with potentially nephrotoxic agents, especially in patients with already impaired renal function. By controlling the dosage in relation to the plasma creatinine, infection can be safely controlled in anuric or grossly oliguric patients, with resulting improvement of renal function (Atuk *et al.*, 1964).

SUPERFICIAL WOUNDS AND BURNS. A cream containing 1 mg. per g. polymyxin has had considerable success in preventing burns becoming colonized by *Ps. aeruginosa* and in some cases the cream exerts curative effect on burns already infected with this organism. Elimination of pseudomonas from infected burns has also followed the intramuscular use of sulphomethyl colistin (Jones *et al.*, 1966).

Since the development of resistance to polymyxin is not a problem, and the antibiotic does not appear to damage healing wounds, it can be used as a spray, powder or cream, for the treatment of any superficial infection with *Ps. aeruginosa* such as superficial wounds, ulcers or otitis externa.

MENINGITIS. Polymyxins have been successfully used in the treatment of meningitis due to *H. influenzae* and *Ps. aeruginosa*. Polymyxins do not ordinarily reach the C.S.F. so that it is necessary to give the drug intrathecally and in some cases the injections have been followed by an increase in cells in the fluid (after it had become sterile) with signs of meningeal irritation, and a cauda equina lesion after intrathecal treatment with polymyxin has been recorded.

CHEST INFECTION. Some success has been claimed in the treatment of pulmonary infections with sulphomethyl polymyxins but the results are frequently unimpressive. We have been more successful in eradicating pseudomonas from the bronchi with inhalation therapy (it is essential to use a nebuliser which generates an aerosol of particles small enough to penetrate the bronchi) but Pines *et al.* (1970) found such therapy useless.

GASTRO-INTESTINAL INFECTIONS. Since polymyxin is not absorbed from the intestinal tract it can be administered orally without fear of toxic symptoms. Some success has been claimed in the treatment of dysentery due to *Shigella flexneri* and *sonnei* (Swift, 1963) and in enterocolitis due to enteropathic escherichia (Diamond, 1962). Polymyxin is of doubtful value in the treatment of salmonella infections. Gotoff *et al* (1965) found very wide differences in the concentrations of polymyxin in the faeces of their patients. Only in those with the highest concentrations (1-2 mg. polymyxin per g. faeces) were salmonella eradicated for the whole period of follow up.

Polymyxin in combination with a drug which will attack the Gram-positive intestinal flora, *e.g.* bacitracin, has been investigated for suppression of the gut flora prior to surgical procedures (Shidlovsky *et al.*, 1960).

GENERALISED INFECTION. By the time *Ps. aeruginosa* can be isolated from the blood-stream, infection is usually overwhelming and death occurs rapidly. In addition, such infections occur terminally in patients with severe underlying diseases or in those treated with immuno-suppressive agents. Post-mortem studies show extensive invasion of the small arteries and veins of many organs, particularly the lungs, with enormous numbers of bacilli. As might be expected, treatment of such cases is often of no avail. Fekety *et al.* (1962), Murdoch (1964) and Jones *et al.* (1966) were successful in treating some of their cases of pseudomonas septicaemia with sulphomethyl polymyxins and Holloway and Scott (1963) successfully treated septicaemia due to bacteroides and coliform bacilli.

Polymyxin treatment may also be life-saving in Gram-negative septicaemia complicating urological procedures (Hewitt *et al.*, 1965).

PHARMACEUTICAL PREPARATIONS AND DOSAGE

COLISTIN SULPHATE (Polymyxin E Sulphate; Colomycin,* *Pharmax*; Coly-Mycin, *U.S.A.*)
   UNIT=0·00005128 mg. British Standard (1965)=19,500 units per mg.
Tablets: 250,000 units; B.P. 1·5 mega units; Syrup: 250,000 units per 5 ml.
Dose: oral: 9-18 mega units, daily in divided doses.

COLISTIN SULPHOMETHATE SODIUM (Sodium colistimethate, U.S.P., Colo-mycin* Injection, *Pharmax*, Colo-Myçin Injectable, *U.S.A.*)
   UNIT=0·00008 mg. British Standard (1965)=12,500 units per mg. Injection 0·5 and 1·0 mega units; U.S.P. equiv. 30 and 50 mg. colistin. Dose: i/m, i/v infusion: 3-9 mega units; Intra-thecal: 500-1,000 units per kg. per day in single dose.

POLYMYXIN B SULPHATE (Aerosporin *Burroughs Wellcome*) (Polymyxin M Sulphate, *U.S.S.R.* is similar)
   UNIT=0·000127 mg. International Standard=7,874 units per mg. Tablets, U.S.N.F.: 250,000 and 500,000 units. Dose: 1-2 mega units per day. Injection, B.P.C., B.N.F.: 500,000 units. Dose: i/m: 500,000 units, 8 hourly.

SULPHOMYXIN SODIUM (Polymyxin B sodium methane sulphonate; Thiosporin, *Burroughs Wellcome*)
   Injection: equiv. 500,000 units polymyxin B sulphate. Dose: i/m: up to 500,000 units, 6 hourly.

* NOT Colimycin, *U.S.S.R.*—an aminoglycoside.

REFERENCES

AINSWORTH, G. C., BROWN, A. M. & BROWNLEE, G. (1947). *Nature (Lond.)*
   160, 263.
ASBOE-HANSEN, G. & CLAUSEN, J. (1964). *Amer. J. med.* **36**, 144.
ATUK, N. O., MOSCA, A. & KUNIN, C. (1964). *Ann. intern. med.* **60**, 28.
BAINES, R. D. & RIFKIND, D. (1964). *J. Amer. med. Ass.* **190**, 278.
BARBER, M. & WATERWORTH, P. M. (1964). *Brit. med. J.* **2**, 603.
BARNETT, M., BUSHBY, S. R. M. & WILKINSON, S. (1964). *Brit. J. Pharmacol.*
   23, 552.
BENEDICT, R. G. & LANGLYKKE, A. F. (1947). *J. Bact.* **54**, 24.
BEVERIDGE, E. G. & MARTIN, A. J. (1967). *Brit. J. Pharmacol. Chemother.*
   29, 125.
BISWAS, K. & MUKERJEE, S. (1967). *Proc. Soc. exp. Biol. N.Y.* **126**, 103.
BODANSZKY, M. & ONDETTI, M. A. (1964). *Antimicrob. Agents Chemother.*
   1963, 360.
BRUMFITT, W., BLACK, M. & WILLIAMS, J. D. (1966). *Brit. J. Urol.* **38**, 495.
COMAISH, J. S. & CUNLIFFE, W. J. (1967). *Brit. J. clin. Pract.* **21**, 97.
CURTIS, J. R. & EASTWOOD, J. B. (1968). *Brit. med. J.* **1**, 484.
DAVIS, N. A. & DAVIS, G. H. G. (1965). *J. Path. Bact.* **89**, 380.
DIAMOND, E. F. (1962). *Arch. Pediat.* **79**, 170.
DUBOS, R. J. (1939). *J. exp. Med.* **70**, 1.
DUBOS, R. J. & HOTCHKISS, R. D. (1941). *J. exp. Med.* **73**, 629.
EICKHOFF, T. C. & FINLAND, M. (1965). *Amer. J. med. Sci.* **249**, 172.
ELWOOD, C. M., LUCAS, G. D. & MUEHRCKE, R. C. (1966). *Arch. intern.
   Med.* **118**, 326.
FEKETY, F. R. JR., NORMAN, P. S. & CLUFF, L. E. (1962). *Ann. intern. Med.*
   57, 214.
GARROD, L. P. & WATERWORTH, P. M. (1956). *Brit. med. J.* **2**, 61.
GAUSE, G. F. & BRAZHNIKOVA, M. G. (1944). *Nature (Lond.)* **154**, 703.
GOTOFF, S. P., LEPPER, M. H. & FIEDLER, M. A. (1965). *Amer. J. med. Sci.*
   249, 399.

HEWITT, C. B., OVERHOLT, E. L., FINDER, R. J. & PATTON, J. F. (1965). *J. Urol. (Baltimore)* **93**, 299.

HIRSCH, H. A., MCCARTHY, C. G. & FINLAND, M. (1960). *Proc. Soc. exp. Biol. (N.Y.)* **103**, 338.

HOLLOWAY, W. J. & SCOTT, E. G. (1963). *J. Urol. (Baltimore)* **89**, 264.

JOHNSON, B. A., ANKER, H. & MELENEY, F. L. (1945). *Science* **102**, 376.

JONES, R. J., JACKSON, D. M. & LOWBURY, E. J. L. (1966). *Brit. J. plast. Surg.* **19**, 43.

KAWAMATA, J. & NAKAJIMA, K. (1966). *Antimicrob. Agents Chemother.* 1965, p. 403.

KAYE, J. J. & CHAPMAN, G. B. (1963). *J. Bact.* **86**, 536.

KOYAMA, Y., KUROSASA, A., TSUCHIYA, A. & TAKAKUTA, K. (1950). *J. Antibiot. (Tokyo)* **3**, 457.

KUBIKOWSKI, P. & SZRENIAWSKI, Z. (1963). *Arch. int. Pharmacodyn.* **146**, 549.

LAWSON, J. S. & HEWSTONE, A. S. (1964). *Med. J. Aust.* **1**, 917.

LEVY, L. (1967). *Arch. int. Pharmacodyn.* **165**, 92.

LINDESMITH, L. A., BAINES, R. D., BIGELOW, D. B. & PETTY, T. L. (1968). *Ann. intern. Med.* **68**, 318.

MACAULAY, M. A. & CHARLES, D. (1967). *Clin. Pharmacol. Ther.* **8**, 578.

MACKAY, D. N. & KAYE, D. (1964). *New Engl. J. Med.* **270**, 394.

MUELLER, P. & RUDIN, D. O. (1967). *Biochem. Biophys. Res. Commun.* **26**, 398

MURDOCH, J. McC. (1964). *Proceedings of the 3rd International Congress of Chemotherapy*, Stuttgart, p. 319.

NAIMAN, J. G. & MARTIN, J. D. Jr. (1967). *J. surg. Res.* **7**, 199.

NOON, G. P., BEALL, A. C. Jr., JORDAN, G. L., RIGGS, S. & DE BAKEY, M. E. (1967). *Surgery* **62**, 73.

NORD, N. M. & HOEPRICH, P. D. (1964). *New Engl. J. Med.* **270**, 1030.

O'GRADY, F. & PENNINGTON, J. H. (1967). *Postgrad. med. J. Suppl. (March)* **43**, 72.

PERKINS, R. L. (1964). *J. Amer. med. Ass.* **190**, 421.

PERLMAN, D. & BODANSZKY, M. (1966). *Antimicrob. Agents Chemother.* 1965, p. 122.

PINES, A., RAAFAT, H., SIDDIQUI, G. M. & GREENFIELD, J. S. B. (1970). *Brit. med. J.* **1**, 663.

RAMACHANDRAN, L. K. (1963). *Biochemistry* **2**, 1138.

RAMOS, L., RAMOS, A. O., OEHLING, R. & CORBETT. C. F. (1963). *Chemotherapia* **7**, 85.

RODGER, K. C., NIXON, M. & TONNING, H. O. (1965). *Canad. med. Ass. J.* **93**, 143.

ROY, C., MRIDHA, K. & MUKERJEE, S. (1965). *Proc. Soc. exp. Biol. N.Y.* **119**, 893.

RUTTENBERG, M. A., KING, T. P. & CRAIG, L. C. (1965). *Biochemistry* **4**, 11.

SCHRÖDER, VON E. & LÜBKE, K. (1963). *Experientia* **19**, 57.

SCHWARTZ, W. S. (1967). *Amer. Rev. resp. Dis.* **94**, 858.

SEBEK, O. K. (1967). In *Antibiotics I: Mechanisms of Action.* p. 142. Ed. Gottlieb, D. and Shaw, P. D. New York.

SHIDLOVSKY, B. A., FETZER, V. & PRIGOT, A. (1960). *Antibiot. Chemother.* **10**, 640.

SIEWERT, G. & STROMINGER, J. L. (1967). *Proc. Nat. Acad. Sci. (Wash.)* **57**, 767.

SLADE, N. & LINTON, K. B. (1965). *Brit. J. Urol.* **37**, 73.

STANSLY, P. G., SHEPHERD, R. G. & WHITE, H. J. (1947). *Bull. Johns Hopk. Hosp.* **81**, 43.

STREAMER, C. W. and numerous others (1962). *Amer. J. Dis. Child.* **104**, 157.

SUZUKI, T., HAYASHI, K., FUJKAWA, K. & TSUKAMOTO, K. (1964). *J. Biochem* **56**, 335.

SWIFT, P. N. (1963). *Clin. Med.* **70**, 76.

SWIFT, P. N. & BUSHBY, S. R. M. (1951). *Lancet* **2**, 183.

SYMPOSIUM (1949). *Ann. N.Y. Acad. Sci.* **51,** 875, 879, 891, 897, 909, 952.
TALLGREN, L. G., LIEWENDAHL, K. & KUHLBÄCK, B. (1965). *Acta med. scand.* **177,** 717.
VAN DIJK, P., VANDERHAEGHE, H. & DE SOMER, P. (1957). *Antibiot. Chemother.* **7,** 625.
VAZQUEZ, D. (1962). *Biochim. Biophys. Acta* **61,** 849.
VINNICOMBE, J. & STAMEY, T. A. (1969). *Invest. Urol.* **6,** 505.
VOGLER, K. & STUDER, R. O. (1966). *Experientia* **22,** 345.
WOLF-JURGENSEN, P. & ZACHARIAE, H. (1965). *Acta derm-venereol.* (*Stockh.*) **45,** 207.
YAMAGUCHI, H. & TANAKA, N. (1964). *Nature* (*Lond.*) **201,** 499.

CHAPTER XII

VARIOUS ANTI-BACTERIAL ANTIBIOTICS

HERE follow accounts of antibiotics not classifiable among the main groups described in other chapters. Those of some of the less important are necessarily brief, but some mention of them may be more helpful than none at all. Only those are included which have been used in human therapeutics (bacteriocines being an exception); we do not, for example, include tylosin, a macrolide, or nisin, a peptide, for which the only uses have been non-medical. Other exceptions are antibiotics used exclusively in tuberculosis, which are referred to in Chapter XXV.

ACTINOSPECTACIN

Actinospectacin, a product of *Streptomyces spectabilis,* was originally described by Mason and his colleagues (1961). It shows a moderate degree of *in vitro* activity (M.I.C. for most sensitive species of the order of 5-10 μg. per ml.) against a wide range of bacteria, both Gram-positive and Gram-negative (Lewis and Clapp, 1961). Staphylococci can become resistant to it fairly rapidly, but this capacity is not shared by other organisms. Administered by injection, it is more effective against various infections in mice than its *in vitro* activity would suggest. There are several reports on its clinical use, not only in urinary tract infections (Lindemeyer *et al.,* 1962), but in other infections including septicaemia and pneumonia (Romansky *et al.,* 1962). The conclusion appears to have been reached that although effective, it is no more so than other antibiotics, and its clinical use, except for gonorrhoea (p. 427) has been abandoned. Under the name spectinomycin it is now being used for growth promotion and the treatment of certain infections in farm stock.

REFERENCES

LEWIS, C. & CLAPP, H. W. (1961). *Antibiot. Chemother.* **11,** 127.
LINDEMEYER, R. I., TURCK, M. & PETERSDORF, R. G. (1962). *Amer. J. med. Sci.* **244,** 478.

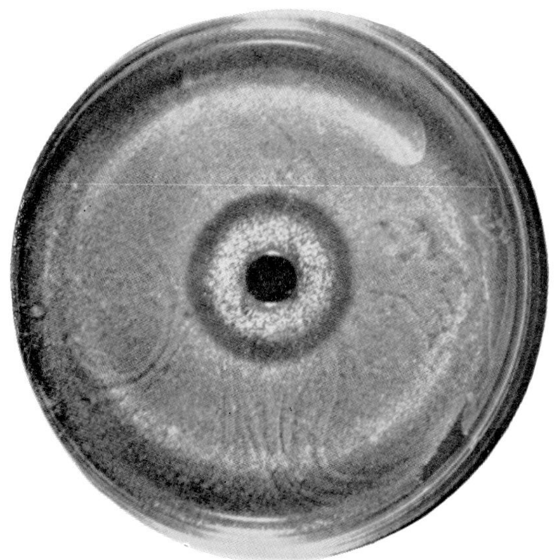

FIG. 17A

A. Appearance of culture made from a suspension of staphylococci (mixed colonies from a primary culture), the central cup containing streptomycin solution. It consists, in fact, of two strains of *Staph. aureus,* one being resistant to streptomycin but sensitive to a staphylococcine formed by the other which is sensitive to streptomycin.

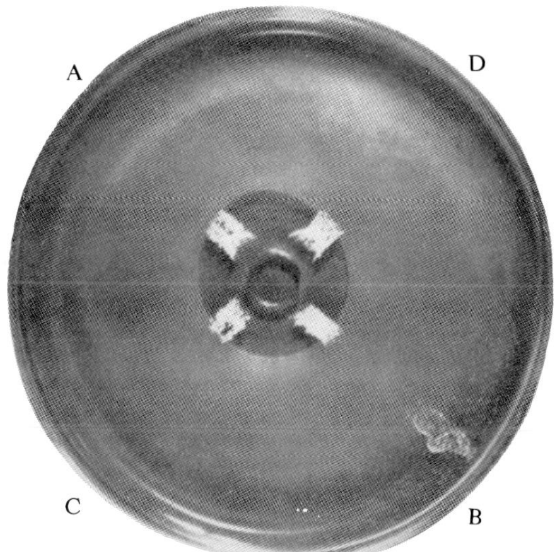

FIG. 17B

B is the proof of this. A pour plate was made of the sensitive strain, and a thin layer of uninoculated medium was poured over it. The cup contains streptomycin. A suspension of the streptomycin-resistant staphylococcus was streaked from A to B before incubation, and from C to D after incubation for $1\frac{1}{2}$ hours. The growth of this organism is inhibited except over the zone where that of the sensitive (staphylococcine-forming) staphylococcus is itself inhibited.

facing p. 202

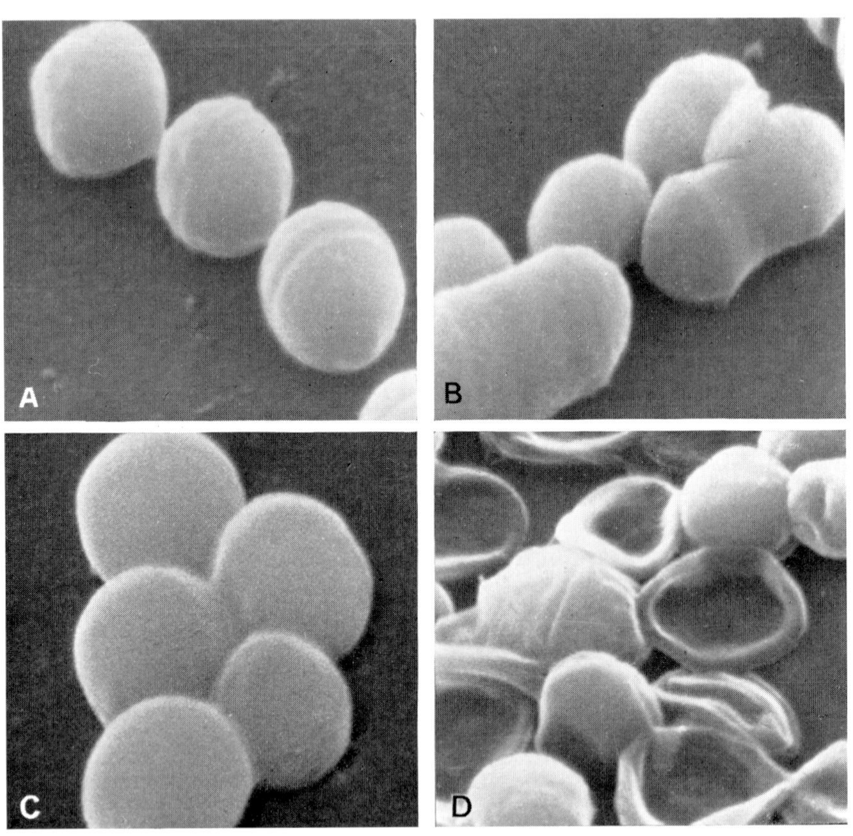

FIG. 18

Streptococcus pyogenes (A) before (B) after 90 min. exposure to 100 µg. ampicillin per ml.

Staphylococcus aureus (C) before (D) after 2½ hr. exposure to 3 µg. fucidin per ml.

(Stereoscan electron micrographs × 30,000 by David Greenwood.)

MASON, D. J., DIETZ, A. & SMITH, R. M. (1961). *Antibiot. Chemother.* **11,** 118.
ROMANSKY, M. J., WALTERS, E. W., JOHNSON, A. C. & PECK, F. A. (1962). *Antimicrob. Agents Chemother.* 1961, p. 524.

BACTERIOCINES

These interesting substances differ from antibiotics, and offer no known therapeutic possibilities, but some mention of them, however brief, seems called for.

Bacteriocines are substances formed by bacteria which inhibit the growth of other strains of the same or related species, an effect best demonstrated by cross-streaking on plates. A variable proportion of strains of a given species may be found to form such a substance: others form none. The bacteriocines formed by different strains are not identical: another strain may be inhibited by some and not by others. The best known and most extensively studied are the colicines, formed by *Esch. coli*, the existence of which was first detected by Gratia in 1925. Staphylococcines were described by Fredericq in 1946. Since then they have been observed in other enterobacteria, including *Salmonella* spp. (Agarwal, 1964; Hamon and Peron, 1966), enterococci (Brock *et al.*, 1963) group A streptococci, in which Kuttner (1966) found the property to be constant in strains of types 12, 4 and 49 derived from cases of nephritis, and a variety of other bacteria, including *Cl. welchii* and *Listeria monocytogenes.*

These substances are of practical interest in two directions. Their multiplicity within a species and different patterns of susceptibility to them afford an opportunity of identifying individual types among strains of the organism: examples are the colicine typing of *Sh. sonnei* and the pyocine typing of *Ps. aeruginosa.* Secondly, they may give rise to very puzzling appearances in diagnostic cultures, as when two staphylococci, one forming a staphylococcine to which the other is susceptible, are present together: the combined effect of the staphylococcine and of the antibiotic in a disc may be to produce a double zone of inhibition (Waterworth, 1956; see Fig. 17).

What part bacteriocines play in nature is almost unknown. Such evidence as there is of their activity within the body concerns only colicines. By repeated cultures of the faeces of five individuals during six months Branche *et al.* (1963) found that strains of *Esch. coli* forming colicines tended to persist, whereas non-colicine forming strains were frequently replaced by others. Friedman and Halbert (1960) showed that the growth of *Sh. flexneri* in the mouse peritoneum was antagonized by the addition of a colicine-producing *Esch. coli* to the inoculum. Braude and Siemienski (1965) injected colicine subcutaneously in mice and found their serum strongly bactericidal: these authors go so far as to suggest that colicines absorbed from the bowel or even the infected urinary tract may ' contribute to the heat-resistant bactericidal property of normal blood '.

REFERENCES

AGARWAL, S. C. (1964). *Bull. Wld Hlth Org.* **30,** 444.
BRANCHE, W. C. JR., YOUNG, V. M., ROBINET, H. G. & MASSEY, E. D. (1963). *Proc. Soc. exp. Biol. N.Y.* **114,** 198.
BRAUDE, A. I. & SIEMIENSKI, J. S. (1965). *J. clin. Invest.* **44,** 849.
BROCK, T. D., PEACHER, B. & PIERSON, D. (1963). *J. Bact.* **86,** 702.
FRIEDMAN, D. R. & HALBERT, S. P. (1960). *J. Immunol.* **84,** 11.
HAMON, Y. & PERON, Y. (1966). *Ann. Inst. Pasteur* **110,** 389.
KUTTNER, A. G. (1966). *J. exp. Med.* **124,** 279.
WATERWORTH, P. M. (1956). *J. med. Lab. Technol.* **13,** 385.

CYCLOSERINE

Cycloserine is a product of *Streptomyces orchidaceus* and other organisms, and has also been synthesized. Chemically it is D-4-amino-3-isoxazolidone, with a molecular weight of only 102, and thus perhaps the simplest known substance possessing antibiotic activity. A fairly wide range of bacteria, both Gram-negative and Gram-positive, including *Myco. tuberculosis,* are sensitive to it. Early studies of *in vitro* activity, such as those of Welch, Putnam and Randall (1955) produced discouraging results, but these were carried out before it was recognized that the action of cycloserine is specifically antagonized by D-alanine, a fact which provides the clue to its mode of action. Determinations in a medium free from this amino acid produce more realistic results. A majority of strains of *Esch. coli* were inhibited and some were killed, in such a medium by 25·5 μg. per ml. (Hoeprich, 1964): this paper contains similar observations on a variety of other bacteria.

MODE OF ACTION. At an early stage of cell wall synthesis L-alanine is converted to D-alanine, and two D-alanine molecules are linked together (Fig. 4, p. 57). Both these sequential processes are inhibited by cycloserine which is a structural analogue of D-alanine and competitively inhibits the two enzymes concerned (Strominger, 1962). There is a clear similarity between certain faces of the cycloserine and D-alanine molecules (Richmond, 1966). Cycloserine also inhibits a number of amino acid transaminases and as a result inhibits protein synthesis. It appears at present, however, that it is the interference with cell wall rather than with protein synthesis which is the major effect of cycloserine.

Cycloserine is well absorbed after oral administration, attaining high and well sustained concentrations in the blood and being excreted unchanged in the urine (Anderson *et al.*, 1956). Its principal use is as a second-line drug for the treatment of tuberculosis, but it requires mention here because it also has advocates as a remedy for urinary tract infection including Hoeprich (1963) in the United States and Murdoch and his colleagues (Syme *et al.*, 1961; Gray *et al.*, 1967) in this country. *Esch. coli* infections are the most susceptible, *Proteus* less so and some others not at all. The dose commonly given is 250 mg. three times a day: Hoeprich advises up to 15-20 mg. per kg. daily in patients under 45, but at ages greater than this or if renal function is impaired it must be reduced. All authors advise blood assays to ensure that the concentration attained shall not exceed 20-25 μg. per ml. Of the two British papers cited, the first reports the results of 14-day courses for the treatment of existing infections, and the second those of long-term treatment with 250 mg. every other day for the prevention of recurrences, in which considerable success is claimed.

Cycloserine passes all toxicity tests in animals, and produces none of the side effects associated with other antibiotics in man, but a drawback to treatment with full doses is the possibility of effects on the central nervous system, ranging from headache and drowsiness to convulsions. The risk of these can be reduced by careful regulation of dosage, and no permanent damage appears to be caused.

CYCLOSERINE ('Seromycin' *Lilly*; 'Oxamycin' *Merck*).
  Capsules or Tablets of 250 mg. For dosage see text.

REFERENCES

ANDERSON, R. C., WORTH, H. M., WELLES, J. S., HARRIS, P. N. & CHEN, K. K. (1956). *Antibiot. Chemother.* **6**, 360.

Gray, J. A., Geddes, A. M., Wallace, E. T. & Murdoch, J. McC. (1967). *Symposium on Pyelonephritis, Edinburgh,* 1966, p. 33. Edinburgh, E. & S. Livingstone.
Hoeprich, P. D. (1963). *Arch. intern. Med.* **112,** 405.
Hoeprich, P. D. (1964). *Amer. J. clin. Path.* **41,** 140.
Richmond, M. H. (1966). *Symp. Soc. gen. Microbiol.* **16,** 301.
Strominger, J. L. (1962). *Fed. Proc.* **21,** 134.
Syme, J., Sleigh, J. D., Richardson, J. E. & Murdoch, J. McC. (1961). *Brit. J. Urol.* **33,** 261.
Welch, H., Putnam, L. E. & Randall, W. A. (1955). *Antibiot. Med.* **1,** 72.

FUSIDIC ACID

Chemistry. Several antibiotics from different sources have proved, rather surprisingly, to possess the basic cyclopentenophenanthrene structure of steroids. Three have received a fair amount of study: cephalosporin P_1, helvolic acid and fusidic acid. Their structures are shown in Figure 19. They have in common a narrow antibacterial range, synergic activity with penicillin and some other agents, and ready emergence of resistant mutants on passage *in vitro*. Their principal interest lies in their activity against penicillinase-producing staphylococci. Fusidic acid is about 10 times as active as the others and is the only one commercially available.

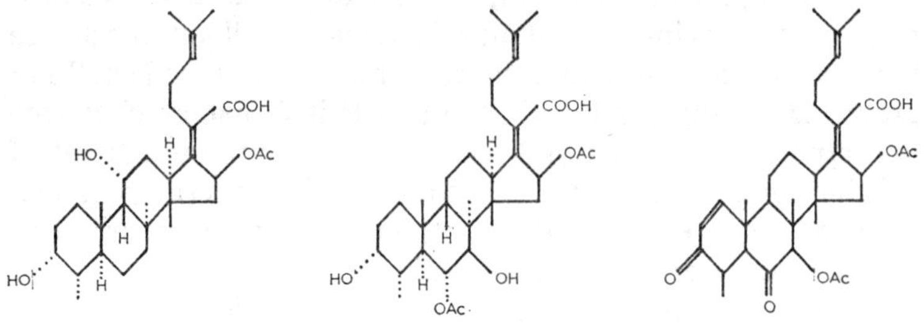

FUSIDIC ACID[1] CEPHALOSPORIN P_1[2] HELVOLIC ACID[3]

Fig. 19
Structure of steroid antibiotics.

[1] Gotfredsen, W. O., *et al.* (1965). *Tetrahedron* **25,** 3505.
[2] Halsall, T. G., *et al.* (1966). *Chem. Comm.*—1966, p 685.
[3] Okuda, S., *et al.* (1964). *Chem. Pharm. Bull.* (Japan) **12,** 121.

Fusidic acid is a colourless crystalline compound sparingly soluble in water, isolated from a strain of *Fusidium coccineum*. Fucidin is the sodium salt and is readily soluble in water (Godtfredsen *et al.,* 1962). The relationship between the structure of fusidic acid and its antibacterial activity has been studied by Godtfredsen *et al.* (1966).

ANTI-BACTERIAL ACTIVITY. Fucidin is active against species of Gram-positive bacteria and the Gram-negative cocci. Nearly all strains of *Staph. aureus,* regardless of their sensitivity to other antibiotics, are outstandingly sensitive to fucidin, and are inhibited by from 0·03 to 0·12 μg. per ml. It is bactericidal for many strains in concentrations close to the MIC (although a proportion of the cells, increasing with inoculum size, always remains) and has been shown by stereoscan electron microscopy to exert a marked destructive effect on staphylococci (Fig. 18). *N. gonorrhoeae, N. meningitidis, Corynebacterium diphtheriae* and many strains of *Clostridia* are also highly sensitive, and a few strains of *Myco. tuberculosis* have been shown to be partially inhibited by from 1·0 to 3·0 μg. per ml. Streptococci and pneumococci are relatively resistant and coliform bacilli and fungi are highly resistant (Table XXXII). The

TABLE XXXII

Minimum Inhibitory Concentrations of Fucidin
in μg./ml.

*Staph. aureus**	0·03-0·16
Str. pyogenes	4·2-16·0
Str. viridans	1-6
Str. pneumoniae	2·0-16·0
Str. faecalis	1·0-5·0
N. meningitidis	0·06-0·25
N. gonorrhoeae	0·03-1·0
C. diphtheriae	0·004-0·005
Bacillus spp.	0·06-1·7
Clostridium spp.	0·016-0·59
Myco. tuberculosis	0·5-1·6
Kl. pneumoniae	4·0-160·0
Enterobacteria	>100

* Including penicillin-resistant strains.
Godtfredsen *et al.,* 1962; Barber and Waterworth, 1962.

difference in sensitivity between streptococci and staphylococci has been utilized by Lowbury *et al.* (1964) in preparing a selective medium for the isolation of haemolytic streptococci.

Fucidin is believed to interrupt protein synthesis like erythromycin by inhibiting translocation on the ribosome (p. 101).

ACQUIRED RESISTANCE. A large inoculum of most strains of *Staph. aureus* contains a very small number of resistant mutants (Barber and Waterworth, 1962; Hilson, 1962) and this appears to be responsible for the effect of inoculum size on the efficacy of fucidin. As would be expected from this, fucidin-resistant strains of *Staph. aureus* emerge rapidly *in vitro* and sometimes during clinical therapy. The growth rate, coagulase, haemolysin and penicillinase production of these mutants appears to be un-impaired (Taylor and Bloor, 1962). There is cross-resistance between fucidin and cephalosporin P_1.

In some strains resistance appears to be very unstable and in poly-resistant strains reversion to the sensitive state on sub-culture may be accompanied by recovery of sensitivity to other agents (Evans and Waterworth, 1966) suggesting that the multiple resistance was plasmid-borne (p. 253). In 50 per cent serum the MIC may increase 50-100-fold. Fucidin is slightly more effective at pH 6-7 than at pH 8 (Stewart, 1964).

SYNERGY. Synergy has been described with erythromycin, novobiocin and with penicillin, but the effect of penicillin is of an unusual kind also seen when combinations of peni-cillin and erythromycin are tested against strains showing the dissociated (p. 170) type of resistance (Waterworth, 1963). It is not seen with highly active penicillinase-producing strains but only with those that inactivate penicillin relatively slowly. The majority of the cells are inhibited by the fucidin, while the smaller number of resistant mutants which are always present, are too few to exert a significant penicillinase effect, and are destroyed by the penicillin (Waterworth, 1963; McDonald, 1965). The effect is therefore not a true synergy since the two drugs are acting on different members of the population: the fucidin inhibits the greater part of the population preventing destruction of the penicillin, and the penicillin acts on the fucidin-resistant mutants, preventing their emergence. In con-trast, fucidin can often be shown to be antagonistic *in vitro* (at least in certain concentration ratios) to the bactericidal action of benzyl penicillin against penicillin-sensitive staphylo-cocci and also to that of methicillin or cloxacillin for penicilli-nase-producing strains (Waterworth, 1963).

PHARMACOLOGY. Fucidin is well absorbed after oral administration, a single dose of 500 mg. in the adult producing peak plasma levels at about 4 hours of 15-20 μg./ml. In children the absorption is more rapid. About 95 per cent is reversibly bound to plasma protein. Milk appears to delay absorption, peak concentrations not being reached for 4-8 hours. Because of slow elimination, considerable accumulation of the drug occurs on repeated administration of doses above 250 mg.: 500 mg. t.d.s. for four days produced plasma concentrations of 11-41 μg. per ml. after 24 hours and 30-144 μg. per ml. after 96 hours. On doses of 3 g./day (40 mg./kg.) Saggers *et al.* (1968) found plasma levels of 45-200 μg./ml. An intravenous form of the drug is available for the treatment of patients in whom oral therapy is impossible.

Fucidin is well distributed in the tissues and most organs of the body, but does not reach the cerebro-spinal fluid. Inhibitory levels are obtained in muscle, kidney, lungs and pleural exudate. Levels of 4-8 μg./ml. were found in bone (Stewart, 1964) and the drug has been detected in brain, milk and placenta which it crosses to reach the foetus. In patients treated with 1·5 g. per day, levels of 0·08-0·84 μg./ml. were found in the aqueous humour after one day and 1·2-1·28 μg./ml. after 3 days' treatment (Williamson *et al.*, 1970). Chadwick and Jackson (1969) found levels up to 2·0 μg./ml. and in contrast to other agents (p. 387), levels in the vitreous were 2-3 times as high. It is excreted and concentrated in the bile and about two per cent. of the administered dose can be recovered in active form in the faeces. Little or no active antibiotic is excreted in the urine. After four days' treatment less than 1 per cent was recovered from the urine producing concentrations of only 0·8 μg. per ml. Studies with radioactive material have shown that a large proportion of the dose is converted to a microbiologically inactive form in the body (Godtfredsen *et al.*, 1962) partly in the liver.

SIDE EFFECTS. When given by mouth fucidin appears to be well tolerated and apart from mild gastro-intestinal disturbance and occasional rashes no untoward symptoms have been reported.

The steroid structure of fusidic acid has excited speculation about possible metabolic effects unrelated to its antibacterial activity. It differs from the steroid hormones in that the methyl group at C13, and the C11 oxygen of the glucocorticoids, are missing and the side chain at C17 is different. Wynn (1965) has clearly shown that no profound metabolic changes follow fucidin administration. It has a protein catabolic effect which is milder than that of tetracycline (Edwards *et al.*, 1970) and unlikely to lead to clinical difficulty.

A number of workers have been sufficiently impressed by the rate at which staphylococcal infections heal to suggest that fucidin might exert a beneficial effect on healing, unrelated to its effect on the infection, but the experimental evidence is conflicting (Calnan and Fry, 1962; Cowan, 1965).

CLINICAL APPLICATION. Fucidin is a useful addition to the antistaphylococcal armoury. It has been successfully used for the treatment of a variety of severe staphylococcal infections often after other potent antistaphylococcal agents have failed. Several authors have reported outstanding success with combinations of fucidin and penicillins and although fucidin and penicillinase-resistant penicillins may show antagonism *in vitro* (p. 208), methicillin or cloxacillin delays the emergence of fucidin-resistant mutants, and Jensen and Lassen (1969) found no evidence in treated patients that a combination of fucidin and methicillin was antagonistic. Nevertheless, the possibility of antagonism should be borne in mind when treating severe infections such as endocarditis. An imperfect response from this cause can only convincingly be demonstrated by improvement on withdrawal of one or other agent. Particular benefit has been claimed for fucidin treatment of bone and joint infections in both the acute and intractable chronic forms of the disease (Rowling, 1970).

Drug-resistant mutants which emerge so easily *in vitro* have appeared in some patients but have not generally proved a problem in treatment. The serious consequences of the spread of resistant strains, however, makes it desirable to limit their emergence as far as possible and for this reason fucidin should generally be given in combination with a penicillin.

PHARMACEUTICAL PREPARATIONS AND DOSAGE

SODIUM FUSIDATE (Fucidin, *Leo Laboratories*)

Capsules, B.P., B.N.F.: 250 mg. Mixture, B.N.F.: equiv. 175 mg. per 5 ml. Dose: 1·5 g., daily in divided doses.

Paedriatic suspension (Diethanolamine salt) equiv. 35 mg. fucidin/ml. Dose: 20-30 mg./kg./day in 3 equal doses. Intravenous (Diethanolamine salt) 500 mg.+50 ml. sterile buffer. Freshly dilute in 500 ml. saline, administer over 2-4 hours. Dose: not more than 1·5 g./day.

REFERENCES

BARBER, M. & WATERWORTH, P. M. (1962). *Lancet* **1**, 931.
CALNAN, J. & FRY, H. J. R. (1962). *Brit. J. Pharmacol.* **19**, 321.
CHADWICK, A. J. & JACKSON, B. (1969). *Brit. J. Ophthal.* **53**, 26.
COWAN, A. (1965). *Irish J. med. Sci.* (6th Series), p. 125.
EDWARDS, O. M., HUSKISSON, E. C. & TAYLOR, R. T. (1970). *Brit. med. J.* **1**, 26.
EVANS, R. J. & WATERWORTH, P. M. (1966). *J. clin. Path.* **19**, 555.
GODTFREDSEN, W., ROHOLT, K. & TYBRING. L. (1962). *Lancet* **1**, 928.
GODTFREDSEN, W. O., ALBRETHSEN, C., V. DAEHNE, W., TYBRING, L. & VANGEDAL, S. (1966). *Antimicrob. Agents Chemother.*, 1965, p. 132.
HILSON, G. R. F. (1962). *Lancet* **1**, 932.
JENSEN, K. & LASSEN, H. C. A. (1969). *Quart. J. Med.* **38**, 91.
LOWBURY, E. J. L., KIDSON, A. & LILLY, H. A. (1964). *J. clin. Path.* **17**, 231.
MCDONALD, F. (1965). *Med. J. Aust.* **1**, 969.
ROWLING, D. E. (1970). *J. Bone Jt Surg.* **52-B**, 302.
SAGGERS, B. A., HARWOOD, H. F. & DAY, B. H. (1968). *Brit. J. clin. Pract.* **22**, 429.
STEWART, G. T. (1964). *Pharmacother.* **2**, 137.
TAYLOR, G. & BLOOR, K. (1962). *Lancet* **1**, 935.
WATERWORTH, P. M. (1963). *Clin. Med. Winnetka.* **70**, 941.
WILLIAMSON, J., RUSSELL, F., DOIG, W. M. & PATERSON, R. W. W. (1970). *Brit. J. Ophthal.* **54**, 126.
WYNN, V. (1965). *Brit. med. J.* **1**, 1400.

LINCOMYCIN

Lincomycin was isolated in the laboratories of the Upjohn Company from the fermentation products of a previously undescribed soil streptomycete, *Streptomyces lincolnensis* var. *lincolnensis* (Mason *et al.*, 1963).

Chemistry

Lincomycin is chemically unlike any other major antibiotic. Its structure is shown in Figure 20. The closely related celesticetin has only about 25-30 per cent of the antibacterial activity of lincomycin *in vitro*, and about 5 per cent *in vivo*. A number of derivatives of lincomycin have been prepared, the majority of which are less active than the parent compound but 7-chloro-7-deoxy-lincomycin (Magerlein *et al.*, 1967) is substantially more active (Phillips *et al.*, 1970) and is now commercially available (p. 217).

Lincomycin is monobasic and is usually supplied as the hydrochloride ('Lincocin') which is very soluble in water, soluble in methanol and ethanol, but relatively insoluble in less polar solvents. The free base is soluble in water and most organic solvents except hydrocarbons. The dry crystalline hydrochloride stored at 70°C. for six months showed no deterioration (Herr and Bergy, 1963).

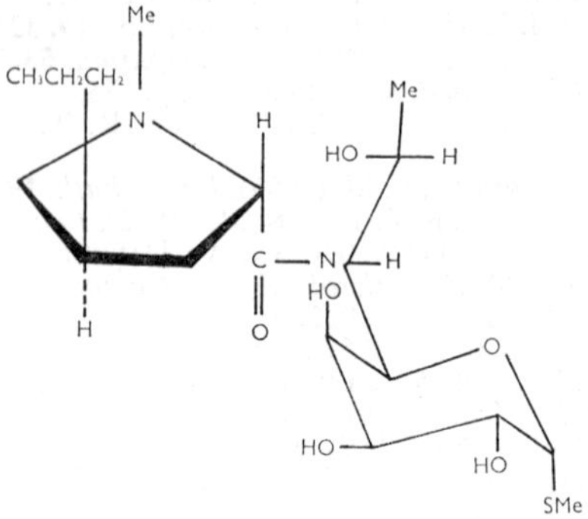

FIG. 20

LINCOMYCIN

Hoeksema, H. *et al.* (1964). *J. Amer. chem. Soc.* **86,** 4223.

Antibacterial Activity

Lincomycin closely resembles erythromycin in its activity against Gram-positive organisms, notably staphylococci, haemolytic streptococci and pneumococci. It also closely resembles the macrolides in showing a characteristic variety of cross-resistance (p. 170). How substances of such different chemical structure come to share these biological properties has yet to be elucidated. There are also some interesting differences. The enterobacteria are resistant to both lincomycin and the macrolides, but haemophilus and neisseria, which are sensitive to erythromycin, are resistant to lincomycin. The behaviour of neisseria is particularly interesting since despite their Gram-negative staining they generally respond to antibacterial agents like Gram-positive organisms. *Streptococcus faecalis* is unusual amongst Gram-positive organisms in being resistant to lincomycin, but on the other hand, the faecal Gram-negative anaerobic bacilli (bacteroides) and anaerobic cocci (veillonella) are all sensitive. The minimum inhibitory concentrations of lincomycin for various species are shown in Table XXXIII. The activity of lincomycin was not inhibited by the presence of up to 50 per cent serum (Lewis *et al.*, 1963).

TABLE XXXIII

Minimum Inhibitory Concentrations of Lincomycins
(µg. per ml.)

	Lincomycin	Clindamycin*
Staph. aureus	0·36-2·8	0·1-1·5
Str. pyogenes	0·04-0·72	0·01-0·2
Str. pneumoniae	0·08-0·72	0·03
Str. viridans	0·17-0·92	0·03-0·06
Str. faecalis	1·4-46·0	0·06-50
B. anthracis	0·25-8·0	
Clostridium spp.	0·36-25·0	
A. israeli	0·12-0·6	
N. gonorrhoeae	10·0-40·0	0·4-3·0
N. meningitidis	>32	
H. influenzae	4·0-16	3·0-12
Enterobacteria	>100	64-100
B. fragilis	2-4	0·03-0·12
Veillonella spp.	<0·1-0·3	

Lewis, Clapp and Grady (1963); Barber and Waterworth (1964); Finegold *et al.* (1966). Magerlein *et al.* (1967); Garrison *et al.* (1968); Lerner (1968).
* 7-chloro-7-deoxy-lincomycin.

Resistance

There have been wide geographical variations in the frequency with which lincomycin-resistant staphylococci have been found. In several series, 15-20 per cent of recently isolated, previously unexposed *Staph. aureus* have been resistant to lincomycin (Nunnery and Riley, 1965) yet Phillips *et al.* (1970) were impressed with the infrequency with which lincomycin-resistant staphylococci had been encountered in their hospital over a 4-year period. Lincomycin resistance is relatively easily induced by passage (Barber and Waterworth, 1964) especially in erythromycin-resistant strains, and has certainly been observed to emerge in the course of treatment when such strains often show the dissociated resistance (p. 170) typical of macrolides (Duncan, 1968). There have also been reports from various parts of the world of lincomycin-resistant haemolytic streptococci and pneumococci and these strains are commonly also resistant to erythromycin (Weisblum, 1967; Lowbury and Kidson, 1968).

Mode of Action

It is believed that the immediate cessation of protein synthesis which follows exposure of staphylococci to lincomycin

TABLE XXXIV

Serum Levels of Lincomycins in Man

Route	Dose	Peak		Half life hr.
		Hour	μg. per ml.	
LINCOMYCIN				
Oral	500 mg. 250 mg. 6 hourly 500 mg. 6 hourly	4	2-7 0·8-1·1 4·6-7·0	4-6
I.M.	200 mg. 600 mg.	1-2	3·5-4·2 8·0-18·0	4-6
I.V.	300 mg.	0	8·0-22·0	3-5·5
CLINDAMYCIN				
Oral	120 mg.	1-2	4·7-7·9	2-3

Ma *et al.* (1964).
Reinarz and McIntosh, (1966).
Vavra *et al.* (1964).

results from interference with amino-acyl translocation analogous to that which is brought about by macrolides (p. 101). The incidence of part-shared and part-separate cross-resistance between lincomycin and the macrolides may result from partly specific binding sites (Apirion, 1967).

Pharmacology

Lincomycin is readily absorbed when given by mouth. The drug is also promptly and completely absorbed from intramuscular sites. The serum levels obtained by various authors following administration by different routes are given in Table XXXIV. Several authors have commented that constant, near maximum levels can be maintained on 4-6 hourly schedules. Much the same results have been obtained in children (Nunnery and Riley, 1965). Food significantly delays and decreases absorption of the oral dose, the mean peak serum level from a dose given immediately after a meal being only about half the fasting levels (McCall, Steigbigel and Finland, 1967).

The drug is widely distributed in the body. Ma *et al.* (1964) found its distribution space to approximate to the total body size. It does not appear to be concentrated in any particular organ (Meyer and Lewis, 1964). Medina *et al.* (1964) found low levels in C.S.F. (up to 1·2 μg. per ml.), and levels of 1·5-6·9 μg. per ml. in cord serum and amniotic fluid 2-4 hours after 600 mg. intramuscularly. Six hours after the last of 2×6 hourly doses of 0·5 g. they found levels in human milk of 0·5-2·4 μg. per ml. Holloway *et al.* (1964) found 1·1-6·6 μg. per g. of bone in patients successfully treated for osteomyelitis. The corresponding serum levels were 6-16·5 μg. per ml.

Excretion

Most workers have found the urinary levels of the drug to be low except after intravenous injection. (Vavra *et al.*, 1964; Ma *et al.*, 1964; Medina *et al.*, 1964). After oral administration only 3-5 per cent of the dose appeared in the urine over the next 24 hours but after intravenous injection up to 57 per cent was recovered. That renal excretion is of some importance is shown by the finding that in patients with severe renal disease serum levels were 3-4 times normal and high levels persisted for over 24 hours. Lincomycin appears to be virtually non-dialysable since its half life in dialysed and undialysed azotaemic patients was approximately the same (Reinarz and McIntosh, 1966).

Finegold *et al.* (1966) found 0·9-6·8 μg. lincomycin per g. faeces after 1·5 g. orally and 1·6-9·6 μg. per g. after 4 g. orally. In the rat part of the unabsorbed drug is broken down in the

8

caecum presumably as a result of bacterial action. In non-azotaemic patients with liver disease, Bellamy *et al.* (1967) found that the peak plasma level after a single intramuscular dose of 600 mg. was somewhat depressed (7·2-12·8 μg./ml.) and the plasma half-life increased from the 4·85 hr. found in their normal subjects to 8·96 hr.

Toxicity

Lincomycin appears to be an innocuous compound. Most authors have reported no side effects apart from diarrhoea which has commonly affected about 10 per cent of the patients and many more in some series (Price *et al.*, 1968). It has occasionally been so severe that therapy has had to be withdrawn. Much of the difference in incidence of diarrhoea may be explained by varying relation of drug administration to meals. If given with food much more of the drug remains unabsorbed to disturb the gut. Brown and Cunningham (1965) reported a single case of granulocytopenia developing during lincomycin therapy in a negro woman, but concluded that it was coincidental. White (1966) concluded from experimental studies that lincomycin is of low antigenicity. Lincomycin chemically coupled to bovine albumin produced antibodies in the rabbit only to the albumen.

Clinical Use

Lincomycin has been used for the treatment of streptococcal pharyngitis, and for Gram-positive coccal otitis, pneumonia and pyoderma with very satisfactory results in both adults and children (Anderson *et al.*, 1968; Bentley and Pollock, 1968). It has also been satisfactorily used in more serious infections including diphtheria and staphylococcal septicaemia. Because of its penetration into bone, it has been particularly commended for the treatment of both acute and chronic osteomyelitis (Herrell, 1968).

Its antibacterial range, low toxicity, and clinical efficacy make lincomycin a suitable substitute for penicillin in Gram-positive coccal infections where penicillin is contraindicated—circumstances in which erythromycin might otherwise be used. Whether lincomycin possesses sufficiently different and desirable features to oust the better established agent in fields other than osteomyelitis remains to be seen (Sanders, 1969).

In the meantime, the frequency of existing and induced resistance strongly suggests that lincomycin should not be widely used for conditions for which there are a number of satisfactory alternatives and that in the treatment of staphylococcal infection it should be combined with another anti-staphylococcal agent.

CLINDAMYCIN

This synthetic modification of lincomycin, involving only the loss of an O and H and the addition of Cl, is, to give its full chemical name, 7-chloro-7-deoxylincomycin hydrochloride hydrate, and is known in the United States as Clinimycin and in this country as ' Dalacin C ' (a somewhat misleading term, since there are no other dalacins) or ' Clindamycin '.

It appears from such studies as those of Wagner *et al.* (1968) and McGehee *et al.* (1968) to be many times more active than lincomycin against staphylococci and pneumococci, and either more active or at least equally active against all other sensitive species (Table XXXIII). Moreover it is better absorbed than lincomycin, producing substantially higher blood levels (Table XXXIV), and this advantage is accentuated when doses are taken after a meal which impairs the absorption of lincomycin but merely slows that of the new derivative.

No countervailing disadvantages have been reported, and the available facts suggest that 7-chlorolincomycin should simply replace lincomycin in therapy, but both continue to be available. It should at least be recognized that 7-chlorolincomycin is not a new antibiotic, as its nomenclature and description suggest, but only a slight modification of an old one.

PHARMACEUTICAL PREPARATIONS AND DOSAGE

LINCOMYCIN HYDROCHLORIDE (Lincocin, *Upjohn*, Mycivin, *Boots*)
   Capsules: Equiv. 500 mg.; Syrup equiv. 125 mg. per 5 ml. Dose: 500 mg., 6-8 hourly, between meals. Injection: 600 mg. in 2 ml. Dose: i/m 300-600 mg., 12 hourly; i/v infusion: 600 mg., 8-12 hourly in 250 ml. saline over 30 minutes.

CLINDAMYCIN (Dalacin C., *Upjohn*)
   Capsules of 150 mg. and 75 mg. (paediatric).
   Doses 150-300 mg. 4 times a day, but can be increased.
   (Also known as CLINIMYCIN in U.S.A. In the U.K. this name refers to a brand of oxytetracycline).

REFERENCES

BARBER, M. & WATERWORTH, P. M. (1964). *Brit. med. J.* **2,** 603.
ANDERSON, R., BAUMAN, M. & AUSTRIAN, R. (1968). *Amer. Rev. resp. Dis.* **97,** 914.
APIRION, D. (1967). *J. molec. Biol.* **30,** 255.
BROWN, E. B. & CUNNINGHAM, C. E. (1965). *J. Amer. med. Ass.* **194,** 668.
BELLAMY, H. M., BATES, B. B. & REINARZ, J. A. (1967). *Antimicrob. Agents Chemother.*—1966, p. 36.
BENTLEY, J. F. R. & POLLOCK, D. (1968). *Arch. Dis. Child.* **43,** 58.
CURTIS, J. R. & EASTWOOD, J. B. (1968). *Brit. med. J.* **1,** 484.
DUNCAN, I. B. R. (1968). *Antimicrob. Agents Chemother.*—1967, p. 723.
FINEGOLD, S. M., HARADA, N. E. & MILLER, L. G. (1966). *Antimicrob. Agents Chemother.*, 1965, p. 659.
GARRISON, D. W., DE HAAN, R. M. & LAWSON, J. B. (1968). *Antimicrob. Agents Chemother.*—1967, p. 397.
HERR, R. R. & BERGY, M. E. (1963). *Antimicrob. Agents Chemother.*, 1962, p. 560.
HERRELL, W. E. (1968). *Clin. Med.* **75,** 19.
HOLLOWAY, W. J., KAHLBAUGH, R. A. & SCOTT, E. G. (1964). *Antimicrob. Agents Chemother.*, 1963, p. 200.
JACKSON, H., COOPER, J., MELLINGER, W. J. & OLSEN, A. R. (1965). *J. Amer. med. Ass.* **194,** 1189.
LERNER, P. I. (1968). *Antimicrob. Agents Chemother.*—1967, p. 730.
LEWIS, C., CLAPP, H. W. & GRADY, J. E. (1963). *Antimicrob. Agents Chemother.*, 1962, p. 570.
LOWBURY, E. J. L. & KIDSON, A. (1968). *Brit. med. J.* **2,** 490.
MA, P., LIM, M. & NODINE, J. H. (1964). *Antimicrob. Agents Chemother.*, 1963, p. 183.
McCALL, C. E., STEIGBIGEL, N. H. & FINLAND, M. (1967). *Amer. J. Med. Sci.* **254,** 144.
MAGERLEIN, B. J., BIRKENMEYER, R. D. & KAGAN, F. (1967). *Antimicrob. Agents Chemother.*—1966, p. 727.
McGEHEE, R. F. Jr., SMITH, C. B., WILCOX, C. & FINLAND, M. (1968). *Amer. J. med. Sci.* **256,** 279.
MASON, D. J., DIETZ, A. & DEBOER, C. (1963). *Antimicrob. Agents Chemother.*, 1962, p. 554.
MEDINA, H., FISKE, N., HJELT-HARVEY, I., BROWN, C. D. & PRIGOT, A. (1964). *Antimicrob. Agents Chemother.*, 1963, p. 189.
MEYER, C. E. & LEWIS, C. (1964). *Antimicrob. Agents Chemother.*, 1963, p. 169.
NUNNERY, A. W. & RILEY, H. D. (1965). *Antimicrob. Agents Chemother.*, 1964, p. 142.
PHILLIPS, I., FERNANDES, R. & WARREN, C. (1970). *Brit. med. J.* **2,** 89.
PINES, A., RAAFAT, H., SIDDIQUI, G. M. & GREENFIELD, J. S. B. (1970). *Brit. med. J.* **1,** 663.
PRICE, D. J. E., O'GRADY, F. W., SHOOTER, R. A. & WEAVER, P. C. (1968). *Brit. med. J.* **3,** 407.
REINARZ, J. A. & McINTOSH, D. A. (1966). *Antimicrob. Agents Chemother.*, 1965, p. 232.
SANDERS, E. (1969). *Ann. intern. Med.* **70,** 585.
VAVRA, J. J., SOKOLSKI, W. T. & LAWSON, J. B. (1964). *Antimicrob. Agents Chemother.*, 1963, p. 176.
WAGNER, J. G., NOVAK, E., PATEL, N. C., CHIDESTER, C. G. & LUMMIS, W. L. (1968). *Amer. J. med. Sci.* **256,** 25.
WEISBLUM, B. (1967). *Lancet* **1,** 843.
WHITE, G. J. (1966). *Antimicrob. Agents Chemother.* 1965, p. 398.

LYSOSTAPHIN

The discovery of this interesting substance was made by chance at the University of Texas, Austin (Schindler and Schuhardt, 1964). In some transduction experiments with *Staph. aureus*, a small white colony was seen to be surrounded by an area of growth inhibition. This organism, which itself had the characters of a staphylococcus, was found to form an extra-cellular lysin attacking staphylococci, whether living or killed, with such vigour that suspensions were rapidly cleared and the organisms could be seen microscopically to be reduced to debris within a few minutes. All of 54 strains of *Staph. aureus* examined were susceptible. *Staph. epidermidis* was lysed more slowly and other bacteria not at all.

Harrison and Cropp (1965) examined this substance further, and refer to it both as an antibiotic and as a ' unique bacterial enzyme '. They confirmed its activity against numerous strains of *Staph. aureus*, as did Zygmunt and his colleagues (1965) who found its minimum inhibitory concentration for 20 strains of type 80/81, resistant to penicillin but sensitive to oxacillin, etc. to be between 0·012 and 0·39 μg. per ml. They point out that since the molecule of lysostaphin is about 75 times larger than that of semi-synthetic penicillins to which these strains were sensitive, on a molar basis it exceeds their activity by several hundred-fold.

The best evidence hitherto of *in vivo* activity is provided by the experiments of Harrison and Zygmunt (1967), who gave a single intravenous dose varying from 0·5 to 50 mg. per kg. to mice one hour after intravenous inoculation with *Staph. aureus*, and obtained more effective suppression of renal lesions than that achieved by any of 10 other antibiotics given in the same way. Dixon, Goodman and Koenig (1968) achieved optimum results in this infection with a single dose of lysostaphin followed by 4 daily doses of methicillin. There are no reports of clinical use, in which the possible antigenicity of a substance of this kind may well prove a difficulty.

REFERENCES

Dixon, R. E., Goodman, J. S. & Koenig, M. G. (1968). *Yale J. Biol. Med.* **41**, 62.
Harrison, E. F. & Cropp, C. B. (1965). *Appl. Microbiol.* **13**, 212.

HARRISON, E. F. & ZYGMUNT, W. A. (1967). *J. Bact.* **93**, 520.
SCHINDLER, C. A. & SCHUHARDT, V. T. (1964). *Proc. nat. Acad. Sci.* **51**, 414.
ZYGMUNT, W. A., HARRISON, E. F. & BROWDER, H. P. (1965). *Appl. Microbiol.*
    13, 491.

NOVOBIOCIN

Two apparently new antibiotics, both highly active against the staphylococcus, were reported to the Third Antibiotics Symposium in Washington in 1955 under the names of 'Cathomycin' and 'Streptonivicin'. Cathomycin was isolated from a new species of actinomycete which was given the name *Streptomyces spheroides* on account of its colonial appearance (Wallick *et al.*, 1956). Streptonivicin was isolated from a species of actinomycete with snow-white colonies and thus given the name *Streptomyces niveus* (Smith *et al.*, 1956).

Finland drew attention to the similarity of the anti-bacterial activity of the two compounds at the Symposium and their identity was established by ultra-violet and infra-red absorption studies.

By common agreement the antibiotic was given the generic name novobiocin.

Chemical Properties

Novobiocin is a dibasic acid usually supplied as the calcium or monosodium salt. The calcium salt is soluble at 3 mg./ml.

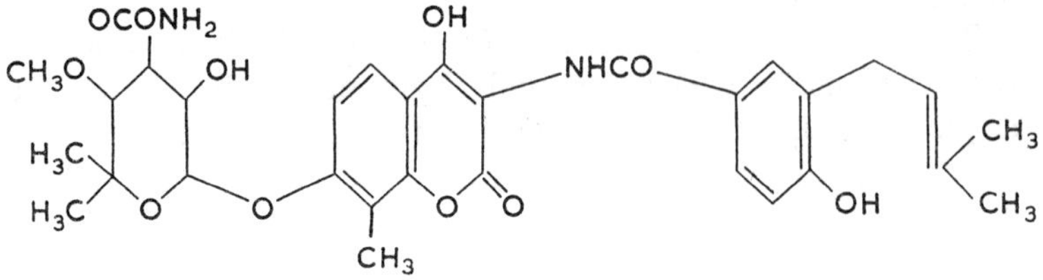

FIG. 21

Structure of novobiocin (Hoeksema *et al.*, 1956, *J. Amer. Chem. Soc.* **78**, 2019; Shunk *et al.*, 1956, *ibid*, 1770).

water and 125 mg./ml. alcohol. The monosodium salt is much more readily soluble in water: 200 mg./ml. water, 140 mg./ml. ethyl alcohol and 350 mg./ml. methyl alcohol. With both salts a 2·5 per cent solution has a pH of 7·0 to 8·5. Both salts are moderately stable if kept dry, stored in the cold and protected from light.

Novobiocin combines with the common basic antibiotics (*e.g.*, streptomycin, neomycin, erythromycin and spiramycin) in stoichiometric proportion to form water-insoluble salts; antibiotics that are neutral, acidic or amphoteric do not form salts with novobiocin.

Anti-bacterial Activity

Novobiocin has a rather unusual anti-bacterial spectrum (Table XXXV). It is outstandingly active against *Staph. aureus,* most strains of which, in the absence of previous contact with the drug, are among the most sensitive bacteria. Other highly sensitive species are *Str. pneumoniae, C. diphtheriae, H. influenzae, N. gonorrhoeae* and *N. meningitidis* and some strains of *Pasteurella.*

TABLE XXXV

Sensitivity of Bacteria to Novobiocin
Usual minimum inhibitory concentration (μg./ml.)

Gram-positive Bacteria		Gram-negative Bacteria	
Staph. aureus	0·1 - 2	*H. influenzae*	0·2 - 0·8
Str. pyogenes	0·5 - 4	*N. meningitidis*	0·5 - 4
Str. pneumoniae	0·2 - 2	*N. gonorrhoeae*	4
Str. faecalis	1 - 16	*Pasteurella*	2 - 16
C. diphtheriae	0·4	*Proteus vulgaris*	2 - 50
		Proteus mirabilis	8 - 100
		Proteus morgani	16 - >100
		Proteus rettgeri	
		Escherichia, Klebsiella, Salmonella, Shigella	>100
		Pseudomonas	

Jones, W. F., Nichols, R. L. and Finland, M. (1956). *J. Lab. clin. Med.* **47,** 783.
Frost, B. M. *et al.* (1956). *Antibiot. Ann.* 1955-56, p. 918.
Schneierson, S. S. and Amsterdam, D. (1957). *Antibiot. Chemother.* **7,** 251.

Streptococci are relatively resistant but occasional strains are moderately or highly sensitive.

Some strains of *Proteus,* particularly of the species *Proteus vulgaris,* are sensitive to moderate concentrations but other enterobacteria are resistant.

Mode of Action

Novobiocin is primarily a bacteristatic drug, but with highly sensitive species a concentration two to ten times that required for bacteristasis has a slow killing effect and may lead to sterilization of the culture in 24-48 hours. Cell wall precursors promptly accumulate when novobiocin is added to staphylococci but there is evidence, both biochemical and from comparative effects on L forms, that it does not operate like penicillin and D-cycloserine solely through inhibition of cell wall synthesis. Its initial effect is to depress DNA and, to a lesser extent, RNA synthesis. Cell-wall and protein synthesis are affected later (Smith and Davis, 1967).

A 500- to 1,000-fold increase in the size of inoculum causes a 4-8-fold increase in the minimum bacteristatic concentration of novobiocin for staphylococci and a much larger increase in the concentration necessary to sterilise the culture in 24 hours. The minimum inhibitory concentration is 8 or more times greater at pH 8·0 than at pH 5·4.

SERUM. The presence of 10 per cent or more serum or blood causes a marked decrease in the anti-bacterial activity of novobiocin. This is because about 90 per cent of the antibiotic is reversibly bound to serum albumin and the bound antibiotic is no longer active against bacteria. Novobiocin may displace other substances from protein binding sites and one possible effect of this is to lower the plasma-bound iodine by displacing thyroxine (Takemura *et al.*, 1966).

Acquired Resistance

Many species of bacteria initially sensitive to novobiocin readily develop resistance to it *in vitro* and a considerable increase in the resistance of the infecting staphylococcus during treatment has been recorded by several investigators. No cross resistance has been recorded with other common antibiotics.

Absorption

Early studies showed that novobiocin is well absorbed from the alimentary tract, producing high blood levels which are long sustained (Table XXXVI). Wagner and Damiano (1968) found the plasma half-life in adults to be almost 3 hours and in children 1·7-4 hours.

After repeated doses there is some accumulation and during treatment with full doses serum levels of 50 to over 100 μg./ml. may be reached.

Absorption from intramuscular injection appears satisfactory, but the injections cause pain, and this route is indicated only when oral therapy is impracticable.

Table XXXVI

Average Serum Concentrations of Novobiocin at Intervals after Single Oral Dose

Dose (g)	Hours after Dose						
	1	*2*	*4*	*6*	*12*	*24*	*36*
0·25	10·9	8·2	5·7	3·7	1·3	—	—
0·5	10·6	14·1	18·8	13·6	6·7	1·0	—
1·0	37·7	42·4	40·0	37·7	16·3	4·8	1·7
2·0	63·5	67·7	65·7	60·4	36·8	11·3	3·8

Wright, W. W., Putnam, L. E. and Welch, H., 1956. *Antibiot. Med.* **2**, 311.

Distribution and Excretion

Organ distribution shows no peculiarities. Concentrations rather lower than that in the blood are found in serous effusions, but all authors are agreed that even when the blood level is high, cerebrospinal fluid contains very little or none.

Whereas most antibiotics are excreted mainly in the urine, novobiocin is an exception, and this largely accounts for the high blood levels attained. The amount found in the urine does not usually exceed three per cent of the dose. It has even been observed that in single specimens of urine the concentration may be considerably lower than that in the blood.

Novobiocin is excreted mainly in the bile, in which the concentration is high. Reabsorption must follow, and a continuous process of biliary excretion and reabsorption is the second important factor in maintaining the high blood levels. Nevertheless much of the antibiotic eventually escapes by this route, and high concentrations are found in the faeces.

Toxicity and side effects

RASHES AND FEVER. Maculopapular, morbilliform or urticarial skin eruptions with or without fever are common if treatment is continued for more than a week with doses of 2-4 g. per day, but uncommon with doses of 1 g. Rashes have appeared on the 6-27th day of treatment often rather characteristically developing about the 9th day. The rashes disappear on stopping the drug but may promptly re-appear if the drug is re-administered. This evidently results from the extensively protein-bound antibiotic acting as a haptene (White, 1966). Shelley (1963) treated 25 volunteers with 1 g. novobiocin daily and found that a third developed basophilia. One subject developed a characteristic generalized pruritic rash on the 9th day. On re-challenge up to 120 days later he showed a prompt and profound fall in circulating basophils indicative of sensitization with reappearance of generalized itching.

GASTRO-INTESTINAL SYMPTOMS. Mild intestinal symptoms consisting of nausea, intestinal cramps and loose stools are common, but rarely necessitate stopping treatment.

BLOOD CHANGES. Eosinophilia has been observed frequently, usually in association with skin eruptions. A moderate degree of leucopenia is occasionally seen but the count may rise again even during continued treatment. Thrombocytopenia which may be severe (Holswade *et al.*, 1964) and haemolytic anaemia (Montgomery, 1963) have also been reported.

LIVER FUNCTION. An increased icteric index and a raised indirect van der Bergh reaction have been recorded in many patients on novobiocin therapy. The significance of this has been questioned, since novobiocin gives rise to a yellow pigment metabolite in the serum, which may give an indirect positive van der Bergh reaction (Lazar, 1962). There is no doubt, however, that novobiocin may exert a profound effect on hepatic excretory function by interfering with uptake of various compounds by hepatic cells, inhibiting glucuronyl transferase—the enzyme concerned with glucuronide conjugation—and suppressing excretion of conjugates into the bile (Hargreaves and Lathe, 1963). Particularly severe effects may occur in the new-born where glucuronide formation is imperfectly developed (London, 1964), and the response of infantile glucuronyl transferase to novobiocin may differ from that of the adult enzyme (Brown and Henning, 1963).

CLINICAL APPLICATION

Novobiocin is an interesting and active compound but it is difficult to define for it a distinctive role amongst currently available antibiotics. Its once useful place as an anti-staphylococcal agent has been overtaken by the penicillinase-resistant penicillins and other agents, which are at least as active, bactericidal and much less liable to produce the troublesome side effects which are a common feature of novobiocin therapy (Holdswade *et al.,* 1964).

Since staphylococci readily develop resistance to novobiocin, it has been suggested that it should be used in combination with another antibiotic for which purpose erythromycin appears suitable. Novobiocin has been found effective in the treatment of pneumococcal pneumonia and fairly satisfactory results have been obtained in haemolytic streptococcal infections: enterococcal infections seem less responsive. In all these conditions other antibiotics are more active, and novobiocin can rarely be the drug of choice.

Several authors found that novobiocin was clinically effective in the treatment of urinary infections due to some strains of *Staph. aureus, Proteus* and enterococci. Although admittedly the tissue effect may be the more important, it seems advisable to use a drug which is capable also of sterilizing the urine itself, and so little of this one is excreted that it must be at a disadvantage from this standpoint.

Combination with Other Antibiotics

It has several times been claimed that novobiocin and tetracycline act synergically (Masson and Kingsley, 1964) and this mixture is available commercially as, for example, 'Albamycin T '. However, Hirsch and Finland (1960) found that not only was there no suggestion of synergy, but when the test staphylococcus was resistant to tetracycline, the action of the combination on it was actually less that that of the same dose of novobiocin given alone. In an unpublished study by one of ourselves, so far from any synergy being demonstrable, the effect of this combination was not even additive, the inhibitory concentration of each remaining the same regardless of the presence of a sub-inhibitory concentration of the other. In training experiments, contrary to the findings of Vavra (1967), a tetracycline-resistant staphylococcus rapidly became resistant to novobiocin when exposed to the mixture: even strains initially sensitive to both could be trained to resistance.

Several reports of the clinical efficacy of this combination have appeared but they have not generally included comparisons of the mixture with its components. In a study from general practice, Seddon *et al.* (1964) concluded that the mixture was advantageous, but there seems no strong reason to believe that this mixture is an exception to the general rule that packaged antibiotic combinations are unlikely to provide the critical concentration relationships which are frequently required for synergic action between pairs of agents.

PHARMACEUTICAL PREPARATIONS AND DOSAGE

NOVOBIOCIN (Streptonivicin, Albamycin*, *Upjohn;* Cathomycin, *Merck, Sharp and Dohme,* Cardelmycin, *U.S.A.;* and other proprietary names) Tablets: B.P., B.N.F.: equiv. 250 mg.; Suspension, U.S.N.F.: equiv. 2·5-3 per cent w/w. Syrup, B.N.F.: 125 mg per 5 ml. Dose: 1-2 g. daily in divided doses.

* NOT Albomycin (*U.S.S.R.*)—a basic peptide antibiotic from *Actinomyces subtropicus.*

REFERENCES

BROWN, A. K. & HENNING, G. (1963). *Ann. N.Y. Acad. Sci.* **111,** 307.
HARGREAVES, T. & LATHE, G. H. (1963). *Nature (Lond.)* **200,** 1172.
HIRSCH, H. A. & FINLAND, M. (1960). *New Engl. J. Med.* **262,** 209.
HOLSWADE, G. R., DINEEN, P., REDO, S. F. & GOLDSMITH, E. I. (1964). *Arch. Surg.* **89,** 970.
LAZAR, H. P. (1962). *N.Y. State J. Med.* **66,** 3590.
LONDON, W. L. (1964). *N. Carolina Med. J.* **25,** 417.
MASSON, E. L. & KINGSLEY, V. V. (1964). *Antimicrob. Agents Chemother.* 1963, 624.
MONTGOMERY, J. R. (1963). *New Engl. J. Med.* **269,** 966.
SEDDON, J. C., STEVENS, E. A. & ABBOTT, B. C. (1964). *Brit. J. clin. Pract.* **18,** 273.
SHELLEY, W. B. (1963). *Arch. Derm. (Chicago)* **88,** 759.
SMITH, C. G., DIETZ, A., SOKOLOSKI, W. T. & SAVAGE, G. M. (1956). *Antibiot. Chemother.* **6,** 135.
SMITH, D. H. & DAVIS, B. D. (1967). *J. Bact.* **93,** 71.
TAKEMURA, Y., YAMADA, T. & SHICHIJO, K. (1966). *Metabolism* **15,** 566.
VAVRA, J. J. (1967). *J. Bact.* **93,** 801.
WAGNER, J. G. & DAMIANO, R. E. (1968). *J. clin. Pharmacol.* **8,** 102.
WALLICK, H., HARRIS, D. A., REAGAN, M. A., RUGER, M. & WOODRUFF, H. B. (1956). *Antibiot. Ann.* (1955-6), p. 909.
WHITE, G. J. (1966). *Antimicrob. Agents Chemother.,* 1965, p. 398.

PRASINOMYCIN

This substance, derived from a strain of *Streptomyces prasinus* recovered from Colorado soil, was first described by Weisenborn *et al.* (1967). It acts exclusively on Gram-positive bacteria and appears of unique interest in that it contains phosphorus and that a single subcutaneous dose protects against inoculation with *Str. pyogenes* for as long as 28 days. Meyers *et al.* (1968) describe it as a diester of phosphoric acid, with a molecular weight of 1600+, and mention that although streptococci and pneumococci are highly sensitive to it, *Sarcina lutea* is resistant. These authors assert that a single large dose renders mice refractory to inoculation with haemolytic streptococci for no less than 2 months, and report other interesting findings on the timing of medication in relation to curative effects in pneumococcal and staphylococcal infection.

It now appears that a similar if not identical phosphorus-containing antibiotic is formed by several other species of *Streptomyces*. Known originally as moenomycin and now as flavomycin, it is proposed for use as a growth-promoting food additive in livestock. The reasons for abandoning the study of this interesting antibiotic as a therapeutic agent have not been made clear.

REFERENCES

MEYERS, E., MIRAGLIA, G. J., SMITH, D. A., BASCH, H. I., PANSY, F. E., TREJO, W. H. & DONOVICK, R. (1968). *Appl. Microbiol.* **16,** 603.
WEISENBORN, F. L., BOUCHARD, J. L., SMITH, D., PANSY, F., MAESTRONE, G., MIRAGLIA, G. & MEYERS, E. (1967). *Nature* **213,** 1092.

RIFAMYCIN

The rifamycins are a family of antibiotics produced by *Streptomyces mediterranei* and studied in the laboratories of Lepetit, Milan. Rifamycin B is the most active, and its molecule has been modified with advantage in various ways, the derivatives recently studied and used in therapeutics being ' rifamycin SV ' and rifamycin B diethylamide (' Rifamide '). The principal account of these antibiotics is by Bergamini and Fowst (1965) who describe their structure, differing from that of other antibiotics, *in vitro* activity, pharmacology and clinical applications.

Extremely low concentrations (0·01 to 0·1 µg. per ml.) are said to inhibit the growth of staphylococci, streptococci (other than *S. faecalis*) and *Myco. tuberculosis*: Gram-negative species require 10-100 µg. per ml. or more. Welsch and Esther (1963) found the concentrations necessary to inhibit the growth of staphylococci and streptococci to be somewhat higher, and that results are affected by inoculum size and length of incubation: they also draw attention to the existence of small numbers of much more resistant cells in populations of staphylococci. The action is also bactericidal, and there is no cross-resistance with other antibiotics.

Rifamycin is little absorbed from the alimentary tract. Intramuscular injection of 500 mg. produces a therapeutic blood level for up to eight hours, but protein binding is extensive: with a blood level of 5 μg. per ml. only 14 per cent is said to be free. Elimination is mainly via the bile, in which a concentration as high as 2·8 mg. per ml. has been observed: some re-circulation occurs, but much is excreted in the faeces and little in the urine. On this account it has been described as ' the only specific antibiotic ' for cholecystitis (Stratford and Dixson, 1966), but it should be recognized that erythromycin and novobiocin are also excreted mainly by this route, and that ampicillin attains high concentrations in the bile, while possessing greater activity than rifamycin against some Gram-negative species likely to occur in the biliary tract.

Therapeutic applications have included the treatment of staphylococcal infections, both systemically and where applicable locally, of biliary tract infections, and of tuberculosis. Apparently the systemic treatment of tuberculosis in combination with other drugs has not been altogether successful, and greater emphasis is placed on local application, including the use of aerosols, intracavitary introduction in patients subjected to Monaldi drainage, and instillation into empyema cavities. A few encouraging results have also been obtained in leprosy. We have no experience of this antibiotic, and feel unable to adjudicate on the now extensive literature, mainly Italian, describing its clinical use.

Rifampicin

This derivative of rifamycin, 3-(4-methyl-piperazinyliminomethyl) rifamycin SV, represents perhaps the greatest advance over the original properties of an antibiotic which has yet been achieved by synthetic modification. It is one of 500 derivatives prepared by Ciba of Basel and Lepetit of Milan in collaboration (Kradolfer, 1968). It has the same spectrum as other rifamycins but much higher activity, the M.I.C. for highly sensitive species being almost incredibly low (*e.g.* for *Staphylococcus aureus* 0·002 µg./ml.). Moreover it is well absorbed after oral administration, a 600 mg. dose producing blood levels of 32 and 2 µg./ml. after 2 and 12 hours respectively (Begg, 1967). Like other rifamycins it is excreted largely in the bile, in which concentrations of 200 µg./ml. or more are attained. After a dose of 150 mg. the amount so excreted much exceeds that in the urine, but with larger doses urinary excretion mounts and biliary does not, the ratio being thus reversed.

It is most important to recognize that large bacterial populations may contain a few resistant mutants. Hence the M.I.C. as determined in a fluid medium with a generous inoculum may be enormously higher than that in the plate dilution method with a light one (Atlas and Turck, 1968; McCabe and Lorian, 1968). A more important consequence is that, at least in treating most infections, rifampicin should never be given alone, but together with another drug to which the organism is sensitive.

Much the most important clinical use of rifampicin is for the treatment of tuberculosis, which is discussed from both experimental and clinical standpoints in Chapter XXIV. Some take the view that it should be reserved solely for this purpose. Among other uses for which it has been tried or examined are the following.

It may exceptionally be indicated in staphylococcal infection. One of us recently found rifampicin and erythromycin to be the most bactericidal of many antibiotic combinations for a strain of *Staph. aureus* from an infection of a patent interventricular septum in a child aged 3. The fact that both drugs could be given orally was welcome at this age, and the infection was rapidly eliminated. Results from a single dose in gonorrhoea were good (Cobbold, Morrison and Willcox, 1968). No benefit was achieved in chronic bronchitis, and *H. influenzae* rapidly became resistant (Citron and May, 1969). Rapidly acquired resistance in enterobacteria originally inhibited by 4-8 µg./ml. was also seen during the treatment of urinary tract infection (Murdoch *et al.*, 1969), from which similar unsatisfactory results are reported by Atlas and Turck (1968). The following studies are only in the experimental stage. Rifampicin is highly active against gas gangrene clostridia, and controls experimental infection by *Cl welchii* and *Cl. septicum* but not by *Cl. novyi* (Schallehn 1969). *Malleomyces pseudomallei* is more sensitive to rifampicin than to any of 11 other antibiotics, and it controls experimental melioidosis, but apparently not much better than tetracycline (Hobby *et al.*, 1969). In all these studies rifampicin was given alone, and might have done better if combined with another appropriate drug. Finally, considerable activity against pox viruses and trachoma agent has been demonstrated (see Chapter XXVII).

PHARMACEUTICAL PREPARATIONS AND DOSAGE

SODIUM RIFAMYCIN B DIETHYLAMIDE: RIFAMIDE (Rifocin M, *Lepetit*)
    Ampoules of 150 mg. in 3 ml.
    Dose i.m. 1 every 6-12 hours.
RIFAMPICIN (Rifadin, *Lepetit*: Rimactane, *Ciba*: Rifampin in U.S.A.)
    Capsules of 150 and 300 mg.
    Dose 600 mg. daily.

REFERENCES

ATLAS, E. & TURCK, M. (1968). *Amer. J. med. Sci.* **256,** 247.
BEGG, R. J. (1967). *Tubercle* **48,** 149.
BERGAMINI, N. & FOWST, G. (1965). *Arzneitmittel-Forsch.* **15,** 953.
CITRON, K. M. & MAY, J. R. (1969). *Lancet,* **2,** 982.
COBBOLD, R. J. C., MORRISON, G. D. & WILLCOX, R. R. (1968). *Brit. med. J.*
    4, 681.
HOBBY, G. L., LENERT, T. F., MAIER-ENGALLENA, J. & DeNOIA-CICENIA, E.
    (1969). *Amer. Rev. resp. Dis.* **99,** 952.
KRADOLFER, F. (1968). *Schweiz. med. Wschr.* **98,** 622.
MCCABE, W. R. & LORIAN, V. (1968). *Amer. J. med. Sci.* **256,** 255.
MURDOCH, J. McC., SPEIRS, C. F., WRIGHT, N. & WALLACE, E. T. (1969).
    Lancet **1,** 1094.
SCHALLEHN, G. (1969). *Schweiz. med. Wschr.* **99,** 1057.
STRATFORD, B. C. & DIXSON, S. (1966). *Med. J. Aust.* **1,** 1.
WELSCH, M. & ESTHER, H. (1963). *Chemotherapia (Basel)* **7,** 269.

VANCOMYCIN

Vancomycin, isolated in 1956 in the laboratories of Eli Lilly Co. from strains of *Streptomyces orientalis,* is now a well recognized antibiotic with very limited if important uses, and calls for only a brief description.

Antibacterial Activity

The 'spectrum' of vancomycin includes only Gram-positive organisms, and only its activity against staphylococci and streptococci is of clinical interest. The findings of various authors on the sensitivity of these and other organisms are shown in Table XXXVII.

The effect exerted is rapidly bactericidal in a concentration not much higher than that required for bacteristasis (Ziegler, Wolfe and McGuire, 1956; Geraci *et al.*, 1957).

Neither inoculum size nor pH within the range 6·5 to 8·0 affects activity, but the presence of 25 per cent horse serum has

TABLE XXXVII

Sensitivity of Bacteria to Vancomycin

	No. of Strains	Minimum Inhibitory Concentration (μg./ml.)
Staph. aureus[1]	10	0·8 - 1·6
Staph. aureus[1]	1	6·2
Staph. aureus[2]	41	0·156 - 1·87
Staph. aureus[2]	2	>10
Staph. aureus[3]	10	2·0 - 3·0
Str. pyogenes[2]	24	0·156 - 2·5
Str. pyogenes[3]	8	0·5 - 1·0
Str. pyogenes[2]	4	0·3 - 1·25
Str. pneumoniae[3]	6	0·5 - 1·0
Str. faecalis[2]	2	0·3 - 2·5
Str. faecalis[3,4]	6	2·0 - 5·0
Bacillus spp.[1]	6	0·2 - 3·1
Corynebact. spp.[1]	4	0·4 - 0·8
Clostridium welchii[4]	3	0·39 - 0·625
Clostridium spp.[4]	9	0·625 - 5·0

All species of Gram-negative bacteria, Mycobacteria and fungi are resistant.

[1] McCormick *et al.* (1956).
[2] Griffith and Peck (1956).
[3] Kirby and Divelbiss (1957).
[4] Geraci *et al.* (1957).

been shown to cause a two-fold increase in the bacteristatic concentration (Kirby and Divelbiss, 1957) and a two-fold increase in the bactericidal concentration (Geraci *et al.*, 1957).

Acquired resistance does not appear to be a problem. Early studies (McCormick, *et al.*, 1956; Griffith and Peck, 1956) recorded a few strains of *Staph. aureus* which were naturally resistant to five or more μg./ml. vancomycin but initially sensitive strains do not readily acquire resistance (Ziegler *et al.*, 1957; Garrod and Waterworth, 1956; Geraci *et al.*, 1957).

Pharmacology

Vancomycin is not absorbed from the alimentary tract, and intramuscular injection causes pain and necrosis. Administration has therefore to be intravenous. Kirby and Divelbiss (1957) studied the blood levels after single and repeated intravenous injections of vancomycin. After a single dose the following levels were obtained:

Dose	μg./ml. in Sera at Hours after Dose						
	2	4	6	8	12	24	48
0·5 g.	10	3	3	1	0·5	0	—
1·0 g.	25	10	—	5	3	2	—
2·0 g.	50	33	—	10	10	3	0

When doses were repeated at 6- or 12-hour intervals there was slight accumulation. Therapeutic levels could be maintained by a regimen of 0·5 g. six-hourly, 1·0 g. 12-hourly, or 2·0 g. once a day. A regimen of 1·0 g. 12-hourly appeared to be the most satisfactory from the standpoint of ease of administration and effective blood levels.

In patients with impaired renal function much higher blood levels are obtained, and one such patient had a serum concentration of 5 μg./ml. nine days after vancomycin had been discontinued. Organ distribution shows no noteworthy features, except that little of the antibiotic is found in either cerebrospinal fluid or bile. A very high proportion (about 90 per cent) of a dose of vancomycin administered intravenously is excreted in the urine.

Clinical Applications

The principal indication for vancomycin is the treatment of septicaemia, usually accompanied by endocarditis, caused by staphylococci or streptococci resistant to other antibiotics. This resistance may only be manifested *in vivo*. Vancomycin should be considered as an alternative when other treatment (despite its suitability as indicated by *in vitro* tests) is apparently failing.

The treatment of staphylococcal endocarditis has been most extensively studied at the Mayo Clinic (Geraci *et al.*, 1958; Geraci *et al.*, 1962), where divided intravenous doses totalling 2 g. daily have usually been given for up to three or four weeks, although a shorter course may sometimes be adequate. Enterococcal endocarditis has also been successfully treated (Romansky and Holmes, 1958) and occasionally *Str. viridans* infection clinically resistant to other treatment.

Another use recently reported on very favourably is oral administration for acute staphylococcal enterocolitis, usually resulting from treatment with other antibiotics. Wallace *et al.* (1965) successfully treated 7 such patients by giving 0·5 g. in 30 ml. water or fruit juice at 6-hour intervals. Khan and Hall (1966) gave the same dose at 4- or 6-hour intervals to 45 patients with uniform success.

Toxic Effects

Thrombophlebitis and febrile reactions are common but the most serious risk is that of producing deafness. As usual with ototoxicity, the excessively high blood levels responsible are liable to be attained in patients with impaired renal function, and this unfortunately sometimes exists in patients requiring this treatment. Dosage should be controlled by blood assays: the aim should be to keep the level at between 5 and 25 μg./ml. Dutton and Elmes (1959) describe a rapid method for this purpose. The vancomycin level in the blood is little affected by renal dialysis (Lindholm and Murray, 1966); in spite of dialysis once or twice weekly 3 μg. per ml. was found in the blood three weeks after a 1 g. dose in a patient with ' end-stage kidney disease '.

PHARMACEUTICAL PREPARATION

VANCOMYCIN (Vancocin, *Lilly*).
  Vials of 500 mg. for solution for intravenous injection. Dose: see text.

REFERENCES

DUTTON, A. A. C. & ELMES, P. C. (1959). *Brit. med. J.* **1**, 1144.
GARROD, L. P. & WATERWORTH, P. M. (1956). *Brit. med. J.* **2**, 61.
GERACI, J. E., HEILMAN, F. R., NICHOLS, D. R., WELLMAN, W. E. & ROSS, G. T. (1957). *Antibiot. Ann.* 1956-7, p. 90.
GERACI, J. E., HEILMAN, F. R., NICHOLS, D. R. & WELLMAN, W. E. (1958). *Proc. Mayo Clin.* **33**, 172.
GERACI, J. E., NICHOLS, D. R. & WELLMAN, W. E. (1962). *Arch. intern. Med.* **109**, 507.

GRIFFITH, R. S. & PECK, F. B. JR. (1956). *Antibiot. Ann.* 1955-6, p. 619.
KHAN, M. Y. & HALL, W. H. (1966). *Ann. intern. Med.* **65,** 1.
KIRBY, W. M. M. & DIVELBISS, C. L. (1957). *Antibiot. Ann.* 1956-7, p. 107.
LINDHOLM, D. D. & MURRAY, J. S. (1966). *New Engl. J. Med.* **274,** 1047.
MCCORMICK, M. H., STARK, W. M., PITTENGER, G. E., PITTENGER, R. C. &
    McGUIRE, J. M. (1956). *Antibiot. Ann.* 1955-6, p. 606.
ROMANSKY, M. J. & HOLMES, J. R. (1958). *Antibiot. Ann.* 1957-8, p. 187.
WALLACE, J. F., SMITH, R. H. & PETERSDORF, R. G. (1965). *New Engl. J. Med.*
    272, 1014.
ZIEGLER, D. W., WOLFE, R. N. & MCGUIRE, J. M. (1956). *Antibiot. Ann.*
    1955-6, p. 612.

RISTOCETIN

This antibiotic was described at length in the same chapter as vancomycin in the first edition of this book. There are many similarities between them in range of activity, pharmacological behaviour, and indications for clinical use. Interesting differences between them are that ristocetin is active against *Mycobacteria,* whereas vancomycin is not, and toxic to the bone marrow, causing leucopenia, rather than to the eighth nerve.

We are informed by the discoverers, Abbott Laboratories, that the manufacture of ristocetin (' Spontin ') was discontinued several years ago.

Chapter XIII

ANTI-FUNGAL ANTIBIOTICS

Most of the major antibiotics are produced by fungi, and it is thus not surprising that others should be resistant to them. So resistant are they that quantities of penicillin and streptomycin enough to inhibit any bacterial growth can be added to culture media used for the isolation of pathogenic fungi: this is a useful proceeding in dealing with, for instance, material from secondarily infected lesions of histoplasmosis.

There is a single exception to this in the only systemic mycosis commonly occurring in Great Britain. *Actinomyces israeli* is usually highly sensitive to penicillin, and sufficiently so to several other antibiotics (Garrod, 1952; Blake, 1964). Actinomycosis in all its forms will usually respond to penicillin given in adequate doses for long enough: tetracyclines are the second choice, and their efficacy has been demonstrated, although not on the same scale.

All other mycoses, systemic or surface, are susceptible only to certain highly specialized antibiotics or other drugs, which in general have no anti-bacterial action. These have different specificities among the fungi themselves, very different pharmacological properties, and hence quite separate indications. Several are polyenes, but they now include two other antibiotics and two synthetic compounds.

Cycloheximide

This antibiotic, originally known as actidione, is β-[2-(3,5,-dimethyl-2-oxocyclahexyl)-2-hydroxyethyl] glutarimide, and is produced, usually together with other antibiotics, by several *Streptomyces* species. It is active against fungi but not bacteria, and has also some anti-protozoal and anti-tumour activity. It has been used with some success in a few cases of systemic mycotic infection, but toxic effects are a severe limitation: it has numerous applications in the control of plant diseases (Waksman and Lechevalier, 1962).

POLYENES

Nystatin

Originally named fungicidin, this antibiotic was the product of a soil survey by members of the staff of the New York State Department of Health (Hazen and Brown, 1951), and this is the derivation of its present name. It is formed by *Streptomyces noursei,* the original strain of which came from dairy farm soil in Virginia, and has a tetraene structure which is not very fully elucidated.

The very low solubility of nystatin has compelled investigators to work with suspensions prepared in various ways. Its discoverers used them not only to demonstrate *in vitro* activity, which is highest against yeast-like fungi, but therapeutically in animals by subcutaneous injection. In their experiments and those of Campbell *et al.* (1954, 1955) some effect was observed in infection by *Histoplasma capsulatum, Cryptococcus neoformans* and *Coccidioides immitis.* Drouhet (1955) not only had similar success from parenteral treatment of *Candida albicans* infection in rabbits, but good results from *oral* administration in 25 patients, some of whom had systemic infections. In human infections the primary and most extensive lesions are usually in the alimentary tract, where they are directly accessible, and it seems possible that when the organism is destroyed in these, the task of its elimination from inaccessible sites may become easier. How much of a systemic effect can be obtained with nystatin is now of less practical interest since the effect is certainly inferior to that obtainable with the more recently discovered amphotericin and perhaps with other drugs.

The local action of nystatin in controlling candidiasis involving any part of the alimentary tract from the mouth to the anus is now so generally familiar as to call for no further discussion. The only aspect of it on which there can be two opinions is whether or when it should be given together with tetracyclines as a preventive, since this class of broad spectrum antibiotic, with its suppressive action on the normal flora, is now probably the commonest cause of intestinal candidiasis. This question is discussed later (p. 240) Nystatin is available in suitable form for the local treatment of *Candida* infections elsewhere (skin, vagina, etc.).

Full purification of nystatin is impracticable, and it is usually prescribed in units, an average dose for candidiasis of the alimentary tract being 500,000 units administered three times a day: 3,500 units is the activity of 1 mg. of the pure substance.

Amphotericin B

This is the more useful of two antibiotics formed by a strain of *Streptomyces nodosus* found in soil from Templadora on the Orinoco river. It is a heptaene of not yet fully ascertained structure, insoluble in water but forming salts with a low solubility. It has a satisfactorily low acute toxicity in animals, and inhibits the growth of all yeast-like fungi causing systemic mycoses in a concentration not exceeding and sometimes considerably less than 0·5 μg./ml. Filamentous fungi are also susceptible: bacteria are not.

In early studies amphotericin B was shown to be effective in various mycotic infections in mice, including some caused by filamentous (*e.g. Aspergillus fumigatus, Rhizopus oryzae*) as well as yeast-like fungi. The intravenous route was chiefly used, but there is some evidence of an effect from much larger doses given orally. That there could be such an effect is shown by the human pharmacological studies of Louria (1958), who gave oral doses of 1·6 - 5·6 g. daily and found amounts up to 0·3 μg./ml. in the blood: on the other hand, an intravenous dose of about 1 mg./kg. gave blood levels of 0·5 to 3·5 μg./ml. and these were found still to be 0·5 to 1·5 μg./ml. 20 hours later, indicating very slow elimination. Very small amounts were found in the cerebro-spinal fluid, and urinary excretion accounted for only a small fraction of the dose given. An ingenious and highly sensitive method was used for these assays, depending on the difference between counts of *C. albicans* in known concentrations of the antibiotic with and without addition of the fluid to be tested.

Treatment by the intravenous route has now been shown to be effective in histoplasmosis, coccidioidomycosis, North American blastomycosis, and cryptococcal meningitis, for which additional small (0·5 mg.) intrathecal doses are advisable. Intravenous treatment is begun with doses of 1, 5 and 10 mg. increased to 1 mg./kg. on alternate days, continued if possible until 3 g. have been given (Andriole and Kravetz, 1962). More recently the antibiotic has been solubilized with sodium desoxycholate: in this form it is both more effective, giving higher blood levels, and more toxic. Various toxic effects are common, including fever and nausea and vomiting (which are usually mitigated by also giving aspirin and an antihistamine), local thrombophlebitis resulting from the injection, anaemia, hypokalaemia and a rise in blood urea. The latter is usually said to be ' reversible ', but Sanford *et al.* (1962) who performed renal biopsies on three successfully treated cases of coccidioidomycosis, found proliferative changes in glomeruli, degenerative tubular changes and interstitial deposits of calcium, indicative of some degree of permanent damage.

A conference at the National Institutes of Health, Bethesda (Utz *et al.,* 1964) on the toxic effects of amphotericin B includes two contributions in which effects on the kidney are fully described, in both patients and experimental animals. It is emphasized that some effect is invariable if a certain total dose is exceeded. A rise in blood urea and decreased clearance of creatinine may occur without albuminuria. In this paper and another from the same source (Tynes *et al.,* 1963) hydrocortisone is commended for reducing the frequency of immediate reactions such as fever and vomiting: its effect on actual tissue changes was not examined.

This is the only antibiotic used in the treatment of microbic infections of which so small a total dose can have such effects. It is therefore clear that this treatment should not be undertaken except in certainly diagnosed cases, and when, as in coccidioidomycosis, the severity of the infection is variable, only in the more severe and disseminated form.

Amphotericin B may also be indicated for systemic candidiasis. Its value for this has also been proved: indeed there are now several recorded instances of cure of *C. albicans* endocarditis, a condition which formerly was invariably fatal. Drouhet (1963) describes the treatment of 7 personal cases of *Candida* septicaemia, with successful results in 5.

The efficacy of this treatment is unquestioned but the course is difficult to administer, arduous for the patient, and not without risk. It will be interesting to see to what extent the use of several more recently discovered drugs, to be described later, can replace it.

Other Polyenes

Over 50 polyene antibiotics have now been discovered, a few of which have come into clinical use, although so far exclusively as local applications and principally for the treatment of candidiasis.

CANDICIDIN, a heptaene, formed by *Streptomyces griseus*, is more active than nystatin against *Candida* spp., but has been little used in therapeutics until recently, when good results have been obtained in vaginal candidiasis (Waksman *et al.,* 1965).

HAMYCIN, a heptaene from *Streptomyces pimprina* recovered from local soil in the Research Laboratories of Hindustan Antibiotics, is also said to be more active than nystatin against *Candida* (Thirumalachar *et al.,* 1961). *Aspergillus niger* is also sensitive, but *A. fumigatus* is resistant. Otomycosis due to *A. niger* was successfully treated by Atre *et al.* (1961). Maniar and Mavdikar (1963) have shown that repeated oral administration results in levels of 1-3 μg. per ml. in the blood and various organs of mice, and the same authors (1966) report that 100 or 200 mg. per kg. daily for 10 days eliminates *Cryptococcus neoformans* from the lungs of intravenously inoculated mice. Divekar, Vora and Khan (1966) contest some of the statements of the foregoing authors about the properties of hamycin, and claim themselves to have shown that it is indistinguishable from trichomycin. Several studies (*e.g.* that by Williams *et al.,* 1966) have shown that hamycin even when administered orally, is toxic, the main lesions being in the kidneys.

PIMARICIN, a tetraene, so-called because *Streptomyces natalensis* forming it was derived from soil near Pietermaritzburg, (Struyk *et al.,* 1958) has been successfully used in vaginal candidiasis and has some effect also on trichomoniasis (Korteweg *et al.,* 1963). Bronchopulmonary aspergillosis and candidiasis were treated successfully in 7 out of 10 cases by inhalations (Edwards and La Touche, 1964).

TRICHOMYCIN, a heptaene, so-called because of its activity against *Trichomonas vaginalis,* a product of *Streptomyces hachijoensis,* was discovered in Japan (Hosoya *et al.,* 1952). This property, together with the usual susceptibility of *Candida* to a polyene, enables this antibiotic to be used successfully for the treatment of both common forms of vaginitis (Magara *et al.,* 1954). Efficacy in vaginal candidiasis has been confirmed in the United States (Smith *et al.,* 1963) although only an 80 per cent cure rate is claimed, and some of the patients were also given trichomycin orally, whether in expectation of some systemic effect or merely to prevent re-infection from the bowel is not clear.

Prophylactic use of Polyenes

Several preparations are on the market in which a polyene, usually nystatin, is mixed with a tetracycline, with the object of preventing overgrowth of *Candida* in the alimentary tract. The merits of this combination require to be considered, and particularly the pros and cons of its regular use, as suggested by some manufacturers. This question was discussed at length in the previous edition, and the arguments now need only be summarized.

There are three objections to this practice. The first is that it usually fails to achieve any useful object. Almost all observers (*e.g.* Smits *et al.,* 1966) are agreed that giving the usual dose of 250,000 units of nystatin along with 250 mg. of tetracycline reduces the numbers of *Candida* in the bowel, but with a single exception (Larkin, 1959) no such study has revealed any difference in the frequency of side effects (Metzger *et al.,* 1957; Rein *et al.,* 1957). This lack of effect was confirmed in a more recent study (Report, 1968), an interesting feature of which is that in patients treated with tetracycline only, *Candida* was grown from rectal swabs in 37 and 38 per cent respectively of those with and without gastro-intestinal symptoms. In fact the common assumption that the ordinary side effects result from the proliferation of *Candida* is baseless. More extensive proliferation and actual tissue invasion can occur in debilitated patients, and in them only does the treatment appear to be indicated.

The second objection is one which applies to the indiscriminate and unnecessary use of any antibiotic: that it may lead eventually to increased microbic resistance. This has not yet been seen in clinical isolates of *Candida albicans,* but Hebeka and Solotorovsky (1965) trained this organism to a 60-fold increase in resistance to amphotericin B. There is evidence of cross-resistance among polyenes: Bodenhoff (1968) trained 5 strains of *Cryptococcus neoformans* to resistance to nystatin and amphotericin B, and with one exception the cultures resistant to one antibiotic were also resistant to the other. It has been pointed out (Medical Letter, 1961) that only a small increase in resistance to amphotericin B would be disastrous, since the margin between the present inhibitory concentration and the maximum achievable blood levels is dangerously narrow, and the efficacy of the only effective antibiotic for systemic candidiasis could thus be lost. The conclusion reached is that ' the routine prophylactic use of antifungal agents along with tetracyclines cannot be justified '.

A different objection applies to preparations, the first of which was intended only for administration to children, which contain tetracycline and amphotericin B. These have been shown to reduce the *C. albicans* population of the bowel, and are said to cause no ill effects (Stough *et al.*, 1959). On the other hand, amphotericin B is the most toxic antibiotic in therapeutic use: the studies of Louria (1958) already cited show that it is absorbed when administered orally, and therapeutic action from oral administration has been reported by Drouhet (1958) and O'Grady and Thompson (1961). The organ most likely to suffer damage is the kidney, and such damage would be undetected, since in discussing the nephrotoxicity of this antibiotic Butler (1964) states: ' Proteinuria . . . has been described in only a few patients, and is not considered characteristic.' In view of this possibility, however remote, and of the fact that severe forms of candidiasis are almost unheard-of in children, the advisability of using this preparation is questionable.

ANTI-MYCOTIC DRUGS OTHER THAN POLYENES

These include one antibiotic, griseofulvin, which is now a well established remedy solely for dermatomycoses, and three other recently discovered drugs, one being an antibiotic and two synthetic, the value of which cannot yet be fully assessed.

Saramycetin

This antibiotic, originally known as X-5079C, is a peptide with a high sulphur content, unique among peptides in having anti-fungal and no anti-bacterial activity (Grunberg, Berger and Titsworth, 1961). Emmons (1961) found it to be of low toxicity, highly effective in experimental histoplasmosis, rather less so in blastomycosis and coccidioidomycosis and ineffective in cryptococcosis. The first report on its clinical use by Utz, Andriole and Emmons (1961) concerns 27 patients, whose further progress together with results in 12 more, is reported on by Witorsch *et al.* (1966). The drug was injected subcutaneously at 6-hour intervals, 3-5 mg./kg. daily being usually given to a total dose of about 20 g. Of 16 patients with North American blastomycosis, 14 responded both clinically and with negative cultures, but 8 relapsed, and of 13 with histoplasmosis 6 failed to respond or relapsed. Both sporotrichosis and aspergillosis responded in 2 out of 3 patients. Treatment failed in patients with coccidioidomycosis and in 3 severe *Candida* infections, 2 with endocarditis. To set against these unpromising or equivocal results is the fact that saramycetin is far better tolerated than amphotericin B, and could perhaps safely be given with better effect in larger doses.

5-Fluorocytosine

That this substance has a systemic anti-fungal action was reported by Grunberg, Titsworth and Bennett (1963) but the earlier literature on it is somewhat uninformative, and the best account of its properties is that by Shadomy (1969), although the main object of this paper is to point out that the action of the drug is neutralized by constituents of ordinary culture media. In a ' completely synthetic ' medium it inhibits *Cryptococcus neoformans* in concentrations of 0·46-3·9 µg./ ml. and kills it at 3·9-15·6 µg./ml. *Candida albicans* is about equally sensitive. Since the drug can be given in doses of 100 mg./kg. daily, and then attains concentrations in the blood and cerebro-spinal fluid of 10-30 and 8-20 μg./ml. respectively, an effect in these two infections is to be expected, and this has been confirmed clinically. *Histoplasma capsulatum* and *Blastomyces dermatitidis* are resistant.

The main clinical report on this treatment, by Utz, Shadomy and McGehee (1969) is regrettably only an abstract, but records successful results in all but 4 of 15 cases of cryptococcosis, 2 with meningitis. Doses of 1-6 g. daily were given for from 14 to 42 days. It is mentioned, without details, that drug resistance in the organism may accompany relapse. Tassel and Madoff (1968) treated *Candida* septicaemia in a diabetic successfully by giving 4 g. daily for 17 days, and a cryptococcal meningitis which had resisted treatment with amphotericin B. This patient was at one stage given 2·25 g. at 6-hour intervals, which produced a C.S.F. level of '100 mg./ml.' (presumably 100 μg./ml.). Since doses of this order can be tolerated, there is evidently scope for further study of what they can achieve.

Clotrimazole (BAYb 5097)

This compound, bis-phenyl-(2-chlorphenyl)-1-imidazole methane, one of a long series of tritylimidazole derivatives prepared in the Bayer laboratories, is fully described by Plempel *et al.* (1969). It has no anti-bacterial activity, but inhibits all the principal fungi causing systemic infections in concentrations of the order of 1 μg./ml. It is well absorbed from the alimentary tract. Blood levels are well sustained, and toxicity is very low. Some of the drug in the blood and that excreted in the urine is an inactive metabolite. Efficacy has been demonstrated in mice in *Candida, Histoplasma* and *Aspergillus* infections. Clinical results in three patients are reported by Oberste-Lehn, Baggesen and Plempel (1969). A pulmonary aspergilloma (*A. nidulans*) shrank and sputum culture became negative during a long course of oral treatment at the rate of 60 mg./kg. daily. Treatment with the same dose relieved a *Candida krusei* bronchial infection in an asthmatic, and a 15-day course sufficed to cure a sycosis barbae due to *C. albicans*, which was also eliminated from the faeces.

Griseofulvin

This antibiotic was discovered as a product of *Penicillium griseofulvum* by Oxford, Raistrick and Simonart (1939), who found it to be $C_{17}H_{17}O_6Cl$ and provisionally ascertained its structure, which has since been confirmed. It was re-discovered some years later as the product of a *Penicillium* in soil at Wareham Heath, Dorset, in which conifers grew poorly because of its action on mycorrhizal fungi: from its effect on these organisms it was called 'curling factor'. Its identity with a sample of griseofulvin supplied by Raistrick was verified by Grove and McGowan (1947). Its anti-fungal action was then further examined and exploited in the field of plant pathology. Clinical use was at first considered inadvisable because of the observation of an anti-mitotic effect, but this was produced by large doses given intravenously in animals, and there is not now believed to be any risk of such an effect from the doses employed clinically.

The highest activity of griseofulvin is against dermatophytes: yeast-like fungi are less susceptible, although O'Grady and his colleagues (1963), by giving large doses to mice, obtained a reduction in the size of *Candida* lesions in the mouse thigh, possibly by some indirect mechanism. A curative effect was first demonstrated in experimental *Microsporum canis* infection in guinea-pigs by Gentles (1958) who was also responsible (Gentles *et al.,* 1959) for showing that the antibiotic is actually in the hair of treated animals, some of it being only extractable with methanol. The fact that griseofulvin when administered orally is actually incorporated in keratin as it is formed explains its unique activity in fungus infections of the hair and nails.

The reader can now be referred to works on dermatology for details of clinical use. The results in *Microsporum audouini* and other infections of the scalp hair are uniformly good, and this treatment is now preferred to X-ray epilation. A good account of results in onychomycosis is given by Davies, Everall and Hamilton (1967). Treatment was continued for up to 2 years, 0·5 g. being given 3 times a day for one month and thereafter twice daily. Finger nail infections responded better than those of the toes, and *Trychophyton rubrum* infections better than *T. mentagrophytes,* the former being the more sensitive organism.

The antibiotic is better absorbed when in finely divided form, and its absorption is also said to be promoted by fat in the diet (Crounse, 1961). Blood levels are much reduced by administration of phenobarbitone, which apparently enables the liver to break down griseofulvin more rapidly (Busfield *et al.,* 1964). Other systems of dosage have been proposed for short courses. Atkinson *et al.* (1962) contest the suggestion made by others that scalp ringworm can be cured by a single massive dose, and showed that divided doses give higher blood levels than a single daily dose. Grin and Nadazdin (1965) observed effects by microscopy of hairs plucked at intervals, and confirmed that a single large dose is ineffective, but achieved economy by initial large doses (50 mg. per kg. daily) for five days followed by only 6·25 mg. per kg. daily for the remainder of a 28-day course.

Even long courses of treatment are usually well tolerated. Rashes, headache and gastric discomfort are uncommon and rarely severe. The disturbance of porphyrin metabolism and liver damage produced by large doses in mice (De Matteis and Rimington, 1963) appear to have little or no counterpart in patients given conventional doses.

PHARMACEUTICAL PREPARATIONS AND DOSAGES

NYSTATIN (' Fungicidin ', ' Mycostatin ', *Squibb*)
Tablets 500,000 units: usual dose 1 t.d.s. Also in form of ointment, suspension, pessaries, etc.

AMPHOTERICIN B (' Fungizone ', *Squibb*)
Vials containing 50 mg.+sodium desoxycholate and buffer for intravenous infusion: usual dose 0·1 mg. rising to 1 mg. per kg. body weight daily.

PIMARICIN (' Natamycin ', ' Myprozine ', ' Pimafucin ', *Brocades*)
Sterile 2-5 per cent aqueous suspension for intrabronchial administration as aerosol: 2·5 mg. have been given t.d.s. Also as ointment, enteric-coated tablets and vaginal tablets.

GRISEOFULVIN (' Grisovin ', *Glaxo;* ' Fulcin Forte ' *I.C.I.*)
Tablets of 125 or 250 mg.: usual dose 250 mg. 4 times a day.

REFERENCES

ANDRIOLE, V. T. & KRAVETZ, H. M. (1962). *J. Amer. med. Ass.* **180,** 269.
ATKINSON, R. M., BEDFORD, C., CHILD, K. J. & TOMICH, E. G. (1962). *Antibiot. Chemother.* **12,** 225.
ATRE, W. G., WAKANKAR, P. S. & PADHYE, A. A. (1961). *Hindustan Antibiot. Bull.* **3,** 172.
BLAKE, G. C. (1964). *Brit. med. J.* **1,** 145.

BODENHOFF, J. (1968). *Acta Path. Microbiol. scand.* **73**, 572.
BUSFIELD, D., CHILD, K. J. & TOMICH, E. G. (1964). *Brit. J. Pharmacol.* **22**, 137.
BUTLER, W. T. (1964). *Ann. intern. Med.* **61**, 344.
CAMPBELL, C. C., HODGES, E. P. & HILL, G. B. (1954). *Antibiot Ann.* 1953-54, p. 210.
CAMPBELL, C. C., O'DELL, E. T. & HILL, G. B. (1955). *Antibiot. Ann.* 1954-5, p. 858.
CROUNSE, R. G. (1961). *J. invest. Dermatol.* **37**, 529.
DAVIES, R. R., EVERALL, J. D. & HAMILTON, E. (1967). *Brit. med. J.* **3**, 464.
DE MATTEIS, F. & RIMINGTON, C. (1963). *Brit. J. Derm.* **75**, 91.
DIVEKAR, P. V., VORA, V. C. & KHAN, A. W. (1966). *J. Antibiot. (Tokyo) Ser. A* **19**, 63.
DROUHET, E. (1955). *Ann. Inst. Pasteur* **88**, 298.
DROUHET, E. (1958). *Bull. Soc. Path. exot.* **51**, 76.
DROUHET, E. (1963). *Antibiot. et Chemother. (Basel)* **11**, 21.
EDWARDS, G. & LA TOUCHE, C. J. P. (1964). *Lancet* **1**, 1349.
EMMONS, C. W. (1961). *Amer. Rev. resp. Dis.* **84**, 507.
GARROD L. P. (1952). *Brit. med. J.* **1**, 1263.
GENTLES, J. C. (1958). *Nature (Lond.)* **182**, 476.
GENTLES, J. C., BARNES, M. J. & FANTES, K. H. (1959). *Nature (Lond.)* **183**, 256.
GRIN, E. I. & NADAŽIN, M. (1965). *Bull. Wld Hlth Org.* **33**, 183.
GROVE, J. F. & MCGOWAN, J. C. (1947). *Nature (Lond.)* **160**, 574.
GRUNEBERG, E., BERGER, J. & TITSWORTH, E. (1961). *Amer. Rev. resp. Dis.* **84**, 504.
GRUNBERG, E., TITSWORTH, E. & BENNETT, M. (1964). *Antimicrob. Agents Chemother.*—1963, p. 566.
HAZEN, ELIZABETH L. & BROWN, RACHEL (1951). *Proc. Soc. exp. Biol. (N.Y.)* **76**, 93.
HEBEKA, E. K. & SOLOTOROVSKY, M. (1965). *J. Bact.* **89**, 1533.
HOSOYA, S., KOMATSU, N., SOEDA, M. & SONODA, Y. (1952). *Jap. J. exp. Med.* **22**, 505.
KORTEWEG, G. C., SZABO, K. L. H., RUTTEN, A. M. G. & HOOGERHEIDE, J. C. (1963). *Antibiot. et Chemother. (Basel)* **11**, 261.
LARKIN, R. (1959). *Lancet* **1**, 1228.
LOURIA, D. B. (1958). *Antibiot. Med.* **5**, 295.
MAGARA, M., YOKOUTI, E., SENDA, T. & AMINO, E. (1954). *Antibiot. Chemother.* **4**, 433.
MANIAR, A. C. & MAVDIKAR, S. (1963). *Hindustan Antibiot. Bull.* **5**, 113.
MANIAR, A. C. & MAVDIKAR, S. (1966). *Canad. J. Microbiol.* **12**, 377.
MEDICAL LETTER (1961). *The Medical Letter on Drugs and Therapeutics (N.Y.)* **3**, 33.
METZGER, W. I., STEIGMANN, F., JENKINS, C. J., PAMUKCU, S. F. & KAMINSKI, L. (1957). *Antibiot. Ann.* 1956-57, p. 208.
OBERSTE-LEHN, H., BAGGESEN, I. & PLEMPEL, M. (1969). *Dtsch. med. Wschr.* **94**, 1365.
O'GRADY, F. & THOMPSON, R. E. M. (1961). *Antibiot. Chemother.* **11**, 26.
O'GRADY, F., THOMPSON, R. E. M. & COTTON, R. E. (1963). *Brit. J. exp. Path.* **44**, 334.
OXFORD, A. E., RAISTRICK, H. & SIMONART, P. (1939). *Biochem. J.* **33**, 240.
PLEMPEL, M., BARTMANN, K., BUCHEL, K. H. & REGEL, E. (1969). *Dtsch. med. Wschr.* **94**, 1356.
REIN, C. R., LEWIS, L. A. & DICK, L. A. (1957). *Antibiot. Med.* **4**, 771.
REPORT (1968). *Brit. med. J.* **4**, 411.
SANFORD, W. G., RASCH, J. R. & STONEHILL, R. B. (1962). *Ann. intern. Med.* **56**, 553.
SHADOMY, S. (1969). *Appl. Microbiol.* **17**, 871.
SMITH, A. G., TAUBERT, H. D. & MARTIN, C. W. (1963). *Amer. J. Obstet. Gynec.* **87**, 455.

SMITS, B. J., PRIOR, A. P. & ARBLASTER, P. G. (1966). *Brit. med. J.* **1,** 208.
STOUGH, A. R., GROEL, J. T. & KROEGER, W. H. (1959). *Antibiot. Med.* **6,** 653.
STRUYK, A. P., HOETTE, I., DROST, G., WAISVISZ, J. M., VAN EEK, T. & HOOGERHEIDE, J. C. (1958). *Antibiot. Ann.*, 1957-8, p. 878.
TASSEL, D. & MADOFF, M. A. (1968). *J. Amer. med. Ass.* **206,** 830.
THIRUMALACHAR, M. J., MENON, S. K. & BHATT, V. V. (1961). *Hindustan Antibiot. Bull.* **3,** 136.
TYNES, B. S., UTZ, J. P., BENNETT, J. E. & ALLING, D. W. (1963). *Amer. Rev. Resp. Dis.* **87,** 264.
UTZ, J. P., ANDRIOLE, V. T. & EMMONS, C. W. (1961). *Amer. Rev. resp. Dis.* **84,** 514.
UTZ, J. P., BENNETT, J. E., BRANDRISS, M. W., BUTLER, W. T. & HILL, G. J. (1964). *Ann. intern. Med.* **61,** 334.
UTZ, J. P., SHADOMY, S. & McGEHEE, R. F. (1969). *Amer. Rev. resp. Dis.* **99,** 975.
WAKSMAN, S. A. & LECHEVALIER, H. A. (1962). *The Actinomycetes,* vol. III. London: Baillière.
WAKSMAN, S. A., LECHEVALIER, H. A. & SCHAFFNER, C. P. (1965). *Bull. Wld Hlth Org.* **33,** 219.
WILLIAMS, T. W., Jr., WITORSCH, P., HIGHMAN, B., EMMONS, C. W. & UTZ, J. P. (1966). *Antimicrob. Agents Chemother.* 1965, p. 700.
WITORSCH, P., ANDRIOLE, V. T., EMMONS, C. W. & UTZ, J. P. (1966). *Amer. Rev. resp. Dis.* **93,** 876.

CHAPTER XIV

DRUG RESISTANCE

INTRODUCTION

THE adaptability of bacteria in the presence of poisonous agents has been well known since the early days of bacteriology and a paper on this subject appeared in the first volume of the *Annales de l'Institut Pasteur,* published in 1887, under the patronage of the master himself (Kossiakoff, 1887). Ehrlich, in his pioneer work on chemotherapy at the beginning of this century, appreciated the significance of this and attempted to cure syphilis with a single massive dose. As it affects antibiotics, this problem is of exceptional magnitude, since the degree of abnormal resistance which may appear is often enormously greater than that capable of being acquired to any other type of drug.

CHARACTERISTICS OF DRUG-RESISTANT STRAINS

Nature of Resistance

Drug-resistant bacteria can be divided into two fundamentally different types according to their response to the antibiotic. They are conveniently referred to as *drug-tolerant* and *drug-destroying.*

Drug-tolerant bacteria are capable of growing in the presence of an increased concentration of an unchanged antibiotic. This is the usual type of drug-resistance encountered *in vitro* with all antibiotics, and in clinical practice with all antibiotics except penicillin. Drug-tolerant bacteria may be indifferent to the drug, that is to say, capable of growing equally well in its presence or absence. Other strains, although capable of multiplication in the presence of the drug, grow more luxuriantly in its absence. Conversely in a few instances, particularly with streptomycin, the strain may be completely or partially addicted to the drug and is referred to as *drug-dependent.*

Drug-destroying Bacteria. In clinical practice the most frequently encountered drug-destroying bacteria are penicillinase-producing staphylococci. These strains owe their resistance almost entirely to inactivation of penicillin by penicillinase, and are intrinsically almost as sensitive as a normal strain. The result of a tube dilution test of sensitivity is thus determined by the size of the inoculum: if this is heavy, it contains enough preformed penicillinase to destroy a concentration of penicillin 100 times or more greater than that which will inhibit the growth of a small inoculum.

Penicillin-inactivating enzymes are also produced by many coliform bacilli. *B. anthracis* and some strains of *Clostridia* also produce a penicillinase, but in both cases the individual bacteria, like staphylococci, are sensitive to benzyl penicillin, and in the case of *B. anthracis* so highly sensitive that treatment is fully effective.

Drug-destruction does not play much part in resistance to other antibiotics. An enzyme which hydrolyses chloramphenicol has been reported from several species, including *Esch. coli, Proteus vulgaris* and *B. subtilis,* but the strains were all sensitive to chloramphenicol and production of the enzyme apparently had no relationship to the development of drug-resistance (Smith and Worrel, 1950). More recently Dunsmoor *et al.* (1964) have found that some strains of staphylococci inactivate chloramphenicol by a different mechanism, and that their resistance does depend on their ability to do this. Waterworth (1966) has shown that only naturally occurring resistant variants of normally sensitive species (*Staph. aureus* and *albus* and some enterobacteria) can inactivate chloramphenicol in this way: normally resistant species do not. The presence of an organism of the former type in a mixed culture incorporating a sensitivity test can destroy the antibiotic and make another sensitive organism appear resistant. A streptomycin antagonist of a rather different type has been isolated from *Ps. aeruginosa* (Lightbown, 1954) but no such antagonist has been isolated from streptomycin-resistant variants of other species.

Stability of Resistance

Drug-tolerant Strains. The stability of drug-resistance in drug-tolerant strains is very variable. Streptomycin-resistant organisms, whether isolated from *in vitro* experiments or from clinical infections, are usually highly stable and retain their resistance after prolonged passage in the absence of the anti-biotic. Tetracycline- and chloramphenicol-resistant organisms are also fairly stable, especially when isolated from clinical infections. Erythromycin-resistant strains are often more labile and many, in the absence of the antibiotic, tend to revert to erythromycin sensitivity. Staphylococci trained to penicillin tolerance *in vitro* are highly unstable and rapidly revert to the sensitivity of the parent strain.

PENICILLINASE-PRODUCING STAPHYLOCOCCI. The capacity to produce penicillinase is usually a fairly stable characteristic, but there is a tendency for penicillin-destroying strains to yield a proportion of penicillin-sensitive cells, which completely fail to produce detectable amounts of the enzyme.

Changes in Sensitivity to Other Drugs

CROSS-RESISTANCE. With chemically related drugs there is usually almost complete cross-resistance. Thus bacteria which have developed resistance to one sulphonamide will show a corresponding increase in resistance to all sulphonamides. Similarly there is almost complete cross-resistance between the different tetracycline antibiotics. The erythromycin group are in a special category. Thus strains of staphylococci which have developed resistance by passage in one of the macrolides *in vitro* usually show a similar increase in resistance to all other members of the group. On the other hand, erythromycin-resistant staphylococci isolated from clinical infections are frequently sensitive to spiramycin and oleandomycin. (For a fuller discussion of this see Chapter X.)

Moderate degrees of cross-resistance are sometimes seen with chemically unrelated antibiotics. This has been noted with chloramphenicol and the tetracyclines (Pansy *et al.*, 1950) and chloramphenicol and erythromycin (Barber, Csillag and Medway, 1958). According to Sutherland *et al.* (1964) training *S. paratyphi* B to resistance to either benzyl penicillin, ampicillin, chloramphenicol or tetracycline produces a sub-stantial increase in resistance to all four antibiotics, but not to streptomycin. In similar experiments with other enterobacteria, several behaved in the same way, but others (*Proteus* and *Shigella* spp.) did not. These interesting findings seem so far to be unexplained.

INCREASE IN SENSITIVITY TO OTHER DRUGS. More rarely a resistant variant isolated by *in vitro* passage in one antibiotic may show an increase in sensitivity to other antibiotics. In the best known instance of this, diminished resistance to penicillin in a staphylococcus trained to streptomycin, chloramphenicol or tetracycline resistance is likely to be due either to reduced growth rate with consequent delay in penicillinase formation, or to the presence of non-penicillinase forming variants (Barber, 1953).

Associated Changes

Organisms trained to resistance *in vitro* often have a slower growth rate, with the result that during further transfers in drug-free broth of a mixture of resistant and sensitive cells the latter soon predominate. Accompanying changes may be diminished virulence and altered morphology. Most naturally occurring resistant variants usually show none of these changes: an exception are small-colony variants sometimes seen in cultures resistant to erythromycin and occasionally to other antibiotics.

MODE OF ORIGIN

Abnormal resistance to antibiotics and other drugs as seen in the clinical sphere may arise in at least four different ways.

Therapeutic selection

Here no change in bacteria themselves is involved. The extensive therapeutic use of a drug eliminates sensitive strains of an organism, but favours the spread of an originally very small minority of strains possessing natural resistance. It was thus that sulphonamide resistance in gonococci became prevalent within a few years of the introduction of this treatment. The outstanding example of this mechanism in the antibiotic field is penicillin resistance in staphylococci. An originally very small minority of strains forming penicillinase has multiplied to a majority in hospital environments.

Drug-tolerant Bacteria

In laboratory experiments drug-tolerant bacteria usually arise by a discontinuous process which suggests spontaneous mutation. In the first instance a few drug-resistant cells appear, which if not favoured by the environment are likely to be overgrown. But the presence of the antibiotic has a selective action so that the few resistant mutants are favoured at the expense of the sensitive cells until a pure culture of antibiotic-resistant cells is obtained.

It has been fashionable to attribute all drug resistance in a previously sensitive culture to mutation, and many ingenious methods have been devised to prove that this is so: among these perhaps the most convincing is the use of replica plating by Lederberg and Lederberg (1952) to prove the presence of resistant bacterial cells before exposure to an antibiotic. It should nevertheless be recognized that this proposition is not universally or wholly accepted. Hinshelwood and his colleagues have published a long series of studies, of which some of the latest are by Dean and Hinshelwood (1964) and by Dean and Giordan (1965) providing evidence that increased bacterial resistance to various noxious agents, including some antibiotics, can arise by a process of adaptation.

Whatever the mechanism of the change, the fact remains that exposure to an antibiotic, whether *in vitro* or *in vivo,* may result in increased resistance to it in a bacterial population. The rapidity and extent of the change vary widely among different antibiotics. An organism may become highly resistant to streptomycin overnight (' single step ' mutation), or within a few days to erythromycin or novobiocin, but to most other antibiotics the development of resistance is a more gradual process. In some cases the number of steps involved may be so great, and the increase in resistance with each step so slight, that the development of resistance may appear to be an almost continuous process. To some antibiotics, no substantial degree of resistance can develop at all: these include the peptides and vancomycin. It is also fortunate that in the clinical field no pathogenic species except the gonococcus has yet shown itself capable of becoming resistant to penicillin.

The two remaining processes by which resistance may be acquired involve the transfer of genetic material from a resistant cell to a sensitive.

Transduction

The transmission of capacity to produce penicillinase by a phage to a penicillin-sensitive staphylococcus was first demonstrated by Ritz and Baldwin (1958). Since then the same mechanism has been shown capable of transmitting resistance to streptomycin, tetracycline, chloramphenicol and macrolides. In their study of the latter, Pattee and Baldwin (1962) were able to transduce resistance of both the ' double ' and ' dissociated ' types (Garrod, 1957) to sensitive staphylococci, and offer the first acceptable explanation of the difference between these types. This is that the enzyme system responsible for double resistance (*i.e.* resistance to oleandomycin and other macrolides as well as to erythromycin) is constitutive, whereas that conferring dissociated resistance (resistance to erythromycin only, but also to other macrolides in the presence of erythromycin) is inducible. Transducibility is governed by the phage type of the recipient: it occurs most readily between strains each of group I or group III, is less frequent from one of these groups to the other, and never succeeds from either to a strain of group II (McDonald, 1966). Co-transduction of resistances to two antibiotics can occur, as does that of the two properties of penicillinase formation and mercury resistance, which appear therefore to be genetically linked (Richmond and John, 1964).

There are strong reasons for believing that the elements transduced are plasmids: *i.e.* extra-chromosomal particles of genetic material (Novick and Richmond, 1965), although Asheshov (1966) describes an experiment with one strain in which it seems that the material must have been chromosomal. Transduction has also been achieved *in vivo*. Jarolmen *et al.* (1965) inoculated mice intravenously with a sensitive staphylococcus, followed 6 days later by concentrated transducing phage from a strain resistant to both penicillin and tetracycline. Staphylococci resistant to tetracycline, but not to penicillin, were subsequently recovered from the kidneys, their numbers being increased by tetracycline treatment of the mice. The experiments of Novick and Morse (1967) are even more convincing: they inoculated mice intravenously with cultures of two strains of staphylococcus, a lysogenic strain possessing erythromycin resistance and another resistant to streptomycin, and recovered from the kidneys organisms resistant to both antibiotics, in numbers much greater when the mice were also treated with both. Linked penicillin-erythromycin resistance was also transduced *in vivo*.

Until recently a strain of staphylococcus described by Hashimoto *et al.* (1964) in which penicillinase formation is linked with erythromycin resistance, the two properties being regularly co-transduced (Novick and Richmond, 1965) was believed to be unique, but Evans and Waterworth (1966) have now observed two other such linkages. Among strains of staphylococci resistant to fusidic acid, one also resistant to penicillin lost both resistances together, and a second simultaneously lost resistance to tetracycline and kanamycin as well as to fusidic acid, but remained resistant to penicillin.

It is not certainly known whether and if so to what extent transduction is responsible for antibiotic resistance in clinical isolates of staphylococci, but the probability is very high that it plays a major part.

Drug resistance can also be transduced in various enterobacteria. Owing to the limited host range of phages, such transduction is for the most part intra-species, but the mechanism of transfer now to be described can operate between organisms of many different genera.

Episomal Transference by Conjugation (*Infectious Resistance*)

' Infectious ' resistance of this type was first observed in Japan in 1959 (for review of Japanese work see Watanabe, 1963), and reported in Europe first by Datta (1962) in England and by Lebek (1963) in Germany. Its recognition in the United States came late, the first descriptions (Smith and Armour, 1966; Kabins and Cohen, 1966) appearing in 1966. The earlier studies showed that in a mixed culture of a *Shigella* or *Salmonella* possessing multiple resistance (*e.g.* to sulphonamide, tetracycline, chloramphenicol and streptomycin) and a sensitive *Esch. coli,* this resistance may be transferred to a minority of cells of the latter organism, usually *en bloc* but sometimes in part. This organism can then re-transfer resistance to another pathogen. Clear clinical evidence of such transfer within the human bowel was obtained. It is now known that transfer can occur between organisms of all genera of the *Enterobacteriaceae*, and the transfer of resistance to *Serratia marcescens*, *Vibrio cholerae*, and *Pasteurella pestis* has also been observed.

The elements responsible, and transferred by conjugation, are again extra-chromosomal genetic particles (episomes or plasmids). These determine resistance in the cell possessing them, but can only be transferred to another when a second element is present, the ' resistance transfer factor ' (Anderson, 1965). A full account of studies of the mechanism of transference by conjugation is given by Datta (1965).

INFECTIOUS RESISTANCE IN ANIMALS. Much impetus has been given to the study of this subject by the alarming revelations of Anderson and his colleagues (Anderson and Datta, 1965; Anderson and Lewis, 1965; Anderson 1965, 1968) about the spread of infectious resistance among intestinal bacteria in farm animals and thence to man. Some of these observations concern pigs, but the majority calves, from over 1,000 of which *S. typhimurium* of type 29 has been recovered, all but 2·4 per cent of which were drug-resistant. This organism has also been recovered from 500 human sources. Various patterns of resistance have occurred, embracing sulphonamides, streptomycin, tetracycline, neomycin and kanamycin, ampicillin and (fortunately rarely) chloramphenicol. The frequent existence of multiple infectious resistance in *Esch. coli* from calves and pigs has been reported by Walton (1966) and by Williams Smith (1966) in strains from man, pigs and calves, and (less commonly) lambs and fowls. Some recent strains have been resistant to furazolidone, but this resistance is not transferable.

This picture of the free dissemination of multiple drug resistance, often of a high degree, among intestinal bacteria, is highly disquieting. The worst danger apprehended is the transmission of resistance *via* human *Esch. coli* to organisms of the enteric group, particularly *S. typhi*: should this species become resistant to both ampicillin and chloramphenicol, the treatment of typhoid fever would be reduced to diet and nursing. So far the nearest approach to this disaster has been the transfer of resistance to *S. paratyphi B* only during convalescence (Chabbert and Baudens, 1966).

Recent British investigators blame the excessive use of antibiotics in livestock for this state of affairs, and particularly large-scale administration in the form of feed supplements for growth promotion. On the other hand, it is far from certain how much bacterial resistance is attributable to antibiotic feed supplementation and how much to therapeutic use. That to ampicillin which appeared in 1964 was clearly the result of attempts to control enteritis in calves with therapeutic doses. It should be remembered that the only antibiotics permitted as feed supplements in Great Britain are penicillin and oxy- and chlortetracycline, and these may be given only to poultry and pigs and not to calves, although this is not to say that the regulations are always observed. Moreover the root cause of the present situation, which must be tackled if any permanent improvement is to be achieved, is bad methods of animal husbandry, notably the wholesale trade in very young calves, conducted under conditions strongly favouring the spread of infection.

In so far as the restrictions now proposed—and now brought into force—(Report, 1969) on antibiotic feed supplementation, which exclude all medically useful drugs, are designed to limit the spread of infectious resistance from livestock to man, it would be interesting to know on what scale this really occurs. A pathogen such as *S. typhimurium* can readily establish itself in the human bowel, but for large-scale transfer to occur it would be necessary for commensals such as *Esch. coli* to be capable of this, and the experiments of Williams Smith (1969) suggest that they have very little such capacity. Resistant strains of *Esch. coli* from pigs, oxen and fowls swallowed in large numbers by a human subject often failed to establish themselves at all, although two human strains were recoverable for periods up to 35 days later, and in the few instances in which transfer of resistance from an animal to the native human strain occurred, the resistant variant disappeared within a few days.

INFECTIOUS RESISTANCE IN HUMAN ENTEROBACTERIA. It seems strange that not until 1966 was any serious attempt made to discover how much drug resistance in human intestinal bacteria generally is infectious. From this time onwards a series of studies of strains from various sources has yielded remarkably consistent results. The proportion of drug-resistant strains has varied with both species and source (hospital strains being more often resistant than those from elsewhere), but a constant finding has been that transference has been achieved from over 50 per cent of cultures so tested. The organisms examined include *Salmonella* species (Schroeder, Terry and Bennett, 1967), *Shigella sonnei* (Davies, Farrant and Tomlinson, 1968), *Esch. coli, Klebsiella* and *Proteus* exclusively (Smith and Armour, 1966) or mainly (Aandahl, 1968) from urinary tract infections, and *Esch. coli* both from infections and normal faeces (Gunter and Feary, 1968), from patients in a mental hospital and from a normal population (Lewis, 1968), and from adults (Datta, 1969) and infants (Moorhouse and McKay, 1968) on admission to hospital. The last-named paper also affords evidence suggesting that a free exchange of resistant bacteria takes place between infants in hospital.

It thus appears that most antibiotic and other drug resistance in human enterobacteria is transmissible, and much of it may have arisen by transference rather than by exposure to the drug itself. This vast human reservoir of transmissible resistance must be taken into account in any attempt to assess the importance of transmission of resistant strains from animals.

THE CLINICAL PROBLEM

Staphylococci

The staphylococcus is unlikely to show a change in sensitivity to a drug administered for a single short course unless the mutation rate to resistance to that drug is very high, as is the case with streptomycin and erythromycin. This, however, is not the whole story, since in hospitals where staphylococcal infections are nursed in large open wards, cross-infection is likely to occur. If in such a ward a given antibiotic is used extensively, the staphylococcus is in fact passaged from patient to patient in the presence of the antibiotic. Under these conditions staphylococci of enhanced virulence, resistant to all the extensively used antibiotics, have emerged *in vivo*.

PENICILLIN. It is known that rare strains of *Staph. aureus* isolated before the introduction of penicillin formed penicillinase. The increasing prevalence of such strains in the hospital environment after penicillin had come into general use was first described by our late co-author Mary Barber: the frequency of their occurrence was 14, 38 and 59 per cent in the successive years 1946-48 (Barber and Rozwadowska-Dowzenko, 1948). During the next few years similar reports followed from hospitals all over the world and by about 1950 the majority of staphylococcal infections in most general hospitals were penicillin-resistant. Resistance has since then become commoner than before in strains from the general population.

OTHER ANTIBIOTICS. Resistance has subsequently appeared in certain staphylococci to all the major antibiotics. Streptomycin and tetracyclines were first affected: triple resistance to these two and to penicillin has been common in epidemic strains, and resistance to tetracycline came to be regarded as the hall mark of a dangerous strain. Chloramphenicol resistance also appeared early, but diminished in frequency when consumption diminished following recognition of marrow toxicity (Kirby and Ahern, 1953). Resistance to erythromycin can develop rapidly, and according to Lepper *et al.* (1954) resistant strains can spread very rapidly in a hospital where the antibiotic is much used: more gradual spread is described by Maccabe *et al.* (1961) and by Forfar *et al.* (1966). Resistance is also readily produced to novobiocin, but it is not often seen because this antibiotic is little used.

It is not to be supposed that any staphylococcus can acquire these characters. Multiple resistance is largely confined to a few notorious types in phage groups I and III which are also those commonly responsible for epidemics of staphylococcal sepsis (for distribution of these types in epidemics, see Williams, 1959). Multiple resistance is also linked with mercury resistance (Moore, 1960) and with high penicillinase production (Richmond *et al.*, 1964). The selective effect of the therapeutic use of other antibiotics as well as penicillin has in fact been to bring into prominence what must have been an originally very small minority of staphylococci of a few phage types.

From time to time other resistances appear. That to methicillin and other penicillinase-resistant penicillins is discussed in Chapter IV. In 1963 an apparently new strain, described as of type 'A', appeared in Scotland and the north of England, possessing multiple antibiotic resistance, including resistance to neomycin and kanamycin, and said to be of exceptional virulence (Temple and Blackburn, 1963; Mitchell, 1964). Neomycin resistance has also been reported from elsewhere (see Chapter VII).

A progressive diminution in the frequency of antibiotic resistance in staphylococci during the past few years has been reported by Bulger and Sherris (1968) in Seattle and by Thabaut and Canayer (1969) of the French Army Medical Service in Germany. The frequency of multiple resistance has also diminished in strains isolated in St. Thomas' Hospital, London (Ridley *et al.*, 1970). All these authors attribute this change, at least in part, to suitably restricted and more rationally directed antibiotic therapy.

Streptococci

Strains of both *Str. pyogenes* and *Str. pneumoniae* resistant to sulphonamides were beginning to interfere with the efficacy of treatment and to cause grave apprehension for the future when penicillin came to the rescue. Neither species appears capable of developing resistance to penicillin, but resistance to tetracycline now occurs in both. *Str. viridans* is very variable in the degree of its natural resistance to penicillin: a moderate increase in this may occur during prolonged treatment for endocarditis.

STR. FAECALIS, although fairly constant in its moderate degree of sensitivity to penicillin, is liable to be abnormally resistant to streptomycin, tetracycline and other antibiotics.

Neisseria spp.

N. GONORRHOEAE. Sulphonamide resistance in this organism, a product of selection, has eventually been followed by the development of some degree of resistance to penicillin, evidently by a different mechanism, since resistant strains were unknown for many years: resistance to other antibiotics has also been observed. The therapeutic problem posed by these changes is discussed in Chapter XXVI.

N. MENINGITIDIS. For many years cerebrospinal fever remained the only acute bacterial infection for which treatment with sulphonamides remained equal or superior to that with antibiotics. Sulphonamide resistance of a degree precluding successful treatment was first reported in 1963 (Millar *et al.*) in a Naval Training Depot in California. A report from the same State (Leedom *et al.*, 1965) extends these observations to civilians. Of 106 strains isolated from patients with meningococcal infections in the Los Angeles County General Hospital, 35 (33 per cent) were inhibited only by 10 mg. sulphonamide per 100 ml. or more, whereas 59 were inhibited by 0·5 mg. per 100 ml. or less, only 12 giving intermediate results. A majority of strains from a large epidemic at Fort Lamy (Tchad) in 1968 were sulphonamide-resistant (Lefevre *et al.*, 1969). Resistant strains have also been found in Norway (Holten *et al.*, 1969) and several other countries, but further information about their distribution is highly desirable.

All the Los Angeles strains were sensitive to penicillin and to ampicillin, with which the patients were treated. It is not to be expected that this alternative treatment will remain effective indefinitely. Miller and Bohnhoff (1947, 1948) showed long ago that meningococci could be trained to a high degree of penicillin resistance, not only *in vitro* but in experimentally infected mice. With the gonococcus as an example, resistance may be expected in the meningococcus at some time in the future.

Gram-negative Bacilli

Coliform bacilli form a group among which apparently increasing antibiotic resistance presents difficulties only exceeded by similar changes in staphylococci. No purpose would be served by reviewing the extensive and confused literature of this subject. Several processes have evidently been at work. Many authors have found that isolates in successive periods of the normally more drug-sensitive species, notably *Esch. coli*, show an increasing frequency of resistance. Secondly, the therapeutic use of antibiotics has favoured the survival and spread of organisms possessing a high degree of natural resistance, notably *Aerobacter, Pseudomonas,* and some species of *Proteus.* It seems impossible to determine whether organisms of this kind are more drug-resistant now than they were originally, but this seems highly probable. Thirdly, it now seems that a good deal of multiple resistance in intestinal bacteria may have been acquired by contact with other species (infectious resistance). However this situation may have arisen, Gram-negative infections, particularly those complicating other disease, and involving wounds, the bronchial tree or the blood-stream, are now among the most difficult to treat successfully. As they occur in the alimentary and urinary tracts, they are considered elsewhere (Chaps. XXI and XXIII).

Mycobacterium tuberculosis

This is another organism in which drug resistance menaces successful treatment, and has so far as possible to be prevented (see Chap. XXV).

PREVENTION OF BACTERIAL RESISTANCE

Some measures by which an increase in the frequency of bacterial resistance may at least be discouraged are described on page 274.

REFERENCES

AANDAHL, E. H. (1968). *Acta Path. Microbiol. scand.* **74,** 26.
ANDERSON, E. S. (1965). *Brit. med. J.* **2,** 1289.
ANDERSON, E. S. (1968). *Brit. med. J.* **3, 333.**
ANDERSON, E. S. & DATTA, N. (1965). *Lancet* **1,** 407.
ANDERSON, E. S. & LEWIS, M. J. (1965). *Nature (Lond.)* **206,** 579.
ASHESHOV, E. H. (1966). *Nature (Lond.)* **210,** 804.
BARBER, M. (1953). *J. gen. Microbiol.* **8,** 104.
BARBER, M., CSILLAG, A. & MEDWAY, A. J. (1958). *Brit. med. J.* **2,** 1377.
BARBER, M. & ROZWADOWSKA-DOWZENKO, M. (1948). *Lancet* **2,** 641.
BULGER, R. J. & SHERRIS, J. C. (1968). *Ann. intern. Med.* **69,** 1099.
CHABBERT, Y. A. & BAUDENS, J. G. (1966). *Antimicrob. Agents Chemother.* 1965, p. 380.
DATTA, N. (1962). *J. Hyg. (Lond.)* **60,** 301.
DATTA, N. (1965). *Brit. med. Bull.* **21,** 254.
DATTA, N. (1969). *Brit. med. J.* **2,** 407.
DAVIES, J. R., FARRANT, W. N. & TOMLINSON, A. J. H. (1968). *J. Hyg. (Lond.)* **66,** 471, 479.
DEAN, A. C. R. & GIORDAN, B. L. (1965). *Proc. roy. Soc. B.* **161,** 571.
DEAN, A. C. R. & HINSHELWOOD, C. (1964). *Nature (Lond.)* **202,** 1046.
DUNSMOOR, C. L., PIM, K. L. & SHERRIS, J. C. (1964). *Antimicrob. Agents Chemother.,* 1963, p. 500.
EVANS, R. J. & WATERWORTH, P. M. (1966). *J. clin. Path.* **19,** 555.
FORFAR, J. O., KEAY, A. J., MACCABE, A. F., GOULD, J. C. & BAIN, A. D. (1966). *Lancet* **2,** 295.
GARROD, L. P. (1957). *Brit. med. J.* **2,** 57.
GUNTER, A. C. & FEARY, T. W. (1968). *J. Bact.* **96,** 1556.
HASHIMOTO, H., KONO, K. & MITSUHASHI, S. (1964). *J. Bact.* **88,** 261.
HOLTEN, E., VAAGE, L., NEESS, C., MIDTVEDT, J. & JYSSUM, K. (1969). *Scand. J. infect. Dis.* **i,** 185.
JAROLMEN, H., BONDI, A. & CROWELL, R. L. (1965). *J. Bact.* **89,** 1286.
KABINS, S. A. & COHEN, S. (1966). *New Engl. J. Med.* **275,** 248.
KIRBY, W. M. M. & AHERN, J. J. (1953). *Antibiot. Chemother.* **3,** 831.

KOSSIAKOFF, M. G. (1887). *Ann. Inst. Pasteur* **i**, 465.
LEBEK, K. (1963). *Zbl. Bakt. I. Abt. Orig.* **188**, 494.
LEDERBERG, J. & LEDERBERG, E. M. (1952). *J. Bact.* **63**, 399.
LEEDOM, J. M., IVLER, D., MATHIES, A. W., THRUPP, L. D., PORTNOY, B. & WEHRLE, P. F. (1965). *New Engl. J. Med.* **273**, 1395.
LEFEVRE, M., SIROL, J., VANDEKERKOVE, M. & FAUCON, R. (1969). *Bull. Wld Hlth Org.* **40**, 331.
LEPPER, M. H., MOULTON, B., DOWLING, H. F., JACKSON, G. C. & KOFMAN, S. (1954). *Antibiot. Ann.* 1953-54, p. 308.
LEWIS, M. J. (1968). *Lancet* **1**, 1389.
LIGHTBOWN, J. W. (1954). *J. gen. Microbiol.* **11, iii.**
MACCABE, A. F., GOULD, J. C. & FORFAR, J. O. (1961). *Lancet* **2**, 7.
McDONALD, S. (1966). *Lancet* **2**, 1107.
MILLAR, J. W., SIESS, E. E., FELDMAN, H. A., SILVERMAN, C. & FRANK, P. (1963). *J. Amer. med. Ass.* **186**, 139.
MILLER, C. P. & BOHNHOFF, M. (1947). *J. infect. Dis.* **81**, 147.
MILLER, C. P. & BOHNHOFF, M. (1948). *J. infect. Dis.* **83**, 256.
MITCHELL, A. A. B. (1964). *Lancet* **1**, 859.
MOORE, B. (1960). *Lancet* **2**, 453.
MOORHOUSE, E. C. & McKAY, L. (1968). *Brit. med. J.* **2**, 741.
NOVICK, R. S. & MORSE, S. I. (1967). *J. exp. Med.* **125**, 45.
NOVICK, R. S. & RICHMOND, M. H. (1965). *J. Bact.* **90**, 467.
PANSY, F. E., KHAN, P., PAGANO, J. F. & DONOVICK, R. (1950). *Proc. Soc. exp. Biol. (N.Y.)* **75**, 618.
PATTEE, P. A. & BALDWIN, J. N. (1962). *J. Bact.* **84**, 1049.
REPORT (1969). *Joint Committee on the Use of Antibiotics in Animal Husbandry & Veterinary Medicine.* London: Her Majesty's Stationery Office.
RICHMOND, M. H. & JOHN, M. (1964). *Nature (Lond.)* **202**, 1360.
RICHMOND, M. H., PARKER, M. T., JEVONS, M. P. & JOHN, M. (1964). *Lancet* **1**, 293.
RIDLEY, M., BARRIE, D., LYNN, R. & STEAD, K. C. (1970). *Lancet* **1**, 230.
RITZ, H. L. & BALDWIN, J. N. (1958). *Bact. Proc.* p. 40.
SCHROEDER, S. A., TERRY, P. M. & BENNETT, J. V. (1967). *J. Amer. med. Ass.* **205**, 903.
SMITH, D. H. & ARMOUR, S. E. (1966). *Lancet* **2**, 15.
SMITH, G. N. & WORREL, C. S. (1950). *Arch. Biochem.* **28**, 232.
SUTHERLAND, R., SLOCOMBE, B. & ROLINSON, G. N. (1964). *Nature (Lond.)* **203**, 548.
TEMPLE, N. E. I. & BLACKBURN, E. A. (1963). *Lancet* **1**, 581.
THABAUT, A. & CANAYER, H. (1969). *Rev. Hyg. Méd. Soc.* **17**, 563.
WALTON, J. R. (1966). *Lancet* **2**, 1300.
WATANABE, T. (1963). *Bact. Rev.* **27**, 87.
WATERWORTH, P. M. (1966). *J. med. Lab. Technol.* **23**, 96.
WILLIAMS, R. E. O. (1959). *Lancet* **1**, 190.
WILLIAMS SMITH, H. (1966). *J. Hyg. (Lond.)* **64**, 465.
WILLIAMS SMITH, H. (1969). *Lancet* **1**, 1174.

PART II

Chapter XV

GENERAL PRINCIPLES OF TREATMENT

Not one of the drugs with which this book is concerned can be administered without some risk of ill effects. Many of them are costly, and many will preserve their value only if they are used with discrimination. For these and other reasons it is unjustifiable to prescribe a powerful anti-bacterial drug for most trivial infections. It is impossible to be fully dogmatic on this point, because admittedly some specially predisposing factor may convert a minor into a major infection unless steps are taken to prevent this. Such situations are exceptional, and it must regretfully be admitted that much prescribing for minor conditions goes on unnecessarily. If figures of consumption in relation to population were available, it would doubtless be found that some countries sin more gravely in this way than others.

Prescribing habits are revealed in a brilliant and tragic light in reports of fatalities from the administration of antibiotics. An astonishing proportion of deaths from penicillin shock have followed an injection given for what seems an inadequate indication, including even a common cold, toothache and a sprained toe. Likewise, some deaths from marrow aplasia have been caused by chloramphenicol administered for minor catarrhal conditions: in some instances this has even been self-administration from a left-over bottle kept in the bath-room. These are extreme examples, but they can be supported by thousands of others in which more harm than good has been done, and by untold millions in which the drug has merely been wasted because the condition treated is by nature insusceptible to it.

263

Clinical Diagnosis

Successful chemotherapy must be rational, and rational treatment demands a diagnosis. This may only be provisional, and it may later be proved wrong, but the treatment chosen should be based on some explicit assumption as to the nature of the disease process. This may or may not carry with it an implication that the cause is a particular micro-organism.

Bacteriological Diagnosis

This is in a sense more important, because treatment, to be successful, must be aimed at the micro-organism and not at the disease as such. There are fortunately many diseases which have only one microbic cause: if a clinical diagnosis of erysipelas, scarlet fever, typhoid fever, typhus or anthrax can be made, the microbic diagnosis is implicit in the clinical, and furthermore all the organisms concerned here are regularly susceptible to certain antibiotics. On the other hand pneumonia, meningitis, urinary tract infections and wound infections can be caused by any of a number of different bacteria, and the most astute clinician may sometimes be wrong if he has to guess with which of these he is dealing.

It is here that any writer on this subject is faced with his greatest difficulty. Given a patient in a hospital with a good laboratory service, a bacteriological diagnosis should soon be forthcoming. Where laboratory facilities are distant or even non-existent, how is treatment to be directed? It must be insisted that in the more serious of these infections of multiple causation, certainly in meningitis, suspected septicaemia or severe pneumonia, a bacteriological diagnosis must at all costs be made, but for the patient whose life is not in danger, it may often be necessary to dispense with laboratory aid. The choice of treatment may then be based on past experience in similar situations or on bacteriological guesswork. Some attempt will be made in this book to point to probabilities in the commoner of these situations.

Sensitivity Tests

A simple bacteriological diagnosis is not always enough. If the organism is a staphylococcus or one of the tougher coliform bacilli, there is no guarantee that it will be sensitive to the drug of obvious choice or indeed to any of those which would naturally be preferred for their usual efficacy, ease of administration and freedom from toxicity. Here again it may be a counsel of perfection to advise that an appropriate range of sensitivity tests be carried out, but there can be no certainty of effect unless this is done. Fortunately not all pathogenic bacteria are so unpredictable, and it is helpful to the clinician to know which should regularly be susceptible and which he should mistrust.

Choice of Drug

This depends in the first place on the causative organism being sensitive to the drug chosen. A comprehensive statement of normal sensitivities is given in Table XXXVIII.

There are few diagnoses which point unequivocally to a single drug for treatment. There is usually a choice, and it may be of either of two kinds.

Some conditions, such as pneumococcal pneumonia, are susceptible to several different treatments: sulphonamides, penicillin (in various forms), tetracyclines and erythromycin have all in their turn been shown to be efficacious. There is a similar wide range of choice for haemolytic streptococcal infections. A commonsense view of this choice would be that because of the certainty and rapidity of its action, its harmlessness (except in sensitized patients), and incidentally its cheapness, penicillin is to be preferred for these purposes. Sulphonamides are more slowly acting, but easily administered, cheap and almost equally innocuous: there is a good case for their use, particularly in less severe infections. Other antibiotics may be indicated because of intolerance to either of the foregoing, or because there is a suspicion of a mixed infection: the broader cover afforded by a tetracycline might then be helpful.

The second kind of choice is between a relatively harmless but less efficacious drug and one which is more potent but also more potentially toxic. This choice must take into account the severity of the condition, since naturally in a desperate situation risks not otherwise justifiable may rightly

Sensitivity of Important Pathogenic Bacteria to the Principal Antibiotics
Usual Minimum Inhibitory Concentration (μg./ml.)

	Benzyl penicillin	Methicillin	Cloxacillin	Ampicillin	Carbeni-cillin	Cephalo-ridine	Erythro-mycin	Linco-mycin	Novobiocin	Vanco-mycin	Fucidin	Tetra-cycline	Chloram-phenicol	Strepto-mycin	Kanamycin	Gentamicin	Polymyxin
Staph. aureus (a)	0·03	2	0·12	0·06	0·5	0·12	0·12	0·5-2	0·12-1	1	0·06	0·12	4-8	2	0·5	0·12-1	32
*Staph. aureus (b)	R	2	0·25	R	R	5	0·12	0·5-2	0·12-1	1	0·06	0·12	4-8	2	0·5	0·12-1	R
Str. pyogenes	0·015	0·12	0·06	0·03	0·25	0·01	0·03	0·12	0·5	0·5	4-8	0·25	2	32	128	16	R
Str. faecalis	2	32	32	2	25	16	0·5	4-16	1-16	1	4	0·5	2	64	64-128	8-16	R
Str. pneumoniae	0·015	0·25	0·25	0·06	0·5	0·03	0·03	0·5	0·5	0·5	8	0·25	2	64	128	16-32	R
Cl. welchii	0·12	1	1	0·25	0·25	0·4	2	0·5-2	1	1	0·25	0·03-0·25	4	R	R	R	R
B. anthracis	0·015	0·12	0·25	0·06	0·25	0·1	0·25	0·25-8	1	4	0·5	0·12	4	1	1	0·06	R
Ery. insidiosa	0·03	0·5	0·25	0·12	0·5	0·2	0·06	4	>64	>64	0·12	0·12	8	16	>128	>64	R
L. monocytogenes	0·25	1-4	2-4	0·12-0·5	1-2	1	0·06-0·25	2-4	2	1-2	16	0·25	4-8	1-2	0·5	0·03-0·12	R
A. israeli	0·06	4	0·25	0·06		0·015	0·12	0·06	2	2	0·5	2	2	16	16		R
Myco. tubercu-losis	R	R	R	R	R	10	R	R	R	R	64	10	30	1	5	5	R
N. gonorrhoeae	0·015	0·06	0·5	0·12	0·03-1	0·25-4	0·06	32	1-4	R	0·5	1	1	4	8	1-2	R

Bord. pertussis	1	16	16	0.5	0.25	16	0.06	8	2	>32	0.25	2	2	4	2	1	0.5
*Esch. coli	16-R	R	R	8	4	4	64	R	R	R	R	1	2-8	4	1-4	1-4	0.25
*Klebsiella-Aerobacter spp.	4-R	R	R	4-R	1-R	1-R	64-R	R	R	R	R	0.5-R	1-R	2-R	1-R	0.5-4	0.25
*Pr. mirabilis (a)	16-32	R	R	4	1	4	R	R	8-32	R	R	32-64	4-16	4-8	4-8	2-8	R
*Pr. mirabilis (b)	R	R	R	R	R	4	R	R	8-128	R	R	32-64	4-16	4-R	4-8	2-8	R
*Pr. vulgaris	R	R	R	64	2-128	128-R	R	R	2-128	R	R	4-32	4-8	2·8	1-4	1-4	R
*Pr. rettgeri	4-R	R	R	2-R	1-32	4-R	R	R	R	R	R	64-R	16-R	2-R	1-2	1-8	R
*Pr. morgani	R	R	R	128	1-8	R	R	R	16-R	R	R	4-64	4-64	4-R	2-4	1-4	R
Salmonella spp.	2-16	R	R	2	2-16	1-4	64-R	R	R	R	R	1	2	8	2-4	0.25-1	0.12
Shigella spp.	16	R	R	4	2-8	4-8	8-128	R	R	R	R	0.5-2	1-8	8	4	1-2	0.12
Ps. aeruginosa	R	R	R	R	16-256	R	R	R	R	R	R	20-R	R	16-64	64-128	1-8	0.5
Br. abortus	2-8	>32	>32	1-4	4-16	8-16	32	>32	2-16	>32	4-16	0.25-1	1	1-2	0.5-2	0.25-0.5	8-16
Past. septica	0.5	1-4	0.5-8	0.5	2	1-4	1	4-16	1	>32	1-8	0.5	0.5	2	1	1-4	0.5
Bact. fragilis	8->64	>32	32	4-16	8-16	32	4	2	>64	>32	1-32	0.5-2	8	>64	>64	>64	>16

* Strains of these species show large variations in sensitivity and should therefore always be tested.
R = Resistant; (a) = non-penicillinase-producing; (b) = penicillinase-producing.

be taken, and secondly the likelihood that toxic effects will be produced. A vital factor in this is renal function: to the extent that this is already impaired, so do the chances increase of further renal damage by nephrotoxic drugs and of damage to the eighth nerve by those which are ototoxic. Adequate laboratory control of treatment, referred to in Chapter XXVIII, can be a valuable safeguard against these effects.

Dosage and Route of Administration

The object of systemic treatment is to attain a drug concentration in the blood and tissues which is calculated to exert the effect desired, and to maintain this, either continuously or with only short intermissions, until the infection has been overcome. To devise effective treatment it is necessary to know (1) the minimum concentration of the drug necessary to inhibit or kill the infecting organism; (2) the concentration attained in the blood after a given single dose (which should exceed (1) by several-fold for most of the time between one dose and the next), and (3) the rate of elimination of the drug, on which the frequency of dosage must depend. This question therefore involves two other large subjects, the sensitivity of different microbic species, and the pharmacological behaviour of the drugs concerned, both of which are dealt with elsewhere in this book.

When there is a choice between the oral and parenteral routes of administration (as there is, for instance, for sulphonamides, penicillin and tetracyclines) the latter may be preferred in severely ill patients for the greater certainty of its effect, since the whole dose must be absorbed, whereas the whole of an oral dose never is; or to initiate treatment, since its effect is immediate. If the oral route only is used, a ' loading ' dose larger than those which follow may be advantageous, particularly with drugs which are more slowly and incompletely absorbed.

Necessary Accompanying Treatment

There are many kinds of condition in which chemotherapy cannot be expected to do the whole job of getting the patient well. It is most successful in acute uncomplicated infections, and least in those predisposed to by some structural abnormality. An obstructive lesion of the urinary tract or the bronchial dilatation and mucosal changes of bronchiectasis will cause the infection to recur unless they can be dealt with surgically. Chemotherapy does not obviate the necessity for draining an abscess or removing sequestra or calculi. General causes of diminished resistance to infection—nutritional, metabolic or due to disorders of blood formation—also require attention.

A minor example of accessory treatment which is often neglected is the control of urinary pH at the optimum for the drug administered in urinary tract infections. This is fully discussed in Chapter XXIII.

Laboratory Control of the Effects of Treatment

Whether treatment is succeeding is best judged by clinical criteria, but it is also useful to know whether the infecting organism has been eliminated: this is particularly helpful in deciding how long treatment should continue. Repeated cultures are therefore sometimes indicated if facilities for them are available. They are more decidedly called for when treatment is *not* succeeding, because one cause of failure is the replacement of the original sensitive organism by a resistant one requiring a different drug.

A more difficult service perhaps not within the competence of every laboratory is the assay of antibiotics in body fluids. This may be desirable to verify either that the concentration attained is adequate, or that it is not excessive. In the blood the level may prove inadequate if absorption from the alimentary tract is poor, or if long intervals between injections are adopted: in the cerebro-spinal fluid in meningitis treated without intrathecal injections it is reassuring to know that enough antibiotic is diffusing into the infected area. It is no less important to know that the blood level of a potentially toxic drug is not excessive: this possibility should be borne in mind when streptomycin, gentamicin, kanamycin or vancomycin have to be given to a patient with impaired renal function.

Treatment with Drug Combinations

There are five alleged indications for prescribing two antibacterial drugs together:

1. As a temporary expedient during the investigation of an obscure and serious illness.
2. Mixed infections.
3. To permit reduction in dose of a potentially toxic drug.
4. To prevent the development of bacterial resistance.
5. To achieve a synergic effect.

Of these the first three are the least valid: the blind treatment of (1) may obscure the diagnosis and so ultimately be detrimental: (2) is a purpose (exemplified by peritonitis due to perforation of the lower bowel) better served by a tetracycline, and (3) is simply untrue if the dictum be accepted that in combined treatment each drug should be given in its normal independent dose.

The importance of combined treatment in delaying the emergence of bacterial resistance has been amply verified in tuberculosis. This is a special case, because treatment must be so prolonged: the argument from it applies little to acute self-limited infections, and of course not at all to those caused by bacteria, such as haemolytic streptococci and pneumococci, treated with an antibiotic such as penicillin, to which they do not become resistant. The main question here is how far this principle applies to the treatment of infection by staphylococci. There is some evidence that it does. Lowbury (1957), working in a burns unit where sepsis is almost inevitable and cross-infection very difficult to prevent, found that when erythromycin and novobiocin were used together, the appearance of strains resistant to either was delayed, although not indefinitely prevented. A clinical experiment involving an entire hospital is described by Barber *et al.* (1960): here the adoption of a general policy of combined treatment was followed by a substantial reduction in the frequency of multiple antibiotic resistance in staphylococci isolated from all sources. Other measures taken at the same time to combat cross-infection may have contributed to this.

Types of Combined Effect

The attainment of a synergic effect, when this is possible, may be the most important indication of all. This is only one of three possible types of combined action, according to the law formulated by Jawetz and Gunnison (1952) which distinguishes between combinations according to whether each component is bactericidal (*e.g.* penicillin, streptomycin, neomycin, kanamycin) or only bacteristatic (chloramphenicol, tetracycline, erythromycin, novobiocin). The law in simple terms is that:

> Bacteristatic + bacteristatic is simply additive.
> Bactericidal + bacteristatic may be antagonistic.
> Bactericidal + bactericidal may be synergic.

BACTERISTATIC + BACTERISTATIC. Some degree of additive effect is usual when bacteristatic antibiotics are combined, but is not invariable. Synergy is very rare, although a clear example of it is the combined action of the two components of peptolide antibiotics (ostreogricin, pristinamycin, etc.). On the other hand, if synthetic drugs are included, some with perhaps not a purely bacteristatic effect, several types of combined action may be seen.

The best way of studying combined bacteristatic action is to add a series of concentrations of each drug to broth in every possible combination and to inoculate the tubes with a sensitive organism ('carré' method). Four representative results from such tests are shown in Table XXXIX. 'A' shows the result of a test with tetracycline and novobiocin acting on *Staph. aureus,* which is also referred to on p. 225. Each antibiotic behaves as if the other were not there, making no contribution to its effect whatever. 'B' is a hypothetical result showing an additive effect: the same total amount in four different proportions has the same effect as each drug acting alone. 'C' illustrates synergy: the total amount of sulphafurazole + trimethoprim required to inhibit growth is less than that of either drug acting alone. 'D' is an example of antagonism: the action of nitrofurantoin on *Proteus* spp. over a wide range of concentrations is quantitatively neutralized by nalidixic acid.

BACTERICIDAL + BACTERISTATIC. The explanation of antagonism is that bactericidal antibiotics kill only multiplying bacteria, and if growth is prevented by a bacteristatic agent, the

TABLE XXXIX

Results of Three Actual and One Hypothetical Tests of Combined
Bacteristatic Action by the Carré Method
All concentrations in μg./ml.   + = growth.   − = no growth.

TETRACYCLINE

NOVOBIOCIN	0.5	0.25	0.12	0.06	0.03	nil
0.5	−	−	−	−	−	−
0.25	−	−	−	−	−	−
0.12	−	−	+	+	+	+
0.06	−	−	+	+	+	+
0.03	−	−	+	+	+	+
nil	−	−	+	+	+	+

A

	x	x/2	x/4	x/8	x/16	nil
y	−	−	−	−	−	+
y/2	−	−	−	−	+	+
y/4	−	−	−	+	+	+
y/8	−	−	+	+	+	+
y/16	−	+	+	+	+	+
nil	+	+	+	+	+	nil

B

TRIMETHOPRIM

SULPHAFURAZOLE	16	8	4	2	1	nil
4	−	−	−	−	−	+
2	−	−	−	−	−	+
1	−	−	−	−	−	+
0.5	−	−	−	−	+	+
0.25	−	−	−	−	+	+
nil	−	+	+	+	+	+

C

NALIDIXIC ACID

NITROFURANTOIN	32	16	8	4	2	1	nil
128	−	−	−	−	−	−	−
64	−	+	+	+	+	+	+
32	−	−	+	+	+	+	+
16	−	−	+	+	+	+	+
8	−	−	−	+	+	+	+
4	−	−	−	+	+	+	+
2	−	−	−	−	+	+	+
1	−	−	−	−	+	+	+
nil	−	−	−	−	−	+	+

D

A—Indifferent. Tetracycline and novobiocin v *Staph. aureus.*
B—Additive. The two drugs have an equal effect in all proportions as
the same concentration of each acting alone.
C—Synergic, Trimethoprim and sulphafurazole v *N. gonorrhoeae.*
D—Antagonistic. Nitrofurantoin and nalidixic acid v *Proteus mirabilis.*

condition requisite for this action is removed. Such interference is readily demonstrable in experimental infections, and a clear clinical example of it is the much higher mortality in pneumococcal meningitis observed by Lepper and Dowling (1951) when chlortetracycline was given in addition to penicillin. That chloramphenicol also interferes with the bactericidal of penicillin in meningitis is shown by the experimental studies of Wallace *et al.* (1967). Giving chlortetracycline in addition to penicillin for the treatment of streptococcal pharyngitis apparently interfered with the elimination of the organism from the throat, although therapeutic results were satisfactory (Strom, 1955). It is better in general to avoid administering any penicillin (and particularly methicillin) together with a tetracycline or chloramphenicol.

BACTERICIDAL + BACTERICIDAL. The synergy which may be exerted by such a combination is chiefly important for its total bactericidal effect on organisms, particularly *Str. faecalis* or other penicillin-resistant streptococci, causing bacterial endocarditis. Whatever definition of synergy may be preferred, an effect so different as total sterilization from the partial bactericidal action of the two components must surely deserve this description. These combinations are discussed in connection with the treatment of endocarditis in Chapter XVII, where it is pointed out that staphylococcal as well as some streptococcal infections may call for this kind of treatment. Whenever it is proposed to use a combination for so serious a purpose as this its effect should be verified by appropriate *in vitro* test, and others should be examined if the effect is inadequate.

COMMERCIAL COMBINATIONS. The claims made for most commercial combinations are exaggerated, and the use of these preparations is in general to be discouraged. Many consist of penicillin and streptomycin, and although this has an important use just described, no one is likely to use such a commercial combination for treating endocarditis, since the proportions of the two constituents are wrong for this purpose: that of penicillin needs to be higher. These products are mainly used for purposes which often do not require such a combination at all, whether the 'blind' treatment of infection of unknown nature, or as cover for surgical operations, including those for which no such precaution should be necessary. Many patients have quite unnecessarily suffered eighth nerve damage from streptomycin or dihydrostreptomycin in such combinations administered in this way: such damage is most likely to occur in those with unrecognized impairment of renal function, who fail to excrete the antibiotic at the normal rate. Naumann (1966) who roundly condemns these combinations for the reasons given here, adds information about the frequent present-day resistance of Gram-negative species to streptomycin which deprives the combination of its expected broad spectrum effect.

Most other commercial combinations contain bacteristatic antibiotics, and there is no evidence in the extensive studies of Finland and his colleagues (reviewed by Garrod, 1965) that any of these exert an effect superior to that of the more active of their constituents. In a separate category are mixtures of tetracyclines with anti-fungal antibiotics, the merits of which are discussed on p. 240.

Concerted Policies in Antibiotic Prescribing

This chapter has hitherto been concerned with the welfare of the individual patient. The community has also to be considered, since it has been abundantly proved that the more some antibiotics are used, the less useful do they become, because the frequency of bacterial resistance to them increases correspondingly. To counter this tendency, policies in prescribing have been adopted in hospitals or hospital groups, in areas, and in one instance at least, throughout an entire country. They are of four kinds: (1) *restriction,* the use of an antibiotic being reserved for cases in which nothing else will serve; (2) *rotation,* an antibiotic being used until resistance appears and then replaced by another with similar action: while the second is being used, resistance to the first will diminish again; (3) *diversification,* or the prescribing of a wide variety, no single antibiotic being used enough to provoke frequent resistance; (4) *combinations,* an apparently successful application of which has already been cited.

These measures were mainly designed to ensure that there shall always be an effective antibiotic for treating severe staphylococcal infections. There are now so many antibiotics available for this purpose, including the new penicillins un-affected by penicillinase, that the danger of having to stand with folded hands before the bed of such a patient has receded into at least a fairly distant future. The deliberate adoption of any of these policies may now therefore seem less urgent, although the danger of selecting staphylococci of high virul-ence by the process which selects drug-resistant strains (see p. 258) must be borne in mind. However, none of them can rival in the importance of its effects a general restriction of the antibiotics, particularly in prophylaxis, to really necessary purposes.

An altogether new situation has been created by the discovery that drug resistance, often multiple, can readily be transferred by contact between various Gram-negative bac-teria, notably from *Esch. coli* to intestinal pathogens. It so happens that in this country this mode of acquiring resistance has been most actively studied in *S. typhimurium* in farm animals, whence infection by resistant strains has spread on a considerable scale to man (see Chap. XIV). It has been suggested that this menacing situation demands a review of the use of antibiotics in animals and perhaps the imposition of restrictions on this. These have already been applied to the use of medical antibiotics for growth promotion. In view of the fact that animal pathogens are much more able than commen-sals to colonise the human bowel, steps to limit the indiscrimin-ate and often ineffective use of antibiotics for treating enteritis in farm animals might be helpful.

REFERENCES

BARBER, M., DUTTON, A. A. C., BEARD, M. A., ELMES, P. C. & WILLIAMS, R. (1960). *Brit. med. J.* **i**, 11.
GARROD, L. P. (1965). *S. Afr. med. J.* **39**, 607.
JAWETZ, E. & GUNNISON, J. B. (1952). *Antibiot. and Chemother.* **2**, 243.
LEPPER, M. H. & DOWLING, H. F. (1951). *Arch. intern. Med.* **88**, 489.
LOWBURY, E. J. L. (1957). *Lancet* **ii**, 305.
NAUMANN, P. (1966). *Dtsch. med. Wschr.* **91**, 1152.
STROM, J. (1955). *Antibiot. Med.* **1**, 6.
WALLACE, J. F., SMITH, R. H., GARCIA, M. & PETERSDORF. R. G. (1967). *J. Lab. clin. Med.* **70**, 408.

Chapter XVI

DOSAGE

NORMAL doses are specified in appendices to earlier chapters, and some indications for increasing these are mentioned in the text. We are here concerned with situations in which normal dosage needs to be modified, and with other problems of administration.

DOSAGE IN CHILDREN

In general dosage may be related to that for the adult on a body weight basis. Calculation based on body surface area has been suggested for younger children, but this system is not widely accepted. Different considerations altogether apply in the first few weeks of life, when excessive or even moderate doses of antibacterial drugs such as chloramphenicol, streptomycin and sulphonamides can have disastrous effects. Nyhan (1961), who discusses these dangers and the reasons for them, makes a plea for fuller study of ' neonatal pharmacology '. The main reasons for these effects is the elementary state of development of both hepatic and renal function. The liver cannot conjugate drugs which are normally so disposed of at the usual rate, notably chloramphenicol and sulphonamides. The kidneys have a poorly developed capacity to excrete all drugs, with the result that they attain much higher levels in the blood, falling more slowly.

The difficult task of studying this behaviour of antibiotics in the neonatal period has been tackled recently in Germany and the United States. Von Harnack *et al.* (1964, 1965) administered single doses of oxacillin to infants of different ages, older children and adults, and found that in the first week of life a standard dose based on body surface area produced blood levels 4 times higher than those attained in older children: at 2-4 weeks the level attained was already lower. Boe *et al.* (1967) found the blood levels attained after a dose of methicillin based on body weight to be very high in the first 24 hours of life, falling progressively at 4-5, 8-9, 13-15 and 26-30 days. An even more rapid increase in the capacity to excrete benzyl penicillin was demonstrated by Abramowicz *et al.* (1966), with differences between the findings in 12 hours, 13-14 hours, 26-62 hours and thence to 7 days. Axline, Yaffe and Simon (1967) determined the half-life of ampicillin in infants aged 2-7, 8-14, 15-30 and 31-68 days to be 4·0, 2·8, 1·7 and 1·6 hours respectively. Similar results were obtained with methicillin, oxacillin and neomycin, but not with colistin, the half-life of which remained unchanged throughout the neonatal period.

Since penicillins are non-toxic, even at this age, this slow elimination is an advantage: shortly after birth a 12-hour interval between doses will give a sustained effect, shortened through 8- and 6-hours to the usual 4-hourly schedule at 4 weeks of age (Boe *et al.*, 1967). Reduced daily doses are naturally imperative for antibiotics causing toxic effects. Most of the authors responsible for these studies have included premature infants in their tests, and found, as would be expected, that elimination in them is even slower.

DOSAGE IN RENAL DISEASE

It is frequently necessary to administer anti-bacterial drugs to patients with renal disease, either for the treatment of that disease itself or when other disease has impaired renal function. It has then to be considered whether deficient elimination will lead to dangerous accumulation if ordinary doses are given. Several factors determine the answer to this question.

STABILITY IN THE BODY. Most antibiotics and other anti-bacterial drugs are highly stable and persist almost indefinitely if elimination is prevented. On the other hand, cephalothin (in contrast to cephaloridine), oxacillin and to a lesser extent cloxacillin, are unstable, and their half-lives remain short even in advanced renal failure. Since their degradation products are apparently non-toxic, little reduction in the dose given may be necessary.

BILIARY EXCRETION. Not more than 5 per cent of a dose of novobiocin or erythromycin is excreted in the urine, the main excretory route being in the bile. Much of a dose of any rifamycin derivative follows the same path. Hence defective renal excretion demands little or no alteration of dosage.

DEGREE OF TOXICITY. The factor by which the usual blood level must be increased to produce toxic effects is vital. For some drugs this is small, but for penicillins it is very large, and there is a corresponding latitude in permissible concentrations. We are aware of no record of overdosage of methicillin or ampicillin, and in treatment with carbenicillin for a systemic pseudomonas infection poor renal function is a positive advantage in enabling the necessary very high blood levels to be more easily maintained. Effects of overdosage with benzyl penicillin (p. 63) have certainly been seen, but this is the only antibiotic of which such a daily dose as 60 g. (*i.e.* 100 mega units) is ever thought to be indicated, and the simple avoidance of such excessive doses will often be a sufficient precaution.

There are thus many important antibiotics which can safely be given in ordinary doses to patients with renal disease. Among those outside this category, another factor has to be considered: apart from any other toxicity they possess, can they enhance pre-existing damage to the kidney itself?

NEPHROTOXICITY. Polymyxins, bacitracin, kanamycin and to some extent other aminoglycosides and amphotericin B are directly nephrotoxic, and should be used with caution in severe renal disease for this reason. Cephaloridine should probably be placed in the same category. Methicillin has occasionally caused renal damage, but this risk is probably too remote to be a contra-indication even to giving large doses. Tetracyclines cause no direct renal damage, but by their anti-anabolic effect increase the work load on the kidney, and a rise in blood urea results: their use is better avoided.

CONTROL OF DOSAGE. Reduction in dosage may be required, not only to avert further renal damage but to guard against other effects, notably the ototoxicity of the aminoglycosides and vancomycin. Schemes for regulating the doses of two aminoglycosides according to the degree of impairment of renal function have been proposed: for kanamycin Sørenen *et al.* (1967) and for gentamicin by Gingell and Waterworth (1968). Reduction is achieved by prolonging the interval between doses rather than by reducing the dose itself. Control by assays of blood content is highly desirable.

This subject was well reviewed in a paper by Kunin (1967) in which many items of information bearing on it are extensively tabulated. In the present state of knowledge there must still be many gaps in such a table, and in particular, estimates of the degree of retention and of necessary prolongation of inter-dose intervals are so dependent on the degree of renal damage that no single figure for them is valid. In practice lesser and unrecognized impairment of function is almost more important than overt renal disease: there are innumerable reports of ototoxic effects from aminoglycosides in such patients.

DIALYSIBILITY. It may be important to know whether excessive blood levels can be reduced by haemodialysis. Information on this is incomplete and sometimes contradictory, but some important facts are well established, notably that all the aminoglycosides (streptomycin, kanamycin, gentamicin) can be removed in this way. Vancomycin, another ototoxic drug, cannot. Other antibiotics of which the levels can be reduced are cephaloridine, cycloserine (by peritoneal dialysis), tetracyclines and chloramphenicol. Penicillins, including methicillin (Bulger *et al.*, 1964) and ampicillin (Ruedy, 1966) appear to be little affected, but according to Eastwood and Curtis (1968) haemodialysis reduces the level of carbenicillin. Lincomycin is unaffected. Findings with regard to polymyxins are contradictory: Goodwin and Friedman (1968) found haemodialysis ineffective and peritoneal dialysis effective in lowering the blood level of sodium colistmethate whereas Curtis and Eastwood (1968) report precisely the opposite.

Antibiotics are sometimes added to peritoneal dialysis fluid for the prevention or treatment of peritonitis. Not only a local but a systemic effect can be secured by this proceeding (Bulger, Bennett and Boen, 1965; Buck and Cohen, 1968).

INCOMPATIBILITIES

In a patient under treatment with two anti-bacterial drugs, it is necessary to know whether they can be mixed for intramuscular injection or added together to an intravenous infusion fluid. Compatibility with the constituents of such a fluid and with other ingredients such as heparin has also to be considered.

A recent series of publications (Meisler and Skolaut, 1966; Patel and Phillips, 1966; Fowler, 1967; Webb, 1969; Lynn,

10

TABLE XL

Compatibility chart (triangular half-matrix). Both axes carry the same list of substances; each cell gives the compatibility of the row substance with the column substance. C = compatible; − = incompatible; Ct = compatible for a limited time; * = see footnote.

Column (and row) key:

1. Ampicillin sodium
2. Carbenicillin sodium
3. Cephalothin sodium
4. Cephaloridine
5. Chloramphenicol succinate
6. Cloxacillin sodium
7. Colistimethate
8. Erythromycin lactobionate
9. Fucidin (as diethanolamine fusidate)
10. Gentamicin sulphate
11. Kanamycin sulphate
12. Lincomycin hydrochloride
13. Methicillin sodium
14. Novobiocin sodium
15. Penicillin G
16. Polymyxin B sulphate
17. Streptomycin sulphate
18. Tetracycline hydrochloride
19. Vancomycin hydrochloride
20. Heparin sodium
21. Hydrocortisone sodium succinate
22. Isotonic saline solution
23. 5% Dextrose in water
24. Amino acid solution
25. Lactated Ringer's solution

	2	3	4	5	6	7	8	9	10	11	12	13	14	15	16	17	18	19	20	21	22	23	24	25
1. Ampicillin sodium	C	C		C	−		−	−	−	C		−	C	−							Ct	*		
2. Carbenicillin sodium		C	−		C	−		C	C	−		C		−	−						Ct	Ct	−	C
3. Cephalothin sodium			C	−		−	−		−	−	−	C		C	−		−				C	C	−	C
4. Cephaloridine				C	C		C	−	C			C	C		C	C		C	C		C	C		C
5. Chloramphenicol succinate					C	C	−	C	C	−		C		C	−		−				C	C	−	C
6. Cloxacillin sodium						−	−		−	−	−	C	C		C	−		−			C	C		C
7. Colistimethate							C	*	C		C	C	−		C		−				C	−		C
8. Erythromycin lactobionate								−	−	C	C	−	−		−	C		−	C		C	C	−	C
9. Fucidin (as diethanolamine fusidate)									C	C	−								C		C			C
10. Gentamicin sulphate										−	−	C	C	−	−		−	C			C	C	−	C
11. Kanamycin sulphate											−	−	C	C		C		−	C		C	−		
12. Lincomycin hydrochloride												C	C	−	−	C	C	C		C		C	C	−	C
13. Methicillin sodium													C	−	−	C	C	C		C	−	Ct	Ct	−	C
14. Novobiocin sodium														C	C	C	−	−		C	−	C	C	−	C
15. Penicillin G															C	−	−		−	C	−	C	C	−	C
16. Polymyxin B sulphate																−	−		−	C	−	C	C	−	C
17. Streptomycin sulphate																	−		−	C		C	C		C
18. Tetracycline hydrochloride																		−		C	−	C	Ct	−	C
19. Vancomycin hydrochloride																			−		−	C	C	−	C
20. Heparin sodium																				−		C	C	−	−
21. Hydrocortisone sodium succinate																						C	C	−	−

1970) provides much information about the compatibilities of anti-bacterial and many other drugs: some of these findings together with data from Martindale (1967) and with information kindly supplied to us by manufacturers* are condensed in Table XL. Published data are based largely on the physical effects of mixing solutions, and a more subtle change than the formation of a visible precipitate cannot always be excluded. Thus Lynn (personal communication, 1970) determined the effect of mixing solutions of methicillin and kanamycin by actual assays of antibiotic activity, and found that although kanamycin was unaffected, there was rapid loss of methicillin activity (20-30 per cent in 15 minutes). The data in Table XL, although extensive, are incomplete, but they may serve as some guide to what is possible and what should be avoided.

It has recently been reported by Simberkoff *et al.* (1970) that penicillins lose activity rapidly in solutions containing glucose, sucrose or dextran together with bicarbonate.

LOCAL ADMINISTRATION

It may be good practice to introduce a solution, usually of an antibiotic, into an infected cavity, such as a thoracic empyema. A special instance of such treatment is intrathecal injection, the pros and cons of which are discussed in describing the treatment of meningitis (*q.v.*). Different considerations apply to the local treatment of a superficial infected surface. The application of sulphonamide powders to wounds, and of antibiotic creams to burns and areas of dermatitis, has been abandoned by some because such application is believed to carry a special risk of causing sensitization. It is therefore advised that only antibiotics which are unlikely to be employed systemically should be applied in this way, and those often chosen are bacitracin, neomycin and polymyxin. (It should not too lightly be assumed that any of these, and polymyxin in particular, will never be needed for systemic use.)

Assuming that this idea of a special reactivity in the skin is correct, does it also exist in other epithelial surfaces? Penicillin and other antibiotics can be used locally for the treat-

* We are indebted for this to Aspro-Nicholas Ltd., Beecham Pharmaceutical Division, Eli Lilly & Co., Glaxo Research Ltd. and Upjohn Ltd.

ment of conjunctivitis (or the prevention of ophthalmia neonatorum), and they have been sprayed into the nose and the bronchi. Penicillin pastilles were first recommended for the treatment of Vincent's and other infections in the mouth by MacGregor and Long (1944): penicillin chewing gum is now strongly advocated for this purpose by Emslie *et al.* (1962). Should applications like these also be frowned on because of a risk of sensitization? The idea that they should derives largely from an emphatic statement by Guthe, Idsøe and Willcox (1958) in a paper concerned with reactions to penicillin in patients treated for venereal disease. They say: ' Its topical use should be abandoned. The inclusion of penicillin in toothpaste, chewing gum and similar substances is indefensible.' In so far as this refers to preparations like toothpaste freely available to the public, everyone will agree with this statement, but as a general condemnation of all legitimate topical use it may be disputed. In the overwhelming majority of patients sensitized to penicillin there is a history of previous parenteral treatment, and the few examples cited by these authors in which there was a history of local application have little evidential value. Unless evidence can be produced that topical use sensitizes more often than parenteral it seems unjustifiable to prohibit some unquestionably useful forms of topical therapy. Some inquiry also seems advisable into the relative degrees of sensitizing effect of application to different kinds of body surface. If mucous membranes are to be equated with the skin, then presumably all oral administration should come under the same ban.

REFERENCES

ABRAMOWICZ, M., KLEIN, J. O., IGNALL, D. & FINLAND, M. (1966). *Amer. J. Dis. Child.* **111**, 267.

AXLINE, S. G., YAFFE, S. J. & SIMON, H. J. (1967). *Pediatrics* **39**, 9.

BOE, R. W., WILLIAMS, C. P. S., BENNETT, J. V. & OLIVER, T. K. (1967). *Paediatrics* **39**, 194.

BUCK, A. C. & COHEN, S. L. (1968). *J. clin. Path.* **21**, 88.

BULGER, R. J., BENNETT, J. V. & BOEN, S. T. (1965). *J. Amer. med. Ass.* **194**, 1198.

BULGER, R. J., LINDHOLM, D. D., MURRAY, J. S. & KIRBY, W. M. M. (1964). *J. Amer. med. Ass.* **187**, 319.

CURTIS, J. R. & EASTWOOD, J. B. (1968). *Brit. med. J.* **1**, 484.

EASTWOOD, J. B. & CURTIS, J. R. (1968). *Brit. med. J.* **1**, 486.

EMSLIE, R. D., CROSS, W. G. & BLAKE, G. C. (1962). *Brit. med. J.* **112**, 320.

FOWLER, T. J. (1967). *Amer. J. Hosp. Pharm.* **24**, 450.

GINGELL, J. C. & WATERWORTH, P. M. (1968). *Brit. med. J.* **2**, 19.

GOODWIN, N. J. & FRIEDMAN, E. A. (1968). *Ann. intern. Med.* **68,** 984.
GUTHE, T., IDSØE, O. & WILLCOX, R. R. (1958). *Bull. Wld Hlth Org.* **19,** 427.
KUNIN, C. M. (1967). *Ann. intern. Med.* **67,** 151.
LYNN, B. (1970). *J. Hosp. Pharm.* **28,** 71.
MACGREGOR, A. B. & LONG, D. A. (1944). *Brit. med. J.* **2,** 686.
MARTINDALE, [W]. (1967). *The Extra Pharmacopoeia,* Ed. R. G. Todd, 25th
   Ed. London Pharmaceutical Press.
MEISLER, J. M. & SKOLAUT, M. W. (1966). *Amer. J. Hosp. Pharm.* **23,** 557.
NYHAN, W. L. (1961). *J. Pediat. (St. Louis)* **59,** 1.
PATEL, J. A. & PHILLIPS, G. L. (1966). *Amer. J. Hosp. Pharm.* **23,** 409.
RUEDY, J. (1966). *Canad. med. Ass. J.* **94,** 257.
SIMBERKOFF, M. S., THOMAS, L., MCGREGOR, D., SHENKIN, J. & LEVINE, B. B.
   (1970). *New Eng. J. Med.* **238,** 116.
SØRENEN, A. W. S., SZABO, L., PEDERSEN, A. & SCHARFF, A. (1967). *Postgrad.
   med. J.* Suppl. May, 37.
VON HARNACK, G. A., NAUMANN, P., BLUNCK, W., MAI, K. & WINTZER, G.
   (1964). *Dtsch. med. Wschr.* **89,** 2321.
VON HARNACK, G. A., NAUMANN, P., MAI, K. & BLUNCK, W. (1965). *Dtsch.
   med. Wschr.* **90,** 1433.
WEBB, J. W. (1969). *Amer. J. Hosp. Pharm.* **26,** 31.

CHAPTER XVII

SEPTICAEMIA AND ENDOCARDITIS

THERE has been a profound change in the bacterial aetiology
of septicaemia in recent years. Blood-stream infection by
haemolytic streptococci, formerly common, is now very rarely
seen, because of the complete control which penicillin exerts
over the earliest stages of infection by this organism. Staphylococcal infections have not been so well controlled, and in the
experience of Finland *et al.* (1959) at the Boston City Hospital,
there has been a large increase in septicaemia due to various
coliform bacilli. The nett result of these changes, and of the
substitution of infections more refractory to treatment for those
prevalent before, has in Finland's experience been an actually
higher mortality from septicaemia than that recorded in 1935.

In proposing treatment for septicaemia, everything depends
on an exact bacteriological diagnosis, and much on the sensitivities of the organism, which should be accurately determined
to individual appropriate antibiotics and if necessary to combinations. The following are provisional suggestions for each
causative organism, some of which can only be tentative, since
optimum treatment must be based on laboratory studies of the
individual strain.

STREPTOCOCCUS PYOGENES (A). This now most uncommon
infection should always respond to benzyl penicillin.

STAPHYLOCOCCUS AUREUS. Treatment should be begun
with cloxacillin as soon as the diagnosis is verified or even
strongly suspected, since the strain is likely to be penicillin-
resistant. Should it subsequently prove sensitive, it is better to
change to benzyl penicillin. Should the patient not respond,
treatment directed as for *Staph. aureus* endocarditis (q.v.) is
advisable.

COLIFORM INFECTIONS. These, unless transitory and inci-
dental to an infection of the urinary tract from which recovery
is possible, tend to occur in patients gravely ill from other

causes, and the prognosis is consequently poor. For each type of organism which may be responsible there are alternative treatments, and experience with some of these is so far too limited for assessment of their relative merits. Degrees of bacterial sensitivity to some of these drugs are not constant (*e.g.* sensitivity to ampicillin in *Esch. coli* varies considerably), and all the resources of the laboratory should be mobilized to provide accurate information as soon as possible. Among antibiotics, those likely to be indicated are for : —

Esch. coli—ampicillin, cephaloridine, kanamycin, polymyxin.

Proteus—ampicillin, cephaloridine (in each case for some species or strains only), kanamycin.

Klebsiella—polymyxin, cephaloridine (some strains only), kanamycin (also variable).

Pseudomonas—polymyxin, gentamicin, carbenicillin.

Serratia—gentamicin (Wilfert, Barrett and Kass, 1968; Martin *et al.*, 1969).

The combination of trimethoprim and a sulphonamide has also been successfully used in the first two of these infections.

A special variety of this type of infection is ' *bacteriaemic shock* ', severe hypotension of sudden onset assumed to be produced by endotoxin from large numbers of bacteria in the circulation. It occurs most commonly after surgical interference with an already infected urinary tract, often transurethral prostatic resection, but sometimes no more than cystoscopy or the blockage or removal of a catheter (Talbot, 1962). Among other procedures, pelvic operations are a cause. In the extensive series reported by Weil, Shubin and Biddle (1964) shock accompanied 169 out of 692 cases of Gramnegative bacteriaemia, with a mortality of 82 per cent. The commonest infecting organism is *Esch. coli; Klebsiella Aerobacter* spp. come next, then *Proteus* spp.; *Ps. aeruginosa* is a rare cause. This condition calls for immediate anti-bacterial treatment even before verification by blood culture, and the most appropriate antibiotic is kanamycin, of which 2 g. should be administered daily for the first two days, pending laboratory results. Its bactericidal effect on most of the commonly causative bacteria commends it in preference to chloramphenicol and oxytetracycline, which are suggested by Weil *et al.* on the basis of static sensitivity tests on their strains. Polymyxin may be given in addition to afford even broader cover. Gentamicin is a possible alternative to kanamycin.

CANDIDA ALBICANS. Septicaemia is sometimes caused by this organism, usually in patients in whom its overgrowth in the respiratory or alimentary tract has followed treatment with tetracyclines. Some good can be done by the application of nystatin to the primarily infected surface, but a systemic effect can best be exerted with amphotericin B.

Acute Endocarditis

This condition is liable to complicate almost any uncontrolled septicaemia, and much that has already been said therefore applies to it. Since it will be necessary to kill all the bacteria embedded in vegetations, the choice of a bactericidal drug is even more imperative, and treatment will need to be longer continued. Gonococcal and pneumococcal endocarditis, not hitherto mentioned, were sometimes classified as acute: they are now very rarely seen. Each of these infections and the endocarditis sometimes complicating 'chronic' meningococcal septicaemia, should respond to benzyl penicillin, again with the proviso that in the treatment of endocarditis the course of treatment must be greatly extended.

Subacute Endocarditis

Antibiotics have transformed the outlook in this disease more than in any other. Formerly invariably fatal, the infection can now be cured in most patients by well-directed treatment, although severe residual damage to valves may limit the period of survival.

The diagnosis must be verified, if possible, by blood culture, and the organism found should be exactly identified. Further, this is a disease in which something more than ordinary antibiotic sensitivity tests is called for. If penicillin appears to be the antibiotic of choice, its minimum inhibitory concentration should be determined by a tube dilution test with no more than two-fold differences. If this concentration proves to be unduly high, it cannot be assumed that penicillin will be fully bactericidal, and tests should be undertaken to determine how such an effect can be achieved: a combination will often be necessary (Chap. XXVIII).

Consideration in further detail must be in relation to the causative organisms.

STREPTOCOCCUS VIRIDANS. This is not really a species, but a highly heterogeneous group of streptococci having little else necessarily in common except the property of alpha-haemolysis. In addition an endocarditis may be caused by streptococci, presumably derived from the mouth, which are non-haemolytic or have some other peculiar character: some, for instance, are micro-aerophilic. What follows refers to any streptococcus which is neither *Str. pyogenes* nor *Str. faecalis*.

Such organisms are usually highly sensitive to penicillin. Of 339 strains quantitatively tested in the extensive collaborative study reported on by Cates and Christie (1951), 291 were not more than twice as resistant as the Oxford staphylococcus: *i.e.,* they were inhibited by about 0·05 unit (0·03 μg.) per ml. or less. Penicillin alone has served well for the treatment of such infections. The total dose of 2 mega units daily suggested by these authors seems modest by present-day standards, and is now often exceeded. The interval between doses is as important as the total dose, and should probably not exceed six hours if ' soluble ' penicillin is used, since it is almost certainly advisable to maintain a continuous effect.

Systems of treatment which attain lower maximum blood concentrations have also been shown to succeed in fully sensitive infections. Either an adequate dose (say 1 mega unit) of procaine penicillin can be given twice daily, or an acid-resistant penicillin may be given orally. If this is done, the activity of the chosen penicillin against the patient's streptococcus should be tested: it cannot be assumed that this will be the same as that of benzyl penicillin. Phenoxymethyl penicillin should be given in doses of at least 1-2 mega units four-hourly : gastric intolerance sometimes results and injections may then have to be substituted. Propicillin was successful in nine out of ten patients treated by Gray *et al.* (1964) in doses not exceeding 2·5 g. daily, but reinforced in some patients with probenecid, an additional treatment which seems always to be advisable when the maintenance of an adequate blood concentration is in any doubt. Such well tolerated treatment should perhaps always be continued for six weeks.

It is maintained by some that streptomycin should always be given in addition to penicillin even for these fully penicillin-sensitive infections. This is certainly questionable when there is any impairment of renal function and consequent risk of ototoxicity. It is doubtful even apart from this consideration, unless it be accepted that a course of such combined treatment can safely be shorter—some say only two weeks—and this is held to be an important advantage in an individual case. The pros and cons of these alternatives are well discussed by Dormer (1960).

Strains of these streptococci which are somewhat more resistant than this to penicillin may be dealt with adequately by increasing the dose, but it is advisable to verify that the concentration reached in the blood is fully bactericidal *in vitro*. Higher degrees of resistance bring the organism into the same therapeutic category as the following species.

STREPTOCOCCUS FAECALIS. Endocarditis due to this organism has been said to occur in women of 25 and men of 60, the respective sources of infection being the uterus after abortion and the urinary tract, and our experience tallies closely with this statement. It occurs occasionally in other kinds of patient, including even children. The antibiotics to which the streptococcus is most sensitive *in vitro* are almost always the tetracyclines, but treatment with these, or with erythromycin or chloramphenicol, almost invariably fails. These are bacteristatic drugs, and it should be an axiom that for the treatment of endocarditis generally a bactericidal antibiotic or combination is essential. Unless the vegetation is sterilized—even if a single coccus remains, damaged but viable—relapse is likely to follow.

Penicillin in optimal concentration (6 μg./ml.) is bactericidal, but not completely so: some survivors remain (Jawetz, 1952). In a recent paper Jawetz and Sonne (1966) report that penicillin was totally bactericidal for two out of ten strains, but support this with no clinical evidence: all their nine patients were treated with combinations of penicillin and other antibiotics. Two out of nine cases described by Toh and Ball (1960) were successfully treated with penicillin alone, but the sensitivity of these strains to penicillin was so exceptional (M.I.C. 0·1 and 0·05 μg./ml.) that they must have been highly

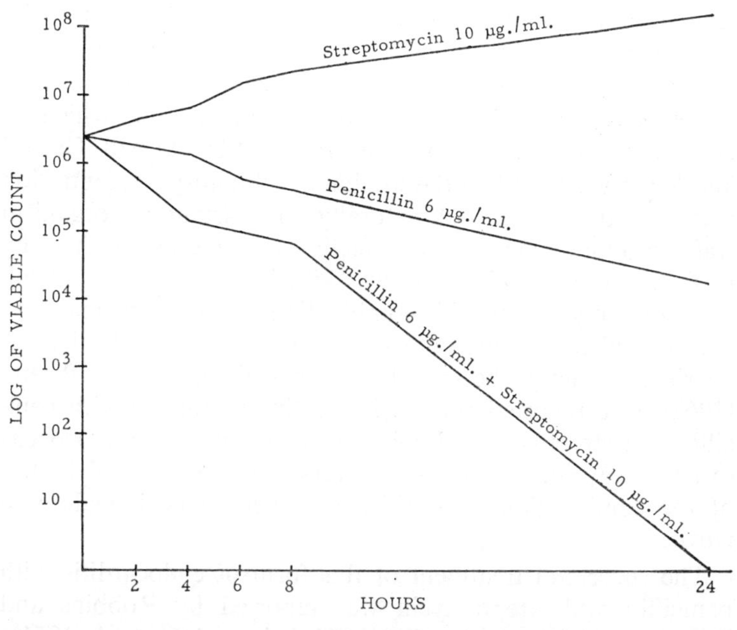

FIG. 22

Viable counts in broth containing an optimal concentration of penicillin (6 μg./ml.), streptomycin (10 μg./ml.) or both, and inoculated with a strain of *Str. faecalis* (G.F.) from the blood of a patient with bacterial endocarditis. Penicillin causes only a slow fall in the viable count. Streptomycin fails to prevent growth (M.I.C. was 16 μg./ml.): the combination sterilizes the preparation. This combination was used successfully in treating not only the original attack of endocarditis but a recurrence eight months later.

atypical. The experience of others has been that penicillin alone will not eradicate this infection. It appears that the same is true of ampicillin, to which the organism is rather more sensitive (a difference of about two-fold). Gray *et al.* (1964) refer to it as ' the penicillin of choice ' for this infection, but of their two patients treated with it, one was also given erythromycin throughout, and the other relapsed and had to be re-treated with ampicillin + streptomycin.

It is now well recognized that in contrast to the limited bactericidal activity of penicillins, penicillin and streptomycin acting together are truly synergic, in the sense that they do something of which neither alone is capable under any conditions: they totally exterminate the organism (Fig. 22). This is true even if the concentration of streptomycin used is incapable when acting alone even of inhibiting growth, as is shown in this figure. The limiting degree of sensitivity to streptomycin is not known, but there is one beyond which no effect can be expected. In a case reported by Havard, Garrod and Waterworth (1959) the minimum inhibitory concentration was 50,000 μg./ml. and naturally so resistant an organism was no more affected by penicillin + streptomycin than by penicillin alone. This strain was killed *in vitro* only by penicillin + neomycin, and this combination was used in treatment with complete success, but at the cost of almost total loss of hearing. It should be added here that Tompsett and Pizette (1962) have reported success in treating two cases with penicillin and streptomycin despite resistance of the streptococcus to streptomycin, in one case of very high degree, and failure of the combination to sterilize a rather heavy inoculum *in vitro*.

The successful treatment of this form of endocarditis with penicillin and streptomycin was reported by Robbins and Tompsett (1951) and by Cates, Christie and Garrod (1951): experience at St. Bartholomew's Hospital reported in the second of these papers has been verified in numerous further cases since then. At least 10 mega units of penicillin daily should be given, perhaps reinforced with probenecid: the daily dose of 4 g. of streptomycin originally given is excessive, and 0·5 g. four times a day should be enough. Even less may be advisable, particularly if there is any impairment of renal function. If this combination is not totally bactericidal *in vitro*, others should be tested; penicillin + kanamycin proved an effective alternative for Case 8 of Garrod and Waterworth (1962a), and in contrast with the patient referred to above who had to be treated with penicillin + neomycin, achieved recovery with no loss of hearing. Combinations including erythromycin and/or bacitracin as well as penicillin were required for and successful in three of the patients described by Jawetz and Sonne (1966).

STAPHYLOCOCCUS AUREUS. Endocarditis caused by this organism is of two kinds. An acute form is a complication of uncontrolled septicaemia and can probably attack normal valves. The subacute form occurs only in patients with pre-disposing rheumatic or congenital lesions, and may be of more insidious onset, the source of the infection being sometimes a trivial lesion such as a boil, although it usually runs a more rapid course with higher fever than a true ' endocarditis lenta '.

Penicillin, if the strain is sensitive to it, methicillin, an isoxa-zolyl penicillin or cephalothin (see p. 90) if not, should be the mainstay of treatment, but since a total bactericidal effect is often not achieved even by an antibiotic to which the strain is fully sensitive, full tests of bactericidal action by single antibiotics and combinations should be carried out. It may well be found that the addition of, for instance, streptomycin or kanamycin to the penicillin will convert incomplete bacteri-cidal effect to complete, and if so this combination should unhesitatingly be used. For a methicillin-resistant strain such a combination is essential, and Bulger (1967) has shown that kanamycin together with methicillin or cephalothin exerts a synergic effect against such organisms.

Among additional antibiotics to be considered is fucidin, which was successfully used by Jensen and Lassen (1964) in combination with methicillin for staphylococcal septicaemia, although the combination failed in two patients actually diag-nosed as having endocarditis.

STAPHYLOCOCCUS ALBUS. This is an infection the existence of which may be overlooked because the organism in a blood culture is taken for a contaminant. A helpful sign that the finding is significant is flocculent growth, due to the action of agglutinin which has always been formed by the time a culture is made: we have rarely seen uniform turbidity in a genuinely positive blood culture, even one containing *Esch. coli*.

This infection occurs in two types of patient. It has always been recognized as an uncommon variety of endocarditis of usually unknown origin in predisposed subjects. Recently it has also been seen as a direct sequel of open heart operations, most often mitral valvotomy, when it may be supposed that implantation occurs during the operation itself. Infections so produced are also sometimes due to *Staph. aureus*. Quinn and Cox (1964) describe 16 *Staph. albus* infections, nine of the first type and seven of the second. In all the idiopathic cases the staphylococcus was sensitive to penicillin, and penicillin, usually with streptomycin, cured the eight treated. From the ' post-cardiotomy ' cases six of the seven strains were penicillin-resistant, and despite a variety of antibiotic treatments, three of these patients died. No series has hitherto been published which enables optimum treatment for a penicillin-resistant *Staph. albus* infection to be defined. Each case demands full laboratory investigation on the lines already indicated.

A peculiar form of infection commonly caused by *Staph. albus* is the colonization of Spitz-Holter valves. Bruce *et al.* (1963) saw 19 patients with persistent bacteriaemia among 300 subjected to ventriculo-caval shunt operations employing this device. *Staph. albus* was cultivated from the blood in eight, *Staph. aureus* in six patients in whom the valve had become exposed by pressure necrosis, and *Serratia marcescens* in four : how this exceptional organism was introduced could not be determined. Despite treatment which sterilizes the bloodstream and is calculated to deal with infection involving any living tissue, bacteria persist in the valve, and the only effective treatment is its removal. Even intra-ventricular injection of methicillin is ineffective (Callaghan, Cohen and Stewart, 1961).

HAEMOPHILUS spp. *H. influenzae,* or, it is said, more usually *H. parainfluenzae,* is an uncommon cause of endocarditis, and not enough cases have been reported in recent years for it to be possible to define optimum treatment. Ampicillin, as a bactericidal antibiotic to which these organisms are usually highly sensitive, if necessary combined with streptomycin, would be a logical first choice.

MISCELLANEOUS INFECTIONS. Those due to *Neisseria* spp. and *Erysipelothrix rhusiopathiae* should respond to penicillin

The treatment of *Brucella* endocarditis is as for undulant fever, but with a longer course and perhaps higher dosage. Coliform infections are usually fatal: antibiotics likely to be indicated are mentioned in the section on Septicaemia at the beginning of this chapter. Fowle and Zorab (1970) cured an *Esch. coli* endocarditis with trimethoprim-sulphamethoxazole after appropriate antibiotics had failed. *Candida albicans* endocarditis should be treated with amphotericin B: several successes have been recorded.

COXIELLA BURNETI is now being increasingly recognized as a cause of endocarditis. This occurs mainly in rheumatic subjects and at varying intervals after an attack of Q fever. Males preponderate and the aortic valve is that usually affected. A high titre of complement-fixing antibody for phase 2 antigen of *C. burneti* enables the diagnosis to be made (Marmion, 1962). Treatment with tetracycline delays the progress of the infection, but does not eradicate it. Surgical treatment becomes essential, and replacement with a prosthesis is preferable to a homograft (Kristinsson and Bentall, 1967): four patients undergoing this operation were successfully treated thereafter with tetracycline to prevent recurrence, this having continued in one of them for two years at the time of reporting.

CAUSE UNKNOWN. Repeatedly negative blood cultures in the face of strongly suspicious clinical features present a difficult problem. According to Griffith and Levinson (1949) it can be of little use to go on repeating blood cultures: in their series of 140, 129 were positive at the first and all but two of the remainder at the second attempt. Nevertheless one should perhaps not be content with less than 8-10 cultures made over a period of several days before admitting defeat. It is assumed that all appropriate laboratory tricks have been tried, including the use of liquoid, pour plates, anaerobiosis and extra CO_2.

The response to penicillin in 34 patients with negative blood cultures in Cates and Christie's (1951) series was poor. Probably the best ' blind ' treatment for a supposed bacterial infection would be with penicillin and streptomycin, but this would be without effect on a rickettsial infection, for which serological tests should be carried out in any suspicious case

It is often extremely difficult to obtain a positive culture in a patient who has had inadequate preliminary treatment with penicillin, as by a practitioner before hospital admission: the two gravest sins committed in connection with this disease are to ignore the possibility of it despite strongly suggestive signs until it is far advanced, and to start treatment before attempting to verify the diagnosis by blood culture. After a full course of treatment cultures may also be negative at first although relapse is taking place.

Treatment of Penicillin-sensitive Patients

Penicillins play at least an important part in the optimum treatment of almost all forms of endocarditis, and nothing can fully replace them. If a patient with endocarditis is said to be penicillin-sensitive, this should first be verified by a cautious test dose, and may be proved untrue. If the condition is verified, there are two alternatives. One is to find a substitute. Most other bactericidal antibiotics, such as streptomycin and the neomycin group, have an inadequate effect on streptococci when acting alone, but may serve in combination with erythromycin or cephaloridine in *Str. viridans* infections. The second, and in our view preferable, course is to administer penicillin and protect the patient against reaction to it, either with antihistamines, as originally advocated by Maslansky and Sanger (1952) or with steroids. Prednisone in doses not exceeding 60 mg. daily served to protect three patients described by Raper and Kemp (1965) during courses of treatment with penicillin or ampicillin. Green, Peters and Geraci (1967) describe extensive experience with these methods.

An alternative is treatment with vancomycin, which may also be resorted to because other treatment has failed. Friedberg, Rosen and Bienstock (1968) report six successfully treated cases, four infected with *Str. faecalis,* two treated from the outset with vancomycin because of penicillin sensitivity and the remainder because reactions occurred to initial treatment with penicillin and streptomycin: in some of them this treatment must at least have contributed to recovery. Mandell, Lindsey and Hook (1970) demonstrated strong synergy between vancomycin and streptomycin in their action on *Str. faecalis,* but do not discuss the advisability or otherwise of combining two ototoxic drugs.

Laboratory Control of Treatment

Blood cultures should be repeated if the response to treatment is inadequate, although they are likely to remain positive only if the antibiotic is singularly ineffective, as in the staphylococcal infection treated with cephaloridine described by Burgess and Evans (1966).

If any system of treatment is being used which justifies doubt about the attainment of adequate blood levels, the antibiotic should be assayed in the blood, preferably at times when maximum and minimum levels are to be expected. This doubt is most likely to arise during oral treatment, when appropriate times would be at one and four hours after a dose—*i.e.* at the peak following absorption and immediately before a further dose is due. Assays are also required to determine that excessive levels, particularly of streptomycin, kanamycin or vancomycin, are not being maintained in patients with possibly impaired renal function. If administration is at six-hour intervals and blood is taken at the end of this period, the level of either of these antibiotics should have fallen to not >10 μg./ml.

A third control procedure, largely employed in the United States but less commonly in this country and deserving more frequent use, is to determine the maximum dilution in which the patient's serum retains a bactericidal effect on his own organism. A method for doing this is described in Chapter XXVIII.

Prophylaxis

Dental extraction, tonsillectomy and other operations causing bacteriaemia should not be undertaken in predisposed patients (*i.e.*, past sufferers from rheumatic fever or those with a known predisposing congenital abnormality) without antibiotic ' cover '. The object of this is to destroy bacteria which enter the circulation before they can colonize a valve, and penicillin, which kills the great majority of a susceptible bacterial population within four hours, is very suitable for the purpose. Penicillin should therefore be given at such a time that the maximum concentration in the blood after the first dose is being reached at the time of the operation: appropriate intervals are a few minutes before if 'soluble' penicillin is given, or one to two hours for procaine penicillin. A single dose containing both these forms of penicillin, such as Fortified Procaine Penicillin Injection B.P. (300 mg. procaine penicillin and 60 mg. benzyl penicillin) given immediately before extraction provides both an immediate high level and a persistent effect, and should not require repetition.

Some have taken the view that the object should be so far as possible to sterilize the area of operation (mouth, throat, etc.) to which end penicillin administration is begun several days beforehand. This is an extremely dangerous policy, because the effect of such treatment is to eliminate the sensitive streptococci from the mouth and to permit a small minority of much more resistant strains to multiply in their place. These highly resistant streptococci are constantly present in the saliva of patients having penicillin treatment, and appear within two days of its being started. Garrod and Waterworth (1962b) who report these findings, which have since been verified by Naiman and Barrow (1963) and by Tozer, Boutflower and Gillespie (1966), also describe two cases of endocarditis due to such organisms, one immediately following dental extraction which was preceded by several days of penicillin 'cover', the other an evident reinfection following dental extraction during a full course of treatment for an endocarditis caused originally by a sensitive streptococcus. It is often said that suspicious teeth are best extracted during a course of treatment for endocarditis because this treatment affords protection: if these findings and their interpretation are accepted this belief must be abandoned. It is better that a full dental examination and any necessary treatment should be carried out as soon as the diagnosis is suspected and while positive blood cultures are awaited.

If dental extraction is necessary in patients receiving small doses of penicillin for the prophylaxis of rheumatic fever, cover may be afforded by an injection of 1 mega unit of penicillin + 0·5 g. streptomycin, a combination which is usually bactericidal for the moderately resistant streptococci found in the mouths of such patients. If large doses of penicillin are being given, and particularly if streptomycin is being given in addition, as in the actual treatment of endocarditis, it seems from the findings of Tozer *et al.* (1966) that cover is best afforded by an injection of 0·5 g. cephaloridine. This can be repeated, or followed by a short course of erythromycin. This proceeding may also be preferred for patients on low prophylactic doses. It should also be employed in patients who have had a therapeutic course of penicillin at any time during the preceding six weeks, since the reversion of the mouth flora from penicillin resistance to sensitivity is a slow process.

Vancomycin, originally suggested by Garrod and Waterworth (1962b) should also be effective according to the findings of Tozer *et al.*, but is much more inconvenient to administer.

Antibiotic cover is also required for proceedings in other parts of the body. Outstanding among these are operations on the heart itself, including mitral valvotomy and the insertion of artificial valves. A five-day course of penicillin + streptomycin is commonly given, and should be capable of eliminating any staphylococci, but has apparently not always succeeded. Holswade *et al.* (1964) tried five different antibiotic combinations in 300 open-heart operations, and conclude by recommending methicillin alone (1 g. six-hourly). Some strains of *Staph. albus* are resistant to methicillin, and might not be disposed of by this treatment. Nelson *et al.* (1965) obtained their best results with the combination of penicillin, streptomycin and oxacillin. The best method of protecting these patients has perhaps yet to be defined.

In predisposed subjects various forms of surgical interference with the urinary tract, including even dilatation of a urethral stricture, may be followed by *S. faecalis* endocarditis. Penicillin + streptomycin should afford appropriate cover.

Undulant Fever (Brucellosis)

The subject of this and the succeeding section are included here for the possibly inadequate reason that both diseases are accompanied by bacteriaemia.

Early specific treatment of *Brucella* infections with, first, sulphonamides and then with streptomycin, was only partially successful: combined treatment with both was more so. The advent of the broad spectrum antibiotics altered the outlook profoundly, because thenceforth an easily administered treatment regularly brought about defervescence within a few days, usually with relief of all symptoms and apparent cure. Unfortunately relapse was common, but usually responded to a further course.

The tetracyclines are the antibiotics of choice: opinions differ only on which to use and for how long, and in particular on whether streptomycin should be given in addition. Spink (1960), whose experience few can rival, advises a 21-day course of tetracycline or oxy- or chlortetracycline, 500 mg. being given six-hourly, 1-2 g. of streptomycin daily by intramuscular injection being also given for 14 days in more severe cases. This second recommendation is noteworthy, since he has not been among the more enthusiastic advocates of combined treatment. On the other hand, Farid *et al.* (1961), who treated 94 cases of *Br. melitensis* infection in Cairo, observed slightly fewer relapses after treatment with a larger dose of tetracycline alone than after two forms of combined treatment. The courses given, all of 21 days, were (1) 1 g. tetracycline six-hourly, (2) 0·5 g. tetracycline six-hourly and 0·5 g. streptomycin 12-hourly, (3) 1 g. erythromycin six-hourly and 0·5 g. streptomycin 12-hourly. The last group had much the highest incidence of gastro-intestinal side-effects.

There appears to be no distinct preference for any one of the older tetracyclines, but two authors commend demethylchlortetracycline, each having successfully treated a series of cases of *Br. melitensis* infection none of which is mentioned as having relapsed. Chavez Max (1960) treated nine cases in Mexico, giving 1,200 mg. daily for the acute and 900 mg. for the subacute form of the disease, each for 40 days. Bruno and Palazzotto (1961) report 33 cases in Sicily, given only 150 mg. six-hourly, reduced to eight-hourly four days after defervescence and continued only until an average total dose of about 7 g. had been given. Most of them left hospital early, and the fact that none returned is the evidence of freedom from relapse.

Chloramphenicol has been much less used, but was the antibiotic given to the majority of 186 patients treated by Tuszkiewicz and Szewczykowski (1962) in Poland. Novobiocin is strongly commended by Torres Gost (1958), and Farid *et al.*

(1963) confirm its efficacy, but deprecate its use because 50 per cent of their patients developed rashes.

According to Lal *et al.* (1970) although *Br. abortus* is only moderately sensitive to trimethoprim, it is highly so to its combination with sulphamethoxazole (M.I.C. 0·05 and 1·0 μg./ ml. respectively of the two drugs together). They treated four cases of acute *Br. abortus* infection with this combination with successful results, although the outcome was doubtful in one who for a time was given trimethoprim alone because of a sulphonamide rash. The possibilities of this treatment evidently deserve further study.

Tularaemia

This disease responds well to streptomycin, a course lasting about seven days eradicating the infection. Chloramphenicol or tetracyclines have a similar immediate effect, but with some tendency to relapse. The fact that streptomycin, by virtue of its bactericidal action, eliminates the organism, whereas chloramphenicol only suppresses it, has been shown by preventive administration to volunteers inoculated subcutaneously. A report by Overholt *et al.* (1961) concerns 42 cases occurring in laboratory staff at Fort Detrick despite previous vaccination: the infection was acquired by inhalation, and was therefore of the ' typhoidal ' type with pulmonary lesions, although of very varying severity. A streptomycin-resistant strain was responsible for 75 per cent. Treatment with 2 g. tetracycline daily for 10 days or more was followed by relapse in five out of 15 cases treated during the first week, but in none of 16 in whom it was begun after this time, suggesting that an adequate immune response combines to render tetracycline alone effective. On the other hand, Knothe and Helpap (1965) in patients treated with tetracycline during an epidemic in Schleswig-Holstein, obtained good results when the antibiotic was given early and less satisfactory when it was delayed. These authors' poor results with streptomycin may have been due in some patients to inadequate dosage, but it also seems possible that American and European strains of *Br. tularensis* differ in their drug susceptibility.

REFERENCES

BRUCE, A. M., LORBER, J., SHEDDEN, W. I. H. & ZACHARY, R. B. (1963). *Develop. Med. Child Neurol.* **5**, 461.
BRUNO, F. & PALAZZOTTO, G. (1961). *Rif. med.* **75**, 874.
BULGER, R. J. (1967) *Lancet* **1**, 17.
BURGESS, H. A. & EVANS, R. J. (1966). *Brit. med. J.* **ii**, 1244.
CALLAGHAN, R. P., COHEN, S. J. & STEWART, G. T. (1961). *Brit. med. J.* **i**, 860.
CATES, J. E. & CHRISTIE, R. V. (1951). *Quart. J. Med.* **20**, 93.
CATES, J. E., CHRISTIE, R. V. & GARROD, L. P. (1951). *Brit. med. J.* **i**, 653.
CHAVEZ MAX, G. (1960). *Antibiot. Annu.* (1959-60), p. 429.
DORMER, A. E. (1960). *Brit. med. Bull.* **16**, 61.
EVANS, A. D., POWELL, D. E. B. & BURRELL, C. D. (1959). *Lancet* **i**, 864.
FARID, Z., MIALE, A. JR., OMAR, M. S. & VAN PEENEN, P. F. D. (1961). *J. trop. Med. Hyg.* **64**, 157.
FARID, Z., OMAR, M. S., MIALE, A. & PRASAD, A. S. (1963). *Lancet* **i**, 334.
FINLAND, M., JONES, W. F, JR. & BARNES, M. W. (1959). *J. Amer. med. Ass.* **170**, 2188.
FOWLE, A. S. E. & ZORAB, P. A. (1970). *Brit. Heart J.* **32**, 127.
FRIEDBERG, C. K., ROSEN, K. M. & BIENSTOCK, P. A. (1968). *Arch. intern. Med.* **122**, 134.
GARROD, L. P. & WATERWORTH, P. M. (1962a). *J. clin. Path.* **15**, 328.
GARROD, L. P. & WATERWORTH, P. M. (1962b). *Brit. Heart J.* **24**, 39.
GRAY, I. R., TAI, A. R., WALLACE, J. G. & CALDER, J. H. (1964). *Lancet* **ii**, 110.
GREEN, G. R., PETERS, G. A. & GERACI, J. E. (1967). *Ann. intern. Med.* **67**, 235.
GRIFFITH, G. C. & LEVINSON, D. C. (1949). *Calif. med.* **71**, 403.
HAVARD, C. W. H., GARROD, L. P. & WATERWORTH, P. M. (1959). *Brit. med. J.* **i**, 688.
HOLSWADE, G. R., DINEEN, P., REDO, S. F. & GOLDSMITH, E. I. (1964). *Arch. Surg.* **89**, 970.
JAWETZ, E. (1952). *Arch. intern. Med.* **90**, 301.
JAWETZ, E., GUNNISON, J. B. & SPECK, R. S. (1951). *New Engl. J. Med.* **245**, 966.
JAWETZ, E. & SONNE, M. (1966). *New Engl. J. Med.* **274**, 710.
JENSEN, K. & LASSEN, H. C. A. (1964). *Ann. intern. Med.* **60**, 790.
KNOTHE, H. & HELPAP, B. (1965). *Dtsch. med. Wschr.* **90**, 2361.
KRISTINSSON, A. & BENTALL, H. H. (1967). *Lancet* **2**, 693.
LAL, S., MODAWAL, K. K., FOWLE, A. S. E., PEACH, B. & POPHAM, R. D. (1970). *Brit. med. J.* **3**, 256.
MANDELL, G. L., LINDSEY, E. & HOOK, E. W. (1970). *Amer. J. med. Sci.* **259**, 346.
MARMION, B. P. (1962). *J. Hyg. Epidem.* (*Praha*) **6**, 79.
MARTIN, C. M., CUOMO, A. J., GERAGHTY, M. J., ZAGER, J. R. & MANDES, T. C. (1969). *J. infect. Dis.* **119**, 506.
MASLANSKY, L. & SANGER, M. D. (1952). *Antibiot. and Chemother.* **2**, 385.
NAIMAN, R. A. & BARROW, J. G. (1963). *Ann. intern. Med.* **58**, 768.
NELSON, R. M., JENSON, C. B., PETERSON, C. A. & SANDERS, B. C. (1965). *Arch. Surg.* **90**, 731.
OVERHOLT, E. L., TIGERTT, W. D., KADULL, P. J. & WARD, M. K. (1961). *Amer. J. Med.* **30**, 785.
QUINN, E. L. & COX, F. (1964). *Antimicrob. Agents and Chemother.*, 1963, p. 635.
RAPER, A. J. & KEMP, V. E. (1965). *New Engl. J. Med.* **273**, 297.
ROBBINS, W. C. & TOMPSETT, R. (1951). *Amer. J. Med.* **10**, 278.
SPINK, W. W. (1960). *J. Amer. med. Ass.* **172**, 697.
TALBOT, C. H. (1962). *Lancet* **i**, 668.

TOH, C. C. S. & BALL, K. P. (1960). *Brit. med. J.* **2,** 640.
TOMPSETT, R. & PIZETTE, M. (1962). *Arch. intern. Med.* **109,** 146.
TORRES GOST, J. (1958). *Lancet* **i,** 191.
TOZER, R. A., BOUTFLOWER, S. & GILLESPIE, W. A. (1966). *Lancet* **i,** 686.
TUSZKIEWICZ, A. R. & SZEWCZYKOWSKI, W. (1962). *Concours Méd.* **84,** 6557.
WEIL, M. H., SHUBIN, H. & BIDDLE, M. (1964). *Ann. intern. Med.* **60,** 384.
WILFERT, J. N., BARRETT, F. R. & KASS, E. H. (1968). *New Engl. J. Med.*
279, 286.

Chapter XVIII

INFECTIONS OF SKIN, SOFT TISSUES AND BONES

In the choice of preparations for topical application for the prevention and treatment of bacterial infections the following points must be borne in mind:

1. Anti-bacterial Activity. The preparation used should have a wide spectrum, since many superficial infections have a mixed bacterial flora. Since the treatment of local infections is very liable to lead to the development of drug-resistance, preparations which are unlikely to lead to the emergence of drug-resistant bacteria should be used. Both these points are best dealt with by combining more than one agent, and even in combinations, agents to which bacteria rapidly become resistant should be avoided.

2. Effect on the Host. The anti-bacterial agent must be non-irritating and non-toxic to leucocytes and other phagocytic cells and granulation tissue. Moreover, those anti-bacterial drugs liable to give rise to hypersensitivity reactions, notably the sulphonamides, penicillin and streptomycin, should not be used for skin infections. It should not be thought that the skin is entirely impervious to topically applied antibiotics. In an experimental system, fucidin penetrated the skin at a rate comparable with that of glucocorticoids (Vickers, 1969). Penicillin, tetracycline and erythromycin penetrated at lower rates and ampicillin very slowly (Knight, Vickers and Percival, 1969).

3. Antibiotics suitable for Systemic Administration should be avoided, so that if drug-resistance or skin hypersensitivity should occur the patient is not thereby deprived of the benefits of a valuable drug for systemic treatment should this become necessary.

4. Choice of Base. Preparations in the form of sprays or insufflation powders are usually more effective than creams or ointments and are less likely to lead to skin sensitization

but they may, on the other hand, be less convenient to apply. Creams in the form of an oil-in-water emulsion are preferable to ointments.

Preparations

Many antibacterial agents are available in proprietary preparations as creams, ointments, powders, lotions and sprays. Neomycin, usually as a 0·5 per cent cream or ointment, has been widely used in local applications, but now suffers two disadvantages: hypersensitivity, which was thought not to occur, has developed in a number of patients; and neomycin-resistant staphylococci have become common in hospital. Currently useful substitutes are:

GENTAMICIN: highly active against both *Staph. aureus* and *Pseudomonas aeruginosa* (page 126). Available as a 0·3 per cent cream and ointment, and

CHLORAMPHENICOL: active against *Staph. aureus* and many enterobacteria. Where its use has not been restricted, resistant strains are common (page 136). Applied to wounds, chloramphenicol is absorbed and there is danger of toxicity (page 139). Available as a 5 per cent dusting powder or cream.

Recommended Combinations

Most of the antibiotic mixtures for use on the skin contain various combinations of bacitracin (or its relatives), neomycin (or its relatives) and polymyxin.

These give wide cover against Gram-positive and Gram-negative bacteria, and are suitable for topical application. If *Ps. aeruginosa* is present polymyxin must be included.

Amongst those commercially available are:

BACITRACIN AND NEOMYCIN.—Neomycin and bacitracin ointment B.N.F. contains neomycin sulphate 5 mg. and bacitracin zinc 500 units per g. Numerous similar proprietary preparations are available some of which e.g. Cicatrin (Calmic: powder and aerosol) contain added amino acids which are said to promote wound healing. Graneodin (Squibb) is a similar preparation in which bacitracin is replaced by gramicidin; in Ecomytrin (Warner) bacitracin is replaced by amphomycin (a peptide antibiotic produced by *Streptomyces canus* principally active against Gram positive cocci). Soframycin (cream and ointment) contains framycetin 1·5 per cent and gramicidin 0·005 per cent.

Bacitracin, Neomycin and Polymyxin

Available as creams, e.g. Polybactrin (Calmic): bacitracin zinc 400 units, neomycin sulphate 3,300 units and polymyxin B 5,000 units per g.; as powders, or as sprays: Polybactrin (Calmic); Rikospray Antibiotic (Riker); Trispray (Pigot and Smith) and others. Framyspray (Fisons) is a similar mixture with framycetin substituted for neomycin.

Several other combinations of neomycin with polymyxin, or bacitracin with polymyxin and many similar mixtures with added corticosteroids are also available.

It may not be widely known that antibiotics are incorporated in some cosmetics and deodorants (Carney, 1963). The presence of neomycin in such preparations may contribute to the development of sensitization and the emergence of resistant strains.

There is, in addition, a very wide choice of antiseptics, singly or in combination, for local application. They include:

Antiseptics

CETRIMIDE (Cetavlon, *I.C.I.*, and numerous other proprietary preparations) B.P., B.N.F.: 0·5 per cent cream.

CHLORHEXIDINE (Hibitane, *I.C.I.*) cream B.P.C., B.N.F.: 1 per cent. Naseptin (*I.C.I.*) contains chlorhexidine hydrochloride 0·1 per cent and neomycin sulphate 0·5 per cent. It is most commonly used for application to the nose in treatment of nasal carriers of staphylococci.

DIBROMO-PROPAMIDINE ISETHIONATE B.P. (Brulidine *M. and B.*); Propamidine isethionate, B.P.C.: 0·15 per cent creams.

POLYNOXYLIN (Anaflex, *Geistlich*) 10 per cent cream and paste.

QUINOLINES: Clioquinol (Vioform, *Ciba*) 3 per cent cream. Halquinol (Quinolor, *Squibb*) 0·5 per cent ointment; Potassium hydroxyquinoline sulphate, B.P.C. (Quinoderm, *Quinoderm Ltd.*) 0·5 per cent cream.

Many preparations for local dermatological use also contain steroids, and numerous warnings have been given about the possible facilitation of superinfection, especially with fungi. While the danger is undoubtedly real and must be watched for, it appears that in the majority of cases the benefits of inflammation control outweigh any deleterious effect on infection (Davis *et al.*, 1968).

SUPERFICIAL INFECTIONS

Impetigo Contagiosa

This is an infection of the superficial layers of the epidermis which occurs in two forms (Dillon, 1968). The commoner is the vesicular, golden-crusted variety which is primarily of streptococcal origin but is commonly superinfected with staphylococci (Markowitz *et al.*, 1965). Less common is the bullous variety, a pure staphylococcal infection, which may occur in hospital nurseries in the severe epidemic form called impetigo (or pemphigus) neonatorum. The streptococci and staphylococci are often of unusual types peculiar to skin infections (Parker and Williams, 1961). Most mild cases respond fairly readily to local treatment. After removal of heavy crusting with warm water the lesions should be treated two or three times a day with ointments or sprays containing neomycin and bacitracin.

In more severe cases, the results of systemic erythromycin therapy (250 mg. 6-hourly for 5 days) are generally superior to those of topical treatment (Hughes and Wan, 1967). Topical erythromycin is ineffective.

Dodge *et al.* (1968) say that mild cases respond to antibacterial soaps and that systemic erythromycin should be reserved for severe cases and those in whom topical treatment fails. Systemic treatment should be supplemented by an antibacterial soap to limit the possibility of relapse.

In some patients with mild crusted impetigo it may be felt that systemic treatment is necessary in order to prevent the sequelae of streptococcal infection. It is currently unsettled whether the rather unusual streptoccocal types involved in superficial skin infections are important in this respect but some patients are evidently infected with nephritogenic strains. Hughes and Wan (1967) had one case of overt glomerulonephritis and three of asymptomatic haematuria amongst those topically treated in their group of 62 children.

Impetigo Neonatorum (*Pemphigus neonatorum*). Milder cases of this staphylococcal infection in the new-born may respond to local treatment as for *Impetigo contagiosa,* but the condition is often very severe, in which case early systemic treatment is essential. Since this is a hospital disease the infecting staphylococcus is likely to be resistant to penicillin and while waiting for laboratory reports treatment should be started at once with cloxacillin, clindamycin or fucidin.

Sycosis Barbae. Mild and early cases usually respond to local treatment as for *Impetigo contagiosa,* but relapses are frequent. The source of infection is sometimes nasal carriage, in which case the nose should be treated as described on page 309. Quinoline derivatives, *e.g.* iodochlorhydroxyquinoline (Vioform) may be helpful in intractable cases. Adult pyoderma (also due to streptococci and staphylococci acting alone or in concert was successfully managed by McMillan and Hurwitz

(1969) with phenoxymethyl penicillin (oxacillin in those infected with penicillin-resistant staphylococci) 500 mg. 6-hourly.

Erysipeloid of Rosenbach (*Erythema serpens*). This is an acute infection of the skin by *Erysipelothrix rhusiopathiae*. The organism is very widely distributed in nature and infection in man usually occurs in those who handle meat, particularly pork, or fish. The disease tends to be limited and in the absence of treatment usually clears up in three or four weeks, but may persist for longer. The condition responds rapidly to benzyl penicillin or the tetracyclines. Sulphonamides and streptomycin are said not to be effective.

Acne Vulgaris

Increasing evidence suggests that normal follicular bacteria, including coagulase-negative staphylococci and *Corynebacterium acnes,* split the triglycerides of sebum liberating free fatty acids causing the inflammation of acne (Freinkel, 1969). Suppression of the lipolytic activity of these organisms may be responsible for the improvement which occurs on tetracycline 250 mg. 6-12 hourly for one or two weeks reduced progressively to the smallest effective maintenance dose. Tetracycline has been shown to lower the fatty acid content of sebum (Beveridge and Powell, 1969) but a placebo effect also occurs and the efficacy and mode of action of tetracycline in this condition are disputed (Juhlin and Liden, 1969). Penicillin, to which the implicated organisms are also sensitive, has no effect on acne and it may be that tetracyclines owe their effect to concentration in the sebaceous glands and follicular epithelium (Marks and Davies, 1969).

Cutaneous Anthrax

B. anthracis is highly sensitive to benzyl penicillin which, like streptomycin, is superior to tetracycline or chloramphenicol in the treatment of experimental infection (Jones *et al.,* 1967). Cutaneous anthrax responds well to penicillin (4-6 mega units per day for 10-12 days). Of 197 cases reviewed by Brachman (1966) 8 died. Penicillin therapy reduced the total inflammation and the systemic symptoms but it did not affect the evolution of the typical local lesion and eschar, even though in the majority of cases the exudate was sterile after 24 hr. Excision of the lesion increased and prolonged both the local and the systemic manifestations and evidently has no place in treatment. Knight, Wynne-Williams and Willis (1969) were dissatisfied with the response in the first 24 hours of one of their two patients to penicillin and added streptomycin for 5 days.

Fungal Infections

Before starting treatment accurate identity of the fungus should be established. Griseofulvin (Blank, 1960), the most important agent for dermatophyte infections, has no effect on *Candida, Malassezia furfur* (the causative organism of pityriasis versicolor), or other non-dermatophytes which occasionally infect the skin.

CANDIDA INFECTIONS

Numerous local agents are available but all are less effective than nystatin (p. 236). This is not absorbed by mouth and is applied locally usually as a cream containing 100,000 units per g. Preparations with added steroids or antibacterial agents are available for use in patients with underlying eczematous conditions or concurrent bacterial infections. Amphotericin B, as a 3 per cent lotion or cream, sometimes succeeds where nystatin has failed. Whiting (1967) describes a method of achieving high local concentrations of amphotericin in the skin with which he successfully treated chromoblastomycosis. On the basis of *in vitro* studies, Caplan and Clabaugh (1969) suggest that the corticosteroids contained in many local dermatological preparations may modify the response to antifungal agents in a complex way.

TINEA CAPITIS. Fungal infections of the scalp hair due to *Microsporum canis, Microsporum audouini* or *Microsporum gypseum* respond well to oral treatment with griseofulvin. This should be given, as the fine particle preparation, in a daily dose of 0·5-1 g. for adults and older children or 0·25 g. for children under four years. Treatment should be continued for 2-3 months. For infections of the glabrous skin three to four weeks is usually sufficient.

Griseofulvin is similarly effective in scalp ringworm due to the trichophyton fungi but recognition of carriers and elimination of the source of infection may be more difficult. In Britain at least epidemics occur more frequently with *Trichophyton tonsurans var. sulphureum* than with the microsporum group. Beare (1960) suggests that in a school where there is an epidemic, all children might be given griseofulvin, in addition to taking energetic measures to eliminate the fungus from the environment.

TINEA PEDIS AND FUNGAL INFECTION OF NAILS. Although early reports suggested that griseofulvin would cure athlete's foot, this has not been borne out by further experience and the same is true of fungal infection involving nails. Clinical improvement may occur but relapses are frequent and the fungus is rarely eradicated, although the finger nails may respond to 6-9 months' treatment. Infection with *Trychophyton rubrum* appears to be particularly intractable. Success may follow treatment for one to two years but some dermatologists doubt whether such prolonged treatment is justified. Local fungicides must be used for these infections whether or not griseofulvin is given.

Two recent preparations tolnaftate (Naph-2-yl-*N*-methyl-*N*-*m*-tolyl thiocarbamate), and pecilocin (an antibiotic obtained from a species of paecilomyces and marketed in an ointment containing 3,000 units per g. under the name Variotin) have both had successful trials (Robinson and Raskin, 1965; Holti *et al.*, 1966) but Wethered *et al.* (1967) were unable to demonstrate any benefit from either substance in the treatment of *Trichophyton rubrum* infection. Neither is active against candida.

Erythrasma

This is caused by *Corynebacterium minutissimum* which appears to possess keratolytic properties (Montes and McBride, 1967). Corynebacteria capable of attacking hair also appear to be the principal occupants of the pigmented incrustations on the axillary hairs in trichomycosis axillaris (McBride *et al.*, 1968). The infected skin in erythrasma shows a striking pink fluorescence when viewed in ultra-violet light. The response to erythromycin 250 mg. 6-hourly for two weeks is striking.

Boils

Boils do not require (or benefit from) systemic antibiotic therapy unless there is evidence of local or lymphatic spread. Local applications of one of the preparations listed on page 303 or of gentian violet paint may be useful in limiting spread to adjacent skin. Infections severe enough to require surgery deserve systemic therapy beginning immediately before operation. Boils on the face should be treated because of the possibility of the grave complication of cavernous sinus thrombosis.

The choice of possible agents is wide. Unless the lesion is sufficiently serious to warrant admission to hospital, oral therapy is obviously desirable. For out-patients, an oral penicillin may well be the drug of choice, although the penicillin sensitivity of the infecting staphylococcus can no longer be relied upon. Erythromycin (250 mg. 6-hourly), cloxacillin (500 mg. 6-hourly), lincomycin (500 mg. 6-hourly), and various other anti-staphylococcal agents have all been successfully used. The drugs should be continued until the lesion heals. Failure to respond is an indication for bacteriological and surgical reassessment.

The danger of the progressive superficial lesion is that it may give rise to septicaemia and metastatic lesions particularly in patients predisposed to infection (for example those with grave blood disorders), but also rarely in otherwise normal patients.

Recurrent Boils

The cropping of recurrent boils can usually only be stopped if vigorous and persistent efforts are made to control the carrier state. Swabs from the usual carrier sites should be taken from the patient and all his family. Positive carrier sites should be treated with naseptin or other suitable cream or spray. Where neomycin-resistant strains are prevalent, or sensitization to neomycin proves troublesome, chlorhexidine, gentamicin, or chloramphenicol may be used. The patient and carriers in the family should substitute for their normal toilet-soap a soap containing hexachlorophene which they should use for all washing and bathing. The patient's underclothes and sheets should be changed at frequent intervals (initially daily), and boiled. A dusting powder containing hexachlorophene ('Ster-Zac') may also be used with advantage. This process should be continued for two months after the last boil has cleared.

In cases troublesome enough to justify this regimen, systemic antibiotic therapy is usually required initially. The choice of available agents is wide; we have been successful with erythromycin or, more recently, clindamycin. In particularly troublesome cases it may be worth giving the patient a small supply of the drug to take as soon as signs of a fresh lesion appear. The interesting state of affairs where some physicians continue to be convinced of the value of staphylococcal vaccines in the absence of any convincing scientific evidence of their value is discussed by Greenberg (1968).

Aerobic Wound Infections

ACCIDENTAL WOUNDS may be infected by one or more of a variety of bacteria of which the most frequent are *Staph. aureus, Str. pyogenes, Esch. coli, Proteus* species and *Ps. aeruginosa*. In healthy individuals the infection is usually only superficial and local treatment with a spray containing one of the combinations of antibiotics recommended at the beginning of the chapter is usually adequate. If deep-seated infection develops, systemic treatment may be necessary, in which case the choice of drug will depend on the sensitivity of the infecting organism or organisms.

OPERATION WOUNDS. The most likely organisms to infect clean operation wounds in hospital are *Staph. aureus, Ps. aeruginosa* and *Esch. coli*. As with accidental wounds local treatment is often sufficient. If infection is deep-seated or becomes generalized appropriate systemic treatment must be given. One superficial infection which has produced septicaemia often enough to cause concern is the entry wound for plastic indwelling intravenous catheters (Moran *et al.*, 1965). Movement of the catheter in the wound facilitates ingress of skin organisms and fixation is one important preventive measure. In addition, the entry site should be cleansed daily and treated with one of the preparations listed on page 303.

Corso *et al.* (1969) discuss the general aseptic management of intravenous catheters.

INFECTION WITH PASTEURELLA SEPTICA. This may follow the bite of cats, dogs or other animals. Constitutional upset is frequent and systemic treatment should be given. Benzyl penicillin, or possibly ampicillin, is the drug of choice. Most strains are also sensitive to the sulphonamides, erythromycin and the tetracyclines.

ANAEROBIC INFECTIONS

Anaerobic infections fall generally into three groups in which the principal organisms are clostridia, bacteroides, and anaerobic streptococci. Bornstein *et al.* (1964) describe the clinical manifestations and general management of these conditions.

Gas Gangrene. This term denotes an acute rapidly spreading myositis with gas formation (detectable by crepitus) caused most often by *Cl. welchii,* and terminating, if unchecked, in a rapidly fatal septicaemia. It is most likely to result from gross trauma, when the wound is contaminated with soil or dirt, as in battle wounds or farm accidents. It very rarely arises in operation wounds, with one exception: amputation through the thigh for obliterating arterial disease; here the source of infection is the skin in the neighbourhood of the anus, and the low oxygen tension in the tissues resulting from the poor blood supply permits spore germination. Nearly all the serious infections reported by Parker (1969) arose in this way. Attention has again been drawn to the dangers of gas gangrene following injection into the buttock of compounds (notably depot adrenaline preparations) which impair the local blood supply (Editorial, 1968).

The most important step in preventing clostridial infection of traumatic wounds is surgical debridement with the removal of foreign material and the excision of grossly traumatized tissue, in which alone the initial multiplication of clostridia can occur in the otherwise healthy subject. Any patient seriously at risk (and this includes patients about to undergo amputations through the thigh or orthopaedic operations between the waist and the knees) should also have the benefit of

11

prophylactic penicillin, the value of which was amply demonstrated in Allied casualties from D-day 1944 onwards. Although all the toxigenic clostridia are sensitive to penicillin, the degree of sensitivity is only about one-tenth of that of a Group A streptococcus; hence at least two million units a day in divided doses should be given for several days, by intramuscular injection. In less severely injured and possibly ambulant patients, phenoxymethyl penicillin in very large oral doses may be substituted. Because of the emergence of resistant strains, tetracycline can no longer be relied upon for this purpose (Johnstone and Cockcroft, 1968) and it appears from one case reported by Parker (1969) that ampicillin should not be used. Erythromycin (250 mg. 6-hourly, if necessary intramuscularly) is generally held to be the best alternative for patients sensitive to penicillin.

It has been repeatedly emphasized that the treatment of clostridial myonecrosis is primarily surgical and that wide excision of the affected tissues or amputation is urgently required. If accumulating experience of hyperbaric oxygen continues to be as favourable, these mutilating procedures may no longer be necessary. The treatment is not without dangers, but with its use a number of authors have achieved high survival rates with limited surgery (Colwill and Maudsley, 1968). Treatment with penicillin, 10-20 mega units a day, is still required and local irrigation with antibiotics and hydrogen peroxide is recommended by some.

Many authors side-step the issue of the place of antitoxin in the treatment of gas gangrene by concluding that it is of questionable value, recounting its dangers and then reciting the dose. We have not recommended the use of antitoxin in the few patients we have seen in recent years and have no reason to believe that the prognosis suffered. We await convincing evidence that it contributes materially to the benefit of the multipronged therapeutic attack which is necessary in this disease.

Bacteroides Infections

These small Gram-negative anaerobic bacilli (the most numerous organisms in normal faeces) are responsible, either alone or in concert with other anaerobic organisms, for infections at numerous sites (Bornstein *et al.*, 1964). Some strains are sensitive to penicillin; occasional strains are resistant to all the common agents. If Gram-stained films of putrid material reveal organisms morphologically resembling bacteroides, clindamycin appears currently to be the drug of choice. The organisms are commonly also sensitive to erythromycin and tetracycline.

Anaerobic Streptococcal Infections

These organisms, which are normal inhabitants of the mouth, gut and vagina, are most frequently responsible for infections around the perineum, but they are important causes of putrid lung abscess, sinusitis and brain abscess, and may cause a myositis clinically resembling gas gangrene. They are also implicated in post-operative synergic gangrene (Meleney's gangrene. This rare condition usually follows abdominal operations (de Jongh *et al.*, 1967). A gangrenous area develops in the vicinity of the wound and rapidly spreads to destroy much of the skin and subcutaneous tissue of the abdominal wall. It is a mixed infection with anaerobic streptococci, *Staph. aureus* and enterobacteria, or sometimes other organisms. Chemotherapy should be instituted as for clostridial myonecrosis but prompt wide excision of the affected tissues has also been essential. Whether this condition will respond to hyperbaric oxygen remains to be seen.

Actinomycosis

Although *Actinomyces israeli* is highly sensitive to many chemotherapeutic drugs (p. 266; Blake, 1964) the chemotherapy of actinomycosis can be difficult, because the granulomatous and fibrotic tissue involved is not readily penetrated. Cervicofacial actinomycosis is relatively amenable to treatment and we, and others (Caron and Sarkany, 1964) have successfully managed this form of the disease with oral phenoxymethyl penicillin (2 g. per day). At least six weeks' treatment is usually necessary. Successful therapy has also been reported with tetracycline (3 g. per day for 28 days; or 3 g. per day for 10 days and 2 g. per day for a further 18 days) and with erythromycin (300 mg. 6 hourly for six weeks).

Thoracic, abdominal, and disseminated actinomycosis (and similar infections with ' anaerobic diphtheroids ') can be very difficult to eradicate. Penicillin is generally regarded as the antibiotic of choice, given in doses of 0·5 to 1·0 mega unit procaine penicillin b.d. for periods of two to three months. There is no advantage in adding sulphonamides (Seabery and Dascomb, 1964). Because of their powers of penetration, fucidin and lincomycin, both of which are highly active against *Actinomyces* (p. 266, Blake, 1970, personal communication) should be considered. It may be that prolonged therapy is more important than high dosage since there have been several reports of relapse after a few weeks' therapy followed by satisfactory response to further treatment with the same dosage. Surgical treatment is necessary to open and drain abscesses or an empyema and to remove infected bone. Excision of tissue may be necessary for diagnosis.

CO-BACTERIA OF ACTINOMYCES. In actinomycotic lesions, the *Actinomyces* is commonly, perhaps regularly, accompanied by small anaerobic Gram-negative bacilli, *Actinobacillus actinomycetem comitans,* and a haemophilus-like organism *Haemophilus aphrophilus.* These may also be found alone as rare causes of endocarditis or of infections arising from the upper respiratory tract (Page and King, 1966). Their therapeutic interest is that they are relatively insensitive to penicillin, but sensitive to tetracycline. It has occasionally been shown that the actinobacillus persists in actinomycotic lesions after treatment with penicillin. The common presence of penicillin-resistant potential pathogens has been used as an argument for treating actinomycosis with tetracycline.

INFECTION IN BURNS

Prophylaxis

It cannot be too strongly emphasised that chemoprophylaxis is not a substitute for physical methods to prevent infection of burns in hospital (Lowbury, 1962). Overwhelming infection remains the greatest threat to the survival of badly burned patients. The organisms most likely to infect burns are *Str. pyogenes, Staph. aureus* or *Ps. aeruginosa.* Of the septicaemias arising from infected burns seen by MacMillan (1967) *Staph.*

aureus was responsible for 6, *Proteus* and other Gram-negative bacilli for 11, and *Pseudomonas* for 29.

From 1960-65 Gram-negative bacilli became increasingly important. Mortality from Gram-positive infections was 50 per cent, and from Gram-negative infection 75 per cent. The importance of preventing burn sepsis is obvious. Most authors agree that systemic antibiotics should not be given prophylactically although several believe penicillin should be given over the first few hours to prevent the establishment of haemolytic streptococci. Larson *et al.* (1966) have shown that penicillin distribution through burned areas is satisfactory.

Interestingly, two abandoned antibacterial agents, silver nitrate and sulfamylon (marfanil) have been resuscitated and proved to be of great benefit in the management of burns. Moyer *et al.* (1965) found that application of 0·5 per cent silver nitrate solution to large burns delayed sepsis and reduced mortality from 81 to 33 per cent. Monafo (1967) found that in patients treated early, *Staph. aureus, Proteus* and *Pseudomonas* were infrequently recovered from the burned areas and nearly 40 per cent were sterile. As treatment progressed, *Klebsiella, Aerobacter,* and *Providentia* appeared and persisted until the wounds healed. *Pseudomonas* appeared only after several weeks' treatment and seldom predominated. In contrast, in patients in whom treatment was delayed, *Pseudomonas* was isolated from every case and was not eliminated; *Staph. aureus* was isolated from all but one, but promptly disappeared on silver nitrate treatment.

The success of this therapy has been confirmed by a number of workers but it has several times been commented that it requires diligent and exact management (Price and Wood, 1966). Sulphamylon, as a 10 per cent cream, has been held to be equally effective and easier to manage. Switzer (1967) reduced the mortality in patients with 30-40 per cent burns from 41·1 to 3 per cent and in those with 40-50 per cent burns from 63·6 to 19 per cent. There was no improvement in patients with more than 60 per cent burns. Still more recently, topical gentamicin has been shown to be equally or more effective (MacMillan, 1969). In a review of the present situation, Moncrieff (1969) concludes that each of the treatments has advantages and disadvantages and that the most important conclusion is that the value of topical antibacterial therapy is now well established.

Treatment

Treatment of a burn already infected must depend on the infecting microbe or microbes and its sensitivity to antibiotics. Since *Str. pyogenes* is not infrequently present in a burn in association with a penicillin-resistant strain of *Staph. aureus,* it is worth pointing out that in such cases benzyl penicillin is liable to be inactivated before it can affect the streptococcus. Thus if penicillin-resistant *Staph. aureus* is isolated in association with *Str. pyogenes* the patient should be given systemic treatment with cloxacillin. This is probably better than methicillin, since it is more active against *Str. pyogenes*.

If a penicillin-resistant *Staph. aureus* is present alone no treatment is necessary unless there are signs of infection. In this case systemic treatment with methicillin or cloxacillin is likely to be the best. In a small study fucidin by mouth was shown to be highly effective in eliminating staphylococci from burns, but resistant mutants were frequent (Lowbury *et al.,* 1962).

In the treatment of *Pseudomonas* septicaemia in burned patients, Stone (1967) found gentamicin more effective than colomycin, but it was essential to combine systemic therapy with local applications of the drug to the burned area.

PYOGENIC INFECTIONS OF BONES AND JOINTS

Acute Osteomyelitis

The infecting organism is nearly always *Staph. aureus*. Haemolytic streptococci and *Salmonella* are each responsible for a few per cent, and *Proteus* and other enterobacteria, *Haemophilus* and other organisms for occasional cases. In the infant, haemolytic streptococci have been the commonest cause, but in the series studied by Lindblad *et al.* (1965) *Staph. aureus* was the only organism isolated. Children with sickle cell anaemia (and perhaps other haemolytic anaemias) appear to be peculiarly susceptible to salmonella infections (Koenig and Rogers, 1962).

Since infection is likely but not certain to be due to staphylococci, attempts should be made to obtain material for bacteriological examination before instituting treatment. In cases not needing surgery this can be obtained by aspiration from the affected metaphysis, from any evident primary focus of infection, often the skin, or blood culture which is positive in a high proportion of early cases.

Prior to antibiotic therapy, up to 50 per cent of the patients died and a high proportion of the survivors were left with chronic discharging sinuses. Of 73 patients treated with penicillin in 3 series between 1945 and 1947, none died and only two developed complications (Gilmour, 1962). Since the advent of penicillin-resistant staphylococci, the situation has to some extent reverted to that of the pre-penicillin era. The incidence of acute osteomyelitis has increased, and while the mortality in patients treated with broad-spectrum antibiotics has remained low, the complication rate has risen and in several series there has been the impression that low grade persistent ' smouldering ' osteomyelitis has become more frequent (Winters and Cahen, 1960; Gilmour, 1962; Tronzo and Dowling, 1962). Of 15 penicillin-sensitive infections treated with penicillin by Meyer *et al.* (1965) none drained spontaneously, required drainage, or relapsed. In contrast, of 14 penicillin-resistant infections treated with appropriate agents, 8 developed chronic osteomyelitis. It has several times been suggested that this imperfect response is the result of using bacteristatic agents such as chloramphenicol or tetracycline.

As soon as adequate specimens have been obtained, treatment should begin with a mixture of benzyl penicillin (which is the most active agent against penicillinase-negative staphylococci) and an agent active against penicillin-resistant staphylococci. The choice lies between cloxacillin, a cephalosporin, fucidin and lincomycin. There has been no extensive direct comparison and their therapeutic efficacy appears to be so similar that there is at present no reason for preferring one to the others. Each has certain theoretical advantages and disadvantages. Cloxacillin and the cephalosporins are the most actively bactericidal *in vitro* and lincomycin the least. Clindamycin is more actively bactericidal than the parent lincomycin but is not yet available in a form suitable for parenteral administration. Both fucidin and lincomycin have the advantage of unusual penetration into bone (Evascus *et al.*, 1969) but the disadvantage that resistant mutants emerge relatively easily, especially to fucidin.

Craven *et al.* (1970) treated six severely ill patients infected with penicillin-resistant staphylococci, four of whom had multiple bone lesions, with trimethoprim-sulphamethoxazole and obtained prompt and satisfactory responses.

If the staphylococcus proves to be penicillin-sensitive the other agent should be discontinued. If the staphylococcus proves to be penicillin-resistant, in a patient treated with cloxacillin and penicillin, the penicillin should be discontinued. With lincomycin and fucidin combined treatment with penicillin should continue since this will be effective against any mutants resistant to the second agent which might appear. Clawson and Dunn (1967) comment on the need to correct anaemia if optimum benefit is to be obtained from antibiotic therapy.

The work of Dawkins and Hornick (1967) suggests that salmonella osteomyelitis should be treated with chloramphenicol. In patients in whom salmonella appears likely—for example those suffering from salmonella infections elsewhere or sickle-cell anaemia—chloramphenicol should be given until the bacteriological diagnosis is established. In patients suffering from osteomyelitis of other etiology the treatment must be guided by the bacteriological findings.

Antibiotics must be given in large doses in order to ensure adequate levels at the site of infection. After the first few days the frequency of injections can be reduced to six- or eight-hourly and after the first week or so oral therapy can be substituted for injections if the response is satisfactory. Benzyl penicillin should be given in a daily dose of 6 mega units, initially as 4-hourly injections or continuous infusion. Cloxacillin should be given in doses of 0·5 to 1·0 g. every four to six hours (children: 25 mg. per kg., 4-hourly). Fucidin and lincomycin should be given in a dose of 500 mg. 6-hourly (children: 50 mg./kg./day). The absorption of lincomycin, which is affected by food, may be uncertain and the drug can be given parenterally over the crucial first 48 hours. Oral therapy may then profitably be continued with the more regularly absorbed and more active clindamycin in a dose of 300 mg. 6-hourly (children: 15 mg./kg./day). The dosage of all drugs may be halved at two-weekly intervals if progress is maintained, but treatment should continue for 3 or 4 weeks after the temperature has become normal (Meyer *et al.*, 1965).

If treatment is started at the onset of disease the response to penicillin is usually obvious within 24 hours. If after 36 hours there is no constitutional response or local pain and swelling persist, surgery must be considered.

In cases where antibiotic treatment is not started for two or three days the response to antibiotics may be slower, and the optimum management is in dispute (Neligan and Elderkin, 1965).

Chronic Osteomyelitis

Chronic osteomyelitis may follow incomplete resolution of acute osteomyelitis or be the sequel to penetrating wounds. The treatment is the same in both instances. Most cases are again due to staphylococci but other organisms, including Gram-negative bacilli, are more frequent and mixed infections are not uncommon (Clawson and Dunn, 1967; Agranat, 1969). Quite apart from complex bacteriology, chemotherapy is difficult, because sequestra have no blood supply and the masses of dense fibrous tissue surrounding the affected bone have a very poor blood supply. There is, however, not the same urgency to begin treatment and as surgery is always necessary, antibiotic treatment can be guided by bacteriological examination.

Where staphylococci are responsible, treatment is along the lines suggested for acute osteomyelitis but protracted treatment rather than initial high dosage is likely to be the key to success.

Septic Arthritis

This condition which may arise spontaneously, as for example in rheumatoid arthritis (Karten, 1969), or complicate trauma, resembles chronic rather than acute osteomyelitis in its bacteriology. *Staph. aureus* is responsible for not much more than half of the cases; streptococci of various kinds, enterobacteria, and mixed infections (sometimes including anaerobes) are all found (Kelly *et al.*, 1965). In children *H. influenzae* is a more common cause than is generally realized (Wall and

Hunt, 1968) and accounted for most of the cases under the age of two reported by Nelson and Koontz (1966).

Aspiration of the joint may be necessary to establish the diagnosis, but blood culture is positive in a high proportion of cases. Open surgical drainage may be preferable to repeated aspiration in the management and is held to be essential in infection of the hip joint (Kelly *et al.,* 1965; Clawson and Dunn, 1967). Following aspiration, the joint should be irrigated with saline and a solution instilled containing 100 mg./ml. each cloxacillin and ampicillin. Systemic treatment with these agents in full dosage should be instituted until the bacteriological diagnosis is established after which the optimum therapy can be planned on the basis of *in vitro* sensitivity tests. There is a division of opinion on the value and wisdom of re-aspirating the joint and instilling anti-bacterial agents whenever exudate re-accumulates. There are potential dangers in aspiration (not the least being super-infection with a resistant organism) and it has been

TABLE XLI

Solutions for Intra-articular Injection

	Units/ml.
Penicillin	100,000
Polymyxin	10,000
	mg./ml.
Ampicillin Cloxacillin Cephaloridine }	100
Streptomycin Kanamycin Neomycin }	50
Gentamicin	5

claimed that many of the antibiotics likely to be useful in this condition reach adequate levels in infected joints on systemic administration (Parker and Schmid, 1968). Unfortunately details of this work are not given and contrary to our experience of its general activity (p. 150) tetracycline is claimed to produce significant bactericidal levels in synovial fluid. In view of the general distribution of fucidin and lincomycin it seems unnecessary to give them directly into the joint but a number of other agents which may be indicated on the basis of *in vitro* sensitivity tests are known not to cross so well into exudates at other sites. Doses in which they may be instilled into joints where this is thought necessary are given in Table XLI.

REFERENCES

AGRANAT, B. J. (1969). *J. oral surg.* **27,** 293.
BEARE, J. M. (1960). *Trans. St. John's Hosp. derm. Soc.* **45,** 61.
BEVERIDGE, G. W. & POWELL, E. W. (1969). *Brit. J. Derm.* **81,** 525.
BLAKE, G. C. (1964.) *Brit. med. J.* **1,** 145.
BLANK, H. (1960). *Arch. Derm.* **81,** 649.
BORNSTEIN, D. L., WEINBERG, A. N., SWARTZ, M. N. & KUNZ, L. J. (1964). *Medicine (Balt.)* **43,** 207.
BRACHMAN, P. S. (1966). *Antimicrob. Agents Chemother.*—1965, p. 111.
CAPLAN, R. M. & CLABAUGH, W. (1969). *J. invest. Derm.* **52,** 247.
CARNEY, R. G. (1963). *J. Amer. med. Ass.* **186,** 646.
CARON, G. A. & SARKANY, J. (1964). *Brit. J. Derm.* **76,** 421.
CLAWSON, D. K. & DUNN, A. W. (1967). *J. Bone Jt Surg.* **49(A),** 164.
COLWILL, M. R. & MAUDSLEY, R. H. (1968). *J. Bone Jt Surg.* **50(B),** 732.
CORSO, J. A., AGOSTINELLI, R. & BRANDRISS, M. W. (1969). *J. Amer. med. Ass.* **210,** 2075.
CRAVEN, J. L., PUGSLEY, D. J. & BLOWERS, R. (1970). *Brit. med. J.* **3,** 201.
DAVIS, C. M., FULGHUM, D. D. & TAPLIN, D. (1968). *J. Amer. med. Ass.* **203,** 298.
DAWKINS, A. T. & HORNICK, R. B. (1967). *Antimicrob. Agents Chemother.*—1966, p. 6.
DE JONGH, D. S., SMITH, J. P. & THOMA, G. W. (1967). *J. Amer. med. Ass.* **200,** 557.
DILLON, H. C. (1968). *Amer. J. Dis. Child.* **115,** 530.
DODGE, B. G., KNOWLES, W. R., MCBRIDE, M. E., DUNCAN, W. C. & KNOX, J. M. (1968). *Arch. Derm.* **97,** 548.
EDITORIAL (1968). *Brit. med. J.* **1,** 721.
EVASKUS, D. S., LASKIN, D. M. & KROEGER, A. V. (1969). *Proc. Soc. exp. Biol. Med.* **130,** 89.
FREINKEL, R. K. (1969). *New Engl. J. Med.* **280,** 1161.
GILMOUR, W. N. (1962). *J. Bone Jt Surg.* **44B,** 841.
GREENBERG, L. (1968). *Bull. N.Y. Acad. Med.* **44,** 1222.
HOLTI, G., LYELL, A., MCCALLUM, D. I. & MORGAN, J. K. (1966). *Brit. J. Derm.* **78,** 661.
HUGHES, W. T. & WAN, R. T. (1967). *Amer. J. Dis. Child.* **113,** 449.
JEFFERSON, J. & MCKNIGHT, A. G. (1969). *Brit. J. clin. Pract.* **23,** 133.
JOHNSTONE, F. R. C. & COCKCROFT, W. H. (1968). *Lancet* **1,** 660.
JONES, W. I. JR., KLEIN, F., LINCOLN, R. E., WALKER, J. S., MAHLANDT, B. G. & DOBBS, J. P. (1967). *J. Bact.* **94,** 609.
JUHLIN, L. & LIDEN, S. (1969). *Brit. J. Derm.* **81,** 154.
KARTEN, I. (1969). *Ann. intern. Med.* **70,** 1147.
KELLY, P. J., MARTIN, W. J. & COVENTRY, M. B. (1965). *J. Bone Jt Surg.* **47(A),** 1005.
KNIGHT, A. G., VICKERS, C. F. H. & PERCIVAL, A. (1969). *Brit. J. Derm.* **81** (Suppl. 4), 88.
KNIGHT, A. H., WYNNE-WILLIAMS, C. J. E. & WILLIS, A. T. (1969). *Brit. med. J.* **1,** 416.
KOENIG, M. G. & ROGERS, D. E. (1962). *J. Amer. med. Ass.* **180,** 1115.
LARSON, D. L., MEYER, J. V., LYNCH, J. B. & LEWIS, S. R. (1966). *Amer. Surg.* **32,** 453.

LINDBLAD, B., EKENGREN, K. & AURELIUS, G. (1965). *Acta paediat. (Uppsala)* **54,** 24.
LOWBURY, E. J. L. (1962). In *Amer. Inst. biol. Sci.* Publication No. 9. Research in Burns, p. 242.
LOWBURY, E. J. L., CASON, J. S., JACKSON, D. M. & MILLER, R. W. S. (1962). *Lancet* **2,** 478.
MACMILLAN, B. G. (1967). *J. Trauma* **7,** 88.
MACMILLAN, B. G. (1969) *J. infect. Dis.* **119,** 492.
MARKOWITZ, M., BRUTON, H. D., KUTTNER, A. G. & CLUFF, L. E. (1965). *Pediatrics* **35,** 393.
MARKS, R. & DAVIES, M. J. (1969). *Brit. J. Derm.* **81,** 448.
MCBRIDE, M. E., FREEMAN, R. G. & KNOX, J. M. (1968). *Brit. J. Derm.* **80,** 509.
MCMILLAN, M. R. & HURWITZ, R. M. (1969). *J. Amer. med. Ass.* **210,** 1734.
MEYER, T. L., KIEGER, A. B. & SMITH, W. S. (1965). *J. Bone Jt Surg.* **47A,** 285.
MONAFO, W. W. (1967). *J. Trauma* **7,** 99.
MONCRIEF, J. A. (1969). *Clin. Pharmacol. Therap.* **10,** 439.
MONTES, L. F., BLACK, S. H. & MCBRIDE, M. E. (1967). *J. invest. Derm.* **49,** 474.
MORAN, J. M., ATWOOD, R. P. & ROWE, M. I. (1965). *New Engl. J. Med.* **272,** 554.
MOYER, C. A., BRENTANO, L., GRAVENS, D. L., MARGRAF, H. W. & MONAFO, W. W. (1965). *Arch. Surg. (Chicago)* **90,** 812.
NELIGAN, G. A. & ELDERKIN, F. M. (1965). *Brit. med. J.* **1,** 1349.
NELSON, J. D. & KOONTZ, W. C. (1966). *Pediatrics* **38,** 966.
PAGE, M. I. & KING, E. O. (1966). *New Engl. J. Med.* **275,** 181.
PARKER, M. T. (1969). *Brit. med. J.* **3,** 671.
PARKER, M. T. & WILLIAMS, R. E. O. (1961). *Acta paediat. (Uppsala)* **50,** 101.
PARKER, R. H. & SCHMID, F. R. (1968). *Arthritis Rheum.* **11,** 503.
PRICE, W. R. & WOOD, M. (1966). *Amer. J. Surg.* **112,** 674.
ROBINSON, H. M. & RASKIN, J. (1965). *Arch. Derm.* **91,** 372.
SEABURY, J. H. & DASCOMB, H. E. (1964). *J. Amer. med. Ass.* **188,** 509.
SOLOMON, S. & BLUEFARB, S. M. (1969). *Indust. Med.* **38,** 54.
STONE, H. H. (1967). *J. Trauma* **7,** 109.
SWITZER, W. E. (1967). *J. Trauma* **7,** 110.
TRONZO, R. G. & DOWLING, J. J. (1962). *Clin. Orthop.* **22,** 108.
VICKERS, C. F. H. (1969). *Brit. J. Derm.* **81,** 902.
WALL, J. J. & HUNT, D. D. (1968). *J. Bone Jt Surg.* (A) **50,** 1657.
WETHERED, R. R., HEELER, W. R. & WARIN, R. P. (1967). *Brit. J. Derm.* **79,** 352.
WHITING, D. A. (1967). *Brit. J. Derm.* **79,** 345.
WINTERS, J. L. & CAHEN, I. (1960). *J. Bone Jt Surg.* **42A,** 691.

Chapter XIX

MENINGITIS

Primary Bacterial Meningitis

THE common causes of bacterial meningitis are *N. meningitidis, H. influenzae,* and *Str. pneumoniae.* In most series, *H. influenzae* is the major cause of meningitis in infants and young children, but rare in older children and adults. The meningococcus is common in children and the main cause of meningitis in the young adult. The pneumococcus is principally represented at the extremes of age. In the neonate, the situation is completely different. Enterobacteria account for most of the cases, and haemolytic streptococci and staphylococci are common, while the principal agents of meningitis in older children are rare (Table XLII).

TABLE XLII

Percentage of Meningitis in Various Age Groups

	Age in Years				
	<1	*<5*	*<30*	*<60*	*60+*
H. influenzae	41	51	7	1	0
N. meningitidis	13	34	16	4	33
S. pneumoniae	16	12	13	31	28

Derived from figures given by Mathies *et al.* (1966).

In most series, no organisms were recovered from the C.S.F. in about a quarter of the patients. Various explanations have been put forward for this of which the most important, from the point of view of ultimate therapy, is pre-treatment. There is no doubt that antibacterial agents given early in the course of unrecognized meningitis may make it impossible subsequently to recover organisms from the C.S.F. This in turn may seriously hinder the management where unusual organisms are concerned, as for example in neonatal or post-traumatic meningitis.

There is, however, no good evidence that in purulent meningitis of common aetiology such pre-treatment makes the prognosis worse (Heycock and Noble, 1964) and in so far as it may represent early treatment with a suitable agent it may make the prognosis better (Harter, 1963).

Secondary Bacterial Meningitis

When meningitis supervenes in chronic ear infections or sinusitis, or follows trauma, operation or lumbar puncture, the infecting organisms resemble those of neonatal meningitis rather than those of acute primary meningitis in older age groups. Staphylococci, streptococci, enterobacteria and pseudomonas are all common, and mixed infections, sometimes including anaerobic organisms, may be found.

Early Diagnosis

In the treatment of bacterial meningitis three principles remain the foundation of success: early diagnosis; early and intensive chemotherapy; and recognition and treatment of complications. As well as early clinical diagnosis, early bacteriological diagnosis is of the utmost importance and an expert opinion on a Gram-stained film of a specimen of cerebro-spinal fluid should be regarded as one of the few bacteriological emergencies. Meningococci can usually be diagnosed with certainty, although a considerable search may be needed to find them in the film. Recognition of scanty organisms, especially in patients who have already received some treament, may be facilitated by immunofluorescent staining (Fox *et al.*, 1969). Similarly, pneumococci, streptococci and haemophilus organisms can in most cases be recognised. If coliform bacilli are seen, although it is impossible to identify the species or even the genus, it is nevertheless a guide in the choice of early chemotherapy.

TREATMENT

Despite the sensitivity of the bacteria commonly causing meningitis to a variety of potent agents, the results of treatment are frequently disappointing. The overall mortality in recent series has been up to 25 per cent, reaching 80 or 90 per cent at the extremes of age. Septicaemic spread not infrequently produces serious secondary infections, notably pericarditis and arthritis, particularly in children but sometimes in adults (Williams and Geddes, 1970) and as many as a third of the survivors may exhibit neurological sequelae (de Lemos and Haggerty, 1969). Factors which have been thought to be important in producing this disappointing response are failure to achieve the requisite high concentrations of drug in the C.S.F., sequestration of infection in intra-meningeal loculi or adjacent structures, antagonism between pairs of simultaneously administered agents and (probably most important of all) delay in diagnosis and the institution of treatment.

Antagonism

The evidence that pairs of drugs may operate antagonistically in the treatment of meningitis is derived from the classic observations of Lepper and Dowling (1951) who found that of 43 patients treated with massive doses of penicillin 13 (30 per cent) died; of 14 patients treated with similar doses of penicillin plus chlortetracycline (previously successfully used alone) 11 (79 per cent) died. Similarly, Mathies *et al.* (1968) found the fatality in patients with bacterial meningitis treated with ampicillin alone to be 4·3 per cent and in those treated with ampicillin plus chloramphenicol and streptomycin 10·5 per cent.

Wallace *et al.* (1966) studied the interaction of penicillin and chloramphenicol against pneumococci and found that both *in vitro* and in the treatment of experimental pneumococcal meningitis in the dog penicillin alone or penicillin given before chloramphenicol rapidly killed the pneumococci while chloramphenicol inhibited growth of the organisms and consequently the action of simultaneously or later administered penicillin, the lethal effect of which is only exerted on growing organisms.

Antibiotic Concentration in C.S.F.

The intrathecal concentrations of antibacterial agents are determined by: (1) Plasma concentration of the agent, (2) diffusion, (3) active cellular transport (in or out of the C.S.F.), (4) entry with other plasma constituents in the course of inflammation, (5) bulk transport (that is to say removal of fluid without change of composition) of the agent in the C.S.F. through the arachnoid villi.

The rapid disappearance of penicillin from the C.S.F. may be due to active transport from the C.S.F. to the blood by a mechanism resembling that of the proximal renal tubule.

Protein binding may be important in both limiting normal diffusion and facilitating access with protein entry in the course of inflammation.

The following are a guide to the percentages of the plasma levels of various agents to be found in the C.S.F. :

Sulphadiazine	40-80
Sulphadimidine	30-80
(Other sulphonamides, except sulphanilamide, less)	
Chloramphenicol	30-50
Tetracycline	10
(Oxy- and chlor-tetracycline less)	
Penicillin	0·5-2 or more
Streptomycin	trace
Polymyxin	nil

Intrathecal Injections

It seems reasonable to attempt to supplement inadequate C.S.F. levels resulting from systemically administered drug by direct intrathecal injection. Unfortunately it appears that the distribution of agents administered in this way is often erratic (Schanker, 1966) and there is no good evidence that the results are significantly improved by these injections. With increasing experience of treating meningitis, several authors have abandoned intrathecal therapy on the grounds that the risks of medullary coning, local toxicity, and the frequency of subdural effusions outweigh the doubtful therapeutic advantage.

It nevertheless appears to us that there is nothing to be lost and possible benefit in instilling a suitable agent at the time of initial lumbar puncture when the C.S.F. is found to be turbid. Benzyl penicillin has been the traditional choice but ampicillin will cover all three common bacterial pathogens. In the management of coliform or *Pseudomonas* meningitis for which *in vitro* testing indicates the use of streptomycin and its relatives, or polymyxins, intrathecal therapy is essential.

If intrathecal injections are necessary, the irritant effect of introducing a foreign substance into the theca must be remembered. The purest available material must be used: the dose must not be higher than necessary to obtain the appropriate bactericidal effect; and the number of injections must be kept to a minimum. The following doses are those usually recommended:

Penicillin	10,000-20,000 units (6-12 mg.)
Streptomycin	50-100 mg.
Polymyxin	10,000-50,000 units; under 2 yr. up to 16,000 units.
Ampicillin	3-5 mg. for children ; 10-40 mg. for adults.
Gentamicin	5 mg., 1 mg. for infants.
Cephaloridine	50 mg., children 25 mg., infants 12·5 mg.

Injections should not be given more than once daily.

Sequestration of Infection

Failure to respond or relapse may be due to re-seeding of the meninges from extra-meningeal sites or to intra-meningeal loculation.

Several authors have felt that results would be improved if intrathecal exudation could be reduced or dispersed ; but corticosteroids administered for this purpose have been disappointing (de Lemos and Haggerty, 1969), and the benefits of fibrinolytic activators or streptodornase appear not to have been dramatic (Newman and Stewart, 1965; Parker *et al.*, 1965).

Initial Treatment

After removal of C.S.F. for laboratory examination, 10 mg. of ampicillin should be instilled, except in neonatal or secondary meningitis where 5 mg. of gentamicin offers wide cover against the likely infecting organisms. An expert opinion on the probable identity of the infecting organism based on examination of the Gram-stained film on the centrifuged deposit of the C.S.F. should be urgently obtained. Initial therapy should be based on this result according to the recommendations given under the individual organisms. If no bacteria are seen but other findings favour the diagnosis of acute bacterial meningitis, initial therapy must cover as far as possible the likely infecting species.

There are two main possibilities. One, which we favour, is to give ampicillin intravenously; the other favoured by those who dislike intravenous therapy and are unimpressed by the risks of marrow aplasia, is to give chloramphenicol. The details of the regimens are given under *H. influenzae* meningitis. There is no evidence that the addition of sulphadiazine enhances the response to either agent and penicillins will exert no bactericidal effect if they are given with chloramphenicol. If organisms are recovered on culture, treatment can be based on the results; if not, initial therapy can be continued. If no organisms are recovered, the general experience of a wide variety of regimens has been that the prognosis is good.

Duration of Treatment

The response to treatment in cases of acute meningitis is usually extremely rapid. Except with coliform infections and tuberculous meningitis (p. 411), if uncomplicated cases are treated early, the cerebro-spinal fluid is often sterile within 24 hours of the onset of treatment and almost invariably within a week. It is rarely necessary for treatment to exceed 10 days. Intrathecal administration is usually needed for a much shorter period. It can be discontinued 24 hours after the cerebro-spinal fluid is sterile, and in many cases this means that only the initial and one subsequent intrathecal injection are necessary.

TREATMENT OF SPECIFIC INFECTIONS

Meningococcal Meningitis

Until recently, meningococcal meningitis was successfully treated with sulphadiazine. Since 1963 when they first appeared, sulphonamide-resistant meningococci have made rapid strides. By 1969, 70 per cent of meningococcal infections in the United States were due to sulphonamide-resistant strains (Artenstein, 1969). Such strains have generally been found to be uncommon elsewhere but they have already been found in several countries (p. 259) and it cannot be hoped that their prevalence will not increase. As a result, sulphonamides can no longer be relied upon for the treatment of meningococcal meningitis. The infection has been shown to respond at least as well to penicillin (150,000 u./kg./day) given as 6-hourly intravenous or intramuscular injections or continuous intravenous infusion plus probenecid (1 g. 6-hourly) and this is now the treatment of choice.

Where no resistant strains have been encountered and constant bacteriological vigilance can be exercised, sulphonamides can still be used. Sulphadiazine has been the traditional choice but sulphafurazole is at least as active (p. 29), and though less well transported into the C.S.F. is much less liable to cause crystalluria. Either should be given intravenously for the first 48 hours changing to oral administration if the response is satisfactory. The initial dose should be 50 mg./kg. followed by a daily dose of 100 mg./kg. given 6-hourly. In infants the dosage should be doubled.

If the organism is sulphonamide-resistant, there is no purpose in adding sulphonamide and even if it is sensitive, there is no good evidence that the results of penicillin treatment are improved by the addition of sulphonamide (Carpenter and Petersdorf, 1962). In the series treated with penicillin plus sulphonamide by Anglin *et al.* (1965) 10·5 per cent died. Of those treated by Mathies *et al.* (1966) with penicillin alone 9·1 per cent died. It is evident both from the *in vitro* sensitivity of the organism and the poor results of treatment that cephalothin should not be used for the treatment of meningococcal meningitis (Southern and Sanford, 1969).

PROPHYLAXIS. Familial spread may occur (Greenfield and Feldman, 1967) and in outbreaks of cerebro-spinal fever in closed communities the treatment of nasopharyngeal carriers must be considered.

Sulphadiazine has been very effective for chemoprophylaxis in contrast to other agents successfully used for the treatment of meningitis which have been largely ineffective in prophylaxis. As a result, the emergence of sulphonamide-resistant strains has posed a considerable problem. It appears that rifampicin is a suitable substitute for sulphadiazine, being markedly more effective than penicillin, ampicillin, tetracycline or erythromycin in controlling the carriage of sulphonamide-resistant strains. Treatment with 600 mg. rifampicin daily for 4 days produced a reduction in carriage rate of 93·3 per cent which was sustained for 4 weeks (Deal and Sanders, 1969). It is, however, arguable whether so valuable a drug to which resistance can easily develop should be used for such a purpose.

Pneumococcal Meningitis

Despite the extreme sensitivity of *Str. pneumoniae* to the agents commonly used in the treatment of meningitis, the mortality from pneumococcal meningitis remains disappointingly high. In most series treated with massive doses of penicillin, with or without sulphonamide, the mortality rate has been 20-30 per cent (Mathies *et al.*, 1966 ; Anglin *et al.*, 1965) ; Wilson and Lerner (1964) contrasted the decline of mortality with improving treatment for all forms of meningitis from 81-37 per cent with that for pneumococcal meningitis from 84-68 per cent. Part of the excess mortality is undoubtedly due to the extreme age, poor general condition and associated diseases of the patients. In Carpenter and Petersdorf's (1962) patients, 60 per cent had concurrent pneumonia and 25 per cent were alcoholic.

Penicillin 150-300,000 units/kg. day should be given by intravenous injection at 2-4 hour intervals or intravenous infusion (changing if preferred to similar intramuscular injections) for not less than 10 days. Several authors report success with cephaloridine 500 mg. intramuscular six-hourly, plus daily intrathecal injections of 50 mg. Love *et al.* (1970) treated 49 patients with an overall mortality of 13·8 per cent, and neurological sequelae in 11·9 per cent of the survivors.

Haemophilus Meningitis

This infection is almost invariably due to *H. influenzae,* Pittman type b. Until recently chloramphenicol was unquestionably the drug of choice. It inhibits the growth of the infecting organism in a concentration of less than 1 μg./ml. and unlike its action on other species it is bactericidal in concentrations which can readily be achieved in the C.S.F.

It then appeared that ampicillin was equally effective (Barrett *et al.*, 1966) and being free from the possible haematological toxicity of chloramphenicol, became the drug of choice. Since then a number of cases have been described in which the initial response was satisfactory but subsequent relapse occurred, apparently because ampicillin penetration into the C.S.F. fell as the inflammatory response subsided (Coleman *et al.*, 1969; Gold *et al.*, 1969).

There are several possible solutions to the dilemma. The dosage of ampicillin may be paradoxically increased as clinical improvement occurs. Treatment which must in any case be instituted with large doses, will then have to be continued with very large doses indeed. Alternatively (and this has been the solution generally employed in the described cases of relapse) treatment can be switched to chloramphenicol when clinical improvement suggests such reduction in meningeal inflammation that ampicillin passage into the C.S.F. is likely to be impaired. Since the majority of patients respond well to ampicillin, there seems no purpose in instituting such sequential treatment routinely but to change to chloramphenicol if progress is not maintained.

Dosage and Administration

Chloramphenicol is given in a dose of 50-80 mg./kg./day, usually as two intravenous or intramuscular doses with appropriate (and important) reductions for younger children (p. 143).

After the first 48 hours oral therapy with the same dosage may be substituted if the response is satisfactory. Treatment should be continued until clinical recovery is complete (usually not more than eight days). Ampicillin is given for a similar period in a dose of 150 mg./kg./day by four-hourly intravenous or intramuscular injections or rapid intravenous infusions (Wehrle *et al.*, 1969). It should be emphasized that the drug must be given parenterally. There are no grounds for believing that oral therapy with ampicillin is adequate.

Cephaloridine should not be used for the treatment of *H. influenzae* meningitis. The organism is relatively resistant to the agent *in vitro* and Walker and Collins (1968) treated three cases with intravenous cephaloridine in doses up to 600 mg./kg. daily without sterilizing the C.S.F.

Enterobacterial Meningitis

Meningitis due to *Escherichia, Salmonella, Proteus,* other enterobacteria and *Pseudomonas* usually complicates septicaemia or infections elsewhere. Most cases are in the new-born (Groover *et al.*, 1961) or in children with abnormalities affecting the spinal cord (Scherzer *et al.*, 1966). In adults, these infections usually follow trauma or surgery, but may be secondary to urogenital (Kunin *et al.*, 1965; Manesis and Stanosheck, 1965) or ear infections (Newlands, 1965). If organisms resembling enterobacteria are seen in the Gram-stained film, treatment should be instituted with intravenous ampicillin as described under *H. influenzae* meningitis (p. 330; 75 mg./kg./day in the first two weeks of life) until the identity and sensitivities of the infecting organism are known. Most of these organisms occur in the neonate or secondary meningitis and in such cases, as recommended on page 327, 5 mg. of gentamicin should be instilled into the C.S.F. at the time of initial lumbar puncture. Sensitivities should be determined to gentamicin, streptomycin, kanamycin, ampicillin, carbenicillin, polymyxin, trimethoprim/ sulphonamide and chloramphenicol. If chloramphenicol is indicated it should be given as described under *H. influenzae* (p. 330). Carbenicillin must be given over the whole period (not less than 10 days) by continuous intravenous infusion of 20 g./day (30 g. day for *Pseudomonas* meningitis). Children should receive 250 mg./kg./day (400 mg./kg./day for pseudomonas infection). The remaining agents cross poorly into the C.S.F. even in the presence of inflammation (see p. 236) and systemic therapy must be supplemented by daily intrathecal injections (despite the deficiencies of this route of administration) in the doses suggested on page 327.

Morzaria *et al.* (1969) describe the successful treatment of neonatal *Escherichia* meningitis with trimethoprim-sulphamethoxazole (20 mg. + 100 mg., 12-hourly) after other agents had failed. Surgical management of underlying or complicating conditions (Burry and Hellerstein, 1966) is, of course, of the greatest importance. Success has been described in the treatment of pseudomonas meningitis in children with polymyxin (Newman and Stewart, 1964; Cooper, 1967) and with gentamicin—1·2 mg./kg./day (Newman and Holt, 1967). With both agents intramuscular therapy must be supplemented by daily instillations of the drug into the C.S.F. in the doses suggested on page 327.

Streptococcal and Staphylococcal Meningitis

Like enterobacterial infections, these may be secondary to trauma, surgery, or ear or sinus infections, or arise *de novo* usually in very young infants (Maher and Irwin, 1966). If the stained film of C.S.F. deposit shows Gram-positive cocci which can be positively identified as streptococci, penicillin treatment, as described under pneumococcal meningitis. should be immediately instituted. If the cocci cannot be identified, or are identified as staphylococci, similar penicillin treatment should be given together with cloxacillin 1 g. 6-hourly (children 100 mg./kg./day) intravenously. When the identity and sensitivities of the infecting organism are known, the inappropriate agent can be stopped or the treatment changed as necessary.

Listeria Meningitis

Although this is undoubtedly an infrequent form of meningitis, it is probably less rare than was previously thought (Moore and Whitmore, 1960). It occurs mainly in the new-born and appears to result from latent genital tract infection in apparently healthy women (Rappaport *et al.*, 1960). The infecting organism is *Listeria monocytogenes* and most strains are sensitive to sulphonamides, penicillin, tetracycline, chloramphenicol and streptomycin, but variation among individual strains has been recorded, particularly in relation to penicillin and chloramphenicol.

According to Seeliger *et al.* (1967) tetracycline has been the antibiotic of choice, but its lack of bactericidal effect and staining action on the teeth are drawbacks. Penicillin is said to be unsatisfactory. Extensive *in vitro* and *in vivo* studies in mice suggest that ampicillin might well be the most useful agent. Weingartner and Ortel (1967) treated 57 infants with listeriosis with twice daily intramuscular injections of 125-250 mg. ampicillin followed by 14 days' oral treatment with nine deaths (16 per cent). The mortality in 82 infants treated with tetracycline, chloramphenicol, or penicillin was

33 per cent. English and McCafferty (1965) successfully treated listeria meningitis in an adult with penicillin 30 mega units/day plus erythromycin 500 mg. four-hourly.

Tuberculous Meningitis

See Chapter XXV.

REFERENCES

ANGLIN, C. S., FUJIWARA, M. W., HILL, D., JAMES, W., McARTHUR, R. & SELIGMAN, G. (1965). *Appl. Ther.* **7**, 1091.

ARTENSTEIN, M. S. (1969). *New Engl. J. Med.* **281**, 678 (Ed).

BARRETT, F. F., EARDLEY, W. A., YOW, M. D. & LEVERETT, H. A. (1966). *J. Pediat.* **69**, 343.

BURRY, V. F. & HELLERSTEIN, S. (1966). *J. Pediat.* **69**, 1133.

CARPENTER, R. R. & PETERSDORF, R. G. (1962). *Amer. J. Med.* **33**, 262.

COLEMAN, S. J., AULD, E. B., CONNOR, J. D., ROSENMAN, S. B. & WARREN, G. H. (1969). *J. Pediat.* **74**, 781.

COOPER, R. G. (1967). *Med. J. Aust.* **1**, 527.

DEAL, W. B. & SANDERS, E. (1969). *New Engl. J. Med.* **281**, 641.

DE LEMOS, R. A. & HAGGERTY, R. J. (1969). *Pediatrics* **44**, 30.

ENGLISH, J. C. & McCAFFERTY, J. F. (1965). *Med. J. Aust.* **2**, 332.

FOX, H. A., HAGEN, P. A., TURNER, D. J., GLASGOW, L. A. & CONNOR, J. D. (1969). *Pediatrics* **43**, 44.

GOLD, A. J., LIEBERMAN, E. & WRIGHT, H. T. (1969). *J. Pediat.* **74**, 779.

GREENFIELD, S. & FELDMAN, H. A. (1967). *New Engl. J. Med.* **277**, 497.

GROOVER, R. V., SUTHERLAND, J. M. & LANDING, B. H. (1961). *New Engl. J. Med.* **264**, 1115.

HARTER, D. H. (1963). *Trans. Amer. neurol. Ass.* **88**, 179.

HEYCOCK, J. B. & NOBLE, T. C. (1964). *Brit. med. J.* **1**, 658.

KUNIN, C. M., BENDER, A. S. & RUSSELL, C. M. (1965). *Arch. intern. Med.* **115**, 652.

LEPPER, M. H. & DOWLING, H. F. (1951). *Arch. intern. Med.* **88**, 489.

LOVE, W. C., McKENZIE, P., LAWSON, J. H., PINKERTON, I. W., JAMIESON, W. M., STEVENSON, J., ROBERTS, W. & CHRISTIE, A. B. (1970). *Postgrad. med. J.* **46** (Suppl. Oct.), 155.

MAHER, E. & IRWIN, R. C. (1966). *Pediatrics* **38**, 659.

MANESIS, J. G. & STANOSHECK, J. (1965). *Arch. Neurol.* **13**, 214.

MATHIES, A. W. JR., LEEDOM, J. M., THRUPP, L. D., IVLER, D., PORTNOY, B. & WEHRLE, P. F. (1966). *Antimicrob. Agents Chemother.*—1965, p. 610.

MATHIES, A. W. JR., LEEDOM, J. M., IVLER, D., WEHRLE, P. F., & PORTNOY, B. (1968). *Antimicrobial Agents. Chemother.*—1967, p. 218.

MOORE, S. & WHITMORE, D. N. (1960). *Brit. med. J.* **2**, 1572.

MORZARIA, R. N., WALTON, I. G. & PICKERING, D. (1969). *Brit. med. J.* **2**, 511 (C).

NEWLANDS, W. J. (1965). *J. Laryngol.* **79**, 28.

NEWMAN, R. L. & HOLT, R. J. (1967). *Brit. med. J.* **2**, 539.

NEWMAN, R. L. & STEWART, G. T. (1964). *Clin. Trials J.* **1**, 11.

NEWMAN, R. L. & STEWART, G. T. (1965). *Arch. Dis. Child.* **40**, 235.

PARKER, R. H., WILCOX, W. D. & DIETRICH, T. S. (1965). *J. Amer. med. Ass.* **192**, 169.

RAPPAPORT, F., RABINOVITZ, M., TOAFF, R. & KROCHIK, N. (1960). *Lancet* **1**, 1273.

SCHANKER, L. S. (1966). *Antimicrob. Agents Chemother.*—1965, p. 1044.

SCHERZER, A. L., KAYE, D., & SHINEFIELD, H. R. (1966). *J. Pediat.* **68**, 731.

Seeliger, H. P. R., Laymann, U. & Finger, H. (1967). *Dtsch. med. Wschr.* **92,** 1095.
Southern, P. M. & Sandford, J. P. (1969). *New Engl. J. Med.* **280,** 1163.
Walker, S. H. & Collins, C. C. (1968). *Amer. J. Dis. Child.* **116,** 285.
Wallace, J. F., Smith, R. H., Garcia, M. & Petersdorf, R. G. (1966). *Antimicrob. Agents Chemother.*—1965, p. 439.
Wehrle, P. F., Mathies, A. W. & Leedom, J. M. (1969). *Pediatrics* **44,** 991.
Weingartner, L. & Ortel, S. (1967). *Dtsch. med. Wschr.* **92,** 1098.
Williams, D. N. & Geddes, A. M. (1970). *Brit. med. J.* **2,** 93.
Wilson, F. M. & Lerner, A. M. (1964). *New Engl. J. Med.* **271,** 1235.

Chapter XX

INFECTIONS OF THE AIR PASSAGES

Acute Nasal Sinusitis

MILDER cases of this kind of infection do not need chemotherapy. In the more severe, especially if some dangerous form of extension is threatened, full doses of penicillin are advisable. No other antibiotic can improve on this for pneumococcal or haemolytic streptoccocal infections, or for the mixed infection of dental origin which may occur in the antrum. Staphylococcal and Gram-negative infections are less common, and the choice of treatment for them should depend on laboratory tests.

Chronic Nasal and Post-nasal Infections

There are several chronic bacterial infections of this area which respond to chemotherapy. The use of combinations of neomycin, bacitracin and/or chlorhexidine as a cream or spray to eliminate staphylococci in carriers is now familiar. Meningococci can be banished from the post-nasal space of carriers by a short course of a sulphonamide unless the strain is resistant. Either this infection or post-nasal catarrh caused by a pneumococcus can be abolished by the use of penicillin-sulphathiazole snuff (5,000 units penicillin per g.). The commonly held view that this kind of local use should be avoided because of a risk of sensitization is disputable (p. 281).

Acute Pharyngitis

This may be largely confined to the tonsils, with a follicular exudate, or more diffuse, with hyperaemia and oedema of the entire fauces, and is characteristically accompanied by fairly high fever. The known cause of this condition is infection by haemolytic streptococci, but these are found in only about 60 per cent of cases corresponding to this description, and the cause of the remainder is unknown, although some (missed unless anaerobic cultures are made) may be due to haemolytic streptococci forming only streptolysin O, and it is a reasonable guess that some types of the very heterogeneous *Str. viridans* are much more pathogenic than they are given credit for.

Either a sulphonamide or penicillin should serve to control most streptococcal infections, the action of the latter being more rapid and more certain. According to Fry (1958) milder cases call for no such treatment: assessing them for severity, he judged penicillin treatment to be necessary in 30 per cent of 286 cases which proved to be infected with haemolytic streptococci and in 19 per cent of 196 in which they were not found. The results were naturally not comparable in the two groups, but were satisfactory. Scarlet fever, on the other hand, should be regarded differently: its exact aetiology is implicit in the diagnosis, and it is more liable to be followed by rheumatic fever or nephritis. Penicillin is usually considered to be indicated for every case: large doses are not necessary, but treatment should be continued for at least seven days, or a second attack may occur, the usual immune response having been interfered with but the organism not eliminated. Jansson and Klemola (1959) from a study of 7,837 cases, treated by different systems of dosage, recommend the inclusion of benzathine penicillin in the material used: its prolonged action was apparently responsible for the lowest second attack rate in the series.

The prevention of streptococcal throat infections in patients subject to rheumatic fever is best achieved with penicillin, although sulphonamides have also given good service for this purpose in the past. Alternatives are a monthly injection of benzathine penicillin, or the oral administration of a small dose (120 mg.) of penicillin V twice a day. The Ministry of Health (1965) gives two daily oral doses of 200,000 units of penicillin G as an alternative, and this is the sole recommendation of the American Heart Association: in one recent study in the United States (Feinstein *et al.*, 1966) only one tablet containing this dose was given daily. Penicillin G given by this route is poorly and irregularly absorbed, and it is clear from the studies of Wood *et al.* (1964) that its protective effect is far inferior to that of monthly benzathine penicillin: in a comparison between these two treatments the streptococcal infection rates per 100 patient-years were 20·7 and 6·1 and the rheumatic fever recurrence rates 5·5 and 0·4 respectively. Corresponding data for penicillin V are not available, but this should be more effective: its drawback is higher cost.

Two other acute throat infections require mention. *C. diphtheriae* is moderately sensitive to penicillin, and large doses have been found helpful in diphtheria: they presumably act both by arresting the activity of the causative organism and by controlling secondary infection. Such treatment does not, of course, remove the need for antitoxin. Vincent's angina (p. 347) and the gingivitis which may accompany it respond well to penicillin and amply justify its use: a very short course and moderate doses are enough.

Acute Otitis Media

In its milder catarrhal form this infection will usually resolve without chemotherapy. Fry (1958) in a study already quoted which also embraced 552 cases of otitis media, judged penicillin treatment to be necessary only in a minority. In the more severe suppurative form, chemotherapy has unquestionably been of great benefit, reducing the incidence of mastoiditis and other and graver complications to a small fraction of those seen in the past. This achievement must be due mainly to the use of penicillin, with some help from sulphonamides: the only question is, how often is the infection of such a nature as to demand other treatment? Two recent studies of the bacteriology of acute otitis media have quite divergent results. Feingold *et al.* (1966) found much the commonest infection in Boston children to be pneumococcal: few were either streptococcal or staphylococcal. Dadswell (1967) in London, dealing with patients of all ages, found haemolytic streptococci, alone or with other organisms, in 36 per cent, pneumococci in 14·2 per cent, and staphylococci in 16·8 per cent (60 per cent penicillin-resistant), of whom many were adults. The only point of exact agreement between the two studies is that *H. influenzae* infections occurred almost exclusively in children below the age of six.

The fact that a majority of infections in both series were either pneumococcal or streptococcal accounts for the continued efficacy of penicillin: these two infections are also those most liable to extend to other structures. It should be necessary to adopt other treatment, preferably on the basis of laboratory findings, in children only if penicillin fails, although perhaps initially in the adult in view of the greater frequency of staphylococcal infection, for which cloxacillin may be indicated.

The best results in a large series of cases treated by Rubenstein *et al.* (1965) were obtained with a single injection of all-purpose penicillin (potassium + procaine + benzathine) together with seven days of a triple sulphonamide. The failure rate was 2·7 per cent: with penicillin alone it was 5·8 per cent and with seven days of tetracycline 10·2 per cent. It may be mentioned also that Trakas and Lind (1966) commend lincomycin for *chronic* otitis media and mastoiditis: discharge cleared and the organism, usually a staphylococcus, was eliminated, in eight out of 14 patients.

Acute Bronchitis

This is most commonly an exacerbation of a chronic infection, and as such is considered in the succeeding section. Occurring in a previously normal subject, it is likely to be primarily a virus infection: if secondary bacterial infection is severe an antibiotic may be indicated (penicillin if pneumococcal, a tetracycline or ampicillin if *H. influenzae* or unknown). A special variety is the acute laryngotracheobronchitis of infants ('croup'); this is primarily a para-influenza virus infection, but secondary *H. influenzae* infection is common, and because of this, of the severity of the condition, and of favourable results reported, treatment with chloramphenicol may be indicated.

Chronic Bronchitis

In many elderly patients this is a progressive and incurable disease, commonly associated with emphysema and terminating eventually in right heart failure. Exacerbations, sometimes leading to bronchopneumonia, are common in the winter. The pathogen credited with the largest share in maintaining the inflammatory process in the bronchial mucosa is *H. influenzae*: second in importance is the pneumococcus. Secondary invaders include staphylococci and species of *Klebsiella* and

Pseudomonas, these two often coming to predominate after prolonged antibiotic treatment.

Anti-bacterial drugs have been given in different ways and with different objects, between which a clearer distinction should be drawn than is often customary. In the main these are three: long-term treatment aimed at reducing the activity of any existing infection and at preventing exacerbations; treatment of exacerbations when they occur; and thirdly, treatment aimed at the temporary suppression of infection in advanced cases with constantly purulent sputum.

LONG-TERM TREATMENT. The benefits obtainable from this have been explored in a series of laborious trials, many conducted in this country, in which the effects were judged mainly by reduction in days off work caused by exacerbations, but also by sputum examination and in other ways. In most of these trials small doses have been given daily throughout the winter, a comparable group of controls receiving an indistinguishable placebo. The results were reviewed at length in the previous edition of this book and by Stuart-Harris (1968) and need now only be summarized. In most studies a reduction in days off work has been achieved, often by diminishing the duration of exacerbations rather than their number. On the other hand tests of respiratory function carried out during two 5-year studies of tetracycline treatment (Report, 1966: Johnston *et al.,* 1969) have shown little or no diminution in the rate of its deterioration.

Of drugs used in this way, sulphonamides have been unsuccessful (but there is evidence of benefit from sulphamethoxazole + trimethoprim); penicillin V has given varied but more often unsuccessful results (the latter not surprising in view of its poor activity against *H. influenzae*); various tetracyclines have been extensively used (the increasing prevalence of resistant pneumococci is a possible threat to their usefulness) ampicillin has also been used, although more often for the following purpose.

TREATMENT OF EXACERBATIONS. An alternative to the foregoing policy is to provide the patient with a stock of the drug to take when he develops a cold or otherwise feels that his bronchial condition may be getting worse. There is some evidence of the value of this method, and its lesser cost is an advantage. Published information relates rather to the treatment of established exacerbations, often of sufficient severity to require hospital admission.

Both tetracycline and ampicillin have also been used for this purpose, the latter often in considerably larger doses. Among recent studies are those of Malone, Gould and Grant (1968) who obtained equal benefit from tetracycline, methacycline and ampicillin, each in a dose of 1 g. daily; Pines *et al.* (1968) who compared daily doses of penicillin 6 mega units + 1 g. streptomycin, ampicillin 4 g. and lymecycline 2·5 g. and found this to be the order of their merit, although with small differences; Hughes (1969), who compared trimethoprim 320 mg. + sulphamethoxazole 1,600, mg. with ampicillin 2 g. to the advantage of the former; and Citron *et al.* (1968) who compared cephaloridine 2 or 4 g. with penicillin 2 mega units + streptomycin 1 g. with indistinguishable results, even the lower dose of cephaloridine being equally effective. In any *H. influenzae* infection cephaloridine may seem an unfortunate choice, its M.I.C. for this organism being usually about 8 μg./ml.: in this series it eliminated *H. influenzae* from the sputum in only 1 out of 10 cases, whereas the other treatment achieved this in 8 out of 11. The most effective antibiotic for this infection is undoubtedly chloramphenicol, and although it has been little studied in such trials because of its toxicity, a short course for a severe exacerbation known to be caused by this organism may be justified.

TREATMENT IN ADVANCED CASES. Among studies in patients with constantly purulent sputum, Pines *et al.* (1967) compared daily doses of penicillin 4 mega units + streptomycin 1 g. with cephaloridine 2, 4 or 6 g. and found the smaller dose inferior and the larger superior to the other treatment. Since coliform organisms were much more often found in the sputum than any other species the main effect of cephaloridine may have been upon them. Pines *et al.* (1970) treated 81 patients with *Ps. aeruginosa* in their sputum with large doses of carbenicillin, with carbenicillin + gentamicin, with gentamicin alone or with colistin. The first two treatments were successful; the two others had little or no effect.

Bronchiectasis

In children this is almost invariably a pure *H. influenzae* infection. It regularly responds to treatment with chloramphenicol by disappearance of the organism from the sputum, which becomes mucoid and much reduced in volume (Franklin and Garrod, 1953). These observations were made before the toxic effect of chloramphenicol was known, and were brought to an abrupt conclusion when one child died of aplastic anaemia. Bronchiectasis in the adult may be of the same nature: in other cases the sputum is liquid and foul-smelling and contains a mixture of bacteria including anaerobes. Anything more than a transient palliative effect is even less to be expected in this condition than in chronic bronchitis. In patients with *Haemophilus* infection only, treatment as for chronic bronchitis may be helpful. Neomycin given by aerosol (0·25 g. twice daily for four days) is strongly recommended by Waisbren (1956). Kanamycin has also been used in this way. It must be remembered that these antibiotics are absorbed from the lungs: over-treatment, especially in a patient with damaged kidneys, has been known to cause deafness.

The staphylococcal bronchial infection common in children with mucoviscidosis is a distinct problem. Of various long-term treatments with anti-staphylococcal antibiotics the combination of fusidic acid and lincomycin has recently given good results (Wright and Harper, 1970). If superinfection with *Ps. aeruginosa* occurs, gentamicin by aerosol appears more likely to be effective than polymyxin.

Pertussis

The antibiotic treatment of this disease has proved somewhat disappointing, possibly because the diagnosis is not often made as early as in other specific fevers, and should probably be reserved for cases selected on the basis of early age, early diagnosis and severity. Oral drugs such as tetracycline or chloramphenicol are liable to be vomited, and Chassagne (1964) for this reason prefers giving penicillin and streptomycin by injection, mainly with the object of preventing secondary infection: he also favours staphylomycin, with or without streptomycin. Nelson, Matteck and McNabb (1966) find

B. pertussis uniformly sensitive to ampicillin, treatment with which eliminated the organism with clinical improvement in four patients. In conflict with this finding are those of Bass *et al.* (1969), who treated 10 carefully observed cases each with ampicillin, chloramphenicol, erythromycin, oxytetracycline and no antibiotics. None of these treatments affected the course of the disease, and ampicillin failed to eliminate the organism, whereas erythromycin achieved this rapidly.

Pneumonia

1. LOBAR. When consolidation is clearly lobar a pure pneumococcal infection may be assumed. This condition has been used to evaluate every drug active *in vivo* against the pneumococcus from sulphapyridine onwards. The later sulphonamides, penicillin in various forms, tetracyclines and erythromycin have all been effective. Penicillin is perhaps to be preferred for the greater rapidity of its effect due to bactericidal action: it may be advisable to begin treatment with a few injections, but at least thereafter oral administration of an acid-resistant form should give adequate levels. This infection is one of the most amenable of all to chemotherapy: it need cause no anxiety unless grafted on serious underlying disease or occurring in debilitated subjects or alcoholics.

In a very small proportion of cases (perhaps 1 per cent) the cause of lobar consolidation is *Kl. pneumoniae* (Friedlander's bacillus). It is important to identify this organism early, because the prognosis is poor and multiple lung abscesses may result. A simple Gram-stained film of the sputum will usually reveal the nature of any untreated infection, and should be made at the earliest possible moment. *Kl. pneumoniae* is usually sensitive to sulphonamides, streptomycin, chloramphenicol and tetracyclines, and some combination of these has been the usual treatment: ampicillin, cephaloridine or trimethoprim + sulphamethoxazole may also be effective, but experience with them is lacking.

2. BRONCHOPNEUMONIA. This may be caused by any of a variety of organisms (apart from the primary virus infection when the condition complicates measles, influenza, etc.) and a guess at the identity of that (or those, since multiple infections

12

occur) concerned is not often likely to be right. The principal species, and their sensitivities to seven antibiotics, are stated in Table XLIII. It is evident from this that sputum examination is highly desirable, although not always conclusive, since in virus infections and perhaps some other cases only a mixed and indifferent flora may be found.

TABLE XLIII

Efficacy of Different Antibiotics against Organisms concerned in Bronchopneumonia

Species of Organism	Antibiotic						
	Penicillins			*Strepto-mycin*	*Tetra-cyclines*	*Ery-thro-mycin*	*Chlor-amphe-nicol*
	Benzyl	*Ampi-cillin*	*Methi-cillin*				
Str. pneumoniae	+	+	(+)	—	±	+	(+)
Str. pyogenes	+	+	(+)	—	±	+	(+)
Staph. aureus	±	±	+	(±)	±	±	(±)
H. Influenzae	(+)	+	—	+	+	+	+
Kl. pneumoniae	—	±	—	+	+	—	+
Psittacosis virus	—	—	—	—	+	—	+
R. burneti	—	—	—	—	+	—	+
Mycoplasma pneumoniae	—	—	—	+	+	+	(+)

+ = full therapeutic effect.
± = variable therapeutic effect.
(+)= lesser therapeutic effect.
— = no therapeutic effect.

Much depends on whether the infection is bacterial, since if not, only a tetracycline or chloramphenicol can have any effect. In the absence of laboratory guidance, tetracyclines have hitherto been regarded as the best choice, since they are more active than chloramphenicol against all the Gram-positive organisms, but now that not only staphylococci, but streptococci and even pneumococci may be tetracycline-resistant, this may no longer be true. A newcomer to the aetiological list is *Mycoplasma pneumoniae*, now known to be the ' Eaton agent ', the cause of primary atypical pneumonia. This organism is more susceptible to demethylchlortetracycline than to other tetracyclines (Jao and Finland, 1967), a difference also found by Newnham and Chu (1965) for strains of *Mycoplasma* from birds and animals, and much the clearest available evidence of therapeutic action in this infection is that of Kingston *et al.* (1961) obtained in an extensive double blind trial of demethylchlortetracycline. The organism is even more susceptible to erythromycin, for which a therapeutic effect has also been demonstrated. Lincomycin, or preferably clindamycin, not included in the Table, is an alternative to erythromycin for pneumococcal and perhaps some other infections.

Staphylococcal bronchopneumonia presents a special problem. In particular it can be a very dangerous complication of influenza, presenting one of the most acute of medical emergencies, and calling for prompt and vigorous treatment of kinds with which we are not concerned here. The staphylococcus is often resistant to penicillin and sometimes to other antibiotics: the only safe course therefore appears to be to use one of the isoxazolyl penicillins at least until laboratory findings are forthcoming.

The reason for failure of therapeutic response may sometimes be revealed in a Ziehl-Neelsen film of the sputum. This should not only never be omitted, but should be repeated on several occasions whenever pneumonia fails to resolve normally.

Colds and Influenza

Colds. The viruses of the common cold are, so far as is known, insusceptible to any anti-microbic drug. On the other hand, it has been represented that the more lingering and objectionable effects are the result of secondary bacterial infection, and some authors find that these can be prevented with antibiotics: Ritchie (1958), for instance, claims success with remarkably small doses of tetracyclines. There are objections to general use of this kind, but it may be justified in patients in whom the complications of a cold are liable to be exceptionally severe.

Influenza. Anti-viral chemotherapy is discussed in Chapter XXVII.

Secondary bacterial infection can be a much more serious complication of influenza than of the common cold, and there appears to be a case for trying to prevent it with antibiotics in patients at special risk and during a severe epidemic. The combination of cloxacillin as an anti-staphylococcal drug with ampicillin to cover other possibilities would be a logical choice if such treatment were thought worth while.

REFERENCES

BASS, J. W., KLENK, E. L., KOTHEIMER, J. B., LINNEMANN, C. C. & SMITH M. H. D. (1969). *J. Pediat.* **75,** 768.

CHASSAGNE, P. (1964). *Presse méd.* **72,** 1597.

CITRON, K. M., EMERSON, P. A., JOYCE, C. R. B., MAY, J. R., SELKON, J. B., SOMNER, A. R. & SPRIGGS, E. A. (1968). *Lancet* **2,** 592.

DADSWELL, J. V. (1967). *Lancet* **1,** 243.

FEINGOLD, M., KLEIN, J. O., HASLAM, G. E., TILLES, J. G., FINLAND, M. & GELLIS, S. S. (1966). *Amer. J. Dis. Child.* **111,** 361.

FEINSTEIN, A. R., SPAGNUOLO, M., JONAS, S., LEVITT, M. & TURSKY, E. (1966). *J. Amer. med. Ass.* **197,** 949.

FRANKLIN, A. W. & GARROD, L. P. (1953). *Brit. med. J.* **2,** 1067.

FRY, J. (1958). *Brit. med. J.* **2,** 883.

HUGHES, D. T. D. (1969). *Brit. med. J.* **4,** 470.

JAO, R. L. & FINLAND, M. (1967). *Amer. J. med. Sci.* **253,** 639.

JANSSON, E. & KLEMOLA, E. (1959). *Brit. med. J.* **1,** 1382.

JOHNSTON, R. N., McNEILL, R. S., SMITH, D. H., DEMPSTER, M. B., NAIRN, J. R., PURVIS, M. S., WATSON, J. M. & WARD, F. G. (1969). *Brit. med. J.* **4,** 265.

KINGSTON, J. R. & nine others (1961). *J. Amer. med. Ass.* **176,** 118.

MALONE, D. N., GOULD, J. C. & GRANT, I. W. B. (1968). *Lancet* **2,** 594.

MINISTRY OF HEALTH (1965). *Prevention of Initial Attacks and Recurrences of Rheumatic Fever,* prepared by Standing Medical Advisory Committee for the Central Health Services Council and the Ministry of Health.

NELSON, J. D., MATTECK, B. M. & McNABB, J. (1966). *J. Pediat.* **68,** 222.

NEWNHAM, A. G. & CHU, H. P. (1965). *J. Hyg. (Lond.)* **63,** 1.

PINES, A., RAFAAT, H., PLUCINSKI, K., GREENFIELD, J. S. B. & LINSELL, W. D. (1967). *Brit. J. Dis. Chest* **61,** 101.

PINES, A., RAFAAT, H., PLUCINSKI, K., GREENFIELD, J. S. B. & SOLARI, M. (1968). *Brit. med. J.* **2,** 735.

PINES, A., RAFAAT, H., SIDDIQUI, G. M. & GREENFIELD, J. S. B. (1970). *Brit. med. J.* **1,** 663.

REPORT (1966). *Brit. med. J.* **1,** 1317.

RITCHIE, J. M. (1958). *Lancet* **1,** 618.

RUBENSTEIN, M. M., McBEAN, J. B., HEDGECOCK, L. R. D. & STICKLER, G. B. (1965). *Amer. J. Dis. Child.* **109,** 308.

STUART-HARRIS, C. H. (1968). *Abstr. Wld Med.* **42,** 649.

TRAKAS, J. C. & LIND, H. E. (1966). *Antimicrob. Agents and Chemother.* —1965, p. 717.

WAISBREN, B. A. (1956). *Practitioner* **176,** 39.

WOOD, H. F., FEINSTEIN, A. R. TARANTA, A., EPSTEIN, J. A. & SIMPSON, R. (1964). *Ann. intern. Med.* **60,** Suppl. 5, 31.

WRIGHT, G. L. T. & HARPER, J. (1970). *Lancet* **1,** 9.

Chapter XXI

INFECTIONS OF THE ALIMENTARY TRACT

The Mouth

STOMATITIS is much more often an indication for stopping antibiotic treatment than for starting it. The condition is produced by the excretion of antibiotics in the saliva with consequent suppression of the normal flora and its replacement by resistant species. This is the only area in which penicillin can cause such a change: the substituted flora is mainly coliform, although it may include *Candida,* and symptoms are uncommon unless very large doses are given or penicillin is employed locally. Tetracyclines, if given in full doses for more than a few days, are more liable to lead to an overgrowth of *Candida albicans*. There are three stages in the resulting process: soreness without visible lesions, redness, and frank thrush. In severe cases this may extend to the fauces and even to the bronchi.

Thrush is in fact the only specific form of stomatitis for which antibiotic treatment is indicated. Nystatin, administered in the form of a suspension which comes in contact with the lesions, is highly effective.

VINCENT'S GINGIVITIS. This otherwise intractable condition merits treatment with penicillin, to which the causative organisms are highly sensitive. Two doses of a mixed potassium and procaine preparation on successive days will usually eradicate the infection. Success has also been claimed for local treatment. This was introduced by MacGregor and Long (1944) who used penicillin in pastilles with a gelatin base. It has been revived by Emslie, Cross and Blake (1962), who strongly advocate the use of a chewing gum containing penicillin, and contest the idea that short-term topical application in the mouth involves any special risk of sensitization (see p. 281). Metronidiazole in doses of 200 mg. three times a day for seven days also gave good results in the hands of

Davies, McFadzean and Squires (1964). It attains concentrations in the saliva as well as in the blood calculated to exert a direct anti-bacterial effect.

Acute Parotitis in its most severe form is usually a staphylococcal infection, and may require surgical treatment. An antibiotic should also be helpful, and methicillin is indicated in the first instance, pending the results of sensitivity tests, particularly in cases arising in hospital. There appears to be no evidence as to the utility of chemotherapy in chronic catarrhal infections of the salivary glands, the secretion in which (only obtainable in suitable form for culture by catheterising the duct) usually contains a pneumococcus.

The Stomach

The main question involved here is whether antibiotic 'cover' is advisable for gastric operations. Several studies of its effects (reviewed by Taylor, 1960) have led to the conclusion that it is actually detrimental, untreated controls having a lower incidence of infection, both at the operation site and in the lungs. The combination of penicillin and streptomycin which has commonly been used also predisposes to staphylococcal enterocolitis (see p. 354). These unfavourable results have followed treatment continued for several days, and a better case can perhaps be made for treatment at the time of operation only. Bernard and Cole (1964) gave three doses only of a mixture of penicillin, methicillin and chloramphenicol, before, during and after gastric and other abdominal operations, and thus reduced the rate of operation site infections from 25 per cent in controls to 5 per cent.

The Biliary Tract

The literature contains numerous reports of the successful use of various anti-bacterial drugs in infections of the bile passages. These are presumably based on symptomatic improvement, since evidence of the nature of the infection and of any effect of treatment on it is only obtainable by duodenal intubation. Moreover, the usual cause of either cholecystitis or cholangitis is obstruction by a gall-stone, and treatment directed merely at the consequences of this can clearly be only palliative. The uncertainty of this subject in its clinical aspects is such that attention is better directed to two aspects which are factual, namely, the nature of the infections concerned, and the concentrations attained by different drugs in the bile, which vary widely.

Bile is a medium congenial to some bacteria, notably the typhoid bacillus, and highly inimical to others, notably the more virulent of the pyogenic cocci, *Str. pyogenes* and *Str. pneumoniae*. Hence most infections in this area are due to coliform bacilli, which are in general bile-resistant: the only Gram-positive organism likely to be found is *Str. faecalis.* Thus, in the absence of direct bacteriological evidence a logical choice would be a drug active against the coliform group.

From the point of view of concentration in the bile, the available drugs are sharply divisible into two classes. Sulphon-amides, chloramphenicol, streptomycin and neomycin are excreted only in low concentrations, usually less than those occurring at the same time in the blood. Others are concen-trated in the bile, some of them owing the maintenance of the blood level after an individual dose to reabsorption after excretion by this route. Antibiotics excreted in larger amounts in the bile but nevertheless mainly via the kidney are tetra-cyclines and penicillins (Harrison and Stewart, 1961), particu-larly ampicillin (Acred *et al.*, 1962): it should be noted that the very high ampicillin bile levels found in experimental animals are not equalled by those in man, and when any obstruction is present they are further reduced even to *nil* (Ayliffe and Davies, 1965; Mortimer, Mackie and Haynes, 1969). Erythromycin and novobiocin are also excreted mainly in the bile.

Much the highest biliary concentrations, according to Acocella *et al.* (1968) are attained by derivatives of rifamycin, and although this antibiotic has only moderate activity against enterobacteria, the high levels attained compensate for this. There are enthusiastic reports of its efficacy in biliary tract infections by Bergamini and Fowst (1965) and Stratford (1966).

The treatment of biliary typhoid carriers is discussed in the following section.

INTESTINAL INFECTIONS

Enteric Fever

The recognized treatment for typhoid fever for over twenty years has been with chloramphenicol. Marmion (1955) recommends a total daily dose (administration being at four- or six-hour intervals) of 50 mg. per kg. until defervescence, and half this dose for a further 14 days. Woodward and Smadel (1964) recommend a dose of 3 g. daily reduced to 2 g. when the temperature falls and continued for 14 days, with the alternative of two five-day courses of this dosage separated by an interval of eight days. In severe cases cortisone or prednisolone may also be given (Rowland, 1961): defervescence is then more rapid and accompanied by a greater sense of well-being.

This treatment has several disadvantages. These are the risk of marrow damage, the frequency of relapse and total lack of bactericidal effect, with the result that a carrier state may persist: it has even been suggested that subsequent carriage is favoured. Moreover it seems that the response of the disease has become slower: Chakraborty (1961) in India and Omar and Wahab (1967) in Cairo both report that the mean period to defervescence, formerly about three days, has more recently extended to about six. It would be interesting to know whether this is attributable to diminished bacterial sensitivity, but in neither of these studies was this possibility examined. Both also report results of treatment with furazolidone, which appears to have been moderately effective.

As an alternative, great hopes were centred on ampicillin, since it is not only more active than chloramphenicol *in vitro* against the typhoid bacillus, but has two additional advantages in being bactericidal and safe to administer in larger doses, but results have been disappointing.

In Sanders' (1965) series given 4 g. ampicillin daily, six out of 10 patients with attacks rated as severe had to be given chloramphenicol 'because their condition was worsening after periods of treatment with ampicillin varying from four to eight days'. Patel (1964) found this necessary in fewer patients, and relates the degree of success with ampicillin to the stage of the disease at which it started: whereas chloramphenicol is effective at any stage, ampicillin brings down fever within a few days only when given early. This difference, and a better effect from ampicillin in mild infections, are evident from the experience of others. Scioli, Giusti and Balestrieri (1964) compared the effect on typhoid fever of 15 days' treatment with either 2 g. of chloramphenicol or 8 g. of ampicillin: the average times to defervescence were 3·6 and 6·1 days. They were also three and six days in patients with paratyphoid B fever given 2 g. chloramphenicol and 6 g. ampicillin by Sleet, Sangster and Murdoch (1964). In a non-comparative trial by Manriquez *et al.* (1965) the results were again judged inferior to those obtained with chloramphenicol. There seems to be no clear evidence that treatment with ampicillin reduces the frequency of relapse, and there is little information about its effect on the subsequent carrier state.

Typhoid fever seems to be the disease *par excellence* in which *in vitro* antibiotic activity is no guarantee of therapeutic success. Dawkins and Hornick (1967) treated experimental disease in prisoners with various antibiotics bactericidal for *S. typhi in vitro* in concentrations lower than that in which chloramphenicol is merely bacteristatic. Cephaloridine, gentamicin and polymyxin E failed even to achieve negative blood cultures. Ampicillin (6 g. daily) produced defervescence in two patients in five and 13 days: in two others chloramphenicol had to be substituted. It must be concluded that, except in infection by a chloramphenicol-resistant strain, ampicillin has no place in the treatment of any but perhaps mild cases of typhoid.

Much more promising results have been obtained from treatment with trimethoprim and sulphamethoxazole, originally reported on by Akinkugbe *et al.* (1968), in whose small series defervescence was more rapid than in cases on chloramphenicol. More recently Kamat (1970) in Bombay studied 220 cases, all with positive blood cultures, treated either with chloramphenicol or with trimethoprim-sulphamethoxazole: mean periods to defervescence were 4·3 and 4·0 days respectively, but there was a much greater difference in the duration of ' toxaemia ' and weakness, which persisted longer in chloramphenicol-treated patients, 10 of whom also had a ' toxic crisis '. There is so far no information about the capacity of this treatment to eliminate the organism, but the bactericidal effect of the combination encourages a hope that excretion may be terminated earlier.

TREATMENT OF CARRIERS. Here ampicillin has had much more success. Whereas tetracyclines or large doses of penicillin have in the past cleared only about 25 per cent of cases, ampicillin has been successful in 80 per cent or more. Christie (1964) cleared seven out of eight by three months' treatment with initially large doses reduced to 3 g. orally daily, together with probenecid and continued for 12 weeks. Münnich, Békési and Uri (1965/66) succeeded in 11 out of 12 cases by giving ampicillin parenterally (500 mg. four times a day) together with oral probenecid for up to six weeks. Simon and Miller (1966) gave 75-100 mg./kg. daily for four weeks or more to 15 cases, clearing 13. These are among the more significant of now numerous reports on this subject, and one conclusion which can be drawn from the last two is that success may be achieved despite the presence of gall stones.

Other Salmonella Infections

The treatment of paratyphoid fever is the same as that for typhoid. Chloramphenicol is also effective in acute *Salmonella* enteritis of the food-poisoning type, but in the previously healthy subject this is a self-limited disease of very short duration, and it is extremely doubtful whether treatment of this nature is necessary or even justified. On the other hand, in infancy or old age or in the presence of other disease, and in infection by a more virulent type such as *S. choleraesuis*, it should be given.

There is strong evidence that unnecessary antibiotic treatment of mild *S. typhimurium* enteritis actually prolongs the subsequent carrier state. This was originally observed by Dixon (1965) and was confirmed in an extensive epidemic reported by Aserkoff and Bennett (1969) in which treatment with various antibiotics not only delayed elimination of the organism but in some cases led to its becoming resistant to one or more drugs, this resistance usually being transferable. A strange episode is reported by Rosenthal (1969): a youth who had recovered from a mild attack of diarrhoea was found to have *S. typhimurium* in his faeces and was given ampicillin, which caused a recurrence much more severe than the original attack. The strain proved to be ampicillin-resistant, and it is suggested that suppression of the normal flora by the antibiotic enabled it to multiply ' unrestrainedly '. Loss of restraint by the normal flora —including that depending on bacteriocine production—may contribute to continued excretion of a pathogen when antibiotics are given.

Acute Infantile Gastro-enteritis

Anti-bacterial drugs are only a part, and probably not the most important part, of the treatment of this condition. For some years the best results have been obtained with neomycin, given orally in a total daily dose of 50-100 mg. per kg., but bacterial resistance, also involving kanamycin, is now not uncommon. Paromomycin (50-60 mg. per kg. daily) is strongly commended by Kahn, Stein and Wayburne (1963) in whose unit at Baragwanath Hospital, Johannesburg, intravenous fluid therapy is given to over 2,000 cases annually, of varied bacterial origin. In a small series intensively studied on the basis of body weight and weight of excreta paromomycin and chloramphenicol, particularly the former, gave results so clearly better than a placebo that this had perforce to be dropped.

In several recent epidemics of *Esch. coli* enteritis the strain has possessed transferable resistance to as many as eight drugs, but there is little or no published information about treatments used and their effects. Those worth considering may be with gentamicin (Valman and Wilmers, 1969) if the strain is sensitive, a polymyxin, or trimethoprim-sulphamethoxazole.

Acute Staphylococcal Enterocolitis

This is a profuse watery diarrhoea, usually with some fever, and leading rapidly to severe dehydration and collapse. Many reported cases have been fatal, and the condition found post mortem is a superficial necrosis of large areas of mucosa in the jejunum and ileum (sometimes also of the colon), the denuded surface being thickly covered with a mass of staphylococci: the intestinal contents, and the faeces during life, contain this organism almost to the exclusion of all others, so that the condition can be instantly recognised by the simple staining of a film.

It occurs mainly in surgical patients, attacking them a few days after operation, and results from treatment with a broad spectrum antibiotic or combination (usually a tetracycline or penicillin + streptomycin). Neomycin used for pre-operative bowel preparation can also be responsible. An empty small intestine is often another factor: gastrectomy predisposes to it presumably for this reason. A third and essential factor is the presence in the environment of a virulent staphylococcus possessing multiple antibiotic resistance. Such an organism, given the opportunity, can cause what amounts to an epidemic of this infection, as described at the Radcliffe Infirmary, Oxford, by Cook *et al.* (1957): many of their cases were due to a single phage type. These authors make the interesting suggestion that in a patient who has become a nasal carrier of such a resident strain, it may be directly conveyed towards the site of infection by a per-nasal gastric tube.

This is an almost wholly preventable condition, the means of prevention being simply the prohibition of broad spectrum antibiotic cover for operations. Exceptions must of course be made, as in the patient already suffering from peritonitis. The treatment of staphylococcal enterocolitis consists of stopping the responsible antibiotic(s), generous fluid replacement, and the administration of an antibiotic to which the staphylococcus is sensitive. Penicillinase-resistant penicillins have been used successfully. Khan and Hall (1966) make a strong case for vancomycin, given orally in 0·5 g. doses every 4-6 hours: in 45 patients so treated there were no deaths from the enterocolitis, whereas in 54 treated with other antibiotics and 10 given none there were eight and three such deaths respectively.

Intestinal Candidiasis

' Superinfection ' of the bowel consequent on suppression of the normal flora by broad spectrum antibiotics is of three kinds, staphylococcal, coliform (resistant strains of *Pseudomonas, Proteus,* etc.), which is rarely accompanied by anything more than mild diarrhoea, and that due to *Candida albicans.* This also is accompanied by diarrhoea which is liable to be more intractable, and by pruritus ani. Oral nystatin may be indicated as a preventive and also affords the best treatment.

Bacillary Dysentery

The average mild infection due to *Sh. sonnei* does not require specific treatment, and it seems inadvisable that routine reports of the isolation of this organism should include information about drug sensitivities, since this may seem to encourage such treatment. Moreover, *Sh. sonnei* is now frequently drug-resistant. This is a species in which multiple transferable resistance has been studied for years, and Farrant and Tomlinson (1966) describe an epidemiological study suggesting that such transference is occurring on a large scale in this country. Almost all strains are now sulphonamide-resistant, and a large majority of strains examined by Scrimgeour (1966) were resistant to ampicillin, although in only a minority possessing a higher degree of resistance was this transferable.

Specific treatment may be required for more severe *Sh. flexneri* infections, and the choice of an antibiotic should depend on laboratory tests either of the patient's own strain or of previous isolates in an epidemic. Chloramphenicol, tetracyclines and ampicillin have all been found clinically effective, and reported results do not seem to justify placing them in any order of therapeutic merit. Unabsorbed antibiotics (polymyxin and the several aminoglycosides) have also been commended, and since some of the cases of infantile gastro-enteritis treated with paromomycin by Kahn, Stein and Wayburne (1963) were apparently *Shigella* infections, such treatment must be accepted as beneficial, at least in infants. Whether it can hasten elimination of the organism from the bowel, or whether perhaps it can even delay this, as has been reported after *Salmonella* enteritis, is uncertain.

Amoebic Dysentery

The consensus of opinion among those more experienced in treating this infection than anyone can be in this country, appears to be that no antibiotic can replace emetine for its action on *E. histolytica* in the lesions, emetine bismuth iodide for eliminating cysts, and chloroquin for treating amoebic hepatitis. Fumagillin is an antibiotic with an unquestionable direct action on the amoeba, but is said to have given disappointing results and is by no means free from toxicity. Good results have been claimed with an astonishing variety of other antibiotics, among which chlor- and oxytetracycline have chiefly been favoured, but their effect is believed to be mainly on the bacterial flora, which contributes to the ulcerative process, and—at least *in vitro*—to the nutrition of the amoeba itself. Whatever the explanation, remarkably rapid healing of the lesions has been observed. Good results have recently been reported with paromomycin (see Chapter VII).

Cholera

Since the publication of the first edition of this book it has been clearly demonstrated for the first time that tetracycline is of value in cholera, although it does not remove the initial need for fluid replacement. Carpenter *et al.* (1964) in India and Greenough *et al.* (1964) in Pakistan have shown that tetracycline in moderate doses, the first few intravenous and thereafter oral, rapidly eliminates *V. cholerae* from the bowel, greatly reduces both stool volume and the requirement for intravenous fluid, and enables patients to be discharged in three days instead of seven. The economy in intravenous fluids and in bed occupancy is important in enabling more patients to be treated in an epidemic. Furazolidone (Chaudhuri *et al.*, 1968; Pierce *et al.*, 1968) is a cheaper and apparently effective alternative.

Therapeutic Suppression of the Normal Bowel Flora

The commonest indication for this is an operation on the colon, which it facilitates by diminishing both gaseous distension and liability to subsequent peritonitis. The less soluble sulphonamides were first used for this purpose, and later tetracyclines: these have a more profound effect, but were abandoned because they predispose to dangerous superinfections. The most popular antibiotic is now neomycin. It is not necessary, and indeed highly undesirable, to give this in large doses or for long periods, as described by Jacobson *et al.* (1960), who found that such treatment caused mucosal changes and malabsorption. Provided that the bulk of the intestinal contents has been reduced by suitable diet and aperients, two days' treatment should suffice. The following regime employed at St. Bartholomew's Hospital has been found satisfactory: initial doses of 4 g. phthalyl sulphathiazole and 2 g. neomycin followed by half these doses at six- and 12-hour intervals respectively for 48 hours. Some authorities prefer neomycin + bacitracin. Kanamycin or paromomycin are alternatives to neomycin. In the hands of Sellwood *et al.* (1969) a combination of neomycin, bacitracin and nystatin was more effective than phthalylsulphathiazole in preventing post-operative infections, and a correspondingly much greater reduction in numbers of the principal bowel flora was demonstrated.

Possibly the only indication for much more prolonged treatment of this kind is hepatic failure, the effects of which can be mitigated by administering an antibiotic, usually neomycin or kanamycin, for considerable periods. This inhibits bacterial activity otherwise responsible for the formation of toxic amines: which of the intestinal flora are responsible for this does not appear to have been established. In patients also suffering from renal failure, the small amounts of antibiotic absorbed may accumulate in the blood and cause damage to the eighth nerve, and possibly further damage to the kidneys (Last and Sherlock, 1960; Kunin *et al.*, 1960). As the less ototoxic, kanamycin may be preferable to neomycin for such patients.

REFERENCES

ACOCELLA, G., MATTIUSSI, R., NICOLIS, F. B., PALLANZA, R. & TENCONI, L. T. (1968). *Gut* **9,** 536.
ACRED, P., BROWN, D. M., TURNER, D. H. & WILSON, M. J. (1962). *Brit. J. Pharmacol.* **18,** 356.
AKINKUGBE, O. O., LEWIS, E. A., MONTEFIORE, D. & OKUBADEJO, O. A. (1968). *Brit. med. J.* **3,** 721.
ASERKOFF, B. & BENNETT, J. V. (1969). *New Engl. J. Med.* **281,** 636.
AYLIFFE, G. A. J. & DAVIES, A. (1965). *Brit. J. Pharmacol.* **24,** 189.
BERGAMINI, N. & FOWST, G. (1965). *Arzneimittel forsch.* **15** (Suppl.), 951.
BERNARD, H. R. & COLE, W. R. (1964). *Surgery* **56,** 151.
CARPENTER, C. C. J., SACK, R. B., MONDAL, A. & MITRA, P. P. (1964). *J. Indian med. Ass.* **43,** 309.
CHAKRABORTY, G. (1961). *Indian J. Pediat.* **28,** 357.
CHAUDHURI, R. N., NEOGY, K. N., SANYAL, S. N., GUPTA, R. K. & MANJI, P. (1968). *Lancet* **1,** 332.
CHRISTIE, A. B. (1964). *Brit. med. J.* **1,** 1609.
COOK, J., ELLIOTT, C., ELLIOT-SMITH, A., FRISBY, B. R. & GARDNER, A. M. N. (1957). *Brit. med. J.* **1,** 542.
DAVIES, A. H., McFADZEAN, J. A. & SQUIRES, S. (1964). *Brit. med. J.* **1,** 1149.
DAWKINS, A. T. & HORNICK, R. B. (1967). *Antimicrob. Agents and Chemother.*—1966, p. 6.

DIXON, J. M. S. (1965). *Brit. med. J.* **2,** 1343.
EMSLIE, R. D., CROSS, W. G. & BLAKE, G. C. (1962). *Brit. dent. J.* **112,** 320.
FARRANT, W. N. & TOMLINSON, A. J. H. (1966). *J. Hyg. (Lond.)* **64,** 287.
GREENOUGH, W. B. III., GORDON, R. S., ROSENBERG, I. S., DAVIES, B. I. & BENENSON, A. S. (1964). *Lancet* **1,** 355.
HARRISON, P. M. & STEWART, G. T. (1961). *Brit. J. Pharmacol.* **17,** 420.
JACOBSON, E. D., PRIOR, J. T. & FALOON, W. W. (1960). *J. Lab. clin. Med.* **56,** 245.
KAHN, E., STEIN, H. & WAYBURNE, S. (1963). *Lancet* **2,** 703.
KAHN, M. Y. & HALL, W. H. (1966). *Ann. intern. Med.* **65,** 1.
KAMAT, S. A. (1970). *Brit. med. J.* **3,** 320.
KUNIN, C. M., CHALMERS, T. C., LEEVY, C. M., SEBASTYEN, S. C., LIEBER, C. S. & FINLAND, M. (1960). *New Engl. J. Med.* **262,** 380.
LAST, P. M. & SHERLOCK, S. (1960). *New Engl. J. Med.* **262,** 385.
MACGREGOR, A. B. & LONG, D. A. (1944). *Brit. med. J.* **2,** 686.
MANRIQUEZ, L., SALCEDO, M., BORGONO, J. M., MARZULLO, E., KRALJEVIC, R., PAREDES, L. & VALDIVIESO, R. (1965). *Brit. med. J.* **2,** 152.
MARMION, D. E. (1955). *Med. ill. (Lond.)* **9,** 214.
MORTIMER, P. R., MACKIE, D. B. & HAYNES, S. (1969). *Brit. med. J.* **3,** 88.
MÜNNICH, D., BÉKÉSI, I. & URI, J. (1965/6). *Chemotherapia* **10,** 253.
OMAR, M. E. S. & WAHAB, M. F. A. (1967). *J. trop. Med. Hyg.* **70,** 43.
PATEL, K. M. (1964). *Proc. IIIrd Int. Congr. Chemother.,* Vol. 1, p. 416. Stuttgart: Thieme.
PIERCE, N. F., BANWELL, J. G., MITRA, R. C., CARANASOS, G. J., KEIMOWITZ, R. I., THOMAS, J. & MONDAL, A. (1968). *Brit. med. J.* **3,** 277.
ROSENTHAL, S. L. (1969). *New Engl. J. Med.* **280,** 147.
ROWLAND, H. A. K. (1961). *J. trop. Med. Hyg.* **64,** 101.
SANDERS, W. L. (1965). *Brit. med. J.* **2,** 1226.
SCIOLI, C., GIUSTI, G. & BALESTRIERI, G. (1964). *Postgrad. med. J.* **40,** (Suppl.) 87.
SCRIMGEOUR, G. (1966). *Mth. Bull. Minist. Hlth Lab. Serv.* **25,** 278.
SELLWOOD, R. A., BURN, J. I., WATERWORTH, P. M. & WELBOURN, R. B. (1969). *Brit. J. Surg.* **56,** 610.
SIMON, H. J. & MILLER, R. C. (1966). *New Engl. J. Med.* **274,** 807.
SLEET, R. A., SANGSTER, G. & MURDOCH, J. McC. (1964). *Brit. med. J.* **1,** 148.
STRATFORD, B. C. (1966). *Med. J. Aust.* **1,** 7.
TAYLOR, G. W. (1960). *Brit. med. Bull.* **16,** 51.
VALMAN, H. B. & WILMERS, M. J. (1969). *Lancet* **1,** 1122.
WOODWARD, T. E. & SMADEL, J. E. (1964). *Ann. intern. Med.* **60,** 144.

CHAPTER XXII

ANTIBIOTICS IN OBSTETRICS

Prolonged Labour

ALTHOUGH the amniotic fluid, placenta, and foetus are normally sterile, the vagina and cervical canal contain a variable bacterial flora which frequently includes potential pathogens (Morris and Morris, 1967).

These organisms are barred from ascent to the uterus by the membranes and provided these remain intact, intrauterine infection is uncommon. The membrane barrier can be involved by vaginal inflammatory disease and breached by premature (including surgical) rupture.

There is no conclusive proof that inflammatory conditions of the lower genital tract allow these organisms to gain access to the foetal membranes but the circumstantial evidence is considerable. Infections of the lower genital tract increase the prematurity rate (Hawkinson and Schulman, 1966) and sometimes reach the foetus either from infected amniotic fluid entering the foetal respiratory tract, or via the umbilical vein to the foetal blood. Such infection may be present without inducing symptoms in the mother.

Ascent of vaginal organisms is facilitated by repeated vaginal examination. The total duration of prolonged labour is less important in determining the risk of infection than the interval between rupture of the membranes and onset of labour.

Both foetus and mother may suffer the consequences of ascending infection and there is a sharp rise in perinatal mortality and maternal morbidity when the membranes have been ruptured for more than 24 hours (Still and Adamson, 1967). Uterine sepsis may develop insidiously, with no evidence of infection beyond a foul or foetid vaginal discharge for as long as 48 hours. The result of untreated sepsis may be a foul-smelling still-birth and, in the mother, bacteraemia with a 30-60 per cent incidence of septic shock.

With such potentially serious consequences, it generally continues to be the practice in premature rupture of the membranes to protect the foetus, as far as possible, by maternal antibacterial prophylaxis. So far, however, convincing evidence is lacking that either systemic treatment of the mother, or the instillation of topical antibacterial agents into the genital tract, significantly reduces the incidence of infections in the amnion or foetus (Brelje and Kaltreider, 1966; Hawkinson and Schulman, 1966).

There is no such doubt about the need and efficacy of antibiotic protection of the mother. The only fatality from streptococcal infection in the puerperium recorded in Britain for some years occurred in a patient in whom this precaution was omitted, in spite of prolonged labour and manual removal of the placenta.

Choice of Agent

In selecting the appropriate antibiotic its antibacterial spectrum and its capacity to pass into the liquor amnii and into the foetal circulation must be borne in mind. The organisms principally concerned are *Escherichia,* other enterobacteria, staphylococci, and streptococci, including some anaerobic strains. *Listeria monocytogenes* is frequently mentioned amongst more exotic organisms likely to infect the foetus, but while its role is indisputable, it does not appear to be an important cause of foetal loss (Ansbacher *et al.*, 1968). Only negligible amounts of streptomycin, the tetracyclines and chloramphenicol reach the liquor amnii, whereas with penicillins and cephalosporins high and prolonged levels result from excretion by the foetal kidneys. Benzyl penicillin has been found to produce levels up to 32 times those in the blood and Blecher *et al.* (1966) have shown that after three 500 mg. doses of ampicillin to the mother, the liquor amnii usually contains 2·5 μg. per ml. or more. Barr and Graham (1967) found that doses of 1 g. of cephaloridine produced levels of 1-8 μg./ml. in both the amnion and the cord serum of the majority of babies, but in 5-10 per cent, the levels were less than 1 μg./ml.

A number of studies comparing antibiotic concentrations in maternal and umbilical blood have shown that penicillin, streptomycin and the tetracyclines administered to the mother

all reach the foetal circulation within about half an hour but
the concentrations are substantially lower than those found in
maternal blood. Chloramphenicol reaches the foetal circulation rather less readily. It appears therefore that the best protection against ascending vaginal organisms is likely to be
afforded by agents which besides being active against the main
incriminated pathogens are concentrated in the liquor.

Cervical swabs should be taken and examined bacteriologically, but while waiting for a report it appears that cover
will probably be provided by ampicillin, or cephaloridine, but
they are not likely to produce adequate foetal blood levels
unless large doses are given.

PUERPERAL PYREXIA

Slight fever in the puerperium without clinical signs should
be observed and not treated with antibiotics in the absence
of positive findings. Observation should include examination
of the urine and high vaginal or cervical swabs. If haemolytic
streptococci of Lancefield groups A, C or G are found in
vaginal or cervical swabs antibiotic treatment must always be
given and penicillin is the drug of choice. The presence of
other organisms in the vagina, even those commonly associated
with puerperal infection, does not necessarily indicate antibiotic
treatment, in the absence of clinical evidence of infection.

Puerperal Infection of the Genital Tract

Patients with severe pyrexia of more than 24 hours' duration
or with clinical signs of genital tract infection should always
be given antibiotic treatment. Infection is still the most important cause of maternal death (Stevenson, 1969). The bacteriological investigation of puerperal infection of the genital tract
is not very satisfactory. In most hospitals reliance is placed on
the high vaginal swab, which is perfectly adequate if the infecting agent is *Str. pyogenes* but in other cases may give misleading results, either because the infecting agent is not isolated
or because the organism isolated is so frequently present in
the vagina of apparently healthy women in the puerperium that
its pathogenic significance is doubtful.

These cases arise in the same way as the ascending infection
which may complicate premature rupture of the membranes.

Cervical swabs and blood cultures should be obtained and treatment instituted with ampicillin or cephaloridine along the lines suggested on page 361. Amongst possible infecting organisms *Staph. aureus* is likely to be resistant to ampicillin, and bacteroides to cephaloridine (some strains are sensitive to ampicillin). As it happens, both of these possibilities can be covered by adding clindamycin to either agent for the first day or two until the nature of the infection is established. The problems of concomitant shock are mentioned on page 363.

Puerperal Bacteriaemia in Patients with Heart Disease

It has been claimed that bacteriaemia can be demonstrated in up to 5 per cent of women during delivery and that there is a corresponding risk of endocarditis in those with heart disease. Baker and Hubbel (1967) found the incidence to be only a tenth of this, with no bacteriaemia after the first 24 hours. They doubt the necessity of giving prophylactic antibiotics during the uncomplicated delivery of women with heart disease.

SEPTIC ABORTION

Infection is liable to occur in cases of incomplete abortion, where all or part of the placenta is retained, or in cases where abortion is illegally performed by the inexpert use of unsterile instruments. Common infecting organisms are *Staph. aureus,* coliform bacilli, anaerobic streptococci and enterococci. After instrumental abortion, particularly if the uterus is ruptured, gas gangrene may occur. More than half of all maternal deaths result from septic abortion. The mortality rate is variously reported as 0·29-3·25 per cent and is especially high in those with septic shock. Moritz and Thompson (1966) emphasize that these patients often appear deceptively well for some time and then suddenly deteriorate. The clinical picture of *Cl. welchii* abortal sepsis, which has a mortality of 53-85 per cent, is described by Decker and Hall (1966). The management of this condition and other anaerobic infections may be revolutionized by the use of hyperbaric oxygen (Parker and Jones, 1966), but large doses of penicillin should certainly still be given.

The antibiotic therapy of septic abortion cannot be separated from other essential parts of the treatment over which there is fundamental disagreement and on which we are in no position to adjudicate. If infection is severe treatment should be started at once and if gas gangrene is suspected the drug of choice is penicillin. In other cases broad cover, for example, with ampicillin plus cloxacillin, or with cephaloridine, should be given pending a bacteriological report. In all cases cervical swabs should be taken for bacteriological examination and in severe cases blood cultures should also be examined.

Some believe that the infected uterus should be curetted or removed at the earliest opportunity (Decker and Hall, 1966); others that surgery should be delayed until intensive antibiotic therapy has rendered the patient afebrile for at least 24 hours (Freel *et al.*, 1969). Some believe that concomitant septic shock should be treated with corticosteroids and vasopressors to restore the blood pressure; others that corticosteroids are useless (except in adrenal failure) and that vasodilators, not vasopressors, are essential to restore failing tissue perfusion. It is plain enough that the most potent antibacterial agents will exert no beneficial effect unless their delivery to the site of infection can be assured by early reversal of the circulatory disorder.

BACTERIURIA IN PREGNANCY

E. H. Kass has been responsible for drawing attention to the frequency with which pregnant women develop symptomless urinary infection (Norden and Kass, 1968). The usual prevalence found has been about 4-6 per cent although both lower and higher figures have been quoted partly perhaps because of the influence of age and social class (Williams *et al.*, 1969). The condition is important because about a quarter or a third of the patients develop clinical pyelonephritis. A number of studies have shown that bacteriuric patients are more likely to suffer abortion or premature labour and to deliver small or dead babies, but this has been disputed (Cavanagh and Sandberg, 1966).

Kass showed that treatment of asymptomatic bacteriuria would prevent the development of pyelonephritis and this has been generally confirmed. Both long-term and short-term treatment has been employed. Successful treatment throughout pregnancy without untoward effect has been achieved with sulphamethoxydiazine (0·5 g. per day) changing after the 13th week to sulphadimidine (1 g. 8-hourly); sulphamethoxypyridazine 0·5 g. per day); ampicillin (500 mg., 8-hourly); nitrofurantoin (50 mg., 6-hourly) and rotational therapy employing sulphafurazole, ampicillin, nitrofurantoin and nalidixic acid (Wren, 1969).

Many of these patients, however, respond to a short course of therapy. Gruneberg *et al.* (1969) cured 75 per cent of their patients with sulphonamide (usually sulphadimidine or sulphafurazole, 2 g. initially, then 1 g. 6-hourly for 8 days) and a further 16 per cent by repeating the course.

It is evident that as in the non-pregnant patient (p. 376) there is a variety of urinary tract infection which responds comparatively readily to treatment, and a variety which is very resistant. In a proportion of these very resistant patients—but by no means all—radiological abnormalities of the renal tract are demonstrable (Gower *et al.,* 1968). In Australia, Kincaid-Smith and Bullen (1965) found that in a third of their patients significant bacteriuria was still present 6 months after delivery. Over half their patients had abnormal pyelograms and it appears that pregnancy may effectively advertise the existence of long-standing renal disease.

Since some patients respond readily to treatment it seems reasonable to give them the chance to do so, thereby avoiding the disadvantage of prolonged medication. Appropriate short-term treatment, as for acute symptomatic urinary infection, is discussed on page 377. Those who fail to respond should be re-treated or given a short course of another agent. Regular follow-up examination is of the greatest importance. Patients who fail to respond may require suppressive therapy throughout pregnancy, and should undergo urological investigation postpartum.

While there has been general agreement that treatment will prevent progression from asymptomatic bacteriuria to clinical pyelonephritis, there has been much less agreement that it significantly influences the foetal loss rates (Wren, 1969).

Trichomoniasis in Pregnancy

Trichomonas infection is usually reported to occur in 10-20 per cent of pregnant patients although figures as high as 50 per cent have been given (Sands, 1966). Despite the efficacy of oral metronidazole (p. 432), there has been reluctance to prescribe it for pregnant patients for fear of foetal toxicity. Rodin and Hass (1966) review the previously published results of treatment during pregnancy and add 78 patients of their own, including 10 treated during the first 8 weeks with the conventional dose of 200 mg. metronidazole 8-hourly for 7 days. In no instance was there any congenital malformation attributable to the drug. This is supported by Sands (1966) who gave 750 mg. metronidazole daily for only three days. Only 2/113 patients failed to respond. There was no foetal abnormality and no maternal disturbance other than a rash in one patient and vomiting in another. He suggests that metronidazole treatment of trichomoniasis in pregnancy is not only safe but necessary because of evidence that inflammatory conditions of the cervix and vagina significantly increase the prematurity rate (Hawkinson and Schulman, 1966).

Vaginal Candidiasis

This is common in pregnancy and readily transferred to the infant during birth producing oral thrush. It may be controlled by vaginal tablets containing 100,000 units of nystatin inserted once, or in severe cases, twice a day. Csonka (1967) cured 9/11 pregnant and all 18 non-pregnant patients with 15 days' treatment, and found that amphotericin B pessaries were no better. Other polyene antibiotics have also been used. Using vaginal tablets containing pimaricin, Don (1967) cured 9/17 pregnant and 29/40 non-pregnant patients. Cameron (1969) claims excellent results without side effects from preparations containing 0·3 per cent candicidin.

BREAST ABSCESS

Breast abscess in the puerperium is invariably due to *Staph. aureus* and the general principles of chemotherapy are the same as those outlined for staphylococcal infection generally in Chapter XVI. If the patient has been delivered in hospital the staphylococcus is likely to be penicillin-resistant and treatment should be started with cloxacillin pending a bacteriological report.

NEONATAL INFECTIONS

Babies born to mothers receiving chemoprophylaxis because of premature rupture of the membranes should continue on treatment. It is also generally felt that because of the high risk and danger of respiratory infection, prophylactic antibiotics should also be given to babies asphyxiated at birth or with the respiratory distress syndrome, or those requiring tracheal intubation or assisted respiration.

Generalised Infection

If an infant is seriously ill with no obvious cause, cultures of blood and urine and swabs from any local lesions, nose, throat and umbilicus should be examined bacteriologically: a lumbar puncture may also be indicated.

Difficulty of localizing infection and rapid deterioration of the new-born not infrequently demand the institution of treatment before the nature of infection is fully established. Cephaloridine (15 mg./kg., 12-hourly) is generally very suitable for this purpose, but some deaths have occurred from cephaloridine-resistant enterobacteria or *Pseudomonas*. The addition of streptomycin (10 mg./kg., 12-hourly) extends the antibacterial range (Burland *et al.*, 1970; Keay and Fleming, 1970) but the combination still cannot be relied upon to be effective against *Pseudomonas*. It seems preferable to add gentamicin (2·4 mg./kg./day) or sulphomethyl polymyxin or colistin (50,000 u./kg./day) rather than streptomycin for the first 24-48 hours until it can be established that *Pseudomonas* is not implicated. Because of potential toxicity, the second agent should be withdrawn as soon as the infecting organisms have been shown to be sensitive to cephaloridine.

Alternative broad cover against enterobacteria, penicillinase-producing staphylococci and streptococci is provided by cloxacillin (100 mg. per kg.) plus ampicillin (15 mg. per kg.) by 6-hourly intramuscular or intravenous injections, but a polymyxin or gentamicin must still be added until pseudomonas infection can be excluded.

The choice between ampicillin plus cloxacillin and cephaloridine should be guided by the local prevalence of strains resistant to these agents.

Thrush

This is usually confined to the mouth and can be treated by local application of gentian violet or nystatin. The lesions sometimes extend down the alimentary tract, in which case nystatin should be given orally in a dose of 100,000 units every six hours. If the infant is having a broad spectrum antibiotic, this should be stopped.

REFERENCES

ANSBACHER, R., BORCHARDT, K. A., HANNEGAN, M. W. & BOYSON, W. A. (1966). *Amer. J. Obstet. Gynec.* **94**, 386.
BAKER, T. H. & HUBBELL, R. (1967). *Amer. J. Obstet. Gynec.* **97**, 575.
BARR, W. & GRAHAM, R. (1967). *Postgrad. med. J.* **43** (Suppl. Aug.), 101.
BLECHER, T. E., EDGAR, W. M., MELVILLE, H. A. H. & PEEL, K. R. (1966). *Brit. med. J.* **1**, 137.
BRELJE, M. C. & KALTREIDER, D. F. (1966). *Amer. J. Obstet. Gynec.* **94**, 889.
BURLAND, W. L., SIMPSON, K. & SAMUEL, P. D. (1970). *Postgrad. med. J.* **46** (Suppl. Oct.), 85.
CAMERON, P. F. (1969). *Practitioner* **202**, 695.
CAVANAGH, D. & SANDBERG, J. R. (1966). *Amer. J. Obstet. Gynec.* **96**, 579.
CSONKA, G. W. (1967). *Brit. J. vener. Dis.* **43**, 210.
DECKER, W. H. & HALL, W. (1966). *Amer. J. Obstet. Gynec.* **95**, 394.
DON, R. A. (1967). *Med. J. Aust.* **1**, 382.
FREEL, J. H., GARDNER, W. M. & GEITTMANN, W. F. (1969). *Amer. J. Obstet. Gynec.* **104**, 651.
GOWER, P. E., HASWELL, B., SIDAWAY, M. E. & DE WARDENER, H. E. (1968). *Lancet* **1**, 990.
GRUNEBERG, R. N., LEIGH, D. A. & BRUMFITT, W. (1969). *Lancet* **2**, 1.
HAWKINSON, J. A. & SCHULMAN, H. (1966). *Amer. J. Obstet. Gynec.* **94**, 898.
KEAY, A. J. & FLEMING, J. G. (1970). *Postgrad. med. J.* **46** (Suppl. Oct.), 81.
KINCAID-SMITH, P. & BULLEN, M. (1965). *Lancet* **1**, 395.
MORITZ, C. R. & THOMPSON, N. J. (1966). *Amer. J. Obstet. Gynec.* **95**, 46.
MORRIS, C. A. & MORRIS, D. F. (1967). *J. clin. Path.* **20**, 636.
NORDEN, C. W. & KASS, E. H. (1968). *Ann. Rev. Med.* **19**, 431.
PARKER, R. T. & JONES, C. P. (1966). *Amer. J. Obstet. Gynec.* **96**, 645.
RODIN, P. & HASS, G. (1966). *Brit. J. vener. Dis.* **42**, 210.
SANDS, R. X. (1966). *Amer. J. Obstet. Gynec.* **94**, 350.
STEVENSON, C. S. (1969). *Amer. J. Obstet. Gynec.* **104**, 699.
STILL, R. M. & ADAMSON, H. S. (1967). *J. Obstet. Gynaec. Brit. Cwlth.* **74**, 412.
WILLIAMS, G. L., CAMPBELL, H. & DAVIES, K. J. (1969). *J. Obst. Gynaec. Brit. Cwlth.* **76**, 229.
WREN, B. G. (1969). *Med. J. Aust.* **1**, 1220.

Chapter XXIII

URINARY TRACT INFECTIONS

About 80 per cent of acute urinary tract infections are caused by *Esch. coli* (Mond *et al.*, 1965; McGeachie, 1966); *Proteus* species (almost all *Pr. mirabilis*) account for another 8-12 per cent. The remainder are *Staph. albus, Str. faecalis,* and other enterobacteria. In chronic infections, *Escherichia* are much less common and various other enterobacteria, notably *Klebsiella,* and *Ps. aeruginosa,* predominate (Gould, 1968). The most important feature shared by these organisms is their resistance to antibacterial agents.

Another important difference is that acute infection is almost always caused by a single bacterial species. In chronic infection, particularly in patients with gross structural or functional abnormalities of the urinary tract, more than one kind of organism is frequently present.

Diagnosis

It was an accepted doctrine until recently that reliable evidence of infection in the female was obtainable only by examining a catheter specimen. Since it is now widely accepted that catheterization actually causes infection in a proportion of patients, the practice has been abandoned for purposes of diagnosis. Various manoeuvres have been devised for collection of urine in the female by midstream techniques. The ease with which this can be achieved outside clinics where urinary tract infection is a special interest appears to have been over-estimated by the enthusiasts. Contamination with vaginal material is the principal difficulty and very much better results can be obtained if a tampon is inserted before the vulva is cleaned. Preliminary cleansing of the orifice should be with water; soap may be helpful, but strong antiseptics should not be used: specimens in which the more aromatic of these are detectable by smell are not unknown.

Such specimens are bound to contain some extraneous bacteria, and if these are left to multiply while the specimen stands in a warm room for hours, a completely false picture results. *All specimens of urine should be either examined within one hour of collection or refrigerated until they can be.*

The difficulties of collection are even greater in children. Specimens obtained by attaching bags or tubes—which others find satisfactory (Normand and Smellie, 1965)—are in our hands frequently contaminated to a degree which makes interpretation impossible. Excellent specimens may be obtained on filter paper strips (Leigh and Williams, 1964) if the child can be stimulated to empty the bladder and the strip held in the stream. Several investigators have described supra-pubic puncture as a safe and reliable way of obtaining uncontaminated specimens (Saccharow and Pryles, 1969).

There are several simple bacteriological tests suitable for use in general practice which will identify the presence of 10^5 or more organisms per ml. of urine generally accepted as the sole criterion of infection (Leigh and Williams, 1964; Mackey and Sandys, 1965; Guttmann and Naylor, 1967).

TREATMENT

Choice of Agent

The choice of suitable agents for the treatment of urinary tract infection is governed by bacteriological and pharmacological factors. The agents must obviously be active against organisms commonly responsible for urinary infection and it is generally felt preferable that they should be bactericidal—though there is no direct evidence that this property materially influences the comparative performance of different agents. As in other infections the toxicity of the compounds should be low—particularly if they are to be used for long-term therapy or in patients with impaired renal function. The mode of handling by the kidney should ensure that adequate concentrations are available at the site of infection.

Obviously they should attain an effective concentration in the urine itself, but is this enough? From time to time a voice is raised maintaining that the site of infection is the tissues and that the drug must act there: in fact that a concentration sufficient at least to restrain bacterial growth must also be attained in the blood.

If this were true, all urinary antiseptics in use before 1936 and one undoubtedly successful one introduced since then (nitrofurantoin) could have no action at all, since they reach anti-bacterially effective levels only when concentrated in the urine. The fact is that in many infections confined to the bladder or perhaps to the renal pelvis it is enough to sterilize the urine itself: as soon as the tissues lining them cease to be bathed in a fluid teeming with bacteria, they can look after themselves. On the other hand, if the substance of the kidney is involved, a drug with a systemic action is imperative, and established pyelonephritis is a notoriously difficult condition to treat by reason of that difference.

Antibacterial Range

The degree of activity against important bacterial species of agents commonly used in the treatment of urinary tract infection is stated in Table XLIV. It will be observed that only *Ps.*

TABLE XLIV

Sensitivity to Drugs of Bacteria causing Urinary Infections

Drug	Con-centration attained in urine (μg./ml.)	Minimum Inhibitory Concentration (μg./ml.)					
		Esch. coli	*Proteus mira-bilis*	*Kl. aero-genes*	*Ps. aeru-ginosa*	*Staph. aureus*	*Str. faecalis*
Sulphonamides	1000	1	8	R	50	4-16	R
Nitrofurantoin	125	16	200	100	R	4	25
Penicillin	250+	20->100	8	R	R	0·02	4
Ampicillin	250+	8	4	R	R	0·04	2
Carbenicillin	2000	5	2·5	250	50	0·5-50	25
Cephaloridine	300	4	4	4-R	R	0·1-5	16
Streptomycin	1000	5	50	5	50	10	100
Kanamycin	300	2	4	2	64	0·5	64
Gentamicin	50	1-4	2-8	1-2	1-8	0·1-1	8-16
Tetracyclines	300	5	100	10	200	0·5	1
Chloramphenicol	30	2	5	5	500	8	5
Polymyxin	50	1	R	1	1	R	R
Cycloserine	250	64	250	64	128	16	128

R=resistant to concentrations attainable.

aeruginosa shows an unpromising degree of resistance, other organisms, both Gram-positive and Gram-negative, being susceptible in sufficient although varying degree.

EXCRETION PATTERNS. Many compounds are excreted in high concentrations in the urine: some, like streptomycin, principally by glomerular filtration; some, like penicillin, are actively secreted by the tubules; some like nitrofurantoin, have complex tubular reabsorption patterns. With some compounds, for example chloramphenicol, a large proportion of the excreted drug is in conjugated and antibacterially inactive forms. These excretion patterns may or may not be much affected by plasma levels of the drug or by such factors as the pH of the urine.

With some compounds, tediously difficult interactions can occur as with nitrofurantoin with which increase of pH increases the concentration excreted in the urine, by lowering non-ionic back-diffusion in the tubule, but depresses the activity of the agent against some bacterial species.

These complex patterns of excretion have received very little detailed study in patients under treatment. There has, however, been considerable concern over the possible effect of different modes of renal handling on the concentration of antibacterial agents at the site of infection in the renal substance. It is possible, at least theoretically, for an agent to be so efficiently transferred from the plasma to the urine that none appears in the interstitial tissue where organisms are established. On the other hand, very small concentrations may diffuse into the interstitial fluid from the plasma, but much larger concentrations may back-diffuse from the tubules where the agent is concentrated.

Tissue Concentrations

The measurement of concentrations of antibacterial agents in the interstitium of the kidney presents considerable technical difficulties. Apart from the fact that important concentration differences may exist in the vicinity of different micro-anatomical structures, homogenates of kidney cannot be used to determine ' tissue concentrations ' because they contain varying quantities of blood and, more important, of urine, the presence of which usually results in grossly high false values.

There have been several different approaches to this problem. Attempts have been made to sweep the rabbit kidney clear of blood and urine by passing gas through the kidney (A. G. Spencer, personal communication). Fluid cannot be used because of diffusion of antibiotics into the perfusate.

Values obtained for tetracycline and ampicillin were:

	Urine	Plasma	Cortex	Medulla
Tetracycline (μg. per ml.)	82-90	1·4-4	9-29	7-35
Ampicillin (μg. per ml.)	700-6,000	0·4-11	4-41	6·71

An elegant method of determining tissue fluid levels is described by Cockett *et al.* (1965) who found that in a proportion of dogs the surface lymphatics arising from the cortex and medulla of the kidney can be separately cannulated. They found 2·5-5·0 μg. per ml. nitrofurantoin in the renal lymph (about twice that in the plasma) with urine levels of 88-200 μg. per ml. 2 hours after 7·5 mg. per kg. In a patient infused with 180 mg. nitrofurantoin over 2 hours, the renal lymph levels were 14-16 μg. per ml. when the plasma level was only 3-4 μg. per ml. Chisholm *et al.* (1968), who discuss the technical difficulties, found renal lymph levels of nitrofurantoin to be about twice those of the plasma in three of their five dogs but similar in the other two. The levels of gentamicin in the renal lymph (2·5-6 μg./ml.) were generally slightly lower than those in the plasma.

It is not only in the kidney that infection may be sequestered. In the adult male, recurrent urinary infection may result from failure to eradicate organisms from the prostate in which the concentration of most agents active against Gram-negative organisms is considerably less than that in the plasma. Winningham *et al.* (1968) argue that to be concentrated in the acid secretion of the prostate, a drug must be basic and lipid-soluble. Amongst commonly used antibiotics only the macrolides fulfil these criteria and they are predominantly active against Gram-positive organisms. Reeves and Ghilchik (1970) show that trimethoprim, a basic, lipid-soluble compound (p. 42), achieves peak concentrations in the prostatic fluid of the dog 2 to 3 times higher than those of the blood. However, sulphamethoxazole, the other component of commercially available trimethoprim-sulphonamide mixtures (p. 48), behaves quite differently in that its concentration in the prostate is only about a third of that in the blood. The antibacterial spectrum of trimethoprim-sulphamethoxazole makes it very suitable for the treatment of bacterial prostatitis but this difference in the pharmacokinetic behaviour of the two components must be taken into account.

Control of Urinary pH

A deliberate alteration of urinary pH may be a necessary prelude to successful treatment. The normal pH fluctuates, rising after meals and falling to its lowest level during the night: the mean of the day's output is about 6.0. If an infected urine is alkaline, the causative organism should be examined for urease formation: this enzyme, formed by *Proteus,* sometimes other coliforms, and *Staph. albus,* splits urea, liberating ammonia, thus producing a urine of constantly high alkalinity. Acidifying drugs will not correct this: if they are pushed, the patient can die of acidosis with his urine still alkaline.

Provided that ammonia is not being formed, the urine can be rendered more acid by giving ammonium chloride or methionine which not only acidifies well but is believed to cause the excretion of a bactericidal acid. Alkalinization can be achieved with sodium bicarbonate, or more rapidly with acetazolamide. When a drug is being used which requires an alkaline medium, administration should not be started until the pH of the first specimen passed on waking is at least 7.0, and it should if possible be verified daily that this reaction is being maintained.

PRACTICAL THERAPY

Preventive

Some kinds of patient are specially susceptible to urinary tract infections by reason of what is done to them in hospital. When these are the result of cross-infection, usually during instrumentation, with a resident and highly resistant strain of organism, not much can be done except by improving sterilizing methods and aseptic technique. On the other hand some patients, notably those whose bladders are being drained, are liable to become infected by bacteria of their own, possibly from the urethral orifice: these have a normal chance of being sensitive to antibacterial drugs, and one of the latter may act as a barrier to their entry.

Two kinds of infection need guarding against: coccal and coliform. Sulphonamides deal adequately only with the latter, and this was well exemplified in the results of a clinical experiment at St. Bartholomew's Hospital. Women with indwelling catheters after operations on the vagina were given sulphanilamide, 0·5 g., t.d.s. As compared with untreated controls, *Esch. coli* infections were much reduced in frequency, but those due to *Str. faecalis* increased in numbers. A later experiment in the same unit using nitrofurantoin had a much more successful result: whereas 86 per cent of control cases became infected with either *Esch. coli*, *Proteus* or *Str. faecalis,* no treated case had any of these infections, the few occurring (10 per cent) being due to resistant or unusual organisms (Williams, Garrod and Waterworth, 1962).

There have been several kinds of approach to the problem of preventing urinary infection during indwelling catheterization in the male, notably after prostatectomy. Systemic prophylactic chemotherapy has not been particularly successful even where agents such as kanamycin or mandelamine with a wide antibacterial range have been used (Kudinoff *et al.,* 1966). Instillations of various antibacterial agents into the bladder have been employed, including continuous lavage with such agents as neomycin and polymyxin through a triple lumen catheter (Cox *et al.,* 1967). Several authors have emphasized the importance of aspects of the management other than the use of antibacterial agents (Bruce and Quirk, 1964; Miller, 1965), and Gillespie and his colleagues (1967) have drawn particular attention to the importance of closed drainage. Although it is clear that substantial reductions in infection rate can be achieved (Marshall, 1967), many urologists still seem to take infection for granted, and minimize its importance. The patients themselves, overjoyed at having cleared the most dangerous hurdle in later male life, make light of discomfort and accept it as a natural consequence of what they have gone through. They would surely be better off if their urine could be kept sterile.

Treatment of Acute Infections

It might be thought that with so common a condition as acute urinary tract infection (about 26 per 1,000 married women per annum, but only 1·8 per 1,000 men per annum, in general practice in this country—Mond *et al.*, 1965) well conducted trials would already have established clearly which agent is best in which circumstances and which regimen and duration of therapy produces the optimum result. This is unfortunately not so for a number of reasons. Generally it has not been easy to arrange adequate bacteriological support for studies from general practice and this has resulted in a preponderance of trials on hospital patients. As an indication of the inapplicability of many of these studies to the acute infection encountered in general practice it is not necessary to look further than the sex ratio : males commonly predominate.

Several hospital trials on women have been based on infections in gynaecological patients. There are reasons for suspecting that these infections, while necessarily peculiar to women, differ in important respects from those arising spontaneously in women in general practice. Much of the recent interest in urinary tract infection arises from the belief that acute infections —at one time regarded as benign conditions of little more than nuisance value—commonly involve the kidney and can be the prelude to chronic pyelonephritis and renal failure. Direct and unequivocal evidence for this in follow-up of large groups of patients over the prolonged period necessary is being actively sought. Meanwhile, amongst patients who had urinary infections following gynaecological operations, follow-up studies after ten or more years have failed to shown any overt cases of pyelonephritis or any excess of hypertension or renal failure (Cattell *et al.*, 1963; Slade *et al.*, 1965).

This suggests (and there is other evidence) that at least in some circumstances acute bacterial cystitis—a diagnosis scorned in some expert circles in recent years—exists, and has a quite different prognosis from acute infections involving the kidney parenchyma both long-term and in its immediate remission rate. It seems prudent, at present, therefore, in attempting to assess optimum therapy for patients outside hospital to base the conclusions on the relatively small number of adequate trials conducted in general practice.

13

Localization of Infection

The full bacteriological study of general practice patients which this demands has revealed an interesting state of affairs. Of the patients presenting with dysuria and frequency, only half have infected urine (Mond *et al.*, 1965; Gallacher *et al.*, 1965). The remainder, whose symptoms suggest some disease of the anterior urinary tract, are said to be suffering from the ' urethral syndrome ' (Editorial, 1968). A chronic urethritis, likened to ' female prostatitis ' also occurs (Moore and Hira, 1965).

It also appears likely that amongst the patients presenting with infected urine in general practice, some are suffering from uncomplicated cystitis. Considerable effort has been made to try to distinguish these patients from those in whom the kidneys are involved in order to identify those at risk from chronic pyelonephritis (Reeves and Brumfitt, 1968). It is also important to make the distinction therapeutically.

If patients are treated on the basis of symptoms alone, the results are extremely satisfactory. Since half of them are not suffering from urinary tract infection and half the remainder are suffering from a condition with a high spontaneous remission rate, very little contribution on the part of the therapeutic agent will raise the success rate above 80 per cent. If, on the other hand, the response of patients demonstrated to be suffering from acute pyelonephritis is examined, the results are much less gratifying. Therapy commonly fails in 5-25 per cent of patients and higher failure rates are not uncommon. It is hard to resist the conclusion that acute urinary tract infection in the female is made up of a group suffering from a benign self-limiting condition which responds promptly to treatment, and a minority group suffering from intractable infection frequently involving the kidney parenchyma.

Similarly in the male the response to treatment differs when infection is confined to the bladder or involves the prostate or kidney. The localization of lower urinary tract infections in the male is discussed by Meares and Stamey (1968).

The distinction between those cases of urinary infection which respond readily to treatment (and may be largely self-limiting) and those which persist or readily recur is always important in assessing the efficacy of treatment, but nowhere more important than in the child where grave renal damage may result from inadequate treatment. The recognition of sub-groups of childhood urinary infection with different prognosis is discussed by MacGregor and Freeman (1968).

INITIAL TREATMENT

Since a substantial proportion of patients with acute urinary tract infection respond readily to treatment, initial therapy should be with a one week course of one of the agents listed at the top of Table XLIV. The doses are given on page 364. There is very little to choose between the agents *provided the infecting organism is sensitive*. The proportion of organisms resistant to different agents varies widely and often in a quite inexplicable manner from one region to another. Where the choice of agent cannot be based on individual sensitivity tests, it must take account of the local prevalence of resistant strains. On the ground of cost, sulphonamide is usually the first choice where resistant strains are uncommon (e.g. sulphafurazole: 2 g. initially plus 1 g. 6-hourly).

The most important part of management is not the choice of agent but the recognition of failure. Whatever agent is used, a proportion of patients will relapse immediately on cessation of treatment or soon become re-infected.

Relapse

The re-appearance of sensitive strains after what should be adequate courses of therapy is usually explained either by failure of antibacterial agent to reach the site of infection, or by indifference of the organism to its action, even though it appears sensitive on conventional *in vitro* testing. Such evidence as we have (p. 372) does not support the idea that deficient overall tissue concentrations are a common cause of failure. This by no means excludes the possibility, however, that mal-distribution of agents within the kidney is responsible. It is likely that it is precisely in those areas where function is deranged by infection that the adequate levels demonstrable in adjoining normal tissue are not reached. Gross examples of this may be found where the ureteric urine is sterilized on the side where renal function has been moderately preserved, but not on the other side, where renal function is grossly deficient.

One example of metabolic indifference of organisms to an agent to which they are sensitive on conventional testing is the production of L-forms (Gutman *et al.*, 1967). Treatment with agents which interrupt cell-wall synthesis can result in the production of protoplasts which are excreted in the urine where their integrity is preserved by the high osmolality. When no longer exposed to the agent, cell-wall is re-synthesized and infection re-appears. L-forms of enterobacteria, unlike the parent organism, may be sensitive to erythromycin, and *Proteus* infection has been eradicated by successive treatment with ampicillin and erythromycin (Guze and Kalmanson, 1964; Gutman *et al.*, 1967).

While this example has the benefit of a demonstrable mechanism, the persistence of organisms in the presence of high concentrations of agents to which they are ' sensitive ' on conventional testing is not restricted to agents which interrupt cell-wall synthesis. It occurs with many (perhaps all) agents when large bacterial inocula are used, presumably because some of the organisms at the time of exposure to the antibiotic are in a ' dormant ' state (Greenwood and O'Grady, 1969). Infected urine frequently contains a fully-grown or near fully-grown culture, and the activity of many agents against such a culture is likely to be seriously over-estimated by determinations of M.I.C. using the small inocula customary in *in vitro* sensitivity tests.

Diuresis and Frequent Micturition

This suggests that success, and particularly the success of agents like sulphonamides which are only feebly active against large inocula (see p. 462), can occur because intrinsic clearance mechanisms are only marginally impaired and will achieve bacterial elimination with relatively little support from an antibacterial agent. It happens that in the urinary tract we have a unique opportunity to manipulate the intrinsic clearance mechanisms.

Diuresis and frequent micturition play a significant part in freeing the urinary tract from infection, and increased fluids (often with some agent to alkalinize the urine) have long been part of the traditional treatment of urinary tract infection and often bring prompt symptomatic relief. The efficacy of diuresis and frequent micturition in diluting and displacing infected bladder urine depends on the volume left after micturition (O'Grady *et al.*, 1968). The importance of even small volumes of residual urine—and hence the therapeutic importance of complete bladder emptying—was shown by the demonstration of Shand *et al.* (1970) that patients whose residual urine volumes were more than the normal 1 ml. were more likely to suffer urinary infection and more difficult to treat.

The diuresis induced by copious drinking dilutes agents excreted in the urine and for this reason it has been held that it should not be used with antibacterial therapy. In fact, the urinary excretion of most agents used for the treatment of urinary infection is such that the degree of dilution produced by water loading will still leave high concentrations (see Table XLIV for the concentrations obtained on normal water intake) and direct comparison has shown that the very rapid fall in bacterial concentration which usually occurs in the first 24 hours of treatment is both enhanced and prolonged by water loading and frequent micturition (Cattell *et al.*, 1968). Such reduction in bacterial counts is likely to be reversed overnight (when both urine flow and frequency of micturition are at their lowest) unless the last dose of antibacterial agent is given immediately before retiring.

Treatment of Relapse

It must first be established that failure is not due to the emergence of a resistant mutant. This is a very uncommon cause of failure except with streptomycin and, in some series, nalidixic acid. Typically the organism remains fully sensitive and some patients respond to re-treatment with a two-week course of the same or another agent to which the organism is sensitive. The response to trimethoprim/sulphonamide has generally been found to be superior to that to sulphonamide alone (Grüneberg and Kolbe, 1969) and the combination is very suitable for the re-treatment of patients who fail to respond to initial sulphonamide therapy.

If the patient again relapses, there is a high chance that radiology will show some abnormality of the urinary tract which may be surgically correctable. Therapeutically there are two approaches which may be useful but have yet to be subjected to extended study. One is to continue conventional dosage with water loading and frequent, complete (if necessary double or triple) micturition for an extended period (6 weeks in the first instance) on the grounds that final clearance of bacteria from the urinary tract is a slow process (O'Grady *et al.*, 1968). The alternative is to treat patients intensively with high dose parenteral therapy in the expectation that inaccessible areas of bacterial survival in the kidneys or elsewhere will be subjected to eradicative levels of antibacterial agent. This must obviously be done in hospital using agents chosen on the basis of *in vitro* sensitivity tests. Suitable agents are ampicillin, cephaloridine or cephalothin, streptomycin or kanamycin (1·5 g. per day for three days). Dosage should be given frequently, preferably by rapid intravenous infusion, and in the case of the penicillins or cephalosporins enhanced by probenecid. If surgery is undertaken (for example for the removal of renal stones) intensive therapy should begin at the time of operation. Patients who fail to respond to these measures require long-term suppressive therapy (p. 381).

Re-infection

Irrespective of the ease with which infection is eradicated some patients become re-infected with a new organism. The management of patients subject to such re-infection depends on the frequency with which infections occur. If new infections occur infrequently (not more than 2 or 3 a year) and respond readily to treatment, each episode is probably best treated as a first infection as described on page 377. If, on the other hand, attacks occur frequently, if asymptomatic attacks are interspersed (as they frequently are), or if infection, once established, is difficult to eradicate, then such patients are probably better managed on long-term prophylaxis.

Infection should be eradicated, if necessary by intensive therapy, and chemoprophylaxis instituted as soon as the initial treatment has been shown to be successful, in order to prevent the establishment of fresh exogenous infection. Using prophylaxis in this way, Smellie and Normand (1968) have shown on prolonged follow-up of a large group of children with recurrent infection (including many with pyelonephritic scarring and reflux) that kidney growth which is halted by infection can commonly be restored. Most of the children were treated with sulphadimidine or sulphafurazole (less than 1 year of age: 0·25 g. daily; 1-5 years: 0·5 g. daily; more than 5 years 1 g. daily). Nitrofurantoin (2·4 mg. per kg. per day) or ampicillin were used in a few children.

Adults with frequent infections have been successfully maintained on prophylactic trimethoprim-sulphonamide for periods (so far) up to 4 years (O'Grady *et al.*, 1969). Dosage was halved at fortnightly intervals (from 12-hourly to nightly, alternative nightly and twice a week) as long as control was maintained.

As with patients who repeatedly relapse, full uro-radiological examination of patients who suffer frequent re-infection may reveal correctable abnormalities.

Long-Term Therapy

Much disagreement about the place and efficacy of long-term therapy results from failure to recognize that such treatment may be used for three distinct purposes: (1) prophylactic, as just described, (2) curative, as described on page 380 and (3) suppressive. Patients who relapse even after prolonged or intensive therapy may benefit from prolonged treatment which keeps the urine ' sterile ' as long as sufficient antibacterial agent is present. Such treatment may provide symptomatic relief and prevent fresh acute attacks but since it is not curative there is a possibility that resolution of symptoms may conceal the progression of urinary tract disease.

Long-term therapy has two main foreseeable disadvantages: toxicity and superinfection with resistant organisms. These hazards may be minimized by choosing the least toxic agent and progressively reducing the dose to the effective minimum; and by accepting only the most compelling reasons for bringing patients into hospital where the most undesirable organisms live. Long-term toxic effects on these regimens must, of course, be constantly watched for, and only time will tell whether such protracted medication is completely safe.

Resistant Organisms and Mixed Infections

In patients treated for recurrent urinary tract infection over prolonged periods the later infections tend to be caused either by resistant species such as *Pr. vulgaris, Klebsiella,* and particularly *Ps. aeruginosa,* or by resistant strains of otherwise sensitive species such as *Esch. coli.* By using selective media it is often possible to show, even when infection appears to be with only one organism, that other species are present in small numbers (Slade and Linton, 1965). These minor members of the bacterial population inevitably come to predominate if they are resistant to an agent effective in suppressing initially more numerous organisms. Better results of treatment are sometimes obtained if these minor species are isolated and an agent chosen for therapy which is active also against them or if suitable combined therapy is instituted.

Such infections are occasionally the cause of failure in patients whose renal tracts are, as far as can be judged normal, but the majority occur in patients with structural and functional abnormalities of the urinary tract. In many, instrumentation in hospital for diagnostic or therapeutic purposes is unhappily responsible for the introduction of resistant organisms. The importance of avoiding such infections, which enormously increase the difficulty of managing these patients, is obvious. The necessary preventive measures, particularly the importance of closed drainage, are discussed by Miller (1965) and Gillespie *et al.* (1967).

Therapeutically, these patients present a series of difficulties which tend to compound one another. The abnormalities of their urinary tracts greatly impair both natural resolution and response to treatment. The resulting need for repeated therapy (plus instrumentation) facilitates the emergence of organisms sensitive only to a few agents, the more potent of which are toxic—the kidney itself being one of the organs affected. Impaired kidney function results both in poor concentrations of administered agents in the renal tract, and where dosage is not scrupulously regulated, to their accumulation in the blood with increased remote toxic effects and perhaps further impairment of renal excretion.

The results of antibacterial therapy in such a group of patients are never particularly encouraging—nor is there any reason to hope that the discovery of some new agent will suddenly make them so—although there is certainly a need for agents less toxic than some of those which must be currently employed.

Because of the extreme resistance of some of the organisms and the need to monitor dosage, these patients cannot be managed without full bacteriological surveillance. As much as possible should be done to rectify anatomical and functional abnormalities. Patients with large residual volumes should be encouraged to empty their bladders at frequent and regular intervals, practising double or, if necessary, triple micturition (McGregor and Williams, 1966).

Renal Failure

A special problem is presented by the need to treat patients—especially with streptomycin and its relatives or with poly-myxins—when the capacity to excrete these agents is impaired. Conventional dosage will cause the drug to accumulate with neurological sequelae and possible further kidney damage. The toxic effects are discussed under the individual agents. Suitable adjustment of dosage can be so successful that renal function improves while the patient is treated with a potentially nephro-toxic agent because of the beneficial effect of controlling infection. Guidance to suitable dosage in relation to the level of renal function is given on page 277.

REFERENCES

BRUCE, A. W. & QUIRK, J. (1964). *J. Urol.* **92,** 523.
CATTELL, W. R., CURWEN, M. P., SHOOTER, R. A. & WILLIAMS, D. K. (1963). *Brit. med. J.* **1,** 923.
CATTELL, W. R., SARDESON, J. M., SUTCLIFFE, M. B. & O'GRADY, F. (1968). In *Urinary Tract Infection,* p. 212, ed. O'Grady, F. and Brumfitt, W. London, Oxford University Press.
CHISHOLM, G. D., CALNAN, J. S. & WATERWORTH, P. M. (1968). In *Urinary Tract Infection,* p. 194, ed. O'Grady, F. and Brumfitt, W. London, Oxford University Press.
COCKETT, A. T. K., MOORE, R. S. & KADO, R. T. (1965). *Brit. J. Urol.* **37,** 650.
COX, F., SMITH, R. F., ELLIOTT, J. P. & QUINN, E. L. (1967). *Antimicrob. Agents Chemother.* 1966, 165.
EDITORIAL (1968). *Brit. med. J.* **2,** 192.
GALLAGHER, D. J. A., MONTGOMERIE, J. Z. & NORTH, J. D. K. (1965). *Brit. med. J.* **1,** 622.
GILLESPIE, W. A., LENNON, G. G., LINTON, K. B. & PHIPPEN, G. A. (1967). *Brit. med. J.* **2,** 90.
GOULD, J. C. (1968). In *Urinary Tract Infection,* p. 43, ed. O'Grady, F. and Brumfitt, W. London, Oxford University Press.
GREENWOOD, D. & O'GRADY, F. (1969). *J. med. Microbiol.* **2,** 435.
GRUNEBERG, R. N. & KOLBE, R. (1969). *Brit. med. J.* **1,** 545.
GUTMAN, L., SCHALLER, J. & WEDGWOOD, R. J. (1967). *Lancet* **1,** 464.
GUTTMANN, D. & NAYLOR, G. R. E. (1967). *Brit. med. J.* **3,** 343.
GUZE, L. B. & KALMANSON, G. M. (1964). *Science* **146,** 1299.

KUDINOFF, Z., FINEGOLD, S. M., KALMANSON, G. M. & GUZE, L. B. (1966). *Amer. J. med. Sci.* **251,** 70.

LEIGH, D. A. & WILLIAMS, J. D. (1964). *J. clin. Path.* **17,** 498.

McGEACHIE, J. (1966). *Brit. J. Urol.* **38,** 294.

MACGREGOR, M. & FREEMAN, P. (1968). In *Urinary Tract Infection,* p. 95, ed. O'Grady, F. and Brumfitt, W. London, Oxford University Press.

MACGREGOR, M. E. & WILLIAMS, C. J. E. W. (1966). *Lancet* **1,** 893.

MACKEY, J. P. & SANDYS, G. H. (1965). *Brit. med. J.* **2,** 1286.

MACNAUGHTON, G., LAURENCE, A. R. & KNOX, J. D. E. (1967). *Practitioner* **198,** 416.

MARSHALL, A. (1967). *Brit. J. Urol.* **39,** 307.

MEARES, E. M. & STAMEY, T. A. (1968). *Invest. Urol.* **5,** 492.

MILLER, A. (1965). *Brit. J. Urol.* **37,** 34.

MOND, N. C., PERCIVAL, A., WILLIAMS, J. D. & BRUMFITT, W. (1965). *Lancet* **1,** 514.

MOORE, T. & HIRA, N. R. (1965). *Brit. J. Urol.* **37,** 25.

NORMAND, I. C. S. & SMELLIE, J. M. (1965). *Brit. med. J.* **1,** 1023.

O'GRADY, F. & CATTELL, W. R. (1966). *Brit. J. Urol.* **38,** 149.

O'GRADY, F., CHAMBERLAIN, D. A., STARK, J. E., CATTELL, W. R., SARDESON, J. M., FRY, I. K., SPIRO, F. I. & WATERS, A. H. (1969). *Postgrad. med. J.* **45** (Suppl. Nov.) 61.

O'GRADY, F., GAUCI, C. L., WATSON, B. W. & HAMMOND, B. (1968). In *Urinary Tract Infection,* p. 80, ed. O'Grady, F. and Brumfitt, W. London, Oxford University Press.

REEVES, D. S. & BRUMFITT, W. (1968). In *Urinary Tract Infection,* p. 53, ed. O'Grady, F. and Brumfitt, W. London, Oxford University Press.

REEVES, D. S., FAIERS, M. C., PURSELL, R. E. & BRUMFITT, W. (1969). *Brit. med. J.* **1,** 541.

REEVES, D. S. & GHILCHIK, M. (1970). *Brit. J. Urol.* **42,** 66.

SACCHAROW, L. & PRYLES, C. V. (1969). *Pediatrics* **43,** 1018.

SHAND, D. G., O'GRADY, F., NIMMON, C. C. & CATTELL, W. R. (1970). *Lancet* **1,** 1305.

SLADE, N. & LINTON, K. B., (1965). *Brit. J. Urol.* **37,** 73.

SLADE, N., MATHER, H. G., LINTON, K. B., LEATHER, H. M. & POWELL, D. E. B. (1965). *Brit. med. J.* **1,** 1278.

SMELLIE, J. M. & NORMAND, I. C. S. (1968). In *Urinary Tract Infection,* p. 123, ed. O'Grady, F. and Brumfitt, W. London, Oxford University Press.

WILLIAMS, D. K., GARROD, L. P. & WATERWORTH, P. W. (1962). *J. Obstet. Gynaec. Brit. Cwlth.* **69,** 403.

WINNINGHAM, D. G., NEMOY, N. J. & STAMEY, T. A. (1968). *Nature (Lond.)* **219,** 139.

Chapter XXIV

INFECTIONS OF THE EYE

THE treatment of serious ocular infections is a highly special-
ised task, and a full account of it would be out of place in a
work of this kind. The following is no more than an outline
of the underlying principles and of the more important
methods employed.

Superficial infections respond readily to various forms of
local treatment, and few of them present any problems. Those
involving the interior of the eye do present a special problem,
that of penetration of the affected area by anti-bacterial drugs.
Since adequate concentrations may only be obtainable there
by the method of sub-conjunctival injection of a substantial
dose in a small volume, the choice is limited by two considerations, solubility and local tolerance. Antibiotics easily
administered for their systemic effect may be excluded from
this special use on one or other of these grounds.

Intra-ocular Concentrations after Systemic Administration

Systemic administration is seldom used in the treatment of
intra-ocular infection but some anti-bacterial drugs diffuse into
the aqueous humour in therapeutic concentrations after administration by the ordinary route: the levels attained in the
vitreous are much lower and often undetectable. This penetration has been studied extensively in both animals and man,
employing a variety of doses including some very large ones.
This and other variables discourage any too concise and quantitative expression of the results. Simmons and O'Rourke (1968)
point out that with the uveal blood flow of about 0·2 ml. per
min. it takes a week for the blood volume to perfuse the eye.
Hence prolonged rather than transiently high blood levels are
necessary if systemic treatment is to be used to control intra-
ocular infection.

SULPHONAMIDES. The concentration of sulphadimidine attained in the aqueous is about 30 per cent of that in the blood

in the rat, and about 60 per cent in the rabbit, 30 minutes after the intravenous administration of a large dose. Experimentally, sulphonamides will control intra-ocular infections due to a fully sensitive organism such as *Str. pyogenes*. No other drugs penetrate with this facility.

PENICILLIN. Benzyl penicillin is useful, despite poor penetration, because of the large doses which can be given and its great intrinsic activity. An intramuscular dose of 1,000,000 units (0·6 g.) produces a concentration in the aqueous of about 0·5 unit per ml.

AMPICILLIN. Kurose *et al.* (1965) found single doses of 250 mg. gave maximum concentrations in the aqueous of 0·16 μg. per ml. after 4 hours. Single doses of 1 or 2 g. gave maximum aqueous concentrations after 6 hours of 0·96 μg. per ml. and 1·6 μg. per ml. respectively. One hour after the last of six hourly doses of 250 mg., the aqueous concentration was 0·12 μg. per ml., and after similar doses eight hourly, 0·18 μg. per ml. They conclude that unless the drug is given 4 to 6 hourly, or in very large doses, intra-ocular concentrations adequate for the treatment of any other than the most sensitive organisms are unlikely to be achieved. Furgiuele (1964) failed to detect ampicillin in the aqueous after 5-10 mg. per pound body weight when the serum concentration was 0·025 to 1·0 μg. per ml.

METHICILLIN. After 20 or 40 mg. per kg. intra-muscularly, Green and Leopold (1965) found 0·2 or 0·8 μg. per ml. in the aqueous of the normal rabbit eye. In the presence of an intense keratitis produced by 0·2 N. HCl. the concentration was considerably increased: after 40 mg. per kg. to 5·7 μg. per ml. Furgiuele (1964) found that oxacillin and nafcillin failed to penetrate the eye after doses of 5 to 10 mg. per kg.

CEPHALOSPORINS. In patients about to undergo cataract operations who were given 1 g. cephalothin by rapid intravenous infusion, Records (1968) found concentrations in the aqueous of 0-2·5 μg./ml. at 15 min. and 0-1·0 μg./ml. after 30 min., the corresponding serum levels being 22-100 and 10-14 μg./ml. Cephaloridine, given in the same way and in the same dose produced considerably higher levels between 1 and 2 hours which persisted to give 2·5-17 μg./ml. after 8 hours (Records, 1969).

FUCIDIN. In 18 patients about to undergo cataract extractions, and treated for three days preoperatively with 500 mg. fucidin three times daily, Chadwick and Jackson (1969) found aqueous levels of 0·8-2·0 μg./ml. with corresponding serum levels of 10-200 μg./ml. On the same regimen and with the last dose given 12 hours before operation, Williamson *et al.* (1970) found aqueous levels around 1·2 μg./ml. with serum levels of 52-72 μg./ml. After only two days' preoperative treatment, the aqueous and serum levels were 1·2 and 18-64 μg./ml., and after one day's treatment, 0·1-0·84 and 4-36 μg./ml. Fucidin was present in the vitreous of three patients whose eyes were enucleated. In two the levels were 2 to 3 times as high as those in the aqueous. In one patient presumably as the result of prolonged inflammation, the vitreous level was 28·8 (aqueous 12·8) μg./ml. and in another patient the vitreous level was still 0·32 (aqueous 0·1) μg./ml. 4 days after the last dose of fucidin.

SULPHOMETHYL COLISTIN. By intra-arterial infusion in dogs with experimental endophthalmitis, Simmons and O'Rourke (1968) produced levels of sulphomethyl colistin in the aqueous of 5-20 μg./ml. and in the vitreous of 0-0·6 μg./ml. when the serum levels were 40-80 μg./ml.

AMPHOTERICIN B. Green *et al.* (1965) were unable to demonstrate amphotericin B in the normal eyes of systemically treated rabbits, but found that in the presence of albumen-induced uveitis, levels of 0·16 to 0·18 μg. per ml. were obtained 6 hours after intravenous doses of 1 mg. per kg. Significantly, the drug penetrated less well when given sub-conjunctivally.

OTHER ANTIBIOTICS. The evidence with regard to streptomycin and chloramphenicol is somewhat conflicting, but it seems that by giving exceptionally large doses concentrations of either antibiotic of the order of 10 μg. per ml. or more can be attained in the aqueous and lower ones in the vitreous. The concentrations obtained by treatment with various agents are shown in Table 46. Furgiuele (1964) found that the intra-ocular concentrations of the agents which he studied were not affected by giving acetazolamide intravenously (7·2 mg. per kg.)

TABLE XLV

Dosage for Injections in the Eye

	Sub-conjunctival	Intra-ocular
Benzyl penicillin	0·5-1 mega unit	1,000-4,000 units
Methicillin	150 mg.	1 mg.
Neomycin	100-500 mg.	2·5 mg.
Streptomycin	50 mg.	—
Kanamycin	10-20 mg.	—
Polymyxin B (or Colistin) sulphate	0·1 mega unit	1,000 units
Bacitracin	10,000 units	500-1,000 units
Chloramphenicol	1 mg.*	1-2 mg.
Tetracycline	2·5-5 mg.	—
Erythromycin	2·5-50 mg.	1-2 mg.

* The more soluble but less active chloramphenicol sodium succinate may be given in doses of 25-50 mg.

TABLE XLVI

Concentrations of Various Agents Achieved in Normal Rabbits' Eyes after Systemic Injection

Agent	Dose	Route	Interval after Last Dose	Concentration μg. per ml.		
				Aqueous	Vitreous	Serum
Chlor-amphenicol	50 mg./kg.	I/v	15 mins.	12	≦6	48
Erythro-mycin	6·5 mg./kg. 8 hrly × 4	I/v	2½ hrs.	0·1	0	0·36
Tetracycline	20 mg./kg. 12 hrly × 3	I/v	2½ hrs.	0·5	0	2-4
Kanamycin	50 mg./kg.	I/v	1 hr.	8-16	0	128-256
	50 mg./kg. hrly × 2	I/m	15 mins.	1·6	0	26
Ampicillin	1 g. 2 g.	Oral	6 hrs.	0·96 1·6	0	—
	250 mg. 8 hrly	Oral	1 hr.	0·08	0	—
Methicillin	20 mg./kg. 40 mg./kg.	I/m	1 hr.	0·8 0·2	0	—
Vancomycin	45 mg./kg. 12 hrly × 3	I/v	2½ hrs.	1·5	0	23

Furgiuele, F. P., *et al.* (1960). *Amer. J. Ophthal.* **50**, 614. Furgiuele (1964). Green and Leopold (1965). Kurose, *et al.* (1965).

Sub-conjunctival Injection

There are several ways of introducing anti-bacterial substances locally, apart from application to the lids or conjunctiva. Injection into the orbit gives poor penetration, and direct injections into the chambers of the eye are not often indicated. The method of choice is sub-conjunctival injection, a fine

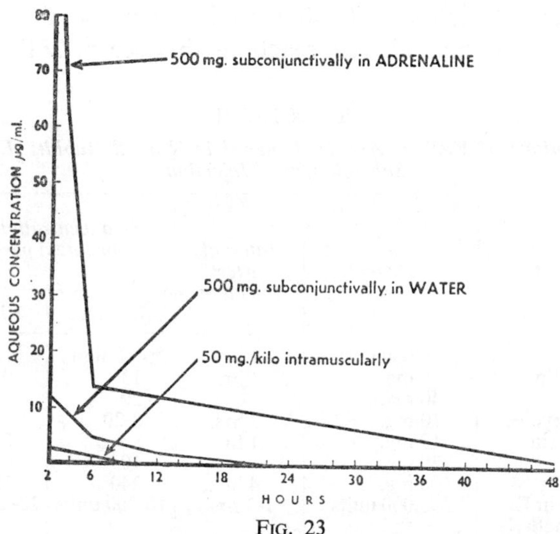

Fig. 23

Aqueous levels of streptomycin after subconjunctival injection in water or adrenaline contrasted with the low level obtained by intramuscular injection of a large dose (Sorsby, A. and Ungar, J., 1960: *Antibiotics and Sulphonamides in Ophthalmology*, Oxford University Press).

needle being inserted between the conjunctiva and the sclera usually below the cornea since the injections are often painful and the patient tends to roll the eyeball up. Up to 1 ml. of solution can be injected. Trapped in this situation, the substance diffuses into the cornea and the chambers of the eye, where concentrations are attained far higher than any to be achieved by systemic administration, and maintained above the therapeutic minimum for as long as 48 hours. It should not be forgotten that antibiotics will be absorbed from this site and there is the possibility of remote toxic effects with such agents as neomycin—which can be given by this route in substantial doses—especially in patients with impaired renal function. The addition of adrenaline to the solution prolongs the effect. The concentrations of streptomycin attainable in the aqueous, contrasted with those obtained by systemic administration are shown in Figure 23.

Antibiotics suitable for administration by this route are:

PENICILLIN is in this situation as in most others the best tolerated: 1,000,000 units (0·6 g.) is often the dose given. Because of possible allergic reactions (but see p. 281) and the

TABLE XLVII

Concentrations of Various Agents Achieved in Normal Rabbits' Eyes after Subconjunctival Injection

Agent	Dose	Interval after Injection	Concentration μg. (or units) per ml.	
			Aqueous	Vitreous
Penicillin	50,000 units	1 hr.	>32 units	17 units
Methicillin	20 mg.	1 hr.	13	0
	40 mg.		20	
Streptomycin	10 mg.	3 hrs.	8-20	—
Kanamycin	10 mg.	1 hr.	8	0-4
	20 mg.		10	0
Neomycin	500 mg.	4 hrs.	240	33
Polymyxin E	250,000 units	1-3 hrs.	10-200 units	20-200 units
Sulphomethyl-polymyxin B	500,000 units	45-120 mins.	95-750 units	—

Sorsby, A. & Ungar, J. (1947). *Brit. J. Ophthal.* **31,** 517.
Gardiner, P. A., *et al.* (1948). *Brit. J. Ophthal.* **32,** 449.
Ainslie, D. & Smith, C. (1952). *Brit. J. Ophthal.* **36,** 352.
Furgiuele, *et al.* (1960).   Ainslie, D. (1965). *Brit. J. Ophthal.* **49,** 98.   Green and Leopold (1965).

inactivity of penicillin against the majority of enterobacteria, treatment is most commonly initiated with neomycin or, where *Pseudomonas* infection is feared, with a polymyxin or gentamicin. According to Delpech (1962) methicillin is much less well tolerated, even considerably smaller amounts being liable to cause chemosis, a fact of some consequence to the treatment of penicillin-resistant staphylococcal infections. Cloxacillin is damaging to the eye and should not be used for this purpose nor as ophthalmic drops.

AMINOGLYCOSIDES. Neomycin is well tolerated in a dose of up to 0·5 g., and produces high and well sustained intra-ocular concentrations. There is clinical confirmation of its efficacy. Framycetin has been used in the same way with naturally corresponding results. Streptomycin and kanamycin behave similarly but smaller doses have generally been recommended (Table XLV). Furgiuele (1970) gave 10 mg. gentamicin in 0·25 ml. subconjunctival injection before cataract extraction and found aqueous levels of 0-4 μg./ml. after 30 minutes and 1·2-9·0 μg./ml. at 1-2$\frac{1}{2}$ hours.

POLYMYXIN. This antibiotic, invaluable for the treatment of one of the most dangerous of eye infections, that due to *Ps. aeruginosa,* is unfortunately much less well tolerated. The assessment of results with it is complicated by the use of two different polymyxins, B. and E (colistin), and of two different salts, the sulphate and the methane sulphonate, of which the latter evidently causes much less local reaction, in the eye as elsewhere (p. 193).

The doses recommended by Leopold (1964) of these and other agents are given in Table XLV. The intra-ocular concentrations of various agents achieved by the sub-conjunctival route are shown in Table XLVII.

The Treatment of Superficial Infections

Cant (1969) emphasizes the simple measures such as removal of a lash or encrusted exudate, and expression of pus from a blocked tear duct, which are essential to success and may be the only therapy necessary. The possibility that continuing or recrudescent inflammation is a reaction to locally applied antibacterial agent must be considered.

Superficial application may take the form of drops or ointment. The former may need very frequent application. Ointments, which obscure vision, are convenient for application last thing at night. Among the sulphonamides, sulphacetamide, as 10 per cent drops or 2·5-6 per cent ointment, has been chiefly used in this way because of its high solubility: it is doubtful whether there is any purpose for which an antibiotic is not more effective. Penicillin is also used in the form of drops containing up to 10,000 units (6 mg.) per ml. The validity of the commonly expressed fear of allergic reactions to such local applications of penicillin is discussed on page 281.

In ointments the antibiotic can be incorporated in the base in solid form, which ensures stability, and a slow process of solution in the lachrymal secretion gives a persistent effect. Penicillin can be used in this way in almost any desired concentration, and an ointment containing 50,000 units (30 mg.) per g. even gives some penetration into the interior of the eye. Ointments containing streptomycin, neomycin, tetracyclines or chloramphenicol are usually made up to contain one per cent. Ointment containing 10,000 and 4,000 units of polymyxin and bacitracin respectively per g. has been found satisfactory for a variety of purposes. Magnuson and Suie (1967) found gentamicin (0·3 per cent) ophthalmic drops and ointment highly effective in 115/131 patients (88 per cent) treated for a week or less, mostly for conjunctivitis, blepharitis or meibomianitis. Out of 50 patients, *Staph. aureus* was recovered from 41. In a double-blind, bacteriologically monitored comparison, Gordon (1970) found gentamicin at least as effective as a mixture of neomycin, bacitracin and polymyxin.

The minutiae of the treatment of various conditions of the eyelids and conjunctiva and of the lachrymal system, which include measures other than the application of anti-bacterial agents, are outside the scope of this book. Apart from the fact that staphylococci, which are responsible for most infections involving the eyelids, may be resistant to penicillin or tetracyclines, the organisms concerned are sensitive to most of the antibiotics mentioned. Even the two Gram-negative species causing conjunctivitis, the Koch-Weeks bacillus (a *Haemophilus*) and the Morax-Axenfeld bacillus, are sensitive to penicillin, as well as to other antibiotics more usually thought of in connection with Gram-negative infections; Delpech (1962) advocates neomycin or colistin for Koch-Weeks infections, and bacitracin, tetracycline or chloramphenicol for pneumococcal, preferring them to penicillin because of the risk of sensitization, although this is the treatment usually advocated.

Gonococcal ophthalmia in the infant is best treated by the instillation of penicillin solution at intervals at first of only one minute, but gradually extended. Systemic treatment may be advisable in addition, and is said to be invariably indicated in the adult.

Pseudomonas Ophthalmia. This dangerous condition has received unwelcome publicity through outbreaks traced to contamination of solutions used for ophthalmic medication. In a controlled trial of various treatments for experimental pseudomonas keratitis, Hessburg *et al.* (1966) found that colistin sulphate irrigation (1 mg. per ml.) was effective, and that the addition of sulphacetamide (1 mg. per ml.) did not significantly improve the results. Furgiuele *et al.* (1965) successfully controlled the condition with local applications of 1 per cent gentamicin drops.

Treatment with daily subconjunctival injections of gentamicin or a polymyxin-neomycin mixture for seven days is also effective (Furgiuele, 1968) but has the disadvantage that some of the potentially toxic agent will be absorbed. To overcome the need to make frequent instillations of drops in human infections, Hessburg (1966) describes a method of continuous corneal lavage. He used lavage, at 6-8 drops per minute, with 0·05 per cent colistin and 0·05 per cent sulphacetamide. He suggests that treatment should be continued for about 14 days, followed by 1 per cent colistin ointment hourly during the day and several times during the night for 3 weeks, followed again by 10 or 15 per cent sulphacetamide eye drops hourly during the day for 3 further weeks.

Fungus Infections of the Eye

In recent years there has been considerable interest in these infections and in the role of broad-spectrum antibiotics and corticosteroids in encouraging their emergence. A great variety of fungi have been identified (sometimes only on morphological grounds) in mycotic keratitis and endophthalmitis. They include both organisms normally regarded as saprophytic, such as cephalosporium and mucor, and some which are conceded more general pathogenic roles such as sporotrichum, aspergillus and candida. Suie and Havener (1963) detail the fungi responsible and review the elective sites of intraocular mycoses. They question the evidence that broad-spectrum antibiotics are responsible for increasing the frequency of fungus infection of the eye, but have no doubt that corticosteroids do so. This appears to be the consensus of opinion on both experimental (Agarwal *et al.*, 1963) and clinical (Rheins *et al.*, 1966) grounds, and numerous warnings have been issued against the indiscriminate use of corticosteroids in the eye. Fungus infection should be suspected wherever purulent corneal ulceration cannot be explained by bacterial infection. Most authors believe that any applications of corticosteroid must be stopped (even though this may result in initial apparent deterioration), but that antibiotics should be continued in order to limit, as far as possible, secondary bacterial invasion. The fully developed clinical picture of ocular mycosis is said to be fairly typical (Theodore, 1964a).

The only agents of proven value are the polyene antibiotics (p. 236). Nystatin is irritating but reasonably safe as ointment (100,000 units per g.). Amphotericin is more effective and can be given as drops containing up to 3 mg. per ml. of the colloidal suspension for injection, in distilled water (not saline) which can be supplemented by subconjunctival injections of 125 μg. Local treatment with amphotericin B is unpleasant and irritating, has often to be supplemented with debridement, and must be continued for months. Newmark *et al.* (1970) obtained good visual results in 7 patients suffering from cephalosporium or fusarium keratitis treated with pimaricin. At hourly intervals, they instilled alternately a 5 per cent suspension of pimaricin and 1 per cent potassium iodide drops. They originally used potassium iodide in the belief that it exerted an antifungal effect but suggest that the benefit is due to the potassium which helps to maintain the physiological state of the cornea and reduce the chance of intraocular sequelae. Treatment was continued for 2 to 4 weeks. The pimaricin suspension was non-irritant and sufficiently viscous to remain in the cul-de-sac for long periods.

The results of treatment of fungal endophthalmitis are very unsatisfactory. There is little intraocular penetration of nystatin or amphotericin from subconjunctival injection, and intraocular injections are not well tolerated so that the final visual result even if the fungus is eliminated is likely to be poor.

Intra-ocular levels of amphotericin are obtained by systemic therapy, but the dangers of this (p. 238) are such that the treatment should only be undertaken in proven cases of fungal infection. Intra-ocular injections of amphotericin are exceedingly irritating but doses of 35-40 μg. in 0·05 ml. distilled water are tolerated (Suie and Havener, 1963; Theodore, 1964a). Injections of 200 units nystatin directly into the aqueous or vitreous are tolerated, but produce inhibitory levels (6-12 μg. per ml) for only 24 hours. Larger or repeated injections cause vitreal degeneration (Suie and Havener, 1963).

Trachoma

Together with inclusion conjunctivitis and inclusion blenorrhoea, trachoma is caused by an organism (TRIC agent) which belongs to the group of *Chlamydia* (p. 447). It has also been suggested that in the trachoma-infected eye, commensal bacteria may function as opportunist pathogens and partly determine the severity of the lesions (Arm and Woolridge, 1966). In keeping with the sensitivity of the causal organism and the possible role of bacterial super-infection, trachoma has been held to respond either to prolonged systemic sulphonamide treatment or to the local application of ointment containing tetracycline. More recent experience has, however, been less encouraging. In 475 cases randomized into three groups: untreated, treated with sulphamethoxypyridazine, or treated with local tetracycline, Foster, Powers and Thygeson (1966) were unable to demonstrate any difference in the cure rates when patients were re-examined after one year. It does not appear that this apparent decline in responsiveness is associated with increased resistance to the antimicrobial agents (Shiao *et al.*, 1967). Grayston (1967) discusses possible reasons for the poor results (including re-infection) and suggests that therapy may have some value in limiting spread of the disease even if it is not curative.

Herpes Simplex Keratitis. This condition, which resolves spontaneously in about 10 per cent of patients, can respond well to idoxuridine (0·1 per cent drops) one-hourly by day and two-hourly by night. Birge (1963) was successful in treating 75/76 of his patients. Idoxuridine (p. 445) has, however, two disadvantages: the effective dose is very close to the maximum permissible so that severe reactions may occur, and resistance develops to it relatively easily. In a general review of the prospects for treating viral infections of the eye, Jones (1967) concludes that idoxuridine offers no advantage over cauterization in the treatment of dendritic ulcers. He suggests that its principal use may be in controlling deleterious effects of steroids on amoeboid ulcers and deep keratitis. Resistance is less likely to develop to cytosine arabinoside which has the added advantage of being very soluble (permitting higher dosage and more efficient steroid antagonism) but is still more toxic.

Post-operative Endophthalmitis

PRE-OPERATIVE PROPHYLAXIS. Opinions differ on the advisability of performing cultures before such operations as cataract extraction when there is no sign of infection. Even when secretion is obtained, as it should be, with a loop from the depths of the lower conjunctival sac, a few *Staph. albus* from the lid may be cultivated, and *C. xerosis* is a normal inhabitant. If a pathogenic organism such as *Staph. aureus* is found, pre-operative treatment with antibiotic drops is indicated. Ointments may enter the eye during operation and are contra-indicated.

POST-OPERATIVE PROPHYLAXIS. The majority view appears to be against routine antibiotic administration, whether systemic or subconjunctival, after clean operations. In 8 cases of post-operative infection reported by Aronstam (1964), 4 had had post-operative sub-conjunctival injections of penicillin plus streptomycin and 4 had not. This treatment delayed both the development and recognition of infection, and the ultimate visual result was poorer in the treated group. In contrast, Kolker *et al.* (1967), who gave alternate patients 100,000 units of penicillin and 66 mg. streptomycin subconjunctivally at the conclusion of operation, found one infection in 480 treated patients and 7 in 494 untreated. Over the next two years, all patients were treated and 2 out of 1,480 developed endophthalmitis. McCoy *et al.* (1968) irrigated the anterior chamber after lens delivery with a solution containing 5 mg. neomycin and 1 mg. polymyxin B per ml. and had no infection in 200 operations and no untoward effects. However, it must be pointed out that the infection rate in the untreated patients described by Kolker *et al.* (1967) is high compared with some other series in which patients receiving no prophylaxis have had very low infection rates (Rollins, 1965). The position is different after removal of an intra-ocular foreign body: the infection which may follow this is usually staphylococcal, and subconjunctival neomycin or cephaloridine is indicated.

TREATMENT OF ESTABLISHED INFECTION. Bacterial endophthalmitis after clean surgery is an unusual and serious complication occuring in most series in about 0·1 to 0·3 per cent of cases. In the series reported by Rollins (1965) there was loss of useful vision in 71 per cent of affected patients. The increased frequency encountered in some series over recent years can be accounted for in part by the increase in fungus infections (Theodore, 1964b). The principal organisms are now *Staph. aureus* and *Pseudomonas aeruginosa* followed by *Klebsiella, Proteus* and *Escherichia*. The classical causes of eye infection, pneumococci and streptococci, appear now to be of much less importance. A bacteriological diagnosis is urgent in such a case. Conjunctival swabs can be misleading by yielding organisms other than those responsible for intra-ocular infection, and several pleas have been made for early anterior chamber aspiration. Gram-stained smears of this material may offer the most valuable guide to therapy since even where organisms are seen they may prove impossible to cultivate.

The aspirate may usefully be replaced by penicillin (5,000 units per ml.) plus streptomycin (5 mg. per ml.). According to Theodore (1964b), higher dosage should not be used. Gentamicin (p. 126) is an even more promising agent for this purpose since it is active against penicillin-resistant staphylococci, *Pseudomonas aeruginosa* and *Proteus,* but intra-ocular injections have so far been little employed. The choice of an antibiotic for subsequent subconjunctival injection in such circumstances must take account of the properties of the four principal antibiotics available as stated in Table XLVIII. Penicillin is clearly indicated for pneumococcal and streptococcal infection. Streptomycin has a wider spectrum, but a strain of any species may be abnormally resistant to it. Polymyxin is active, and to a high degree, against *Ps. aeruginosa, Klebsiella,* and *Escherichia;* but not against *Proteus* or the Gram-positive cocci. Neomycin, on the other hand, has a satisfactory activity against all these problem organisms: staphylococci, whether penicillin-resistant

TABLE XLVIII

Sensitivity to Antibiotics Administrable by Subconjunctival Injection of Bacterial Species causing Ocular Infections

	Penicillin	Strepto-mycin	Neomycin	Polymyxin
Staph. aureus	0·03*	2*	1	R
Str. pyogenes	0·015	32*	>128	R
Str. pneumoniae	0·015	64*	128	R
Ps. aeruginosa	R	50*	50	0·12
Proteus spp.	5-100*	5*	5-50	R
Klebsiella spp.	R	2-R	2	0·25
Escherichia	R	4	8	0·25

Figures are minimum inhibitory concentrations in μg./ml.
* indicates that some strains may be more resistant.
R indicates regular resistance to attainable concentrations.

or not, and both *Ps. aeruginosa* and *Proteus*. It should be the safest choice for treatment before the nature of the infection and the sensitivities of the organism are known.

If the circumstances (for example a series of post-operative infections) or failure to respond to treatment suggest *Pseudomonas* infection, treatment should be supplemented by subconjunctival injections of gentamicin or a polymyxin.

REFERENCES

AGARWAL, L. P., MALIK, S. R. K., MOHAN, M. & KHOSLA, P. K. (1963). *Brit. J. Ophthal.* **47**, 109.
ARM, H. G. & WOOLRIDGE, R. L. (1966). *Med. J. Aust.* **2**, 351.
ARONSTAM, R. H. (1964). *Amer. J. Ophthal.* **57**, 312.
BIRGE, H. L. (1963). *Amer. J. med. Sci.* **246**, 239.
CANT, J. S. (1969). *Practitioner* **202**, 787.
CHADWICK, A. J. & JACKSON, B. (1969). *Brit. J. Ophthal.* **53**, 26.
DELPECH, J. (1962). *Les antibiotiques en Ophthalmologie.* Paris: G. Doin et Cie.
FOSTER, S. O., POWERS, D. K. & THYGESON, P. (1966). *Amer. J. Ophthal.* **61**, 451.
FURGIUELE, F. P. (1964). *Amer. J. Ophthal.* **58**, 443.
FURGIUELE, F. P. (1968). *Amer. J. Ophthal.* **66**, 276.
FURGIUELE, F. P. (1970). *Amer. J. Ophthal.* **69**, 481.
FURGIUELE, F. P., KIESEL, R. & MARTYN, L. (1965). *Amer. J. Ophthal.* **60**, 818.
GORDON, D. M. (1970). *Amer. J. Ophthal.* **62**, 300.
GRAYSTON, J. T. (1967). *Amer. J. Ophthal.* **63**, 1583.
GREEN, W. R., BENNETT, J. E. & GOOS, R. D. (1965). *Arch. Ophthal. (Chicago)* **73**, 769.
GREEN, W. R. & LEOPOLD, I. H. (1965). *Amer. J. Ophthal.* **60**, 800.
HESSBURG, P. C. (1966). *Amer. J. Ophthal.* **61**, 896.
HESSBURG, P. C., TRUANT, J. P. & PENN, W. P. (1966). *Amer. J. Ophthal.* **61**, 49.

Jones, B. R. (1967). *Trans. ophthal. Soc. U.K.* **87,** 437.
Kolker, A. E., Freeman, M. I. & Pettit, T. H. (1967). *Amer. J. Ophthal.* **63,** 434.
Kurose, Y., Levy, P. M. & Leopold, I. H. (1965). *Arch. Ophthal. (Chicago)* **73,** 366.
Leopold, I. H. (1964). *Invest. Ophthal.* **3,** 504.
Magnuson, R. H. & Suie, T. (1967). *J. Amer. med. Ass.* **199,** 427.
McCoy, D. A., McIntyre, M. W. & Turnbull, D. C. (1968). *Arch. Ophthal.* **79,** 506 (c).
Newmark, E., Ellison, A. C. & Kaufman, H. E. (1970). *Amer. J. Ophthal.* **69,** 458.
Records, R. E. (1968). *Amer. J. Ophthal.* **66,** 441.
Records, R. E. (1969). *Arch. Ophthal.* **81,** 331.
Rheins, M. S., Suie, T., Van Winkle, M. G. & Havener, W. H. (1966). *Brit. J. Ophthal.* **50,** 533.
Rollins, H. J. (1965). *Sth. med. J.* **58,** 353.
Shiao, L.-C., Wang, S.-P. & Grayston, J. T. (1967). *Amer. J. Ophthal.* **63,** 1558.
Simmons, R. E. & O'Rourke, J. (1968). *Amer. J. Ophthal.* **66,** 295.
Suie, T. & Havener, W. H. (1963). *Amer. J. Ophthal.* **56,** 63.
Theodore, F. H. (1964a). *Int. ophthal. Clin.* **4,** 861.
Theodore, F. H. (1964b). *Int. ophthal. Clin.* **4,** 839.
Williamson, J., Russell, F., Doig, W. M. & Paterson, R. W. W. (1970). *Brit. J. Ophthal.* **54,** 126.

CHAPTER XXV

TUBERCULOSIS

CHEMOTHERAPY has radically transformed the outlook in this disease. A mortality rate which had been falling by only 3 per cent per annum from 1900 to 1948, fell thereafter by 15 per cent per annum (Fig. 24) and this reduction was even steeper in the lower age groups: total deaths in England and Wales at ages 15-29 were 14,010 in 1930 and only 75 in 1960 (Report, 1962b). The significance of the year 1948 is that it marks the general introduction of streptomycin for treating the disease: various synthetic drugs and other antibiotics have followed.

It is our purpose to describe the properties of these drugs, but to give only a brief account of how they can be used. Needless to say, the treatment of tuberculosis is a speciality, and should be directed only by those experienced in it. Nor do we feel called upon to discuss treatment in ' under-developed ' countries, which is beset by many difficulties not encountered elsewhere.

STANDARD DRUGS

THE three standard drugs used in the treatment of tuberculosis are, in order of their discovery, streptomycin, para-aminosalicylic acid and isoniazid. The general properties of streptomycin are described in Chaper VI and those of para-aminosalicylic acid and isoniazid are summarized below.

Para-Aminosalicylic Acid (PAS)

The anti-tuberculous activity of PAS was discovered in Sweden in 1946 in the course of a systematic study of analogues of salicylic acid and benzoic acid. Of 50 derivatives prepared, *p*-aminosalicylic acid was the most active and caused 50-75 per cent inhibition of the B.C.G. bovine strain of tubercle bacillus in a concentration of 1 in 650,000 (Lehmann, 1946).

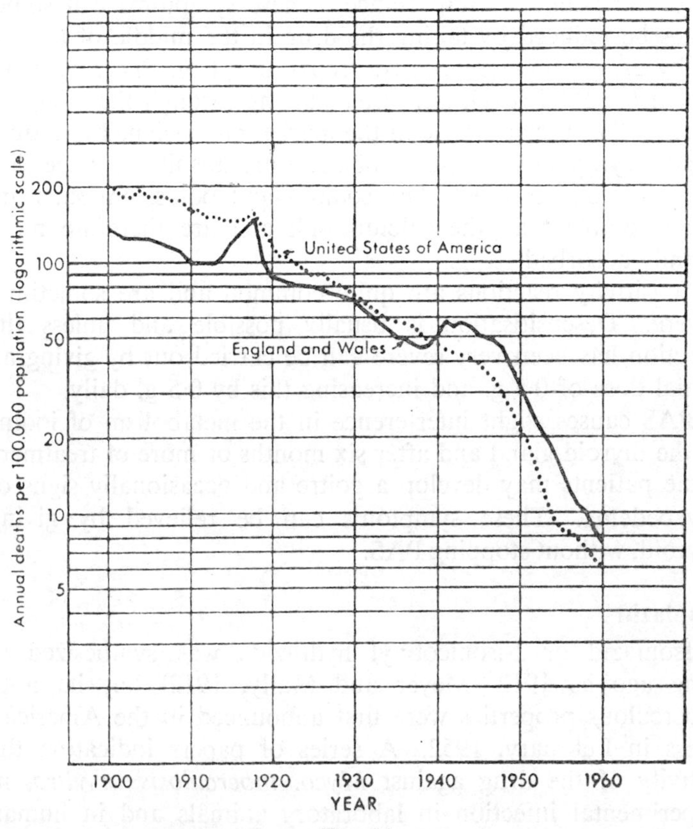

FIG. 24

Annual deaths from Tuberculosis per 100,000 population in England and Wales, and the United States of America 1900-1960.

COMPARATIVE MERITS. In comparison with most other anti-tuberculous drugs the activity of PAS is not very great and it is bacteristatic and not bactericidal. It has the advantages, however, that it is absorbed from the intestinal tract and although not free from side effects these are rarely of sufficient severity to interfere with treatment. To be effective the drug has to be given in very large doses, *e.g.* 10-15 g. daily.

SIDE EFFECTS. Gastric discomfort and nausea, with or without diarrhoea, occur in nearly all patients treated with large doses of the drug. They are seldom intolerable but not infrequently lead patients to discontinue treatment, unless they understand its importance. These symptoms can sometimes be reduced by taking the drug in the middle of a meal or by using an enteric-coated preparation (*e.g. Bactylan*) from which the PAS is released after passing through the stomach. Many other preparations on the market are designed to reduce gastric symptoms, but some of these are unsuitable since they are not well absorbed. The sodium and potassium salts are more soluble than the calcium salt and are therefore more rapidly absorbed.

Sensitivity reactions are quite common and are sometimes severe. Desensitisation is usually possible and unless the reaction has been very severe can be carried out by giving an initial dose of 0·5 g. and increasing this by 0·5 g. daily.

PAS causes slight interference in the metabolism of iodine in the thyroid gland and after six months or more of treatment some patients may develop a goitre and occasionally signs of myxoedema. These symptoms can be relieved by giving thyroid, without stopping PAS.

Isoniazid

Isoniazid or 1-isonicotinyl hydrazide was synthesized as long ago as 1912 (Meyer and Mally, 1912) but its anti-tuberculous properties were first announced in the American press in February, 1952. A series of papers indicating the activity of the drug against *Myco. tuberculosis in vitro,* in experimental infection in laboratory animals and in human infection quickly followed (Grunberg and Schnitzer, 1952; Grunberg *et al.,* 1952; Robitzek *et al.,* 1952) and in March, 1952, the Medical Research Council launched a large controlled clinical trial, which established the value of isoniazid in the treatment of tuberculosis (Report, 1952).

COMPARATIVE MERITS. Isoniazid has an active bactericidal action on *Myco. tuberculosis* and inhibits the growth of most pre-treatment strains in a concentration as low as 0·2 μg./ml. It has the advantage over streptomycin that it is readily absorbed from the intestinal tract, diffuses well into the body tissues and fluids, including the cerebro-spinal fluid, and penetrates into macrophages, so that it is effective against intracellular tubercle bacilli. It is effective clinically in small doses (*e.g.* 200-300 mg. daily) and with this dosage toxicity is very low. It has the disadvantage that tubercle bacilli very readily develop resistance to it. Isoniazid-resistant bacilli are of diminished virulence for guinea-pigs (Mitchison, 1954), but the clinical significance of this is not clear. Resistance affects only some of the cells in the population, and the drug may therefore still have a useful therapeutic effect by its action on the remainder.

METABOLISM. Metabolism of isoniazid in the body has been shown to vary very greatly in different individuals. Broadly speaking most people can be divided into one of two groups, usually referred to as rapid and slow inactivators of isoniazid. Six hours after a dose of 10 mg. per kg. body weight the latter group usually have blood levels of 3-6 μg./ml. whereas with the former group the blood level is less than 2·5 μg./ml. There is some evidence to suggest that isoniazid metabolism is genetically controlled and that the slow-inactivator character is recessive. There is no association between isoniazid metabolism and age or sex (Evans *et al.*, 1960).

EXCRETION. Isoniazid is excreted in the urine in three forms, free drug, its acetyl derivative and hydrazones. The proportion in the latter form is constant: that in the free form is higher in slow inactivators, and that in the form of acetyl isoniazid is higher in rapid inactivators. A determination of this ratio is an alternative to blood assay for distinguishing between the two groups (Short, 1962).

SIDE EFFECTS. Toxic effects are not common with the usual dosage of 200-300 mg. but appear to be more frequent among slow inactivators and also when larger doses are used. The most common side effects are restlessness, insomnia, muscle twitching and difficulty in starting micturition. More serious effects are peripheral neuritis and psychotic upsets. The incidence of toxic symptoms is reduced by the simultaneous administration of pyridoxine.

Resistance to Standard Drugs

Primary resistance to these drugs (*i.e.* resistance in newly diagnosed patients who have had no treatment) has fortunately remained very uncommon in advanced countries. In two extensive surveys in the United States (Report, 1964 : Hobby *et al.*, 1966) the following percentages of strains were found resistant: to streptomycin 2·8 and 2·1, to isoniazid 1·6 and 2·1, and to PAS 0·8 and 3·2. In many under-developed countries in Asia and Africa far higher frequencies of resistance have been found, which are attributed largely to inadequate treatment either of the patient himself or of others from whom infection was acquired. In patients still sputum-positive after a course of treatment resistance is naturally much more frequent, and one or more of the following drugs may then have to be used.

DRUGS OF SECOND CHOICE

These include both antibiotics and synthetic compounds.

Antibiotics

CAPREOMYCIN. This derivative of *Streptomyces capreolus* is a peptide, available as the sulphate. It has little action on species other than mycobacteria. Streptomycin-resistant tubercle bacilli are sensitive to it, but there is some cross-resistance with viomycin and kanamycin. It is an alternative to these two antibiotics, and possibly less toxic than either, although damage both to the eighth nerve (usually auditory) and to the kidney may be caused : reports of the frequency of these effects differ. It has about half the *in vitro* activity of streptomycin against *Myco. tuberculosis,* and in a direct comparison made by Schwartz (1966) who treated patients with 1 g. of either antibiotic together with 12 g. PAS daily, it was less effective in eliminating bacilli from the sputum. The present principal source of information about the clinical use of capreomycin is a Symposium (1966).

CYCLOSERINE. This is a broad spectrum antibiotic, sometimes used for other purposes than this (see Chapter XI). It has a relatively weak action on the tubercle bacillus *in vitro,* but is effective *in vivo,* with the double advantage that resistance to it develops only slowly and that its inclusion in combinations strongly deters the development of resistance to other drugs. The aim should be to administer 0·5 g. twice daily, but the peculiar neurotoxic effects liable to be caused may necessitate reduction of this dose.

KANAMYCIN. The general properties of this antibiotic are described in Chapter VII. It belongs to the same group as streptomycin and has a similar *in vitro* action on *Myco. tuberculosis*. Strains resistant to streptomycin are sensitive to it, although the reverse does not obtain. Its only drawback is ototoxicity, and opinions differ on its merits mainly for this reason. The frequency of hearing loss varies greatly in different reports. Kass (1965) treated 82 patients with 15-20 mg. per kg. daily, varying the dose according to the blood level attained, and in combination with two other drugs, for 4 months: 19 suffered some loss of hearing but 10 of these had previous auditory damage, and in only 4 was deafness complete or severe. It seems likely, although it does not appear to have been proved, that this risk can be reduced by less frequent dosage (*e.g.* 1 g. on alternate days): splitting the daily dose is said to have no advantage (Kreis, 1966b). A good account of the use of kanamycin is given by Kreis (1966a) who prefers it to viomycin both for its greater activity and because should resistance to kanamycin develop, viomycin sensitivity is retained: the converse is not true.

RIFAMPICIN. Earlier derivatives of rifamycin had little success in the treatment of this disease, but rifampicin (see also p. 227) represents an enormous advance on them in two directions. It can be administered orally, attaining high and well sustained blood levels, and it has greatly enhanced antibacterial activity. Apparent activity against *Myco. tuberculosis* varies with the medium used, but in a Tween-albumin medium Hobby, Lenert and Maier-Engallena (1969) found the mean M.I.C. for 20 strains to be only 0·018 μg./ml. As with all rifamycin derivatives, bacterial populations contain a minute proportion of resistant cells which grow out unless this is prevented by the presence of another active drug.

Of now numerous experimental studies the most comprehensive are those of Grumbach, Canetti and Le Lirzin (1969) who treated mice with various combinations of rifampicin and other drugs and different systems of dosage, judging results by quantitative cultures of liver and spleen after 3 and 6 months.

The most effective combination was rifampicin plus isoniazid: daily treatment sterilized the organs of all mice at 6 months. Rifampicin plus ethambutol given daily was almost as effective, but less so when the latter part of the course was intermittent. Isoniazid plus ethambutol was inferior to either of the foregoing. Although the addition of streptomycin to a regime of rifampicin plus isoniazid had little effect, that of an initial one month of rifampicin to a course of isoniazid plus streptomycin had a pronouned effect, particularly on the organ counts at 5 months, *i.e.* long after rifampicin had been discontinued. These authors predict that the use of rifampicin may enable the usual period of clinical treatment to be shortened.

Rifampicin administered alone to advanced cases with multiple resistant bacilli caused a rapid fall in the sputum bacillary count, in some patients to *nil,* with improved appetite and gain in weight (attributed to the patients' having to swallow fewer tablets than before), but bacillary resistance developed in several patients (Hofmann, 1968). In most other trials combinations have been used: Gyselen *et al.* (1968) found rifampicin plus ethambutol the most effective of four regimes in 52 advanced cases. Needless to say, a combination with another drug to which the strain is sensitive should always be used. Some time must elapse before the best ways of using this very valuable drug can be defined. The present view is that it should be reserved for re-treatment of drug-resistant disease. Its high cost is also a factor to be considered.

TETRACYCLINES. These antibiotics have a very weak action against tubercle bacilli, but when given in large doses (2 g. twice a day) in combination with streptomycin or isoniazid appear to prevent the emergence of tubercle bacilli resistant to the two latter. Similarly the tetracyclines in the same dose reduce the incidence of viomycin-resistant organisms when given with viomycin. Administration of tetracyclines does not appear to delay the emergence of strains resistant to pyrazinamide or ethionamide (Crofton, 1960).

VIOMYCIN. This is another antibiotic isolated from a species of *Streptomyces* and similar in many ways to streptomycin, both in its anti-bacterial activity and in its toxicity to the eighth cranial nerve. It also has to be given by intramuscular injection. Unfortunately its anti-bacterial activity is lower than that of streptomycin and its toxicity is higher. With daily treatment for long periods giddiness, deafness and renal damage are frequent, but the incidence of side effects is greatly reduced by giving the drug on only two days of the week, and 1 g. twice a day on each of the two days is the usually recommended dose. There is cross-resistance between viomycin and both streptomycin and kanamycin, but once again it is usually one way, so that strains which have become resistant to streptomycin and kanamycin are often still sensitive to viomycin, but viomycin-resistant strains are usually resistant to both the other two.

Synthetic Compounds

THIOACETAZONE (Conteben: TBI). Thiosemicarbazones were used for the treatment of tuberculosis in Germany as long ago as 1946. They were introduced by Domagk and his colleagues at the Farbenfabriken Bayer Laboratories at Elberfeld, where the anti-bacterial activity of the sulphonamides had been discovered (Domagk *et al.,* 1946). The most active was 4-acetyl-aminobenzaldehyde thiosemicarbazone which was given the name thiacetazone; the proposed name is now thioacetazone. *In vitro* and in experimental infection in laboratory animals, thiacetazone in large doses appears to have an activity greater than that of *p*-aminosalicylic acid and similar or slightly inferior to that of streptomycin.

Thioacetazone is one of the most reliable of the second line drugs, but has a perhaps not wholly deserved reputation for toxicity. Commoner effects are nausea, vomiting and dizziness: fortunately those on the bone marrow, kidney and liver are much less often produced (Moore, 1960). If the daily dose does not exceed 150 mg., a course is usually well tolerated: this was shown in a comparative trial in East Africa (Report, 1960), and again by Miller, Fox and Tall (1966) in a trial embracing 2077 patients in 14 countries, mainly in Asia and Africa. These authors describe the side effects as ' acceptable in the socio-economic circumstances of developing countries ' (where cheapness of the drug is also an advantage) but advise a pilot trial in others, since racial susceptibility to adverse effects may differ.

ETHIONAMIDE. This compound, like isoniazid, is a derivative of isonicotinic acid, with the full chemical name, alpha-ethyl-thioisonicotinamide.

In spite of the structural similarity between isoniazid and ethionamide, tubercle bacilli do not show cross-resistance and ethionamide is fully active against isoniazid-resistant tubercle bacilli. The activity of ethionamide *in vitro* and in experimental infection is about twice that of streptomycin but inferior to that of isoniazid. Like streptomycin and isoniazid the action of ethionamide on tubercle bacilli is bactericidal (Rist *et al.*, 1959). As with isoniazid, ethionamide-resistant tubercle bacilli emerge rapidly, and there is cross-resistance between thioacetazone and ethionamide (Rist *et al.*, 1959).

The full dose, a total of 1 g., daily is liable to cause nausea and anorexia, and may on that account have to be somewhat reduced: neurotoxic effects may also occur (Brouet *et al.*, 1959). Ethionamide has been successfully included in regimes for treating patients whose bacilli were resistant to standard drugs by Chaves, Abeles and Robins (1963), Corpe and Blalock (1965) and Tousek *et al.* (1967).

PYRAZINAMIDE. Following the discovery of the anti-tuberculous activity of nicotinamide a number of nicotinic acid derivatives were synthesized, of which pyrazinamide was the most active (Kushner *et al.*, 1952). Although *in vitro* and in experimental infections in mice and guinea-pigs the activity of pyrazinamide was only moderate, trials in man showed apparently greater activity (Yeager *et al.*, 1952). Moreover, combined treatment with isoniazid and pyrazinamide in experimental infections of mice freed the animals from tubercle bacilli more completely than did any of the standard drugs used singly or together, and early clinical trial suggested that this combination gave better bacteriological and radiographic results than did combinations of any of the three standard drugs (Schwartz and Moyer, 1953; McDermott *et al.*, 1955). Equally good results are not, however, obtained in all cases. This may be partly explained by the fact that a proportion of pre-treatment strains of tubercle bacilli are resistant to pyrazinamide (Riddell *et al.*, 1960).

The disadvantage of pyrazinamide is hepatotoxicity. This was caused in earlier studies mainly by rather large doses, and it seems from the observations of Velu *et al.* (1961) and subsequent experience that a dose limited to 1·5 g. daily is reasonably safe. This dose, divided into three of 0·5 g., was found by Ellard (1969) in a thorough pharmacological study to maintain a blood level about 5 μg./ml. almost continuously. Patients should be under frequent observation, and blood transaminase estimations should be done regularly.

THIOCARBANILIDES. Many studies have been made of the anti-tuberculous activity of substituted thioureas. Many of these have been shown to have therapeutic activity in mice and guinea-pigs, but there is very little correlation between activity *in vitro* and *in vivo*. Clinical trials with one of the most effective compounds in animals, 4-isobutoxy-4'-(2-pyridyl) thiocarbanilide, were disappointing and it was thought that the compound was poorly absorbed from the human intestinal tract. More recently another carbanilide, 4-4'-diisoamyloxythiocarbanilide (isoxyl) has been introduced, and some success was claimed from a combination of this drug in a dose of 500 mg. daily with streptomycin, but recently it has been little used.

ETHAMBUTOL. This is the dextrorotatory isomer of 2.2'-(ethylenediimino)-di-1-butanol. The compound inhibits the growth of human and bovine strains of *Myco. tuberculosis* in a concentration of 1-5 μg./ml. and is effective in the treatment of experimental infection in mice and guinea-pigs (Thomas *et al.*, 1961; Karlson, 1961a and b). It is well absorbed after oral administration in man, and has been found effective both alone and in various combinations: that with pyrazinamide is particularly commended by Bobrowitz and Gokulanathan (1965). Corpe and Blalock (1965) treating 107 patients whose bacilli were almost all resistant to the three major drugs and many to several others, combined it with ethionamide and other drugs and achieved sputum conversion in 84 per cent.

The use of ethambutol has until recently been restricted because it can cause impairment of vision, due to a retrobulbar neuritis, of which the first signs are blurred vision and inability to distinguish colours. Recovery from this seems to have been invariable, and according to the authors cited and to Leibold (1966) it can be prevented by regulating the dose: 25 mg. per kg. for 60 days should then be reduced to 15 mg.

STANDARD TREATMENT

Both standard treatment and that with ' second-line ' drugs are well described by Crofton and Douglas (1969), and only an outline will be given here. The necessity for giving at least two, often three, and sometimes even more than three drugs together has long been recognized, and the evidence that bacillary resistance is thus prevented or at least long delayed is now familiar. Originally furnished by studies with streptomycin and PAS in Great Britain nearly twenty years ago, it has since been extended to many other combinations. Perhaps the principal change in management during recent years has been the recognition that sanatorium treatment is unnecessary for the average patient: provided that drug administration is feasible he can remain at home.

Active Pulmonary Disease

INITIAL TREATMENT. This is usually started with a combination of all three of the standard drugs, streptomycin, isoniazid and PAS (Report, 1962a). The dose for young adults is streptomycin 1 g. daily by intramuscular injection; isoniazid 200 mg. *once* daily (Gangadharam *et al.*, 1961) and PAS 5 g. three times daily, both by mouth. For patients over 40 years the amount of streptomycin should be reduced to 1 g. on three days a week because of the greater risk of vestibular damage in older people (Crofton, 1960).

CONTINUED TREATMENT. Provided sensitivity tests show the infecting tubercle bacillus to be fully sensitive to all three drugs, treatment in younger people can be continued with streptomycin and isoniazid, leaving out PAS. This is undoubtedly the most effective combination. But for older patients the PAS must be continued as the smaller dose of streptomycin is not sufficient to prevent the emergence of isoniazid-resistant tubercle bacilli.

LENGTH OF TREATMENT. For severe pulmonary infection treatment should be continued for from 18 months to two years (Report, 1962a) but once the patient has been discharged from hospital oral treatment as recommended below can be substituted.

For minimal lesions, treatment with the oral drugs alone is probably adequate. The most satisfactory form is cachets containing 5 g. PAS and 100 mg. isoniazid, which are taken twice daily. In this way patients cannot take one drug without the other. Even with mild infection treatment should probably be continued for at least a year.

Patients with no evidence of disease other than an X-ray shadow of uncertain significance present a difficult problem. Oral treatment with isoniazid and PAS may be given for three months, the patient leading his normal life: if then there is radiological improvement it indicates that the disease was active and treatment should be continued for a year. If there is no change and cultures remain negative it can be stopped. A study in Scotland (Report, 1963) in which equal numbers of comparable patients of this kind were treated for 6 months or more and left untreated showed X-ray improvement in 40·3 and 21 per cent and deterioration in 18·1 and 30·5 per cent respectively. Deterioration in the untreated was commoner at ages below 30 and in lesions over 10 sq. cm. in area.

Meningitis

In cases of tuberculous meningitis all three of the standard drugs should be given. Initially the dose should be streptomycin 1 g. daily, or 40 mg./kg. for infants and small children, by intramuscular injection, PAS 10-15 g. daily by mouth; and isoniazid at least 300 mg. daily or 10 mg./kg. by mouth.

Treatment should be continued for at least a year, but after a time the streptomycin injections can be reduced to twice weekly.

With the relatively high dose of isoniazid recommended above adequate levels are obtained in the cerebro-spinal fluid (Fletcher, 1953) and reports from many centres suggest that intrathecal injections of any kind are now unnecessary and possibly undesirable because of the irritant effect (Anderson *et al.*, 1953; Bulkeley, 1953; Report, 1954). A more cautious view is expressed by Lorber (1960) who suggests that intrathecal injections of streptomycin should not be wholly abandoned. He recommends a course of 10 injections and more if the clinical condition or cerebro-spinal fluid findings are unsatisfactory at any subsequent date. The intrathecal dose should not exceed 100 mg. or 50 mg. in young children.

Additional treatment with corticosteroids may be helpful in severe cases. Lorber (1960) recommends this for patients unconscious on admission or for children under one year of age. The dose must be adequate and the duration rarely needs to exceed one month. If intrathecal injections of hydrocortisone are contemplated in desperate cases, special precautions must be taken to prevent secondary infection.

If the infecting tubercle bacillus is resistant to one or more of the standard drugs, treatment with ethionamide should be considered, as this passes from the blood into the cerebro-spinal fluid fairly readily, even in the absence of meningitis (Hughes *et al.*, 1962).

Surgical Tuberculosis

The treatment of this differs in no way in principle, and very little in practice, from that of pulmonary disease. For genito-urinary tuberculosis there is now general agreement that treatment should be continued for two years. The two drugs mainly to be relied on are PAS and isoniazid: since the organism is sometimes of the bovine type and 17 per cent of these are PAS-resistant (Wallace and Webber, 1956), verification of sensitivity is desirable. Some authors have obtained satisfactory results with this combination alone (*e.g.* Band and Murray, 1958): others favour the addition of streptomycin, at least for the first few months (Halkier and Meyer, 1959). In patients with extensive renal disease who are given streptomycin, blood levels should be determined and the dose reduced if these are found to be unduly high. Surgery is now rarely necessary for disease of either the kidney or the epididymis, and lesions of the bladder which formerly led to severe disability now resolve with good restoration of function.

Initial surgical treatment is often still advisable in tuberculosis of bone: chemotherapy follows the same lines as in other forms of the disease.

TREATMENT FOR PATIENTS WITH DRUG-RESISTANT INFECTION

The choice of treatment in such patients is a matter for the expert and can only be briefly discussed here. If the resistance is to only one of the standard drugs treatment with the other two may be satisfactory. If there is resistance to two, the third may be given together with pyrazinamide and ethionamide. A popular combination when there is resistance to all three is ethionamide, pyrazinamide and cycloserine. Ethambutol may be substituted for cycloserine, and an alternative to any of these should intolerance or resistance to it develop is either capreomycin, kanamycin or viomycin: opinions differ on the order of preference among these three antibiotics. Some of the regimes proposed include four reserve drugs, and almost all authors insist that if such multiple treatment is tolerated and faithfully continued the great majority of these long-standing and usually advanced cases can be rendered sputum-negative. The introduction of rifampicin should further improve the prognosis in such patients.

Hypersensitivity to a standard drug presents the same problem as resistance to it, except that de-sensitization by initially very small and frequently repeated doses may be possible.

CHEMOPROPHYLAXIS

Recent contacts should in the first place have a Mantoux test. If this is negative it should be repeated in six weeks.

Those with positive Mantoux tests should have a chest X-ray, and any showing X-ray changes should be treated as cases of tuberculosis on the usual principles. The management of those with positive Mantoux tests and no X-ray changes is debatable; it may be affected by the age of the subject (see below). The use of routine chemoprophylaxis for contacts is another debatable subject. Discussion of it will be found in the reports of two large scale controlled trials of chemoprophylaxis with isoniazid alone, in contacts without signs of tuberculosis, recently carried out by the United States Public Health Service (Ferebee and Mount, 1962; Mount and Ferebee, 1962).

A special case among contacts is the infant with a tuberculous mother. If the infant is vaccinated with B.C.G. segregation is necessary until Mantoux conversion takes place. If the child is protected with chemotherapy during this period the production of immunity is impaired. Canetti (1956) suggested vaccinating the baby with an isoniazid-resistant strain of B.C.G. and treating with isoniazid until Mantoux conversion has taken place. Gaisford and Griffiths (1961) have now reported the successful use of this method of protection, using a vaccine prepared in Glaxo Laboratories (Ungar, Thomas and Muggleton, 1961).

A third group to be considered for prophylactic treatment are children found to be Mantoux-positive. Children under two years with a positive Mantoux reaction should probably always be treated, because of the high morbidity of tuberculous infection in infants. In children of four to ten years treatment is probably unnecessary in the absence of clinical or radiological evidence of disease, but in adolescence the situation may change again. In the Medical Research Council trials of B.C.G. vaccination it was found that the children aged 13 who gave large reactions to three tuberculin units in the pre-vaccination Mantoux test had an exceptionally high morbidity from tuberculosis during the succeeding years. This suggests that it may be wise to give prophylactic chemotherapy to those who in the pre-vaccination tests show high tuberculin sensitivity (Report, 1959).

LEPROSY

If the treatment of tuberculosis is a speciality, that of leprosy is even more narrowly so, and can only briefly be discussed here. Its study has been facilitated by two discoveries which circumvent to some extent the grave handicap imposed by the non-cultivability of *Myco. leprae* and thus the unavailability of the usual methods of testing chemotherapeutic activity in the laboratory.

One of these discoveries is of a method for producing a transmissible infection by the human bacillus in animals. Shepard (1962), inspired by some earlier observations on other mycobacteria by Fenner, inoculated the footpads of CFW mice intradermally with suspensions of bacilli from human lesions. Slow multiplication followed (50-1000 fold in up to 10 months) and serial transmission succeeded. Intra-testicular inoculation was only irregularly successful. The opportunity afforded by this experimental infection of studying the effects of different treatments is obvious. The second observation is one enabling the effects of treatment in man to be assessed, and has already been turned to account. Apparently degenerate forms of *Myco. leprae* in human lesions originally described by Davey have been intensively studied by Rees and his colleagues with a view to defining criteria by which they can be recognized as dead. In their earlier studies with the electron microscope Rees, Valentine and Wong (1960) first showed that the proportion of *Esch. coli* showing certain morphological changes corresponded closely to the proportion shown to be dead by viable counts. Turning to *Myco. leprae* itself they found that the percentages of bacilli from 10 untreated patients showing degenerative changes by electron microscopy and those irregularly stained by Ziehl-Neelsen were almost equal. They were later to show (Rees and Valentine, 1962) by examining individual rat and human bacilli by both methods of microscopy that irregularly stained bacilli were those shown to be degenerate by electron microscopy. These and other observations have made it possible to count the percentage of dead bacilli in films from lesions: thus in a trial in Malaya described by Waters and Rees (1962) and Waters (1963) the percentage of degenerate bacilli increased from 46 to 96 per cent during

9 months' treatment with dapsone. This method of assessing effect is proving a valuable aid to clinical observation.

For many years the standard treatment for leprosy has been with diaminodiphenyl sulphone (dapsone). The doses originally given have been much reduced, and that now recommended is 100 mg. once weekly, continued for 2-4 years, according to the type of disease (Browne, 1967). Among several other more recently introduced drugs this author commends thiambutosine (4-butoxy-4-dimethyl-amino-diphenyl-thiourea; Ciba 1906) the early studies of which were reported by Garrod (1959) and Davey (1960). It is slightly less effective than dapsone, but also considerably less toxic, and is particularly indicated in patients intolerant of dapsone. The dose may be gradually increased to a total of 2 g. daily: this should be divided, since excretion is rapid. Other drugs which have been used are ditophal, diethodithiol *iso*-phthalate; Etisul), a disadvantage of which is its nauseating smell, and B663 (3-*p*-chloranilino)-10-(*p*-chlorophenyl)-2,10-dihydro-2-isopropyliminophenazine), a phenazine dye. Good results have also been obtained with sulphadoxine (sulphormethoxine; Fanasil) usually given in a dose of 1 g. weekly, which is better tolerated than dapsone, and effective in a form of the disease slow to respond to dapsone (Currie, 1966; Gaind, Menor and Ramakrishna, 1966; Price and Fitzherbert, 1966).

One indication for alternative treatment is the development of bacillary resistance to dapsone. This change can now be verified instead of merely deduced, by inoculating the footpads of mice with bacilli from the lesions and treating the mice with different doses of the drug to determine how much is required to prevent multiplication (Pearson, Pettit and Rees, 1968). According to Hastings and Trautman (1968) relapse despite long-continued dapsone treatment is becoming more common: they commend additional treatment with 1 g. streptomycin three times a week in such patients.

It is too early to assess the value of rifampicin in leprosy, but by analogy with its action on *Myco. tuberculosis* much may be expected, and a preliminary study by Rees, Pearson and Waters (1970) is highly encouraging. Even the smallest dose given to mice (0·0025 per cent in the diet) prevented bacillary multiplication in the foot pad. In the lesions of treated patients the morphological index (proportion of bacilli staining normally) fell to *nil* in four weeks: a comparable reduction from dapsone requires 18 weeks. Moreover the infectivity of lesion material for mice was reduced within 3 to 24 days, whereas during dapsone treatment this change occurs only after 69 days. As the authors point out, this is evidence of a bactericidal effect not exerted by other anti-leprotic drugs. Presumably it will be advisable in future clinical use to combine rifampicin with another drug in order to prevent resistance.

PHARMACEUTICAL PREPARATIONS

CAPREOMYCIN SULPHATE (*Dista Products*) vials containing 1 g. of base for solution for intramuscular injection. Usual dose 1 g. daily.
DAPSONE ('Avlosulfon', *I.C.I.*)
Tablets of 50 and 100 mg. Also as powder, suspension, and solution for injection. Usual dose 100-150 mg. once or twice weekly.
DITOPHAL ('Etisul', *I.C.I.*)
Application for inunction. Dose 5 g. three times a week.
ETHAMBUTOL HYDROCHLORIDE ('Myambutol hydrochloride', *Lederle*)
Tablets of 100 and 400 mg. Usual dose (combined with other drugs) 25 mg. per kg. for 60 days, then 15 mg. per kg.
ETHIONAMIDE ('Trescatyl', *May & Baker*)
Tablets of 125 mg. Usual dose 125 mg. four times a day.
ISONIAZID
Tablets of 100 mg. Usual dose up to 300 mg. daily. Also as injection, syrup, and in many combinations with PAS.
KANAMYCIN. See page 129.
PAS ('Para-aminosalicylic Acid')
Tablets of 500 mg. Usual dose 10-16 g. daily. Also available as sodium or calcium salt in sachets, and in numerous combinations with isonizid.
PYRAZINAMIDE
Tablets of 500 mg. Usual dose 500 mg. three times a day.
RIFAMPICIN. See page 230.
STREPTOMYCIN. See page 113.
THIAMBUTOSINE ('Ciba' 1906, *Ciba*)
Tablets of 500 mg. Dose 500 mg. increasing to 2 g. daily.
THIOACETAZONE ('Thioparamizone', *Smith & Nephew*)
Tablets of 25, 50 and 75 mg. Dose up to 150 mg. daily.
VIOMYCIN SULPHATE
Vials containing equivalent of 1 g. of the base for solution for intramuscular injection. Usual dose 1 g. twice in the day on 2 days of the week.

REFERENCES

ANDERSON, T., KERR, M. R. & LANDSMAN, J. B. (1953). *Lancet* **2**, 691.
BAND, D. & MURRAY, W. A. (1958). *Practitioner* **181**, 279.
BOBROWITZ, I. D. & GOKULANATHAN, K. S. (1965). *Dis. Chest.* **48**, 239.
BROUET, G., MARCHE, J., RIST, N., CHEVALLIER, J. & LEMEUR, G. (1959). *Amer. Rev. Tuberc.* **79**, 6.
BROWNE, S. G. (1967). *Trans. roy. Soc. trop. Med. Hyg.* **61**, 265.
BULKELEY, W. C. M. (1953). *Brit. med. J.* **2**, 1127.
CANETTI, G. (1956). *Amer. Rev. Tuberc.* **74**, Suppl. p. 13.
CHAVES, A. D., ABELES, H. & ROBINS, A. B. (1963). *Amer. Rev. resp. Dis.* **88**, 254.

CORPE, R. F. & BLALOCK, F. A. (1965). *Dis. Chest,* **48,** 305.
CROFTON, J. (1960). *Brit. med. J.* **2,** 370, 449.
CROFTON, J. & DOUGLAS, A. (1969). *Respiratory Diseases.* Oxford: Blackwell.
CURRIE, G. (1966). *Lep. Rev.* **37,** 205.
DAVEY, T. F. (1960). *Trans. roy. Soc. trop. Med. Hyg.* **54,** 199.
DOMAGK, G., BENISCH, R., MIETZSCH, F. & SCHMIDT, H. (1946). *Natur-wissenschaften* **33,** 315.
ELLARD, G. A. (1969). *Tubercle* **50,** 144.
EVANS, D. A. P., MANLEY, K. A. & MCKUSICK, V. A. (1960). *Brit. med. J.* **2,** 485.
FEREBEE, S. H. & MOUNT, F. W. (1962). *Amer. Rev. resp. Dis.* **85,** 490.
FLETCHER, A. P. (1953). *Lancet* **2,** 694
GAIND, M. L., MENOR, C. V. & RAMAKRISHNA (1966). *Leprosy Rev.* **37,** 167,
GAISFORD, W. & GRIFFITHS, M. I. (1961). *Brit. med. J.* **1,** 1500.
GANGADHARAM, P. R. J., DEVADATTA, S., FOX, W., NAIR, C. N. & SELKON, J. B. (1961). *Bull. Wld Hlth Org.* **25,** 793.
GARROD, J. M. B. (1959). *Leprosy Rev.* **30,** 210.
GRUMBACH, F., CANETTI, G. & LE LIRZIN, M. (1969). *Tubercle* **50,** 280.
GRUNBERG, E., LEIWANT, B., D'ASCENSIO, I. L. & SCHNITZER, R. J. (1952). *Dis. Chest* **21,** 369.
GRUNBERG, E. & SCHNITZER, R. J. (1952). *Quart. Bull. Sea View Hosp.* **13,** 3.
GYSELEN, A., VERBIST, L., COSEMANS, J., LACQUET, L. M. & VANDENBERGH, E. (1968). *Amer. Rev. Resp. Dis.* **98,** 933.
HASTINGS, R. C. & TRAUTMAN, J. R. (1968). *Int. J. Leprosy* **36,** 45.
HALKIER, E. & MEYER, J. (1959). *Danish med. Bull.* **6,** 97.
HOBBY, G. L., JOHNSON, P. M., CRAWFORD-GAGLIARDI, L., BOYTAR, V. & JOHNSON, G. E. (1966). *Amer. Rev. resp. Dis.* **94,** 703.
HOBBY, G. L., LENERT, T. F. & MAIER-ENGALLENA, J. (1969). *Proc. Soc. Exp. Biol. (N.Y.)* **131,** 323.
HOFMANN, F. (1968). *Schweiz. med. Wschr.* **98,** 1363.
HUGHES, I. E., SMITH, H. & KANE, P. O. (1962). *Lancet* **1,** 616.
ISRAEL, H. L. (1960). *Amer. Rev. resp. Dis.* **81,** 581.
KARLSON, A. G. (1961a & b). *Amer. Rev. resp. Dis.* **84,** 902, 905.
KASS, I. (1965). *Tubercle (Lond.)* **46,** 151.
KREIS, B. (1966a). *Ann. New York Acad. Sci.* **132,** Art. 2, 912.
KREIS, B. (1966b). *Ann. New York Acad. Sci.* **132,** Art. 2, 957.
KUSHNER, S., DALATIAN, H., SANJWZJIO, J. L., BACH, F. L. JR., SAFIR, S. R., SMITH, V. K. JR., & WILLIAMS, J. H. (1952). *Med. Chem. Sect., Amer. chem. Soc.,* Milwaukee, Wisconsin, April 1st.
LEHMANN, J. (1946). *Lancet* **1,** 15.
LEIBOLD, J. E. (1966). *Ann. New York Acad. Sci.* **135,** Art 2, 904.
LORBER, J. (1960). *Brit. med. J.* **1,** 1309.
MCDERMOTT, W. (1960). *Amer. Rev. resp. Dis.* **81,** 579.
MCDERMOTT, W., ORMOND, L., MUSCHENHEIM, C. & DEUTSCHLE, K. (1955). *13th Conf. Chemother. Tuberc.,* p. 170. Washington: Veterans Administration.
MEYER, H. & MALLY, J. (1912). *Mschr. Chem.* **33,** 393.
MILLER, A. B., FOX, W. & TALL, R. (1966). *Tubercle (Lond.)* **47,** 33.
MITCHISON, D. A. (1954). *Brit. med. J.* **1,** 128.
MOORE, W. (1960). *Tubercle (Lond.)* **41,** 448.
MOUNT, F. W. & FEREBEE, S. H. (1962). *Amer. Rev. resp. Dis.* **85,** 821.
PEARSON, J. M. H., PETTIT, J. H. S. & REES, R. J. W. (1968). *Int. J. Leprosy* **36,** 171.
PRICE, E. W. & FITZHERBERT, M. (1966). *Int. J. Leprosy* **34,** 367.
REES, R. J. W., PEARSON, J. M. H. & WATERS, M. F. R. (1970). *Brit. med. J.* **1,** 89.
REES, R. J. W. & VALENTINE, R. C. (1962). *Internat. J. Leprosy* **30,** 1.
REES, R. J. W., VALENTINE, R. C. & WONG, P. C. (1960). *J. gen. Microbiol.* **22,** 443.

REPORT, MEDICAL RESEARCH COUNCIL (1952). *Brit. med. J.* **2**, 735.
REPORT, MEDICAL RESEARCH COUNCIL (1959). *Brit. med. J.* **2**, 379.
REPORT, MEDICAL RESEARCH COUNCIL (1960). *Tubercle (Lond.)* **41**, 399.
REPORT, MEDICAL RESEARCH COUNCIL (1962a). *Tubercle (Lond.)* **43**, 201.
REPORT, VETERANS ADMINISTRATION (1954). *Trans. 13th Conf. Chemother. Tuberc.*, p. 191. Washington.
REPORT (1962b). *Progress against Tuberculosis.* Office of Health Economics, London.
REPORT (1963). Research Committee of the Scottish Thoracic Society. *Tubercle (Lond.)* **44**, 39.
REPORT (1964). United States Pub. Hlth Cooperative Investigation. *Amer. Rev. resp. Dis.*, **89**, 327.
RIDDELL, R. W., STEWART, S. M. & SOMNER, A. R. (1960). *Brit. med. J.* **2**, 1207.
RIST, N., GRUMBACH, F. & LIBERMANN, D. (1959). *Amer. Rev. Tuberc.* **79**, 1.
ROBITZEK, E. H., SELIKOFF, I. J. & ORNSTEIN, G. G. (1952). *Quart. Bull. Sea View Hosp.* **13**, 27.
SCHWARTZ, W. S. (1966). *Amer. Rev. resp. Dis.* **94**, 858.
SCHWARTZ, W. S. & MOYER, R. E. (1953). *12th Conf. Chemother. Tuberc.*, p. 296. Washington: Veterans Administration.
SHEPARD, C. C. (1962). *Internat. J. Leprosy* **30**, 291.
SHORT, E. I. (1962). *Tubercle (Lond.)* **43**, 33.
SYMPOSIUM, (1966). *Ann. New York Acad. Sci.* **135**, Art. 2, 940.
THOMAS, J. P., BAUGHN, C. O., WILKINSON, R. B. & SHEPHERD, R. G. (1961). *Amer. Rev. resp. Dis.* **83**, 891.
TOUSEK, J., JANCIK, E., ZELENKA, M. & JANCIKOVA-MAKOVA, M. (1967). *Tubercle (Lond.)* **48**, 27.
UNGAR, J., THOMAS, V. & MUGGLETON, P. W. (1961). *Brit. med. J.* **1**, 1498.
VELU, S., ANDREWS, R. H., ANGEL, J. H., DEVADATTA, S., FOX, W., JACOB, P. G., NAIR, C. N. & RAMAKRISHNAN, C. V. (1961). *Tubercle (Lond.)* **42**, 136.
WALLACE, A. T. & WEBBER, W. J. (1956). *Tubercle* **37**, 358.
WATERS, M. F. R. (1963). *Leprosy Rev.* **34**, 173.
WATERS, M. F. R. & REES, R. J. W. (1962). *Internat. J. Leprosy* **30**, 266.
YEAGER, R. L., MUNROE, W. G. C. & DESAU, F. I. (1952). *Trans. 11th Conf. Chemother. Tuberc.* Washington Veterans Administration.

Chapter XXVI

VENEREAL DISEASES AND NON-VENEREAL SPIROCHAETOSES

IT is a remarkable fact that the most sensitive of all micro-organisms to penicillin are those causing the two principal forms of venereal disease. Their treatment is now within the capacity of anyone, but because clinical skill and special laboratory facilities are necessary to verify cure and sometimes even to make a diagnosis, the subject must remain a speciality.

Syphilis

THE degree of sensitivity of *Treponema pallidum* to anti-bacterial agents cannot be measured in the ordinary way *in vitro* since the organism cannot be cultured artificially, but the results of curative tests in rabbits are highly significant. Early experiments showed that four days after the intratesticular or intracutaneous inoculation of rabbits a very small dose of penicillin sufficed to abort the infection, even though administered in a long-acting form giving very low blood levels. At two weeks a dose about seven times larger was required to produce the same effect. These findings indicated the possibility of aborting the disease in man by a single dose of a long-acting preparation administered at an early stage.

The object in treating established syphilis is to maintain a therapeutic level in the blood continuously for a period varying somewhat with the stage of the disease. The most certain way of doing this is to give daily injections of 600,000 units of a suspension of procaine penicillin: such a course should ideally be uninterrupted, even on Sundays, although it is common practice to give 1·2 mega units on Saturday to cover the week-end. Because penicillin therapy may be interrupted by patients defaulting or by the development of allergy, some prefer to give an initial dose of 2·4 mega units of a long-acting penicillin which will itself render the patient non-infectious and may

420

even be curative. Preparations containing benethamine or benzathine penicillin give much more prolonged action, but the levels produced, particularly by benzathine penicillin, are lower and inconstant, the rate of absorption varying with the site of injection and still more with degree of muscular activity. Such treatment appears to be indicated only for those unable to attend for a full course of daily injections. The periods of treatment generally advised are 10-12 days for primary and secondary syphilis, 14 for cardiovascular disease, and 21 for neurosyphilis. It is generally recommended that in her first pregnancy after treatment a woman should receive a further 10-day course although there is no good evidence that this is necessary (King, 1965). Established congenital syphilis is treated with 0·5 mega units per kg. body weight over 10 days, but such delayed treatment may not prevent later development of interstitial keratitis or nerve deafness.

For treatment with long-acting penicillins Slatkin (1965) recommends in primary or latent syphilis with negative C.S.F. procaine penicillin with aluminium monostearate (PAM) 2·4 mega units plus 2 further doses of 1·2 mega units at 3-day intervals; or a single dose of benzathine penicillin 1·2 mega units into each buttock. For asymptomatic cardiovascular or neurosyphilis he recommends PAM 5-6 doses of 1·2 mega units at 3-day intervals; or benzathine penicillin 2-3 doses of 3 mega units at 7-day intervals.

JARISCH-HERXHEIMER REACTION. Within a few hours of starting penicillin treatment, over half the patients with early syphilis develop fever, sweating, malaise and headache, often with exacerbation of their symptoms or signs. Putkonen *et al.* (1966) found a rise in axillary temperature to at least 37·6°C. in 95 per cent of patients with secondary or sero-positive primary syphilis. The incidence falls with increasing duration of the disease. Similar reactions are described in other spirochaetal infections (pp. 435 and 437).

The classical explanation has been that the reaction is due to the liberation of toxic products from the massive destruction of treponemes, and this is in keeping with the reaction occurring most frequently in the primary and early part of the secondary stages when organisms are most numerous. It is, however, an all-or-none response independent of the dose of penicillin, and this and other evidence has led to the suggestion that the reaction has an allergic basis. Skog and Gudjonsson (1966) examined this possibility in 31 patients with early syphilis who developed Jarisch-Herxheimer reactions following the first injection of penicillin. Leucocytosis and lymphopenia regularly occurred, usually before the temperature reached its peak, but there were no constant changes in the thrombocytes or basophils. They were unable to confirm previous claims that histological changes resembling those of focal tuberculin reactions occurred in secondary lesions. Skin tests with various reagents produced non-contributory results and they were generally unable to support the view that the reaction has an allergic origin.

The reaction is harmless in the primary and secondary stages, but the focal reaction can be dangerous in certain cases of gummatous, cardiovascular, or neurosyphilis. It has been traditional to try to avoid the reactions in late syphilis by beginning treatment with bismuth. The efficacy of this has long been doubted, and it has been agreed that this regimen will not suppress the reaction in general paralysis. Knudsen and Aastrup (1965), in a direct comparison of 149 patients treated with penicillin with 184 patients treated with bismuth and neoarsphenamine or arsfenoxyl, found no difference in the course or frequency of Jarisch-Herxheimer reactions in the two groups. De Graciansky and Grupper (1961) reduced the frequency and severity of the reaction by simultaneous treatment with corticosteroids, and C. S. Nicol (personal communication) has been successful for some years with prednisolone 5 mg. 8 hourly for 2 days before and after the first injection. It has been felt wise to treat active general paralysis in hospital under barbiturate sedation in the hope of avoiding the occasional psychosis and epileptiform seizures which may follow the first dose of penicillin.

PERSISTENCE OF TREPONEMES IN TREATED SYPHILIS. Several investigators have claimed that treponemes are recoverable from the tissues of some penicillin-treated patients long after the disease was believed to have been eradicated (Collart *et al.*, 1962). It has been suggested that these surviving organisms may be avirulent but antigenic and responsible for the persistence of a positive T.P.I. reaction after adequate treatment. The possibility of recrudescent infection from these organisms, particularly in patients treated with steroids, has aroused considerable interest. In patients believed to have been adequately treated, Rice *et al.* (1970) demonstrated by darkground and immunofluorescent microscopy the persistence in the aqueous humour and C.S.F. of forms at least some of which were *Treponema pallidum*. It is generally felt, however, that as the clinical results of treatment are excellent and only the moist early lesions are infectious, there is no reason to modify the present treatment regimens.

PENICILLIN ALLERGY. Concern has several times been expressed that the growing frequency of allergic reactions to penicillin is seriously interfering with venereal disease control. Willcox (1964) reviews the reactions to penicillin and ways of preventing them. Amongst more than 74,000 patients receiving a single dose of penicillin, the incidence of reaction was less than 1 per cent. Amongst those receiving multiple injections for the treatment of syphilis, the incidence was 6·6 to 10·2 per cent (less in negroes). On the other hand fatalities were very uncommon.

So far, there has been very little trouble in mass campaigns for the control of treponematoses and the principal threat is in the treatment of adult syphilis in urban communities. In his own series, Willcox (1964) found that a history of allergy contra-indicated the use of penicillin in less than 4 per cent. In the course of multiple injections, 7·5 per cent developed reactions, but by then all but 22 per cent had received curative doses.

Patients so highly sensitized as to prohibit treatment with penicillin have been successfully treated with tetracycline (750 mg. 6 hourly for 15 days) or erythromycin (500 mg. 6 hourly for 10 days: Fernando, 1969). However, South *et al.* (1964) report that a young pregnant girl successfully treated with erythromycin two months before delivery, gave birth to an infant with congenital syphilis which died on the third day of life. A dose of erythromycin adequate for the treatment of maternal syphilis will evidently not eradicate the disease from the foetus.

Galla *et al.* (1965) found cephaloridine as effective as penicillin against rabbit syphilis and superior to tetracycline, chloramphenicol, novobiocin, or streptomycin. Glicksman and Knox (1968) treated 10 patients with primary and 13 with secondary syphilis with 0·5 g. intramuscular cephaloridine for 10 days (omitting Saturday and Sunday) without relapse over at least a year. Two had Jarisch-Herxheimer reactions after the first dose but five patients known to be hypersensitive to penicillin showed no signs of reaction.

Other Treponematoses

Late yaws is now seen relatively commonly in immigrants to this country and bejel may be occasionally encountered (Wray, 1966).

BEJEL (and PINTA) are reported to respond well to a single large dose of a repository penicillin preparation.

YAWS. *T. pertenue* is also highly penicillin-sensitive, and this disease has commonly been treated with a single dose of PAM (procaine penicillin in oil with 2 per cent aluminium monostearate), the dose being 0·6 and 1·2 mega unit in children and adults respectively. Fry and Rodin (1966) emphasize the importance of recognizing the occasional case of infectious yaws, and successfully treated a child from St. Vincent with 0·3 mega units aqueous procaine penicillin daily for 14 days. For adults with palmar and plantar hyperkeratosis and those with late lesions, Gentle (1965) recommends 4-6 mega units aqueous procaine penicillin spread over a period of several weeks. Contacts and latent cases can be treated with 0·6 mega units benzathine penicillin and active cases with 1·2 mega units benzathine penicillin (children under 10 should receive half these amounts). Nicol (1962) emphasizes the difficulty of distinguishing with certainty between yaws and syphilis and recommends that where there is any doubt treatment should be with procaine penicillin 0·6 mega units intramuscularly daily for 10 days. Reports on yaws eradication campaigns emphasize the necessity for treating the entire population of an area, and not merely overt cases, since others may be latent or in the stage of incubation.

Gonorrhoea

The treatment of gonorrhoea has been transformed twice in the past 30 years. The first success, that of sulphonamides, was relatively short-lived, resistant strains of gonococci becoming common within a few years. That of penicillin has been both more dramatic and more prolonged, but is now failing from the same cause.

The gonococcus is the most sensitive to penicillin of all ordinary bacteria. It disappears from the exudate within two hours of a moderate dose being given, and that single dose is usually curative. This rapid destructive action, leaving the organism no time to adapt itself, was believed to be the reason why no resistant strains appeared, although it was very early shown that by careful training resistance could be increased *in vitro* several thousand-fold.

The first unequivocal evidence of the existence of resistant strains was obtained in 1958, when it was evident that treatment failures were becoming rather more frequent. Of 1,984 strains examined in nine centres in England (Report, 1961) 262 (13·2 per cent) were inhibited only by concentrations of 0·125 to 1·0 unit per ml., the normal inhibitory concentration being <0·01 unit per ml. Moreover, it was clearly shown that these strains of higher resistance are associated with treatment failure. During the exclusive use of penicillin for treating gonorrhoea, gonococci have largely reverted to sulphonamide sensitivity. Resistance to streptomycin is so readily developed and of such a degree that it was soon apparent that extensive use could not succeed for long.

Substantial increase in the incidence of gonorrhoea and in the female to male ratio continues (British Co-operative Clinical Group, 1970). In this country there has been no marked increase in penicillin resistance but elsewhere great changes have occurred, and in South East Asia increase in both the incidence and degree of resistance has reached a crisis (Willcox, 1970).

No other infectious disease has been the subject of so many therapeutic trials but despite the ready (and increasing) availability of patients, and the relatively large numbers treated in centres designed for this purpose, the design and conduct of the trials have not always been as impeccable as might be hoped.

Where less sensitive strains have become common, the recommended dose of penicillin has been progressively raised from a single intramuscular injection of 1·2 mega units aqueous procaine penicillin for acute uncomplicated gonorrhoea in the male (repeated the next day for the female) to 4·8 mega units. The size of the injection precludes increase beyond this point but even so there have been 5 per cent or more of failures.

Willcox (1970) reviews the reasons for failure which include not only infection with less-sensitive gonococci, but mis-diagnosis, re-infection, and failure of the anti-bacterial agent to reach adequate levels either in the blood or the site of infection. It has also been suggested that the staphylococci commonly present in the urethra might produce enough penicillinase to interfere with the effect of penicillin on the gonococcus. In fact, both Lagerholm *et al.* (1966) and Tawes (1966) found a good correlation between failure rates and *in vitro* sensitivity of the gonococcus, but no correlation with the presence in the urethra of penicillinase-producing staphylococci.

Despondency engendered by decreasing penicillin sensitivity amongst gonococci is likely to lead to insistence on more exacting schedules for all patients. There is copious evidence that therapeutic success is directly related to the *in vitro* sensitivity of the strain and where sensitive strains predominate, as they currently do in this country, treatment with modest doses of penicillin can still be expected to be curative. At the same time it must be acknowledged that the successful control of gonorrhoea involves other considerations than the sensitivity of the organism. In a more perfectly regulated society (where gonorrhoea might in any case be less common) it would be reasonable to use modest doses for initial treatment and to re-treat the failures. This would, however, permit the spread of less sensitive strains on re-exposure during the interval before re-treatment and there arises a natural demand for near-100 per cent success rates on initial treatment.

This ideal may be approached in two ways: by magnified penicillin therapy or by the use of other agents. Ideal therapy, as Willcox (1970) has reiterated, requires plasma concentrations of drug which rapidly reach a peak sufficient to eliminate the gonococcus and equally rapidly fall so as to avoid a tail of low levels which may foster the emergence of more resistant strains or permit their establishment on re-infection. The desire for instant success and the problem of defaulters in treatment also make it highly desirable that this effect should be achieved by a single injection or at least by treatment of very limited duration.

The peak penicillin level may be improved by giving benzyl penicillin in addition to procaine penicillin, by giving more frequent doses, and giving probenecid and prolonging treatment. Near 100 per cent success rates were achieved by Tawes (1966) with procaine penicillin 0·6 mega units plus benzyl penicillin 0·3 mega units, 12 hourly for two days; and by Borring (1965) with procaine penicillin, 1·2 mega units plus benzyl penicillin 1 mega unit daily for three days. Olson and Lomholt (1969) cured 99 per cent of 832 patients (and the other 1 per cent may have been re-infections) with 5 mega units benzyl penicillin and 1 g. probenecid. The success of Evans (1966) with 2·5 mega units (1·25 mega units each buttock) ' Triplopen ' (benethamine penicillin, procaine penicillin and benzyl penicillin) may be criticized on the ground that the presence of a long-acting penicillin provides a protracted tail of low penicillinaemia which may foster the emergence of less sensitive strains in the occasional failures or on re-infection.

Other Agents. Numerous other agents have been tried. Several have the disadvantage that oral administration must be spread over several days with all the difficulties of inconstant absorption, defaulting, and potential storage and sale by patients of their drug supply. There is also the problem that a proportion of strains more resistant to penicillin are also more resistant to other agents, possibly as the result of previous alternative treatment (Reyn and Bentzon, 1969).

PARENTERAL AGENTS. Because of resistance, streptomycin is no longer suitable for treatment and parenteral tetracycline, because of relatively low blood levels, gives poor results unless supplemented by oral therapy (Willcox, 1970). Actinospectacin (p. 202) has had several very favourable reports. Given as a single dose of 2 g. to 108 males and 28 females, it gave 100 per cent cure in the hands of Cornelius and Domescik (1970) who describe it as one of the most effective agents for gonorrhoea. It is not at present commercially available and has not been tested against the most intractable strains. Kanamycin, as a single intramuscular injection of 2 g., continues to give excellent results with failure rates around 5 per cent (Fishnaller *et al.*, 1968; Farrell, 1969). Intramuscular cephaloridine in a 2 g. dose supplemented by 1 g. the following day was successful in 93·6 per cent of females treated by Jouhar and Fowler (1968).

ORAL AGENTS. Most attention has been given to the possible use of ampicillin, tetracyclines and drug combinations. Groth and Hallqvist (1970) treated 311 patients, males and females infected with penicillin-sensitive strains, with two oral doses of 1 g. ampicillin separated by 5 hours. After exclusion of probable reinfections, the failure rate was less than 1 per cent. In 500 males infected with less sensitive strains, and treated with 2 g. oral ampicillin and 1 g. probenecid, Gundersen *et al.* (1969) had a lower failure rate (1·4 per cent) than that achieved by a single intramuscular injection of a mixture of benzyl and procaine penicillins.

Sokoloff (1965), who claims that an alternative is required less because of the failure of penicillin than because of the increasing numbers of allergic patients, cured all 60 patients treated with demethylchortetracycline (900 mg. initially, plus 150 mg. 6-hourly for 5 days). The problem is to simplify and shorten the effective treatment regimen. In groups of 200 females treated by Enfors and Molin (1970) with a single dose of 1·2 g. demethylchlortetracycline the failure rate was 22·2 per cent (41·2 per cent in rectal infection). However, simply by repeating the dose after 4 to 6 hours, Willcox (1969) reduced the failure rate to the acceptable level of 4·3 per cent. With this or other more recent tetracyclines it may be possible to facilitate tetracycline treatment but it would be optimistic to suppose that with the widespread use of such regimens increasing gonococcal resistance to tetracyclines would be long kept at bay.

Several attempts have been made to improve results by using combinations of agents. Garrod and Waterworth (1967) examined the *in vitro* effects on the gonococcus of three such combinations. Kanamycin and penicillin were indifferent or no more than additive (p. 272). Kanamycin and sulphafurazole were usually additive so that simultaneous treatment with sulphafurazole might allow the dose of kanamycin to be reduced. Trimethoprim and sulphonamide were strongly synergic (p. 272). This combination was very successfully used by Csonka and Knight (1967) and by Carrol and Nicol (1970) who gave four tablets (each 80 mg. trimethoprim plus 200 mg. sulphamethoxazole) as one dose daily for 5 days. Arya *et al.* (1970) gave four tablets 12-hourly and found that 65 per cent of the patients were cured after two doses and 96 per cent after three or four. In contrast, Wright and Grimble (1970) found that the drug given 6-hourly for 5 days failed to cure 38 per cent of 97 men, all but one of whom responded to 0·9 mega unit procaine penicillin daily for three days. The possibility that superior results might be obtained in gonorrhoea by the use of a different ratio of trimethoprim to sulphonamide is discussed on page 48.

Concern has often been expressed that the use of other agents or the increased dose of penicillin necessary to treat less sensitive gonococci will mask the development of concurrent syphilis. It goes without saying that every patient treated for gonorrhoea should undergo serological tests for syphilis six months later. Provided that this is done, cannot the possible effect on incubating syphilis be disregarded? The ordinary dose of penicillin might only be suppressive: larger doses might well be curative of syphilis at that stage. Tetracyclines and erythromycin are also active against *T. pallidum*: streptomycin and kanamycin are not, and this is claimed as an advantage in their use.

RE-TREATMENT OF FAILURES. There is nothing in the clinical status of patients which helps to identify the potential failures, except that more prolonged infections are less likely to respond (Wray, 1965). Previously treated patients in Evans' (1966) series showed no special liability to relapse. The most important single factor in failure is reduced sensitivity of the gonococcus to penicillin. In patients infected with gonococci sensitive to 0·1 unit per ml. or less Rantsalo *et al.* (1964) found a failure rate of 5·4 per cent. Amongst those infected with more resistant organisms the failure rate was 4 times as high. Borring (1965) shows a systematic decline in success rate with decreasing sensitivity of the infecting organism. There is also evidence that organisms with reduced sensitivity both to penicillin and to streptomycin are particularly resistant to penicillin treatment (Rantsalo *et al.*, 1964; Evans, 1966). In heterosexual gonorrhoea the chance is about 90 per cent that treatment which has already failed in the partner will be unsuccessful (Evans, 1966).

In the male, relapse usually occurs in the first week after treatment without the urine having cleared completely. In streptomycin-treated patients, Evans (1966) found that relapse occurred immediately on cessation of treatment but in penicillin-treated patients there was a delay of 2-7 days. In the female, relapse is frequently not detectable without bacteriological examination.

It appears that if oral consumption of the drug can be relied upon (and many venereologists believe that this is not often), the following are suitable for re-treatment: (1) *Oxytetracycline* (250 mg. orally, 6-hourly for 7 days). Some begin with an initial intramuscular injection of 500 mg.; others give in addition an initial oral loading dose of 1 g.—the advantage, like that of giving a large dose of depot penicillin, being that it should render the defaulting patient non-infectious and may be curative (2) *Demethylchlortetracycline*, 1·2 g. repeated after 4-6 hours. (3) *Ampicillin* (250 mg., 6-hourly for 8 days). If continuing oral therapy appears unlikely, *cephaloridine* may be given (single intramuscular injection of 2 g.) or *ampicillin* (1 g. intramuscularly, repeated 5-6 hours later). The clinical results may be more spectacular with tetracyclines because of the simultaneous effect on co-existent non-gonococcal urethritis.

COMPLICATED INFECTIONS. Proctitis is more resistant to treatment than urethritis, as shown by Evans' (1966) finding that in homosexual partners similar doses of procaine penicillin cured urethritis in the active partner but not proctitis in the passive. Proctitis should respond to procaine penicillin 1·2 mega units daily for 3-5 days. Tubal infections require still more active treatment: benzyl penicillin, 1 mega unit 6-hourly for 10 days is recommended. Rees and Annels (1969) begin treatment with penicillin and three days later, when the sensitivity of the gonococcus is known, change the treatment if necessary.

Non-gonococcal Urethritis

The cause of this disease (if there is a single cause) still eludes final demonstration and this, combined with its spontaneous remissions and recurrences, make the assessment of treatment difficult. Currently regarded as likely causes are T-mycoplasma (Csonka and Corse, 1970) and TRIC (trachoma-inclusion conjunctivitis) agents (Dunlop *et al.*, 1965) both of which have the attraction of being sensitive *in vitro* to tetracyclines to which the disease commonly responds. It has also several times been suggested that the condition is an allergic reaction to an unidentified antigen (Weston, 1965). Csonka (1965) convincingly argues that it is a mistake to insist on long term follow-up in assessing the efficacy of treatment because of the accumulation of defaulting and re-infected patients. Response, if any, is immediate and the result after two weeks is the best measure of success. At this time, the difference between tetracycline and placebo treatment is highly significant but later becomes less so, presumably as spontaneous cure occurs.

Morton and Wray (1966) treated 50 patients with methacycline (150 mg. 6-hourly for 4 days) and obtained cures in almost 80 per cent. Wright (1969) was less successful. He found the results no better than those obtained with other tetracyclines, and Andrew *et al.* (1969) say the same for clomocycline. Superior results are claimed for an oral tetracycline phosphate complex given for four days (Wijetunga and Morton, 1969) and Statham and Morton (1968) achieved satisfactory results in 88 per cent of patients treated with intramuscular pyrrolidinomethyltetracycline nitrate, 350 mg. daily for 4 days. However, a number of complaints of systemic reactions and of local pain followed this treatment both in these patients and those treated by Schofield and Masterson (1969).

Results with streptomycin and sulphonamides (short, medium and long-acting), alone and in combination, have been conflicting (Csonka, 1965). Alergant (1964) found that a single dose of streptomycin (0·5 g.) plus sulphamethoxydiazine (1 g.) was slightly more effective than the same dose of streptomycin plus sulphadimidine (1 g., 6-hourly for 5 days). The two regimens had failure rates at 7-14 days of 10·8 and 12·3 per cent, and at 14-28 days of 23·7 and 27·8 per cent. Almost identical results were obtained by Willcox (1968) in 106 patients using erythromycin stearate 250 mg. 6-hourly for 6 days. Csonka and Spitzer (1969) treated 51 patients with oral lincomycin 500 mg. 6-hourly for 5 days and cured only a quarter of the patients—a result equivalent to that obtained with a placebo. Retreatment with erythromycin cured 68 per cent. They argue that this supports the aetiological role of T-strain mycoplasma since this, unlike *Mycoplasma hominis,* is sensitive to erythromycin but resistant to lincomycin (Csonka and Corse, 1970). Trimethoprim-sulphamethoxazole was so unsuccessful in a dozen patients treated by Carroll and Nicol (1970) that they abandoned the trial. Treatment of non-gonococcal urethritis with furazone urethral suppositories and with such anti-viral compounds as have so far been used has been unsuccessful.

Trichomoniasis

Trichomonas vaginalis was found in 513/1,355 (38 per cent) cases of sexually transmitted infection in the female (Wisdom and Dunlop, 1965). On treatment with metronidazole (Flagyl: 200 mg., 8-hourly by mouth for 7 days) 98 per cent of 284 cases were clear immediately after cessation of treatment and 72 per cent of 144 cases three weeks later. The propriety of using the drug early in pregnancy is discussed on page 365. There is no evidence that increased resistance of *Trichomonas* to metronidazole is a cause of failure, or that the presence in the vagina of numerous bacteria which inactivate metronidazole significantly affects the response to treatment (MacFadzean *et. al.,* 1969). There have been a number of disputed claims that metronidazole treatment can precipitate vaginal candidiasis. Oller (1969) discusses the factors influencing this complication and shows that it can be controlled by the use of amphotericin pessaries (50 mg. nightly × 7). Since symptomatic superinfection is generally infrequent, he suggests that such combined treatment should be reserved for high risk patients: in pregnancy, diabetes, or following recent vaginal candidiasis.

Nifuratel, a nitrofuran marketed under the name *Magmilor* is useful in vaginal trichomoniasis when given by combined oral (200 mg. 3 times daily for 7 days) and local (250 mg. pessaries nightly × 10) administration, but is apparently less effective than metronidazole (Fowler and Hussain, 1968). Like other nitrofurans (p. 38) nifuratel has a broad antimicrobial spectrum (it is also active against candida) and Churcher and Evans (1969) point out that before instituting treatment it is important to exclude gonorrhoea which is otherwise likely to be masked by the local antibacterial effect. Trichomonas was found in 93/1,646 (5·6 per cent) cases of non-gonococcal urethritis in the male and was cleared by the same regimen as that used in women from all 71 cases seen immediately after treatment and from 93 per cent of the 41 cases who returned for follow-up 90 days later. *Trichomonas vaginalis* is said to occur much more commonly in negroes. Similar success rates are reported by Schapira (1965) who holds to the view that male infection constitutes the main source of the female disease. Difficulty in persuading male consorts to undergo treatment is increased by the fact that only about 10 per cent of male infections produce symptoms. Some observers claim that the male disease is commonly self-limiting if re-infection is prevented by treatment of the female. The organism may nevertheless underly some chronic infections in the male, and Catterall (1965) successfully managed 27/38 cases of prostatitis, believed to be of trichomonal origin, with metronidazole.

Chancroid

Haemophilus ducreyi has similar sensitivities to other species in this genus, and there is therefore a considerable choice of suitable drugs. Willcox (1965) recommends streptomycin 1-3 g. daily in divided doses for 5 days or tetracycline or chloramphenicol 250-500 mg. 6-hourly for 4-5 days. McDaniel (1964) continues tetracycline therapy for 12 days if the nodes have suppurated. Some prefer sulphonamides (4 g. daily until healing) or streptomycin to tetracyclines because they eliminate the risk of masking syphilis, and on the ground of lesser cost.

Lymphogranuloma Venereum

The nomenclature of this and the following disease is confused: the above is now the accepted name for the undoubtedly venereal disease having a trivial primary lesion and followed by secondary suppurative lymphadenitis going on to fibrosis involving inguinal glands in the male and pelvic in the female. The cause is an agent related to that of psittacosis and susceptible to various chemotherapeutic agents.

When 'aureomycin' was first introduced this disease was claimed to be one of its triumphs: even secondary rectal strictures in the female were said to relax. Some of the effects observed may have been due to an action on secondary bacterial infection. Tetracycline (250 mg. 6-hourly) is given for different periods at various stages of the disease by McDaniel (1964): 2 weeks for the acute inguinal disease, 3 weeks for the acute rectal disease, and 6 weeks or more for chronic disease. Willcox (1965) uses larger doses: up to 500 mg. 6-hourly in the male and more in the female. The prognosis is poor in the most chronic cases. It has been claimed that sulphonamides are as effective as tetracyclines and more so than chloramphenicol. Incision of fluctuant nodes is contra-indicated but aspiration may hasten resolution (Abrams, 1968).

Granuloma Inguinale

This doubtfully venereal disease is due to *Donovania granulomatis*. Most authors are agreed that the choice lies between streptomycin (1 g. 6-hourly for 5 days) or tetracycline (500 mg. 6-hourly for 10-15 days). Goldberg and Bernstein (1964) describe two cases, one on each of these regimens, which resolved within six weeks. Davis (1970) describes 14 cases, all negroes, 7 of whom also had evidence of syphilis; 8 of the 10 males were homosexuals. With one exception, all responded to tetracycline 2 g. per day given until the lesions were completely healed (1-4 weeks). Two patients treated over several weeks with ampicillin (up to 4 g. per day) failed to respond and were subsequently successfully treated with tetracycline.

OTHER SPIROCHAETOSES

RELAPSING FEVER. *Borrelia recurrentis* is sensitive to arsenicals and to various antibiotics. Penicillin, which originally replaced arsenicals, is now generally considered inferior to tetracyclines. Only a short course is necessary, but the dose recommended varies from 1 to 3 g. daily and the duration from three to six days. In fact, very much less tetracycline is effective. Bryceson *et al.* (1970) found that 250 mg. tetracycline given intravenously over 2 to 3 minutes cleared the blood of spirochaetes within $2\frac{1}{2}$ hours. Two intramuscular injections of 150 mg. at an interval of 6 hours were also effective. There was no relapse in 18 patients so treated, nor in 45 patients given a total dose of 4·3-5·5 g. over 4 to 5 days. All patients given an effective dose developed a characteristic Jarisch-Hexheimer-like reaction showing the prodromal, chill and flush phases of endotoxic fever. Cardiorespiratory disturbance in the flush phase may be so severe that patients die. Correction of extra-cellular fluid depletion, cardiac failure and hypoxia may prevent fatalities, but large doses of hydrocortisone did not influence the reaction (Warrell *et al.*, 1970). In patients in whom vigorous reactions might be dangerous (one was pregnant), Bryceston *et al.* (1970) substituted an injection of 20,000 units of benzylpenicillin plus 60,000 units of procaine penicillin for the initial dose of tetracycline. Penicillin is, however, poor at eradicating spirochaetes from the brain, some strains of *Borrelia* are resistant, and relapse on penicillin treatment is common. They recommend therefore that the initial dose of penicillin be followed the next day by 250 mg. tetracycline.

RAT-BITE FEVER. Roughgarden (1965) describes the clinical manifestations, diagnosis and laboratory investigation of the acute illnesses caused by *Streptobacillus moniliformis* and *Spirillum minus*. Penicillin is the drug of choice for both infections, which respond to as little as 0·6 mega units daily. Treatment should be given for not less than 7 days. Streptomycin and tetracycline are also effective, but sulphonamides have uniformly failed. McGill *et al.* (1966) successfully treated two patients in this country with penicillin (0·5 mega units, 6-hourly) plus streptomycin (0·5-1 g., 12-hourly). Bacterial endocarditis due to either organism is said to require 12-15 mega units penicillin per day for three to four weeks; we would continue for six weeks.

Leptospirosis

This infection is in a different category, in regard both to the causative organism and to its response to treatment. Arsenicals are without effect, but *Leptospira* spp. are susceptible in varying degrees to most of the major antibiotics. Nevertheless the evalution of their effect presents unusual difficulties in all three spheres, *in vitro,* in the experimental animal and in the clinical field, and their place in the treatment of this disease is still the subject of a controversy which breaks out in print from time to time.

In vitro studies are complicated by the fact that different degrees of anti-leptospiral activity are exerted by antibiotics over a very wide range of concentrations, and any quantitative result depends on the criterion adopted. Very low concentrations of penicillin, of the order of 0·1 unit per ml., will inhibit the normally slow growth of the organism, but motility is retained, and very much higher concentrations fail to sterilize a culture. The effective concentrations determined by various authors, using different methods, are therefore not comparable or worth quoting.

Animal studies meet another difficulty: the guinea-pig and hamster, although suitably susceptible to the infection, are also uniquely susceptible to a 'toxic' effect not only of penicillin (see p. 64) but of tetracyclines and macrolides, and are liable to succumb to this when adequate doses are given. These drug deaths have interfered with animal studies of the treatment of *L. icterohaemorrhagiae* infection, but several workers have nevertheless satisfied themselves of a curative effect, superior to that of penicillin, from large doses of erythromycin or oleandomycin and of curative effects from streptomycin and tetracyclines. Stalheim (1966) believes that in previous animal studies demonstration of leptospiral survival was attempted too soon after cessation of treatment. In his own studies penicillin, chloramphenicol and erythromycin were ineffective in doses corresponding with those generally used in man: chlortetracycline destroyed most of the renal population of leptospira, but dihydrostreptomycin (and hence presumably streptomycin) was the most effective agent.

The clinical value of antibiotic treatment is difficult to assess (Heath, *et al.*, 1965). It is clearly necessary to distinguish the severe infection caused by *L. icterohaemorrhagiae,* occurring sporadically, the diagnosis of which is often delayed, from those due to other serotypes, which are not only milder, but often because epidemic or endemic are recognized earlier.

Examples of such mild infections, almost never fatal and rarely even causing jaundice, are those caused by *L. australis* in Queensland and *L. bataviae* in Malaya. These appear to respond regularly to about 4 mega units of penicillin daily, which causes a characteristic Jarisch-Herxheimer-type reaction, followed by rapid recovery. Kocen (1962) and others working in Malaya, report a shortened duration of fever from treatment with oxytetracycline and penicillin respectively. The infection caused by *L. canicola* is also comparatively mild, and the review by Pertzelan and Pruzanski (1963) concludes in favour of its treatment with tetracycline.

The proper treatment for *L. icterohaemorrhagiae* infections cannot be so confidently defined. The view has been taken that no antibiotics are of any value, but this may well be, as suggested by several authors, because too little is given too late. It certainly seems that by the time the diagnosis is made in a sporadic case of severe leptospirosis, renal damage may already have reached its maximum, and a curative effect is not necessarily to be expected, whatever the anti-leptospiral activity of the drug. The choice appears to lie between full doses of tetracycline, given at first intravenously, and large doses of penicillin, perhaps preferably reinforced with streptomycin. Sarasin *et al.* (1963) gave 40 mega units of penicillin daily by intravenous infusion and 1 g. streptomycin twice daily to a patient with laboratory-acquired infection, who became afebrile within 24 hours, but early treatment evidently contributed to this happy result.

REFERENCES

ABRAMS, A. J. (1968). *J. Amer. med. Ass.* **205,** 199.
ALERGANT, C. D. (1964). *Brit. J. vener. Dis.* **40,** 266.
AMIES, C. R. (1969). *Brit. J. vener. Dis.* **45,** 216.
ANDREW, G. S., EDWARDS, J. C. & OLLER, L. Z. (1969). *Brit. J. vener. Dis.* **45,** 154.
ARYA, O. P., PEARSON, C. H., RAO, S. K. & BLOWERS, R. (1970). *Brit. J. vener. Dis.* **46,** 214.
BORRING, J. (1965). *Brit. J. vener. Dis.* **41,** 193.
BRITISH CO-OPERATIVE CLINICAL GROUP (1970). *Brit. J. vener. Dis.* **46,** 62.
BRYCESON, A. D. M., PARRY, E. H. O., PERINE, P. L., WARRELL, D. A., VUKOTICH, D. & LEITHEAD, C. S. (1970). *Quart. J. Med.* **39,** 129.
CATTERALL, R. D. (1965). *Brit. J. vener. Dis.* **41,** 302.
CARROLL, B. R. T. & NICOL, C. S. (1970). *Brit. J. vener. Dis.* **46,** 31.
CHURCHER, G. M. & EVANS, A. J. (1969). *Brit. J. vener. Dis.* **45,** 149.
COLLART, P., BOREL, L. J. & DUREL, P. (1962). *Ann. Inst. Pasteur* **103,** 953.
CORNELIUS, C. E., III, & DOMESCIK, G. (1970). *Brit. J. vener. Dis.* **46,** 212.
CSONKA, G. W. (1965). *Brit. J. vener. Dis.* **41,** 1.
CSONKA, G. & CORSE, J. (1970). *Brit. J. vener. Dis.* **46,** 203.
CSONKA, G. W. & KNIGHT, G. J. (1967). *Brit. J. vener. Dis.* **43,** 161.
CSONKA, G. W. & SPITZER, R. J. (1969). *Brit. J. vener. Dis.* **45,** 52.
DAVIS, C. M. (1970). *J. Amer. med. Ass.* **211,** 632.

DE GRACIANSKY, P. & GRUPPER, C. (1961). *Brit. J. vener. Dis.* **37,** 247.
DUNLOP, E. M. C., AL-HUSSAINI, M. K., GARLAND, J., TREHARNE, J. D., HARPER, I. A. & JONES, B. R. (1965). *Lancet* **1,** 1125.
ENFORS, W. & MOLIN, L. (1970). *Brit. J. vener. Dis.* **46,** 209.
EVANS, A. J. (1966). *Brit. J. vener. Dis.* **42,** 251.
FARRELL, L. (1969). *Brit. J. vener. Dis.* **45,** 232.
FERNANDO, W. L. (1969). *Brit. J. vener. Dis.* **45,** 200.
FISCHNALLER, J. E., PEDERSEN, A. H. B., RONALD, A. R., BONIN, P. & TRONCA, E. L. (1968). *J. Amer. med. Ass.* **203,** 909.
FOWLER, W. & HUSSAIN, M. (1968). *Brit. J. vener. Dis.* **44,** 331.
FRY, L. & RODIN, P. (1966). *Brit. J. vener. Dis.* **42,** 28.
GALLA, F., PAGNES, P. & FERRARI, M. (1965). *Chemotherapia (Basel)* **10,** 24.
GARROD, L. P. & WATERWORTH, P. M. (1968). *Brit. J. vener. Dis.* **44,** 75.
GENTLE, G. H. K. (1965). *Brit. J. vener. Dis.* **41,** 155.
GLICKSMAN, J. M. & KNOX, J. M. (1968). *Arch. int. Med.* **121,** 342.
GOLDBERG, J. & BERNSTEIN, R. (1964). *Brit. J. vener. Dis.* **40,** 137.
GROTH, O. & HALLQVIST, L. (1970). *Brit. J. vener. Dis.* **46,** 21.
GUNDERSEN, T., ÖDEGAARD, K. & GJESSING, H. C. (1969). *Brit. J. vener. Dis.* **45,** 235.
HEATH, C. W., ALEXANDER, A. D. & GALTON, M. M. (1965). *New Engl. J. Med.* **273,** 857, 915.
JOUHAR, A. J. & FOWLER, W. (1968). *Brit. J. vener. Dis.* **44,** 223.
KING, A. J. (1965). *Practitioner* **195,** 589.
KNUDSEN, E. A. & AASTRUP, B. (1965). *Brit. J. vener. Dis.* **41,** 177.
KOCEN, R. S. (1962). *Brit. med. J.* **1,** 1181.
LAGERHOLM, B., LODIN, A. & NYSTROM, B. (1966). *Acta derm.-venereol.* **46,** 345.
LEIGH, D. A., LEFRANC, J. & TURNBULL, A. R. (1969). *Brit. J. vener. Dis.* **45,** 151.
MCDANIEL, W. E. (1964). *J. Kentucky med. Ass.* **62,** 281.
MCFADZEAN, J. A., PUGH, I. M., SQUIRES, S. L. & WHELAN, J. P. F. (1969). *Brit. J. vener. Dis.* **45,** 161.
MCGILL, R. C., MARTIN, A. M. & EDMUNDS, P. N. (1966). *Brit. med. J.* **1,** 1213.
MORTON, R. S. & WRAY, P. M. (1966). *Brit. J. vener. Dis.* **42,** 195.
NICOL, C. S. (1962). *Practitioner* **189,** 491.
OLLER, L. Z. (1969). *Brit. J. vener. Dis.* **45,** 163.
OLSEN, G. A. & LOMHOLT, G. (1969). *Brit. J. vener. Dis.* **45,** 144.
PERTZELAN, A. & PRUZANSKI, W. (1963). *Amer. J. trop. Med. Hyg.* **12,** 75.
PUTKONEN, T., SALO, O. P. & MUSTAKALLIO, K. K. (1966). *Brit. J. vener. Dis.* **42,** 181.
RANTASALO, I., SALO, O. P. & WALLENIUS, J. O. (1964). *Brit. J. vener. Dis.* **40,** 273.
REES, E. & ANNELS, E. H. (1969). *Brit. J. vener. Dis.* **45,** 205.
REPORT (1961). *Lancet* **2,** 226.
REYN, A. & BENTZON, M. W. (1969). *Brit. J. vener. Dis.* **45,** 223.
RICE, N. S. C., DUNLOP, E. M. C., JONES, B. R., HARE, M. J., KING, A. J., RODIN, P., MUSHIN, A. & WILKINSON, A. E. (1970). *Brit. J. vener. Dis.* **46,** 1.
ROUGHGARDEN, J. W. (1965). *Arch. intern. Med.* **116,** 39.
SARASIN, G., TUCKER, D. N. & AREAN, V. M. (1963). *Amer. J. clin. Path.* **40,** 146.
SCHAPIRA, H. E. (1965). *J. Urol.* **93,** 303.
SCHOFIELD, C. B. S. & MASTERTON, G. (1969). *Brit. J. vener. Dis.* **45,** 47.
SKOG, E. & GUDJONSSON, H. (1966). *Acta derm.-venereol.* **46,** 136.
SLATKIN, M. H. (1965). *Med. Clin. N. Amer.* **49,** 823.
SOKOLOFF, B. (1965). *Clin. Pharmacol. Therap.* **6,** 350.
SOUTH, M. A., SHORT, D. H. & KNOX, J. M. (1964). *J. Amer. med. Ass.* **190,** 70.
SOUTHERN, P. M. & SANFORD, J. P. (1969). *Medicine (Baltimore)* **48,** 129.

STALHEIM, O. H. V. (1966). *Amer. J. vet. Res.* **27**, 803.
STATHAM, R. & MORTON, R. S. (1968). *Brit. J. vener. Dis.* **44**, 228.
TAWES, R. L., JR. (1966). *Brit. J. vener. Dis.* **42**, 155.
WARRELL, D. A., POPE, H. M., PARRY, E. H. O., PERINE, P. L. & BRYCESON, A. D. M. (1970). *Clin. Sci.* **39**, 123.
WESTON, T. E. T. (1965). *Brit. J. vener. Dis.* **41**, 107.
WIJETUNGA, E. B. & MORTON, R. S. (1969). *Brit. J. vener. Dis.* **45**, 50.
WILLCOX, R. R. (1964). *Brit. J. vener. Dis.* **40**, 200.
WILLCOX, R. R. (1965). *Curr. Med. Drugs* **6** (2), 14.
WILLCOX, R. R. (1968). *Brit. J. vener. Dis.* **44**, 157.
WILLCOX, R. R. (1969). *Acta derm.-venereol.* **49**, 103.
WILLCOX, R. R. (1970). *Brit. J. vener. Dis.* **46**, 217.
WISDOM, A. R. & DUNLOP, E. M. C. (1965). *Brit. J. vener. Dis.* **41**, 90.
WRAY, P. M. (1965). *Brit. J. vener. Dis.* **41**, 117.
WRAY, P. M. (1966). *Brit. J. vener. Dis.* **42**, 25.
WRIGHT, D. J. M. (1969). *Brit. J. vener. Dis.* **45**, 167.
WRIGHT, D. J. M. & GRIMBLE, A. S. (1970). *Brit. J. vener. Dis.* **46**, 34.

Chapter XXVII

VIRAL AND CHLAMYDIAL INFECTIONS

UNTIL very recently it was held that viruses are not susceptible to any of the agents used for the treatment of bacterial diseases. It now appears that some antibacterial agents, albeit in concentrations very much greater than those required to inhibit the growth of sensitive bacteria, exert some antiviral effects. Rifampicin in a concentration about 1,000 times that effective against sensitive bacteria has been shown to inhibit the growth of several poxviruses and an adenovirus (Heller *et al.*, 1969); Subak-Sharp *et al.*, 1969). Fusidic acid and cephalosporin P_1 (p. 206) in concentrations of 25-50 μg. per ml. inhibit rhinoviruses and coxsackievirus A 21 (Acornley *et al.*, 1967). These are encouraging signs that viruses are perhaps not quite so insusceptible to attack as was once feared, but the very high plasma concentrations of these agents which would be required for treatment makes it unlikely that these findings will have any immediate clinical benefit. The *Chlamydia,* which were at one time included amongst the viruses but differ from them fundamentally (p. 447) are sensitive to tetracyclines and some other agents.

The present striking contrast between bacteria and viruses in the availability of effective antimicrobial therapy arises from a number of special difficulties. The metabolism of bacterial pathogens is often sufficiently different from that of the host to make them susceptible to agents which have little or no effect on the host's metabolism. Viral replication, on the other hand, occurs by distortion of normal cellular processes causing the cell to synthesize viral nucleic acids and proteins in place of normal cellular components. This intimate relationship between normal and infected cell processes means that compounds capable of interrupting viral replication will have to show an extraordinary degree of selective toxicity if they are not at the same time to inhibit similar processes crucial to the metabolic needs of normal cells. Nevertheless, any enzymic capacity possessed by the virus itself, for example the RNA-polymerase of the pox viruses (Kates and McAuslan, 1967), or even host enzymes sufficiently modified to subserve the parasite's needs, may well show (just as bacterial enzymes do) different susceptibility to inhibitors from that of the corresponding mammalian enzyme.

One serious therapeutic difficulty is that the signs and symptoms of virus disease often appear after peak viral growth is over, the clinical manifestations being due to inflammatory and other processes. It may be, therefore, that symptomatic control of such infections is more likely to be obtained with compounds which interfere with the host response than with those which interfere with viral growth. It follows that substances which inhibit viral replication are more likely to be of use in prophylaxis than in treatment.

Large and growing numbers of compounds have been shown to exert anti-viral activity both *in vitro* and against experimental infections in animals (Thompson, 1964; Tyrrell, 1969). Amongst those of current interest are benzimidazole derivatives active against poliovirus and certain coxsackie, echo and adeno viruses (O'Sullivan *et al.*, 1969). Whether these antiviral effects can be put to any clinical use remains to be seen. A number of compounds have already risen to trials in man and two, idoxuridine and methisazone, have established a place in current therapeutics.

Interferons

First described by Isaacs and Lindemann (1957), interferons are a family of closely related proteins liberated by cells which are actively synthesizing virus and which act on other cells reducing their susceptibility to viral infection (Finter, 1966). With some exceptions, interferons will protect only the cells of the animal species in which they were manufactured, or those of closely related species. On the other hand, the protection afforded includes not only the inducing virus but a wide variety of unrelated viruses. Interferon production is blocked by actinomycin D which inhibits the synthesis of messenger-RNA and it appears that viral infection of the cell may induce (or de-repress) the production of a messenger-RNA which codes the ribosome to produce interferon (Ho, 1964; Baron and Levy, 1966). They are proteins of molecular weight variously calculated to be between 19,000 and 160,000. They are destroyed by proteolytic but not by other enzymes and are otherwise remarkably stable. Some preparations are said to withstand 72°C. for 1 hour but human interferon is considerably less heat-stable (Glasgow, 1965). They are active against a wide variety of both DNA and RNA viruses but viral sensitivity differs considerably. Their potency is at least comparable with that of antibacterial anti-biotics: partially purified preparations inhibit viral growth in concentrations of about 1 or 2 μg. per ml. Interferons are apparently of low toxicity and very poor antigens. Unlike neutralizing antibody, interferon has no effect on extra-cellular virus and does not prevent virus from penetrating cells. It appears to exert its effect very soon after the virus has entered the cell, interfering with the earliest stages of viral replication. Since they have generally little activity in species unrelated to the one in which they were produced, only human or possibly primate interferon is likely to be of any use for therapy in man. Human placenta or leucocytes are possible rich sources of inter-feron but the danger of transmitting serum hepatitis with such products must obviously be circumvented. Considerable techni-cal difficulties remain over the purification, potency and stan-dardization of interferon.

Monkey interferon has been shown to prevent smallpox vaccination from 'taking' if it is injected at the site 24 hours previously (M.R.C., 1962) but it failed to influence the course of experimental respiratory virus infections in volunteers (M.R.C., 1965). Jones *et al.* (1962) successfully treated 5 patients suffering from vaccinial keratitis with topical monkey interferon.

Interferon Inducers. Of considerable interest is the possibility of treating systemic infections by stimulating endogenous inter-feron production. Petralli *et al.* (1965) showed that injection of avirulent measles virus might be used to stimulate endogenous interferon production in a patient suffering from another virus disease (since interferon is non-specific in its anti-viral activity) but the development of antibody against the stimulating virus would soon render this procedure ineffective.

An assortment of substances has been found to excite the production or release of preformed interferons. It appears that the anti-viral effects of the fungal products helenine (derived from *Penicillium funiculosum*) and statolon (derived from *Penicillium stoloniferum*) are exerted in this way (Rytel *et al.*, 1966) and the mechanism of these effects is of great theoretical interest. Lampson *et al.* (1967) showed that the interferon inducer in helenine is double stranded-RNA. Double- and multiple-stranded RNA is produced in cells infected with RNA viruses and this suggests that the origin of the interferon inducer in statolon and helenine is fungal virus and that the inducer is polystranded RNA (Banks *et al.*, 1968; Kleinschmidt *et al.*, 1968). This raises the possibility of using extracted polystranded RNA or synthetic analogues for therapeutic purposes. Some multi-stranded complexes of synthetic polyisosinic and polycytidinic acids are active inducers of interferons (Field *et al.*, 1967). Park and Baron (1968) found that established experimental herpetic keratitis in the rabbit responded to topical applications, or to anterior chamber or intravenous injections. More information will doubtless be forthcoming about the properties and potential toxicity of these interesting compounds.

Amantadines

These drugs have been fairly extensively investigated and are believed to act by blocking entry of adsorbed virus into the cell (Dickinson *et al.*, 1967). *In vitro* these drugs inhibit influenza A and C and rubella viruses. The effect is not profound and cell-to-cell spread of some strains of virus is prevented only if the infecting dose of virus is small. Some viral strains appear to contain relatively high proportions of more resistant particles, and in one study viral susceptibility was lost after a single passage in the presence of the drug (Sabin, 1967).

Experimental influenza A infection in volunteers was prevented by prophylactic use of the drug in some studies (Togo *et al.*, 1968) but not in others (Tyrrell *et al.*, 1965). Similarly discordant results have been obtained in the prophylaxis of natural infection. Galbraith *et al.* (1969a) found that early prophylactic treatment of the household contacts of index cases reduced the incidence of clinical influenza to less than a quarter of that in placebo-treated contacts, and also significantly reduced the frequency of serological evidence of infection. Yet in a similar trial (Galbraith *et al.*, 1969b), they failed to find any protection against the Hong Kong strain. They suggest that the difference may be accounted for by the greater level of immunity in the first population studied. This is in keeping with Quilligan *et al.* (1966) who found that they could suppress clinical and subclinical influenza A2 infection in children providing they had some pre-existing immunity from previous infection or vaccination.

In terms of the prospects for antiviral chemotherapy, there have been several very encouraging reports of the therapeutic use of amantadines. In natural outbreaks of influenza A2, there was more rapid defervescence of illness in patients treated within about 20 hours of the onset of symptoms with amantadine than in those treated with placebo (Hornick *et al.*, 1969; Togo *et al.*, 1970). No effect was demonstrated on rubella in the 1964 outbreak (Sabin, 1967) and Dickinson *et al.* (1967), using 1-adamantanamine-HCl (Symmetrel) and α-methyl-1-adamantanemethylamine-HCl (Rimatadine) confirmed previous reports that these agents are inactive against influenza B. They also failed to demonstrate any effect on the clinical or immunological response of children having live measles vaccine. Adverse effects have not been a problem. Amantadine hydrochloride has been used for the treatment of Parkinson's disease (Parkes *et al.*, 1970).

Isoquinolines

Larin *et al.* (1968) showed that two isoquinoline derivatives inactivated the infectivity of influenza A and B, parainfluenza and measles viruses, but appeared not to affect viral multiplication. With rhino- and echoviruses there was a suppressive effect on replication but not on infectivity; with rubella both processes were affected and respiratory syncytial virus was suppressed but the mode of action was obscure. Beare *et al.* (1968) compared one of these compounds (UK 2371) with a placebo in volunteers challenged intranasally with influenza B virus. A week's treatment begun the day before challenge halved the incidence of clinical and subclinical infection, but similar activity was not shown in a further trial using the Hong Kong strain of influenza A2 (Reed *et al.*, 1970). In a review of the properties of UK 2054 ('famotine') and UK 2371 ('memotine') Williamson and Jackson (1969) found the evidence for their activity in man inconclusive. In a well-designed and controlled trial, Stark *et al.* (1970) found that prophylactic use of the drug failed to influence the incidence of respiratory viral infection, including influenza, amongst students in a hall of residence during the mild winter outbreak of 1969.

Idoxuridine

This compound (2′-deoxy-5-iodouridine) synthesized by Prusoff (1959) is a white crystalline odourless powder with a molecular weight of 354·1. It is sparingly soluble in water (1 in 500) and alcohol (1 in 400) and even less soluble in chloroform and ether. A 0·1 per cent aqueous solution has a pH of about 6. It is stable when stored dry and the 0·1 per cent ophthalmic solution is said to retain its potency for a year at room temperature but this has been disputed and refrigeration is recommended. The solution is sensitive to light and should be stored in amber bottles. About half the potency is lost on autoclaving at 120°C. for 20 minutes.

Idoxuridine and the corresponding 2′-deoxy-5-bromouridine are thymidine analogues which inhibit the utilization of thymidine in the rapid synthesis of DNA which normally occurs in herpes-infected cells. The possibility of similar effect in uninfected cells and the rapid dehalogenation of these compounds in the body makes them unpromising for systemic use although some success has been claimed in the treatment of herpes encephalitis. Viral resistance to idoxuridine is said to develop relatively easily. It has been used principally for the treatment of herpes keratitis and cutaneous herpes. The beneficial result claimed in both conditions has been disputed.

HERPES KERATITIS. This has usually been treated with 0·1 per cent idoxuridine drops, hourly by day and 2-hourly by night. Several authors reporting large series of cases have been satisfied with the results (Maxwell, 1965) but Jones (1967) takes the view that the results are no better than cauterization in the treatment of dendritic ulcer (p. 395).

CUTANEOUS HERPES. The failure of some workers to enjoy the same success as others in the treatment of recurrent cutaneous herpes may be the result of poor contact between the agent and the infected cells. Juel-Jensen and MacCallum (1965) who had previously failed to influence the disease by local applications of idoxuridine ointment, reduced the average duration of lesions from 8·9-5·5 days, by injecting 0·1 per cent idoxuridine into the affected skin with a spray-gun.

HERPES ENCEPHALITIS. Recovery, but with significant residual defects, has several times been described in patients treated with idoxuridine in whom survival seemed otherwise unlikely. Evans *et al.* (1967) treated an 8-year-old girl with daily infusions over eight hours of 1·5 g. idoxuridine, and Buckley and MacCallum (1967) gave successive daily doses of 100, 100, 200, 200 and 400 mg. as a 0·1 per cent solution over two hours to a 41-year-old woman. They judge that a total dose of 100-200 mg./kg. over five days is probably required.

Methisazone

This compound (N-methylisatin β-thiosemicarbazone) was shown by Bauer *et al.* (1962) to be active against variola following a number of observations over the years that various thiosemicarbazones would inhibit pox viruses in mice and chick embryos. It is a fine orange-yellow powder almost insoluble in water but soluble in acetone (1 in 25) and sparingly in chloroform (1 in 800). Brief exposure to light causes a reversible change, but prolonged exposure causes decomposition and it must be suitably protected. Methisazone is believed to affect a late stage of virus maturation (Easterbrook, 1962).

Anorexia, nausea and vomiting are common in those treated with the drug, occurring in 95 per cent of Landsman and Grist's (1964) cases and 66 per cent of the cases of do Valle *et al.* (1965) despite the use of cyclizine or chlorpromazine. Diarrhoea, rashes and thinning of the hair have also been described. Alcohol may exacerbate the side-effects and it is currently recommended that the drug should not be given to pregnant women or to those with liver or kidney disease.

VARIOLA. By the time lesions have appeared viral multiplication is rapidly declining and at this stage treatment with methisazone has little effect (Marsden, 1962) although some effect is possible in the prodromal stage when active viral multiplication is occurring (Ker, 1962). The principal use of these compounds has been in the contact prophylaxis of small-pox. Several successful trials have been reported in variola major.

Bauer (1965) reported 6 cases with two deaths amongst 2,297 close contacts treated with methisazone and 114 cases with 20 deaths amongst 2,842 similar untreated contacts. Similar success has been described in the prophylaxis of variola minor (do Valle *et al.*, 1965). Using M & B 7714 for the prophylaxis of variola major, Rao *et al.* (1966) were less successful, finding 40 cases with 7 deaths amongst 196 treated contacts and 80 cases with 12 deaths amongst 201 untreated contacts.

VACCINIA. Methisazone given at the time of vaccination depresses the local reaction but also possibly impairs the antibody response (Landsman and Grist, 1964). In an uncontrolled trial, Jaroszynska-Weinberger and Mészáros (1966) vaccinated children with a history of eczema without any developing eczema vaccinatum. Established eczema vaccinatum was favourably influenced by methisazone treatment in 14/24 of Adels' and Oppé's (1966) patients, some of whom also received anti-vaccinial gamma globulin. Progressive vaccinia (vaccinia gangrenosa) which without treatment is almost invariably fatal has been treated by a number of authors (usually together with anti-vaccinial gamma globulin) and half have recovered (Connolly, 1966).

Methisazone should not be used as a substitute for vaccination, which currently remains the best prophylactic, and treatment should not begin before vaccination lest it interfere with the development of immunity. If it is necessary to vaccinate patients at special risk, for example those with exudative skin lesions or any disorder of the lymphoreticular system which impairs immunity, methisazone may be given from the fourth day after vaccination. To reduce the risk of foetal vaccinia in pregnant women, anti-vaccinial gamma globulin, and not methisazone, should be given.

CHLAMYDIA

The organisms responsible for trachoma, inclusion conjunctivitis and inclusion blenorrhoea (TRIC agents), lymphogranuloma venereum and psittacosis have many properties in common and are now grouped together under the name

Chlamydia (Moulder, 1966). Like the viruses, they are obligate intra-cellular parasites of small size, but unlike viruses and like bacteria they multiply by binary fission, they have cell walls resembling those of Gram-negative bacteria, they have ribosomal structures with the susceptibility to antibiotics characteristic of bacterial ribosomes, and those which are sulphonamide-sensitive synthesize folates. Their obligate intra-cellular nature (and perhaps their small size) may be accounted for by their complete, or almost complete, lack of mechanisms for the production of metabolic energy.

There are two groups. The first group, including those causing trachoma and lymphogranuloma venereum, produce compact cytoplasmic inclusions and are sensitive to sulphonamides and cycloserine. The other group, including the psittacosis agent, produce diffuse cytoplasmic inclusions and are resistant to sulphonamides and cycloserine (Moulder, 1966).

It has been the general view for a long time that the diseases caused by *Chlamydia* respond to tetracyclines, but more recent, perhaps more critical, study indicates that the results are far from perfect. The efficacy of tetracyclines (and sulphonamides) in trachoma has been seriously questioned (p. 395) and there is evidence, both in this country (Watson and Gairdner, 1968) and in America, that the effects of neonatal inclusion conjunctivitis are by no means as benign as once thought, and that the tetracycline treatment used to date is, in some cases at least, inadequate (Forster *et al.*, 1970). The results of tetracycline treatment of psittacosis are similarly imperfect (Anderson and Bridgewater, 1968) but Timberger and Armstrong (1969) report a prompt and satisfactory response in a single patient treated with erythromycin 500 mg. 6-hourly. Increasing availability of improved diagnostic methods will no doubt result in more frequent recognition of these diseases and the opportunity to undertake the review of their treatment which is evidently now required.

PHARMACEUTICAL PREPARATIONS AND DOSAGE

IDOXURIDINE (IDU; 5 IDUR)

Ophthalmic solution 0·1 per cent. (Dendrid, *Alcon Laboratories, Vestric Ltd;* ' Kerecid ' and ' Stoxil ', *Smith, Kline and French*) 1 drop hourly by day and 2 hourly by night. Ophthalmic ointment 0·25 per cent. in sterile eye ointment base, B.P.

METHISAZONE ('Marboran', *Burroughs Wellcome*)

Capsules 1·5 g. Optimum dosage schedules not yet established. Cyclizine or chlorpromazine may assist in controlling nausea and vomiting. Connolly (1966) recommends: *Prevention of variola* 3 g.+3 g. 12 hours later. *Prevention of complications of vaccinia* on fourth day after vaccination 100 mg./kg./day followed by 50 mg./kg./day for 3-6 days. *Treatment of eczema vaccinatum or progressive vaccinia* 200 mg./kg. followed by 200 mg./kg./day in divided doses for 2 days.

REFERENCES

ACORNLEY, J. E., BESSELL, C. H., BYNOE, M. L., GOTFREDSEN, W. O. & KNOYLE, J. M. (1967). *Brit. J. Pharmacol. Chemother.* **31**, 210.

ADELS, B. R. & OPPÉ, T. E. (1966). *Lancet* **1**, 18

ANDERSON, J. P. & BRIDGWATER, F. A. J. (1968). *Brit. J. Dis. Chest* **62**, 155.

BANKS, G. T., BUCK, K. W., CHAIN, E. B., HIMMELWEIT, F., MARKS, J. E., TYLER, J. M., HOLLINGS, M., LAST, F. T. & STONE, O. M. (1968). *Nature (Lond.)* **218**, 542.

BARON, S. & LEVY, H. B. (1966). *Ann. Rev. Microbiol.* **20**, 291.

BAUER, D. J. (1965). *Ann. N.Y. Acad. Sci.* **130**, 110.

BAUER, D. J., DUMBELL, K. R., FOX-HULME, P. & SADLER, P. W. (1962). *Bull Wld Hlth Org.* **26**, 727.

BEARE, A. S., BYNOE, M. L. & TYRRELL, D. A. J. (1968). *Lancet* **1**, 843.

BUCKLEY, T. F. & MACCALLUM, F. O. (1967). *Brit. med. J.* **2**, 419.

CONNOLLY, J. H. (1966). *Practitioner* **197**, 373.

DICKINSON, P. C. T., CHANG, T-W. & WEINSTEIN, L. (1967). *Antimicrob. Agents Chemother.*, 1966, 521.

DO VALLE, L. A. R., DE MELO, P. R., DE SALLES GOMES, L. F. & PROENCA, L. M. (1965). *Lancet* **2**, 976.

EASTERBROOK, K. B. (1962). *Virology* **17**, 245.

EVANS, A. D., GRAY, O. P., MILLER, M. H., JONES, E. R. V., WEEKS, R. D. & WELLS, G. E. C. (1967). *Brit. med. J.* **2**, 407.

FIELD, A. K., TYTELL, A. A., LAMPSON, G. P. & HILLEMAN, M. R. (1967). *Proc. Nat. Acad. Sci. (Wash.)* **58**, 1004.

FINTER, N. B. (Ed.) (1966). *Interferons.* Philadelphia, Saunders.

FORSTER, R. K., DAWSON, C. R. & SCHACHTER, J. (1970). *Amer. J. Ophthal.* **69**, 467.

GALBRAITH, A. W., OXFORD, J. S., SCHILD, G. C. & WATSON, G. I. (1969a). *Lancet* **2**, 1026.

GALBRAITH, A. W., OXFORD, J. S., SCHILD, G C. & WATSON, G. I. (1969b). *Bull. Wld Hlth Org.* **41**, 677.

GLASGOW, L. A. (1965). *J. Pediat.* **67**, 104.

HELLER, E., ARGAMAN, M., LEVY, H. & GOLDBLUM, N. (1969). *Nature (Lond.)* **222**, 273.

HO, M. (1964). *Bact. Rev.* **28**, 367.

HORNICK, R. B., TOGO, Y., MAHLER, S. & IEZZONI, D. (1969). *Bull. Wld Hlth Org.* **41**, 671.

ISAACS, A. & LINDEMANN, J. (1957). *Proc. roy. Soc. B.* **147**, 258.

JAROSZYŃSKA-WEINBERGER, B. & MÉSZÁROS, J. (1966). *Lancet* **1**, 948.

JONES, B. R. (1967). *Trans. Ophthal. Soc., U.K.* **87**, 537.

JONES, B. R., GALBRAITH, J. E. K., & AL-HUSSAINI, M. K. (1962). *Lancet* **2**, 875.

JUEL-JENSEN, B. E. & MACCALLUM, F. O. (1965). *Brit. med. J.* **1**, 901.

KATES, J. R. & MCAUSLAN, B. R. (1967). *Proc. Nat. Acad. Sci. (Wash.)* **58**, 134.

KER, F. L. (1962). *Brit. med. J.* **2**, 734.

KLEINSCHMIDT, W. J., ELLIS, L. F., VAN FRANK, R. M. & MURPHY, E. B. (1968). *Nature (Lond.)* **220**, 167.

LAMPSON, G. P., TYTELL, A. A., FIELD, A. K., NEMES, M. M. & HILLEMAN, M. R. (1967). *Proc. Nat. Acad. Sci. (Wash.)* **58**, 782.

LANDSMAN, J. B. & GRIST, N. R. (1964). *Lancet* **1**, 330.
LARIN, N. M., BEARE, A. S., COPPING, M. P., McDONALD, C. R., McDOUGALL, J. K., ROBERTS, B. & SMITH, J. B. (1968). *Antimicrob. Agents Chemother.* —1967, p. 646.
MARSDEN, J. P. (1962). *Brit. med. J.* **2**, 524.
MAXWELL, E. (1965). *Amer. J. Ophthal.* **59**, 42.
MEDICAL RESEARCH COUNCIL SCIENTIFIC COMMITTEE ON INTERFERON (1962). *Lancet* **1**, 873.
MEDICAL RESEARCH COUNCIL SCIENTIFIC COMMITTEE ON INTERFERON (1965). *Lancet* **1**, 505.
MOULDER, J. W. (1966). *Ann. Rev. Microbiol.* **20**, 107.
O'SULLIVAN, D. G., PANTIC, D., DANE, D. S. & BRIGGS, M. (1969). *Lancet* **1**, 446.
PARK, J. H. & BARON, S. (1968). *Science, N.Y.* **162**, 811.
PARKES, J. D., ZILKHA, K. J., MARSDEN, P., BAXTER, R. C. H. & KNILL-JONES, R. P. (1970). *Lancet* **1**, 1130.
PETRALLI, J. K., MERIGAN, T. C. & WILBUR, J. R. (1965). *Lancet* **2**, 401.
PRUSOFF, W. H. (1959). *Biochem. biophys. Acta* **32**, 295.
QUILLIGAN, J. J., JR., HIRAYAMA, M. & BAERNSTEIN, H. D., JR. (1966). *J. Pediat.* **69**, 572.
RAO, A. R., McFADZEAN, J. A. & KAMALASHKI, K. (1966). *Lancet* **1**, 1068.
REED, S., BEARE, A. S., BYNOE, M. L. & TYRRELL, D. A. J. (1970). *Ann N.Y. Acad. Sci.* In the Press.
RYTEL, M. W., SHOPE, R. E. & KILBOURNE, E. D. (1966). *J. exp. Med.* **123**, 577.
SABIN, A. B. (1967). *J. Amer. med. Ass.* **200**, 943.
STARK, J. E., HEATH, R. B., OSWALD, N. C., BOOTH, V., TALL, R., FOX, W., MOYNAGH, K. D. & INGLIS, J. M. (1970). *Thorax.* In the press.
SUBAK-SHARPE, J. H., TIMBURY, M. C. & WILLIAMS, J. F. (1969). *Nature (Lond.)* **222**, 341.
THOMPSON, R. L. (1964). *Adv. Chemother.* **1**, 85.
TIMBERGER, R. J. & ARMSTRONG, D. (1969). *Amer. Rev. resp. Dis.* **99**, 936.
TOGO, Y., HORNICK, R. B. & DAWKINS, A. T. (1968). *J. Amer. med. Ass.* **203**, 1089.
TOGO, Y., HORNICK, R. B., FELITTI, V. J., KAUFMAN, M. L., DAWKINS, A. T., KILPE, V. E. & CLAGHORN, J. L. (1970). *J. Amer. med. Ass.* **211**, 1149.
TYRRELL, D. A. J. (1969). *The Scientific Basis of Medicine Annual Reviews,* 1969, p. 294.
TYRRELL, D. A. J., BYNOE, M. L. & HOORN, B. (1965). *Brit. J. exp. Path.* **46**, 370.
WATSON, P. G. & GAIRDNER, D. (1968). *Brit. med. J.* **3**, 527.
WILLIAMSON, G. M. & JACKSON, D. (1969). *Bull. Wld Hlth Org.* **41**, 665.

Chapter XXVIII

LABORATORY CONTROL

EXCEPT in a few diseases with a single bacterial cause always sensitive to the drug of first choice, ' chemotherapy without bacteriology is guesswork ' (Howie, 1962). The first task of the laboratory is to make a bacteriological diagnosis, and skill and experience in identifying the cause of an infection are even more important to-day than they were in the past. Many of the taunts directed at the proceedings about to be described, because patients have responded to treatment with an antibiotic to which their organisms have been reported resistant, are a reflection not on the method but on its user, who has seen nothing in his cultures but commensals.

No more need usually be done if the organism found is, for instance, a Group A streptococcus or a pneumococcus, which may safely be assumed to be sensitive to penicillin. Such species are unfortunately the exception: most others commonly found, particularly in the kinds of non-specific infection of the air passages, urinary tract, wounds etc., which make up the bulk of infective disease in temperate climates, cannot be depended on to be fully sensitive to a given drug. Hence most bacteriological examinations now include determinations of bacterial sensitivity, at least to certain antibiotics.

The vast number of these tests which must now be carried out in all routine laboratories demand a quick reliable method which will indicate whether the infection is likely to respond to treatment with a given drug rather than the precise amount of the drug required to inhibit growth. Some form of diffusion test is universally used for this purpose, and various methods with innumerable modifications are in use. They cannot be of equal merit: indeed, some are open to severe criticism. In the interests of rationally directed and successful treatment, it is desirable that optimum methods should be standardized and during the past 8 years much work has been done to this end by an International Working Party whose report has now appeared (Ericsson and Sherris, 1971). A further advantage of uniformity in method would be that results obtained in different laboratories should be comparable, and their meaning clear to other workers, which is far from being the case at present.

DIFFUSION TESTS OF BACTERIAL SENSITIVITY

In these tests the antibiotic diffuses from a focus through a solid medium, inhibiting the growth of an organism on or in it to a distance depending, *inter alia,* on the sensitivity of the organism. This focus may be:

1. a *ditch*: a strip of medium on one side of a plate is removed and replaced with medium containing anti-biotic. This method is useful for testing multiple strains against a single drug (*e.g.* streptococci against bacitracin, staphylococci against methicillin) and has the advantage that every plate can be controlled by including a standard organism. A simpler modification is the use of blotting paper strips containing the antibiotic which can be applied to the plate immediately before use (see Fig. 26).

2. a *hole* (cup): a disc of medium is punched out with a cork borer and the resulting hole is filled with antibiotic solution. The method has the advantage that the strength of the solutions can be varied as required but it entails labelling each hole with consequent risk of confusion.

3. a *disc*: a circular piece of blotting paper in which a known amount of antibiotic has been dried is firmly applied to the surface. Both the International Working Party and The Association of Clinical Pathologists Broadsheet (1966) recommend this method (see Fig. 27).

Whichever the method used, its results will be affected by certain basic factors which therefore require control.

Factors Affecting Results of Diffusion Tests

MEDIUM. Plates must be flat-bottomed and poured on a level surface (some laboratory benches do not qualify for this description) and the medium must be of uniform depth. The medium used must support free growth of the organism to be tested. Selective media should not be used. Some constituents of laboratory media affect certain antibiotics. The addition of blood will reduce the inhibition zone of antibiotics heavily protein-bound (*e.g.* fucidin, novobiocin). Reducing substances should be avoided: from time to time peculiar results are reported from tests of anaerobes in media containing thioglycollate, in the presence of which penicillin is unstable and streptomycin, apparently for a different reason, also loses most of its activity. Electrolytes affect many antibiotics: the activity of the aminoglycosides is depressed but others may be enhanced (*e.g.* bacitracin, fucidin and novobiocin, and penicillins against *Proteus* spp.). The M.I.C. of gentamicin varies with the magnesium content of the medium (Garrod and Waterworth, 1969). The addition of a sugar enhances the activity of nitrofurantoin against some organisms (Report, 1965).

The agar used for solidifying medium can affect not only the diffusion of some drugs (polymyxin, Bechtle and Scherr (1958); polymyxin and the aminoglycosides, Kunin and Edmondson (1968)), but may also affect the M.I.C. of gentamicin (Garrod and Waterworth, 1969, see p. 126) and of neomycin, kanamycin and polymyxin (Hanus, Sands and Bennett, 1967).

pH OF MEDIUM. Streptomycin is 512 times more active at pH 8·5 than at 5·5: kanamycin and gentamicin are affected similarly to a lesser degree. The macrolides are also favoured by alkalinity. Tetracyclines and some other antibiotics are more active in an acid medium (see Table XLIX). The pH of the medium should not be altered to favour an antibiotic, but it should be remembered that circumstances which do alter it may affect the result. Thus incubation in CO_2 which lowers the pH, may make an organism which is partially resistant to tetracycline appear sensitive and ' satellitism ' around a resistant colony may have a similar explanation. Growth of most species raises the pH of nutrient agar in the surrounding area, and if the antibiotic is favoured by acidity (*e.g.* fucidin) the change may be sufficient to permit growth on an otherwise inhibitory concentration. If the antibiotic is favoured by alkalinity (*e.g.* erythromycin) the same effect can be produced by adding glucose to the medium. Any organism which ferments this will lower the pH of the surrounding medium. These effects are illustrated in Figure 25.

This would seem to be the explanation of the claim of Wolf and Hamburger (1962) that some strains of penicillin-sensitive staphylococci can be shown to produce penicillinase if tested by the Gots method. Although penicillin is not greatly affected by pH it is favoured by acidity, and as the amount added to

TABLE XLIX

Effect of pH on Antibiotics

Little Affected	Less Active in Acid Medium	Less Active in Alkaline Medium
Penicillin	Streptomycin	Tetracyclines
Chloramphenicol	Neomycin group	Methicillin
Polymyxins	Gentamicin	Cloxacillin
Vancomycin	Lincomycin	Fucidin
	Erythromycin group	Novobiocin
	Cephaloridine	

the medium in the Gots method (1945) is little above the M.I.C. for the test organism only slight loss of activity is necessary to permit growth. In an experiment to illustrate this, it was confirmed that some strains of sensitive staphylococci could produce satellitism in a Gots test in simple nutrient agar, but this did not occur when the medium contained glucose (Waterworth, P. M., unpublished observations).

INOCULUM. The activity of many antibiotics is little affected by the number of bacteria present, but nevertheless all zones of inhibition are reduced if the inoculum increases. The probable explanation of this contradiction is that visible growth appears more quickly if the inoculum is heavy, thus allowing less time for the diffusion of the antibiotic. It should be such as will produce 'dense but not confluent growth' (Fig. 27) and it is also essential that it be uniformly distributed. The best results are obtained by flooding with a suspension of the organism, but this method is not without risk to the operator and should not be used with highly pathogenic organisms. Satisfactory results can be obtained by spreading a drop or loopful of the inoculum with a bent wire or sterile bent glass rod. Whole plates cannot be adequately spread with a wire loop.

but cotton wool swabs, as used in the Kirby-Bauer method (see p. 458) are a possible alternative. Barry, Garcia & Thrupp (1970) have recently suggested a modification for this method which appears to be a great improvement on the use of swabs. They inoculated plates by adding a 0·001 ml. calibrated loopful of culture to 8 ml. of a melted and cooled 1·5 per cent aqueous solution of agar which was mixed well and poured over the surface of a 15 cm. plate of Mueller Hinton agar.

INOCULATION OF PLATES. Using a sterile pasteur pipette, flood the plate with a well shaken suspension containing about 10^5 organisms per ml., drain the excess to the side by tilting and remove with the same pipette. If the inoculum is to be spread, transfer 2 or 3 large loopfuls of a well-shaken suspension containing about 10^6 organisms per ml. to a plate. Spread thoroughly with a bent wire or glass spreader, taking care to reach the edge of the plate.

DILUTION OF CULTURES. A suitable suspension for flooding can be prepared by adding a 2 mm. loopful of a well-grown overnight broth culture to 5 ml. saline, the loop being held vertically. If only plate cultures are available, suspend portions of 5-10 colonies in a small volume of broth to give a similar density to an overnight broth culture and proceed as above. If the inoculum is to be spread, add one small drop of broth culture to 5 ml. saline.

DISCS. There is still no general agreement on the ideal content of discs. Manufacturers usually market 2 strengths of each. Higher strengths can justifiably be used when testing organisms from the urinary tract against drugs excreted in high concentration in the urine. They are also applicable when, for some reason, blood or tissue levels are expected to be unusually high or can be attained by higher doses (*e.g.* penicillin). The exclusive use of discs of high content may mask small but clinically significant increases in resistance and may also give a zone of inhibition with a clinically insensitive organism (*e.g. Esch. coli* with erythromycin). In the United States we understand that the F.D.A. are to recommend the exclusive use of high content discs with the Kirby-Bauer method: the disadvantages of these discs if used with the methods generally employed in Great Britain are discussed on page 460. The most suitable disc contents of those commercially available in Great Britain are given in Table L.

STORAGE OF DISCS. Discs must be stored in the cold and kept dry. On removal from the refrigerator they should be allowed to attain room temperature before being opened, to avoid condensation. Only sufficient for the day's use should be removed and any left over should be discarded.

When applying individual discs each must be pressed firmly in position—diffusion cannot take place unless the disc is in close contact with the medium.

TABLE L

Suitable disc contents (µg.)

	Low	High
*Ampicillin	2	25
*Carbenicillin	25	100
*Cephaloridine	5	25
Chloramphenicol	10	30
Clindamycin	2	30
Erythromycin	10	—
Fucidin	10	—
Gentamicin	10	30
Kanamycin	5	30
Methicillin	10	—
Nalidixic acid	—	30
Nitrofurantoin	—	200
Novobiocin	5	30
Penicillin	—	6
Polymyxin B sulphate	30	—
Streptomycin	10	25
Sulphafurazole	100	500
Tetracycline	10	30
Trimethoprim	2·5	—

*High content discs can be used to test coliform bacilli from specimens other than urine, but the fully sensitive control must be used to make it clear that such infections will respond only to high doses (see p. 458).

PREDIFFUSION. Ericsson (1960), who has studied the whole of this subject with admirable thoroughness, makes a strong plea for a three-hour period of pre-diffusion as giving more significant results. Satisfactory results are obtained without it, and in clinical work the difficulties involved would seem to outweigh any possible advantage.

LENGTH OF INCUBATION—this should be the minimum required for the normal growth of the test organism. If it is prolonged, loss of activity of the drug may permit growth of sensitive organisms which were inhibited though not killed This method is suitable only for organisms of a rapid rate of growth. It should be remembered that anything which reduces the speed of growth (*e.g.* poor or selective medium or lower temperature of incubation) will enlarge the inhibition zones.

Control Cultures

All these sources of error can be eliminated or at least the error recognized by the correct use of control cultures, which are also necessary for the proper interpretation of the test. The method described on page 463 is ideal in this respect as it controls every disc. This is not possible if multiple discs are used and it is then essential that control tests are set up every day for every drug and medium that has been used. Three organisms are necessary, *Staph. aureus* (*e.g.* N.C.T.C. 6571), *Esch. coli* (*e.g.* N.C.T.C. 10418) and *Ps. aeruginosa* (*e.g.* N.C.T.C. 10662). Their correct use is discussed on page 458.

Control cultures should be maintained at room temperature on agar slopes and sub-cultivated once a month. Broth cultures should be made from these once a week and either kept in the refrigerator or sub-cultivated daily in broth.

Interpretation of Results

1. COMPARISON WITH A CONTROL. The most usual method of interpreting disc sensitivity tests in routine diagnostic work in Great Britain, is to use low content discs and compare the zone produced with the unknown organism to that given by a control. The control should be an organism known to respond to treatment with normal doses of the drug concerned, and the Oxford staphylococcus (N.C.T.C. 6571) can be used for all the common drugs except polymyxins, when *Esch. coli* (*e.g.* N.C.T.C. 10418) should be used. If a drug is excreted by the kidneys more resistant infections can be treated in the urinary tract. A more resistant control should then be used, but again it must be one known to respond to treatment, *Esch. coli* (*e.g.* N.C.T.C. 10418) serves well: higher strength discs may also be used. Suitable discs for use with this method are given in Table L.

In either case results are reported as sensitive, moderately resistant or resistant and the generally accepted definition of these terms is:

' *Sensitive* '—zone equal to or larger than that of the control, inferring that the infection should respond to treatment with normal doses.

' *Resistant* '—no zone or one of not more than 2 mm. radius, inferring that clinical response to treatment is unlikely.

' *Moderately Resistant* '—zone radius >2 mm. smaller than that of the control (the inocula must be comparable and both measurements made by the same operator). This may signify:

a. Resistance in a normally sensitive species insufficient to justify the term ' resistant '. Whether the drug should be used will depend on other factors.

b. Usual sensitivity of a species which is more resistant than the control organism but may still respond to treatment with normal dosage (*e.g. H. influenzae* and ampicillin and *Ps. aeruginosa* with gentamicin and carbenicillin) or to high dosage (*e.g. Str. faecalis* and penicillin). This should be made clear in the report by describing it either as normally sensitive for the species or as sensitive to high doses. Abnormal resistance of these organisms is difficult to detect and is of particular importance with *Ps. aeruginosa* where any increase in resistance may jeopardize treatment with either gentamicin or carbenicillin. This difficulty can be overcome by using a sensitive strain of the same species as a control (*e.g.* N.C.T.C. 10662), equal sized zones then infer sensitivity normal *for the species,* and a reduced zone moderate resistance (see Fig. 28B).

With this exception it must be emphasized that the choice of the control depends on the site of the infection and not the species being tested. Urinary pathogens isolated from other parts of the body must be compared to the fully sensitive control and not to the *Esch. coli* : this is particularly important if high content discs are used and is illustrated in Figure 28A.

It must always be remembered that other factors besides the activity of the drug affect the result (*e.g.* diffusibility). The activity of different drugs cannot be directly compared by this method even if the discs contain the same amount.

2. THE ZONE OR NO ZONE METHOD employs both high and low content discs for each drug. Zones are not measured; any inhibition round the low content disc indicates sensitivity, a zone round the high disc only, infers moderate sensitivity and no zone round either indicates resistance. Very misleading results are obtained if only high content discs are used.

3. THE KIRBY-BAUER METHOD (Bauer *et al.,* 1966), defines 3 degrees of sensitivity according to zone diameter. For example, using a 30 μg. tetracycline disc zones of >19 mm. = sensitive.

15-18 mm. = intermediate and ⟨15 mm. = resistant. The break-points for each drug can be obtained from published tables, which have been worked out taking into consideration both the corresponding M.I.C. of the organism and the blood levels attainable with normal dosage, and the distribution of zone sizes among species of known clinical responsiveness. The method uses high content discs, Mueller-Hinton agar in plates 5-6 mm. deep, and carefully standardized inoculum applied with a cotton wool swab, giving confluent growth. It must be stressed that the tables are only applicable if the method is followed *exactly;* full details are given by Anderson (1970).

4. THE ERICSSON METHOD (1960) depends on the fact that for most antibiotics there is a linear relationship between the diameter of the zone of inhibition and the log of the M.I.C. A regression line is prepared by plotting the M.I.C. of at least 100 organisms of widely varying sensitivity against the diameter of the zone produced by a high content disc, both tests being run simultaneously under similar controlled conditions. A regression line prepared by one of us for the International Working Party is illustrated in Figure 29. The zone given by an unknown organism tested in similar conditions can be converted into M.I.C. by reference to this line; M.I.C. are not reported but are translated into 4 categories of susceptibility which are based on M.I.C. and drug levels attainable *in vivo.* In practice regression lines are not referred to, zone diameters being translated directly into one of the four categories. All conditions of the test must be completely standardized. A modification of this method, using Mueller-Hinton agar has been under active study by an International working party as a possible reference diffusion technique.

Both the last two methods require a high degree of standardization if published break-points are to be applicable and it may be questioned whether this is attainable in the average diagnostic laboratory. The break-points must also, to some extent, be a matter of individual opinion. Both methods use Mueller-Hinton agar, a medium almost unknown in Great Britain where many laboratories use their ordinary nutrient agar for their sensitivity tests and indeed often perform them on primary culture.

The use of very high content discs (*e.g.* penicillin 10 μg.) necessitates having them widely spaced (3 cm. apart and 2 cm. from the edge of the plate) and their general adoption would greatly increase the cost of these tests: 15 cm. Petri dishes containing 80 ml. medium are recommended. There is also the risk that if only high content discs are available they will be used for other methods without adequate controls. It must be remembered that the volume of water taken up by the disc is very small and the *concentration per ml.* of the drug in the surrounding medium will greatly exceed the stated disc content, thus discs containing 30 μg. kanamycin may give a 12 mm. zone with an organism having an M.I.C. of 64 μg./ml.

Common Sources of Error

PENICILLINASE-PRODUCING STAPHYLOCOCCI are resistant to penicillin by virtue of their ability to destroy the drug, but they may show quite large inhibition zones round a penicillin disc. These organisms can be identified by their appearance at the edge of the inhibition zone. Colonies are full-sized, giving a heaped-up edge (Fig. 27) in contrast to the smooth edge produced by colonies of diminishing size in the control culture. The same effect is seen with ampicillin. Such organisms should be reported as penicillinase-producing or resistant.

Tube dilution tests with these organisms are much affected by the size of the inoculum. The literature contains hundreds of reports to the effect that strains of resistant staphylococci are inhibited by certain concentrations of penicillin, often without specifying the size of the inoculum: without this information the concentration figure is meaningless.

METHICILLIN-RESISTANT STAPHYLOCOCCI. Cultures of most of these organisms contain only a small proportion of cells capable of appearing resistant if grown on normal medium and incubated at 37°C. for 18 hours, and resistance is often not obvious unless a heavy inoculum is used and incubation continued for 48 hours. It was shown by Barber (1964) that the addition of 5 per cent NaCl enabled the entire population of such cultures to grow on higher concentrations of methicillin. Disc tests on this medium usually give satisfactory results, though Hewitt, Coe and Parker (1969) found some batches relatively inhibitory to resistant strains.

Annear (1968) reported that enhanced and nearly uniform resistance was seen with ordinary medium if cultures were incubated at 30°C. for 18 hours, though this made little or no difference to sensitive strains (see Fig. 26). Hewitt, Coe and Parker (1969), who investigated this problem most thoroughly, concluded that this was the most dependable method and that practically all resistant strains will grow to within 1 mm. of a 10 μg. methicillin disc on nutrient agar, with or without blood, if incubated at 30°C. for 18 hours. Similar observations have been reported by Hallander, Laurell and Dornbush (1970). A heavy inoculum should be used for either method.

Diffusion tests with cloxacillin are unreliable. Only methicillin discs should be used and staphylococci shown to be resistant to methicillin can be assumed to be resistant to all penicillinase-resistant penicillins and also to the cephalosporins.

CEPHALORIDINE RESISTANCE in staphylococci is of a similar nature but the problem of detecting it is even greater. Although cephaloridine is much more resistant to staphylococcal penicillinase than benzyl penicillin, some strains of staphylococci can partially inactivate it, and if tested with a heavy inoculum will appear resistant because of this. There is always cross-resistance between methicillin, cloxacillin and cephaloridine and staphylococci proved to be resistant to either of these penicillins may be assumed to be resistant to cephaloridine.

PROTEUS spp. Much confusion arises from the ability of some strains to swarm into inhibition zones. Organisms taken from inside the zone and re-tested are no more resistant than the parent culture and as long as there is a clear edge to the zone, measurements may be taken from this and swarming disregarded.

CYCLOSERINE activity is depressed by D-alanine (see p. 204). Results will therefore be affected by the content of this amino acid in the medium and the M.I.C. may be high. In a recent experiment using commercial dehydrated medium, M.I.C.'s ranged from 32 μg. per ml. for *Staph. aureus* and *Esch. coli* to 256-512 μg. per ml. for *Proteus* spp. and *Ps. aeruginosa*. The drug is very unstable and solutions must be freshly prepared.

POLYMYXINS diffuse very poorly and though growth up to the disc can safely be taken to indicate resistance, a zone of inhibition is only a very rough indication of sensitivity. Determinations of M.I.C. by tube dilution methods are much affected by the medium; we have found that the most consistent results are obtained using either nutrient agar or peptone water.

SULPHONAMIDES AND TRIMETHOPRIM are much affected by the composition of the medium. Harper and Cawston (1945) showed that many laboratory media contain substances which inhibit the action of sulphonamides and that these could be neutralized by the addition of lysed horse blood. Trimethoprim is similarly affected and Bushby and Hitchings (1968) have shown that this effect is due to the presence of thymidine or end-products of folate metabolism, which enable bacteria to by-pass the action of these drugs. Such media permit growth throughout the zone of inhibition, colonies varying from very small to full size. Oxoid Diagnostic Sensitivity Test Agar is satisfactory for these tests, as are some batches of Mueller Hinton agar, but most media can be rendered suitable for use by the addition of 4 per cent lysed horse blood, though there may be some difference in the size of the zones produced.

Sulphonamides are inactivated by *p*-aminobenzoic acid and sensitivity tests are invalidated by a heavy inoculum (which contains enough *p*-aminobenzoic acid to inactivate the drug). Zones are not just reduced; they disappear completely. If these tests are over-inoculated resistance cannot be assumed; the test must be repeated. Among the more active sulphonamides, it matters very little which is used: results obtained with one apply with little difference to others.

The M.I.C. of trimethoprim for a number of organisms known to respond to treatment covers an unusually wide range and this presents some technical problems. *Esch. coli,* normally used for the more resistant urinary control, is one of the most sensitive species (M.I.C. 0·12 μg./ml.): thus not only are very large zones produced with this organism, but also many potentially treatable organisms (*e.g. Proteus,* M.I.C. 1-2 μg./ml.) must appear significantly more resistant than the control. This can only be overcome either by using a special control for this drug (*e.g. Pr. morgani* or *Klebsiella* with an M.I.C. of 1 μg./ml.), or by modifying the interpretation of the test.

Synergy between trimethoprim and sulphonamide can be demonstrated either by placing discs containing each drug singly about 15 mm. apart, when the zones may coalesce by extension, or by showing that a zone produced by a disc containing both drugs is larger than that given by the same amount of each singly (Fig. 36). It cannot be shown using only one disc containing both drugs. The practical value of such tests is questionable. Synergy will only be seen if the drugs are present in the ratio appropriate for the organism being tested; therefore failure to demonstrate it does not mean that it will not occur. It is preferable to test both drugs separately and report sensitivity to each. Experience suggests that treatment with the combination can be recommended if the organism is fully sensitive to trimethoprim, even if resistant to sulphonamide, or if there is not more than moderate resistance to both drugs.

Further information concerning the *in vitro* activity of trimethoprim can be found in the following papers: Bushby and Hitchings (1968), Darrell, Garrod and Waterworth (1968), Bushby (1969), Waterworth (1969a).

ANTI-FUNGAL DRUGS. As an increasing number of these drugs becomes available there is a greater demand for sensitivity tests. These can best be done by the dilution method and glucose-peptone broth or agar is satisfactory for all except 5-fluorocytosine. This is neutralized by the constituents of ordinary media but tests can be done in yeast nitrogen base (Difco) with 0·15 per cent asparagine and 1 per cent dextrose added and the pH brought to 7·4 (Shadomy, 1969). A sensitive strain of *C. albicans* can be used as a control for tests of most of these drugs except griseofulvin.

SENSITIVITY TESTS IN PRIMARY CULTURES

Diffusion tests can be incorporated in primary culture. The method below was devised by Dr. E. J. Stokes (1968) and has the advantage that each disc has a control, making direct comparison easy and the results more reliable.

Inoculate a broad area across the middle of the plate with the specimen, as evenly as possible. Spread a loopful of diluted control culture over each of the remaining areas, leaving not more than 5 mm. between control and test areas of inoculation. Place 4 discs in these gaps between the 2 inocula, each about 1 cm. from the edge of the plate: inhibition zones will then be formed in both control and test cultures.

The success of the method depends on the even distribution of the inoculum. When spreading with a wire loop this can most easily be achieved by first making a single streak across the centre in one direction and then spreading evenly across this to cover the whole area (Fig. 30). Alternatively, plates can be inoculated with cotton wool swabs.

DILUTION OF CONTROLS. Add 5 drops of a well-shaken overnight broth culture to a 5 ml. tube of broth. Shake. This dilution gives approximately the same inoculum as many specimens: it may be kept in the refrigerator for use throughout the day. Use the Oxford *Staph. aureus*. (N.C.T.C. 6571) to control specimens of pus and sputum and the standard *Esch. coli* (N.C.T.C. 10418) for urine.

Suitable drugs for testing are given in Table LI.

Figure 31 illustrates such a culture. The method has several advantages, of which the foremost are speed and simplicity. The main objection is the difficulty of controlling the size of the inoculum and whilst a number of tests will have to be repeated because the inoculum was too heavy or too light, allowance can be made for small variations and a surprisingly large proportion can be reported the day after receipt of the specimen. These tests also have the advantage that they reveal the presence of small numbers of resistant organisms (Fig. 31): they also often facilitate the identification of organisms present in mixed cultures because of the selective action on different species.

It must be borne in mind that penicillinase-producing staphylococci destroy penicillin and may thus make a sensitive organism also present in a mixed culture appear resistant. Similarly, chloramphenicol may be inactivated by organisms which are resistant to it and other organisms present may then grow on a concentration which is normally inhibitory (Waterworth, 1966). In such cases the test should be repeated on a pure culture.

Rapid Methods on Pure Cultures

To obtain a pure suspension takes at least one day, but the test itself can be made to occupy less time by employing a colour indicator of early growth. In a tube dilution test this may simply be a pH indicator in a medium containing glucose, or methylene blue, resazurin or a tetrazolium salt. Gillissen and Becher (1957) favour the last-named, and define conditions for its use. An alternative is to place antibiotic discs on an inoculated layer of blood agar and cover this with plain agar: growth reduces the haemoglobin except in the zones of inhibition. Fust and Böhni (1961) read the results of such a test after six hours: Davis (1959) claims for his modification of it that a two-hour reading may be possible.

THE CHOICE OF DRUGS TO BE TESTED

The increasing array of chemotherapeutic agents available makes it impossible to test them all and it is better to test a few suitable ones well than to report many unreliably. If primary sensitivity tests are done it is usually sufficient to test 4 as in the Stokes method, further tests being done if the organism is resistant to more than 2. In emergencies 8 or more may be included on the primary culture. The 4 drugs to be tested should be agreed with the clinicians and can be varied to suit individual preferences. Suitable drugs for different types of specimens and bacterial species are given in Table LI.

For sensitivity tests with pure cultures many prefer to use some form of multiple disc, when the choice of drugs is governed by what is available commercially. It must be remembered that hospital use of antibiotics is greatly influenced by laboratory reports and the unnecessary use of potentially toxic drugs should not be encouraged by indiscriminate reporting of sensitivity to them.

The number of tests required can be cut down by testing only one representative of the following closely related groups, within which there is always cross-resistance: tetracyclines (tetracycline), sulphonamides (sulphafurazole), polymyxins (polymyxin B sulphate), cephalosporins (cephaloridine), penicillinase-resistant penicillins (methicillin), rifamycins (rifamide). There are some minor exceptions to these rules: *e.g.* ampicillin-resistant enterobacteria, may sometimes be resistant to cephaloridine and cephalothin but sensitive to cephalexin (Waterworth, 1971). If gentamicin is preferred to kanamycin clinically, there seems little point in testing the latter at all. Drugs inapplicable to the specimen (*e.g.* nitrofurantoin for organisms for any source but urine) or unsuited to the method should not be tested. It was pointed out by Waterworth (1962) that laboratory sensi-

TABLE LI

Choice of Drugs for Sensitivity Tests

	Penicillin	Methicillin	Ampicillin	Carbenicillin	Cephaloridine	Erythromycin	Lincomycin Clindamycin	Fucidin	Tetracycline	Chloramphenicol	Streptomycin	Kanamycin	Gentamicin	Polymyxin	Sulphonamide	Trimethoprim	Nitrofurantoin*	Nalidixic Acid*
Primary Cultures																		
Pus	1					1			1				1					
Sputum			1			2			1	2					1	1		
Urine			1		2				2		2	2	2		1	1	1	1
Sub-culture																		
Staphylococcus	1	1				1	2	2	1	3	2	2	2		2	2		
Streptococcus	1				1	1	1		1									
Haemophilus			1						1	2	2				1	1		
Bacteroides			1			1	1		1	2								
Escherichia			1		2				1	2	1	2	2	2	1	1	1	1
Klebsiella			1		1				2		1	1	1	2	1	1	1	1
Proteus			1	1	1					2	1	2	2		1	1	1	1
Salmonella			1						1	1	1	2	2		1	1		
Shigella			1						1		1	2	2		1	1		
Pseudomonas				1							1		1	1				

* Applicable only to organisms from the urine. Figures indicate order of priority.

tivity tests with methenamine mandelate (Mandelamine) are misleading, because its anti-bacterial activity is dependent on the liberation of formaldehyde, which only occurs in an acid environment. Solutions of methenamine mandelate from which discs are prepared are highly acid, so that disc tests only show the sensitivity of organisms to formalin. Waterworth (1962) found that in such tests, strains of *Proteus* species were among the most sensitive organisms, whereas infections of the urinary tract due to *Proteus* are among the least susceptible to the drug because of the high alkalinity they produce in the urine.

TUBE DILUTION TEST

This method is too time-consuming for general use. Indications for it are:

1. When dosage is to be based on determination of the minimum inhibitory concentration, as in the treatment of bacterial endocarditis.
2. For tests of slowly growing organisms, notably *Myco. tuberculosis* and *Actinomyces israeli*.
3. For demonstrating small degrees of acquired bacterial resistance.

The method is described in the section on bactericidal tests. If many strains are to be tested, dilutions can be prepared in agar plates, when a number of strains can be tested on each. A solid medium also has the advantage that it reveals whether the whole inoculum has grown or only a few cells.

Preparation of Stock Solutions

Tablets and capsules should not be used to prepare solutions: they contain binding materials, ' fillers ' and other materials as well as the antibiotic. The pure substance must be obtained, and is available for many antibiotics in preparations supplied for injection. Many antibiotics are highly soluble: for those which are not there are special preparations for injection and these are suitable for laboratory purposes with the following exceptions:—

CHLORAMPHENICOL. Chloramphenicol succinate has little activity *in vitro*. Chloramphenicol powder is available and should be used but has a solubility of only 2·5 mg./ml. in water.

FUCIDIN AND CYCLOSERINE are not available as injection preparations. The pure substances should be obtained from the manufacturers: both are freely soluble in water.

ERYTHROMYCIN LACTOBIONATE (injection preparation) may be used but if erythromycin base is used this must first be dissolved to give 10 mg. per ml. in ethyl alcohol, after which it may be diluted in water.

NYSTATIN is insoluble in water, but owing to its very fine particle size it can be used as a suspension. It is very unstable and must be freshly prepared.

SULPHONAMIDES, NITROFURANTOIN AND NALIDIXIC ACID all have a low solubility in water but can be brought into solution by raising the pH.

TRIMETHOPRIM is available from the manufacturers. The lactate is soluble in water and the base can be brought into solution by lowering the pH with lactic acid.

POLYMYXINS. The sulphomethyl form of both polymyxin B and colistin (polymyxin E) is unsuitable for sensitivity testing (see p. 194): the sulphate should be used.

SENSITIVITY TESTS FOR MYCO. TUBERCULOSIS

So many drugs are now available for the treatment of tuberculosis that most laboratories either use the ready-made sensitivity sets commercially available or send their cultures to special centres.

Tests are done by the tube dilution method, usually with double dilutions in Löwenstein-Jensen medium. The inoculum must be carefully standardized and a duplicate set of slopes inoculated similarly with H37Rv. Cultures are incubated for 14 days or until a control slope containing no drug shows good growth.

INOCULUM. Standardization of the size of the inoculum is important. About 2 cu. mm. (judged by eye) representative growth from a primary diagnostic Löwenstein-Jensen slope, is transferred with a wire loop to 0·5 ml. sterile distilled water in a ¼ oz. screw-capped bottle containing 6 (3 mm.) glass beads. A suspension is prepared by shaking for 1 minute and a full 3 mm. loopful is then spread over the surface of each slope.

This procedure should only be carried out by trained personnel in a suitably ventilated cabinet. Tests must be done not more than 2 weeks after the culture has become positive and subcultures of H37Rv must not be more than 4 weeks old.

The M.I.C. is taken as the lowest concentration yielding <20 colonies and the result reported as the resistance ratio, obtained by dividing the M.I.C. of the test organism by that of the H37Rv. A ratio of 8:1 indicates resistance; if 4:1 the test should be repeated and if the result is confirmed it should be reported as resistant.

Some drugs are unstable. Clark (1967) found that ethionamide lost activity even when stored at 4°C and at 18°C; isoniazid and cycloserine also deteriorated. All drug-containing media should therefore be supplied marked with an expiry date and it is essential not only that this be observed but also that all tubes used for both test and control bear the same date.

In the Proportion Method, viable counts of a culture of the test organism are done on both drug-containing and drug-free media and the proportion of the culture found to be resistant reported. This method is not recommended for routine laboratories; full details of both this and the resistance ratio method can be found in the paper by Canetti *et al.* (1963).

TESTS OF BACTERICIDAL ACTION

These are chiefly of interest for the purpose of identifying a synergic combination for treating a difficult and serious infection, such as an endocarditis due to a streptococcus relatively resistant to penicillin. Total bactericidal effect must be the aim in such treatment: anything short of this may fail, and merely bacteristatic action, in however low a concentration, is notoriously incapable of eliminating the infection. Sensitivity tests must therefore reveal whether the organism has been killed or merely prevented from growing.

Tests in Liquid Medium with Subculture

Tubes of liquid medium containing antibiotics are heavily inoculated, incubated overnight and sub-cultivated on suitable solid medium to determine whether the inoculum has been killed. Bulger and Nielson (1968) studied the bactericidal action of antibiotic combinations in both Mueller-Hinton broth and human serum with almost identical results. They recommend sub-culturing the test mixtures by preparing a pour-plate from 0·001 ml. delivered by a calibrated loop, after only 4 hours' incubation. The method is most useful for determining the minimum bactericidal level (M.B.C.) of single drugs but may also be used for testing combined action.

The result of the test is much affected by the size of the inoculum: if it is very large nothing will sterilize it, but if too small results will be unduly optimistic The final test mixtures should contain about 10^6 organisms per ml.

DETERMINATION OF M.B.C. Prepare 2 sets of two-fold dilutions of the antibiotic in broth (serum may be added if necessary for the growth of the organism). Inoculate one set with 1 drop of a broth culture of the patient's organism diluted to give about 10^6 organisms per ml. in the inoculated test mixture. Immediately sub-cultivate the control tube containing no antibiotic by spreading 1 loopful evenly over a quarter of a plate of suitable medium. Inoculate the second set of tubes with a similar number of a suitable control organism. Incubate overnight.

Sub-cultivate all tubes showing no growth by spreading a loopful over a quarter of a plate of suitable medium. Incubate at least 24 hours. The M.B.C. is the lowest concentration in broth which yielded no growth. Comparison of sub-cultures yielding growth with that from the control tube before incubation will reveal whether there was some bactericidal activity or whether the action was only bacteristatic.

TESTS OF COMBINED ACTION. Each antibiotic is added to broth singly and in all possible combinations, using a single concentration of each attainable in the blood (conveniently 10 μg. per ml.). If a number of drugs are to be tested, tubes can conveniently be arranged in the form of a 'half chess board' (Fig. 32). Prepare solutions of each antibiotic containing 100 μg. per ml. and pipette 0·5 ml. of each into the appropriate rows of tubes. Add 4 ml. broth pre-inoculated to contain 10^6 organisms per ml. to each tube containing 2 antibiotics and 4·5 ml. to those with only one. Shake well. Plate a control tube containing no antibiotic on suitable solid medium. After overnight incubation plate any tubes showing no growth; incubate at least 24 hours.

Sub-cultures may show:—

1. Growth similar to that from the control before incubation —bacteristatic action only.

2. Small number of colonies—incomplete bactericidal action.

3. Sterility—total bactericidal action.

The disadvantages of the method are:

1. Only one concentration of each drug is usually tested in combination. 2. Only a minute proportion of the original inoculum is sub-cultivated. 3. If the organism is highly sensitive, growth of surviving cells may be inhibited by carry-over on

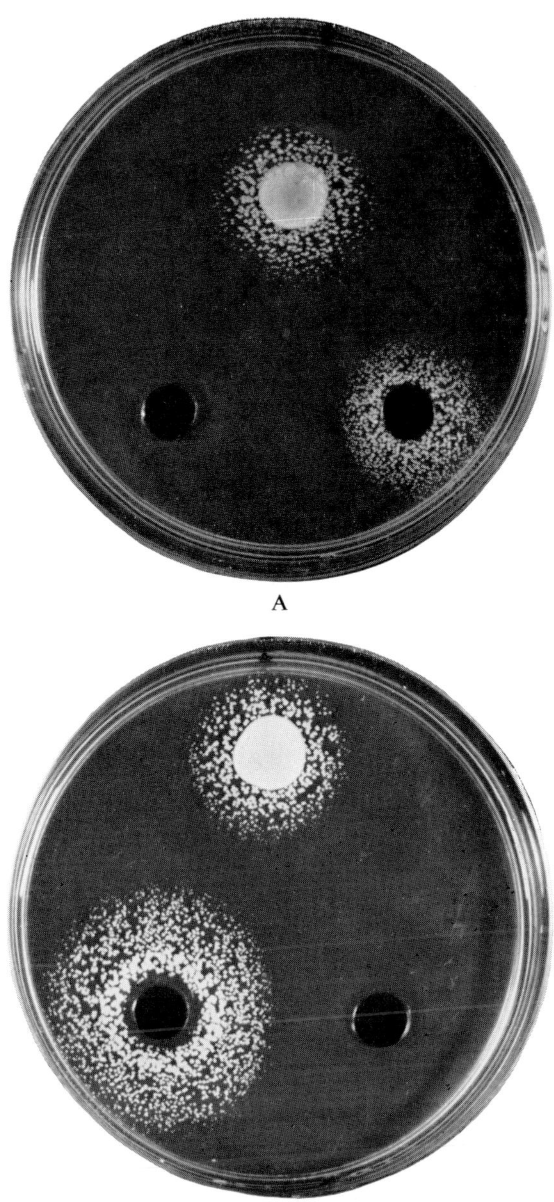

Fig. 25

'Satellitism' produced by a localized change in the pH of the medium.
   A. Nutrient agar containing 0·12 μg. per ml. fucidin.
   B. Glucose agar containing 0·06 μg. per ml. erythromycin.
Both plates were flooded with a suspension of the Oxford staphylococcus and a small area (top centre) of each inoculated with a resistant strain of *Staph. aureus.* Cups contain: left—N/10 HCl; right—N/10 NaOH.
In (A) the Oxford staphylococcus has grown where the resistant organism has raised the pH of the medium, and round the cup containing alkali. In (B) it has grown where fermentation of the glucose by the resistant organism has lowered the pH, and round the cup containing acid.

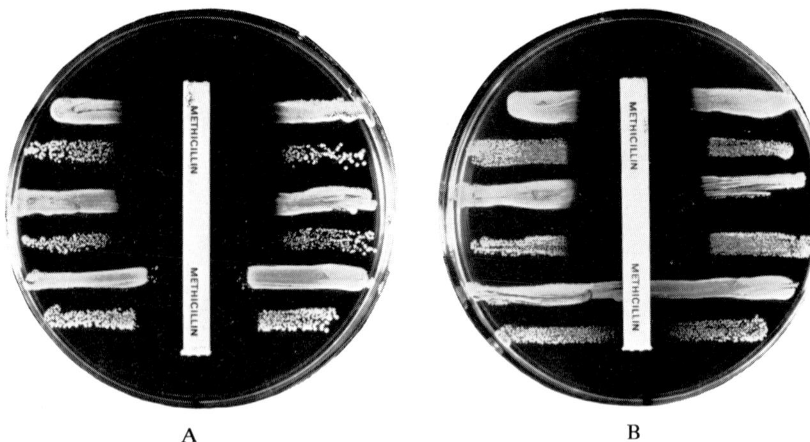

A   B

FIG. 26

The use of blotting paper strips for testing sensitivity to methicillin. Organisms (top to bottom)—Oxford staphylococcus, penicillinase-producing *Staph. aureus* and a methicillin-resistant *Staph. aureus,* with a heavy and light inoculum of each. Strips contain 100 μg. methicillin.

A. Incubated overnight at 37°C. When the inoculum is heavy the zone of the resistant strain is reduced and contains resistant colonies, but when the inoculum is light there is a large zone of inhibition.

B. Incubated overnight at 30°C. The resistant strain grows up to the strip from both heavy and light inocula.

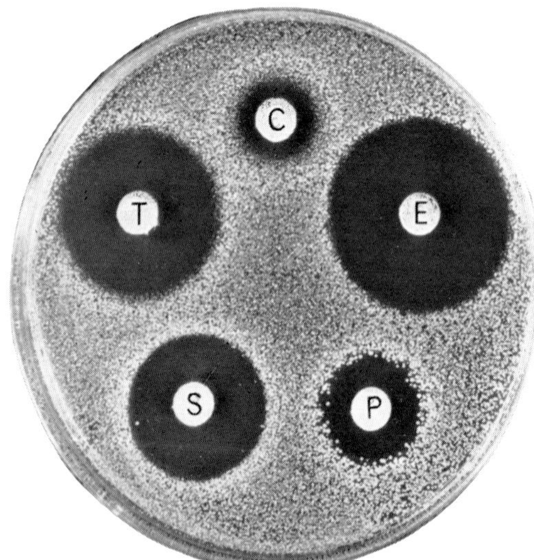

FIG. 27

Disc sensitivity test on a strain of *Staph. aureus* inoculated to give 'dense but not confluent growth'. Colonies at the edge of the zone round the penicillin disc (P) are full-size, making an irregular edge and indicating that the strain produces penicillinase.

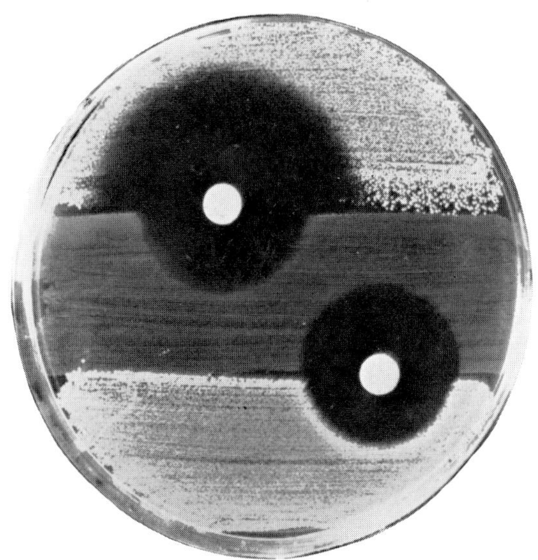

A

FIG. 28

The choice of control for disc tests on organisms of intermediate sensitivity.
A. Sensitivity of *Str. faecalis* (centre) to ampicillin. When isolated from the urine it should be compared to the *Esch. coli* control (bottom), when it will appear fully sensitive and the infection is likely to respond to normal doses. If isolated from other parts of the body it should be compared with the fully sensitive staphylococcal control (top) when it will be seen to be only moderately sensitive and higher dosage will be required.
Discs—ampicillin 25 μg. (Waterworth, 1969b).

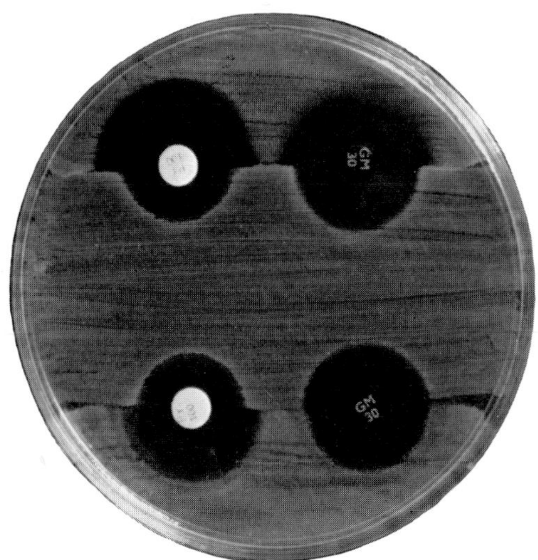

B

B. Sensitivity of *Ps. aeruginosa* (centre) to carbenicillin and gentamicin. If compared to the control *Esch. coli* (top) it appears moderately resistant to both drugs, but when a standard strain of the same species (bottom) is used as a control, the test strain is seen to have *normal sensitivity* to gentamicin but increased resistance to carbenicillin.
Discs—Left—carbenicillin 100 μg. Right—gentamicin 30 μg.

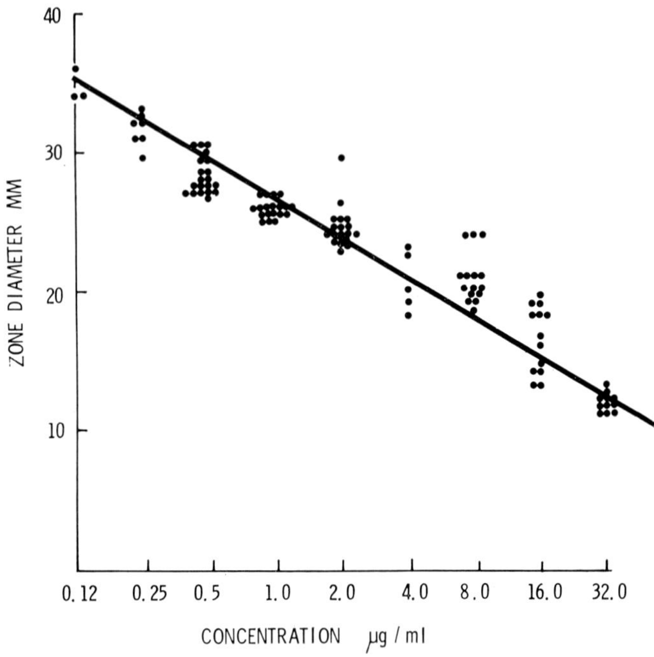

Fig. 29

Regression line for kanamycin prepared by plotting the M.I.C. of
100 organisms against the diameter of the zone of inhibition
produced by a 30 µg. disc.
(The organisms with an M.I.C. of 8 µg./ml. giving points consistently above the line, were Gram-positive cocci isolated from
environmental studies. These usually grow more slowly than most
pathogens and therefore produce larger zones of inhibition.)

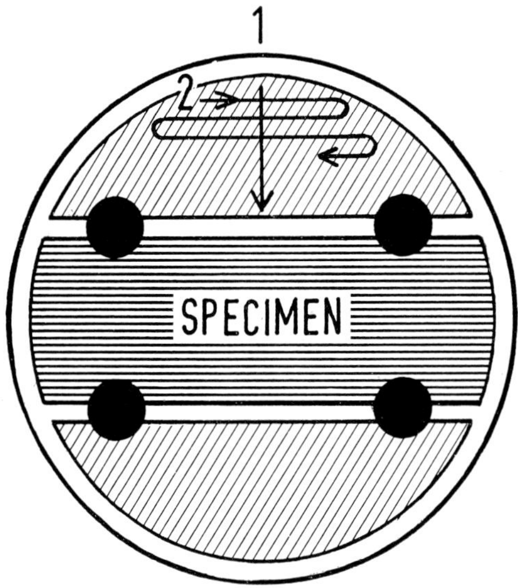

FIG. 30

Diagram showing the preparation of a sensitivity test on a primary culture
by the Stokes method.

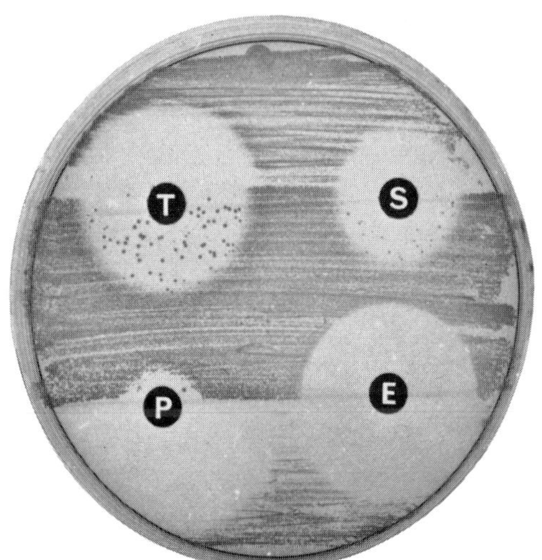

FIG. 31

Sensitivity test on a primary culture of a specimen of pus. Growth consists
entirely of *Staph. aureus* but includes small numbers of a second strain
which can be identified by its resistance to tetracycline (T) and streptomycin
(S). The other antibiotics are penicillin (P) and erythromycin (E).

	Penicillin	Streptomycin	Tetracycline	Erythromycin	Kanamycin
Penicillin	+	−	+ +	+	−
Streptomycin		+ + +	+ +	+	+ +
Tetracycline			+ +	+	+ +
Erythromycin				+	+
Kanamycin					+ +

Fig. 32

'Half Chess Board' bactericidal sensitivity test. Tubes containing each drug singly and in all combinations are arranged as above and results of sub-cultures recorded as follows. Broth itself turbid ' + + + '. Numbers of colonies approximately equal to the original inoculum ' + + '. Marked reduction in the number of colonies ' + '; ' − ' = no growth.

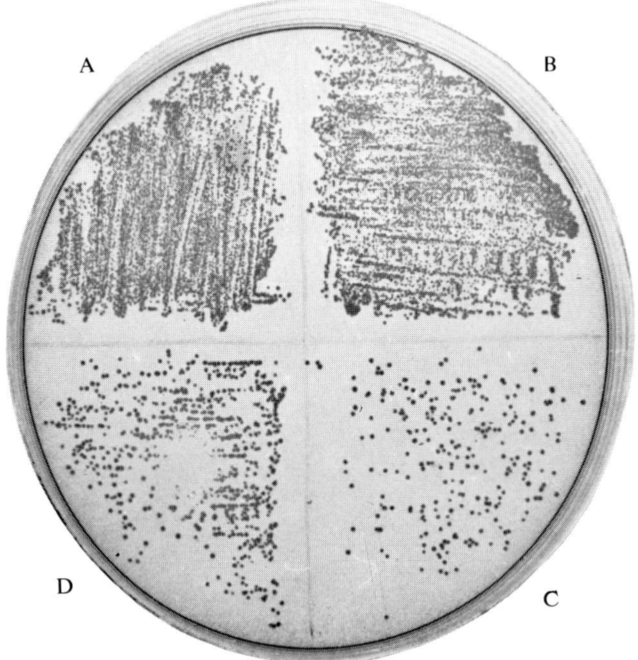

Fɪɢ. 33

Sub-cultures from broth tubes in a ' half chess board ' bactericidal sensitivity
test on a strain of *Staph. albus*.
A. Control tube sub-cultivated before incubation, showing the original inoculum.
B., C. & D. Tubes showing no growth after overnight incubation. B. Growth
similar to A., bacteristasis only. C. Reduced number of colonies—incomplete bactericidal action. D. Incomplete bactericidal effect with an area of
inhibition produced by carry-over.

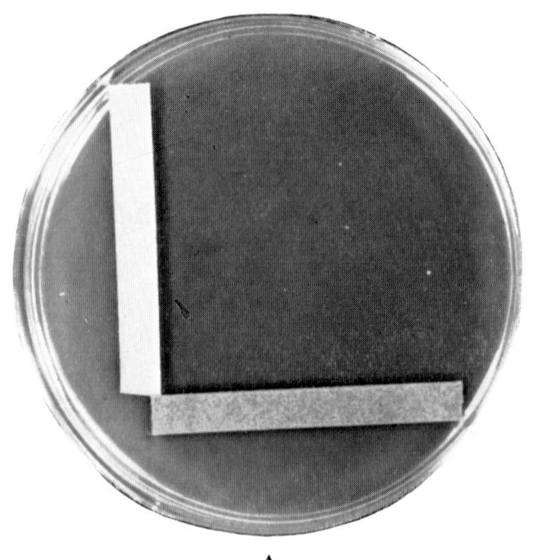

A

B

FIG. 34

The cellophane transfer method.
A. Blotting paper strips containing antibiotic applied to nutrient agar and the antibiotic allowed to diffuse out.
B. Sterile tambour applied to the plate after the strips have been removed.

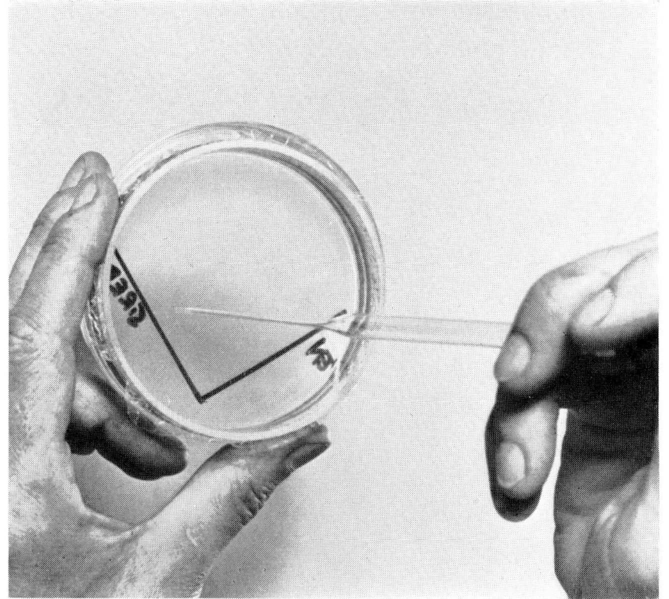

C

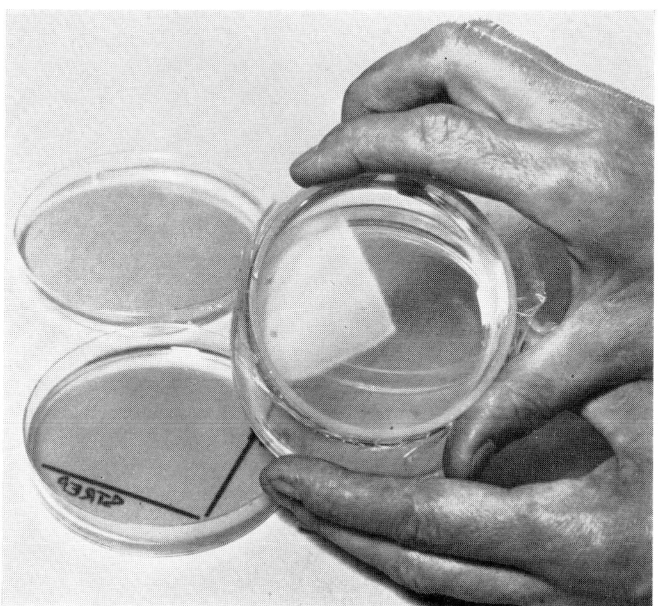

D

Fig. 34

C. The inside of the tambour is flooded with bacterial suspension.
D. After incubation the tambour is transferred to antibiotic-free
medium. Note that the growth is on the cellophane, the plate to
which it had been applied remaining sterile.

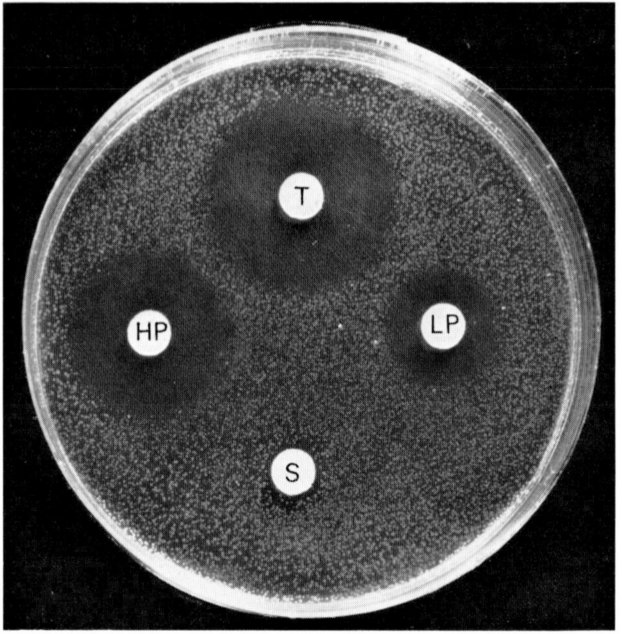

Fig. 35a

Fig. 35 A-D. Disc tests and tests by the cellophane transfer method on a strain of *Str. faecalis* isolated from a patient (G. F.) with bacterial endocarditis.

A. Disc test showing high bacteristatic sensitivity to tetracycline (T), moderate resistance to penicillin (P, LP=1·5 units, HP=5 units) and resistance to streptomycin (S).

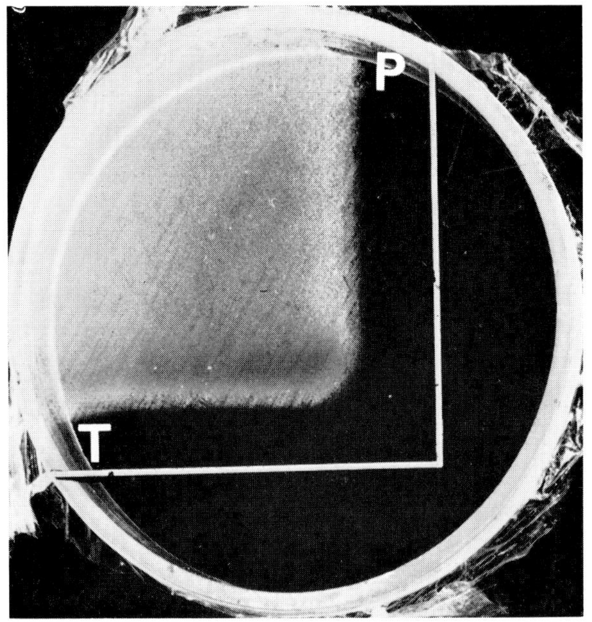

Fig. 35B

B. Tambour after overnight incubation on a plate into which penicillin and tetracycline had been pre-diffused from blotting paper strips. This shows bacteristatic sensitivity.

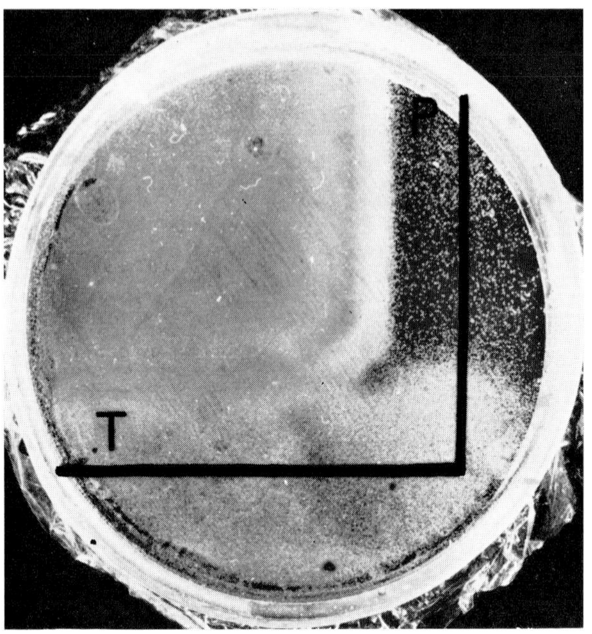

Fig. 35c

C. The same tambour after a further 24 hours' incubation on antibiotic-free medium. Tetracycline alone was purely bacteristatic. Penicillin alone killed most of the inoculum but left some survivors. Where both drugs are present in the area round the angle formed by the strips, the tetracycline has eliminated the bactericidal effect of the penicillin (antagonism).

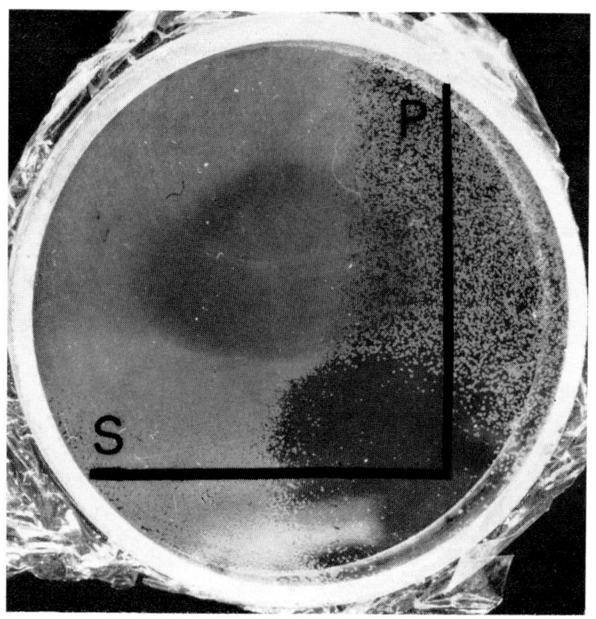

FIG. 35D

D. Tambour after incubation on antibiotic-free medium following exposure to penicillin and streptomycin. Penicillin alone left survivors, streptomycin alone was barely inhibitory. The presence of both drugs sterilized the inoculum (synergy).

This patient, a man of 71, had been ill for 9 months and had received many courses of antibiotics, always relapsing after treatment was stopped. As a result of these tests he made a complete recovery following treatment with penicillin and streptomycin. A re-infection with the same organism 9 months later was again successfully treated with this combination and the patient is alive and well 8 years later.

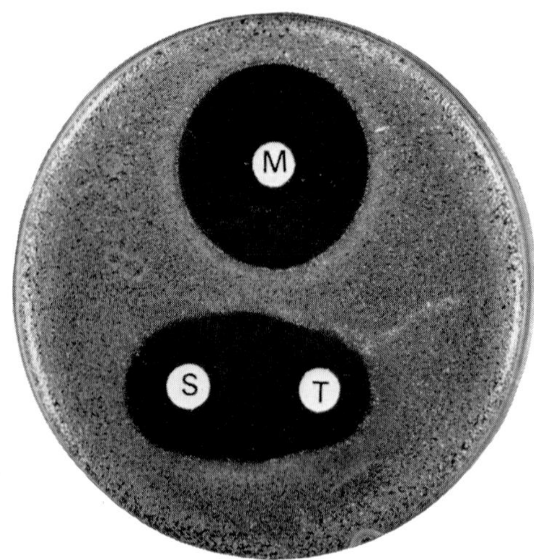

FIG. 36

Bacteristatic synergy between trimethoprim and sulphonamide against a strain of *Pr. morgani*. Discs contain: T—trimethoprim 2·5 μg. S—sulphafurazole 50 μg. M—the same amount of both.

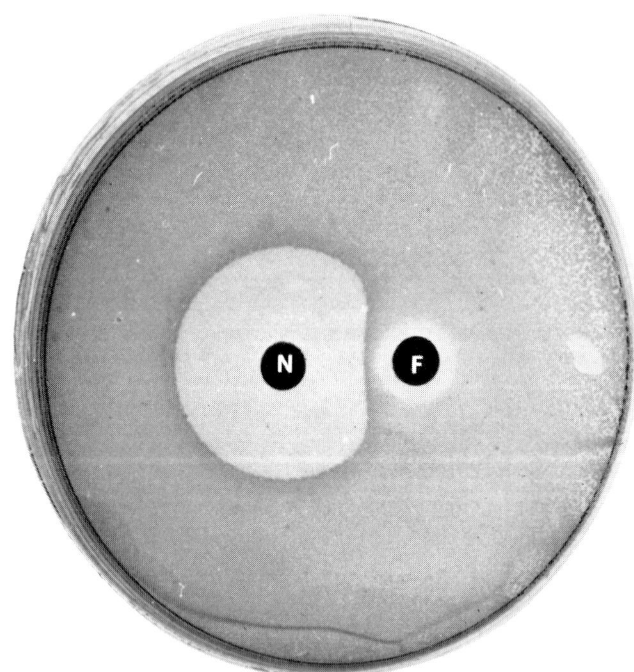

FIG. 37

Bacteristatic antagonism between nitrofurantoin (F) and nalidixic acid (N) against *Pr. rettgeri*.

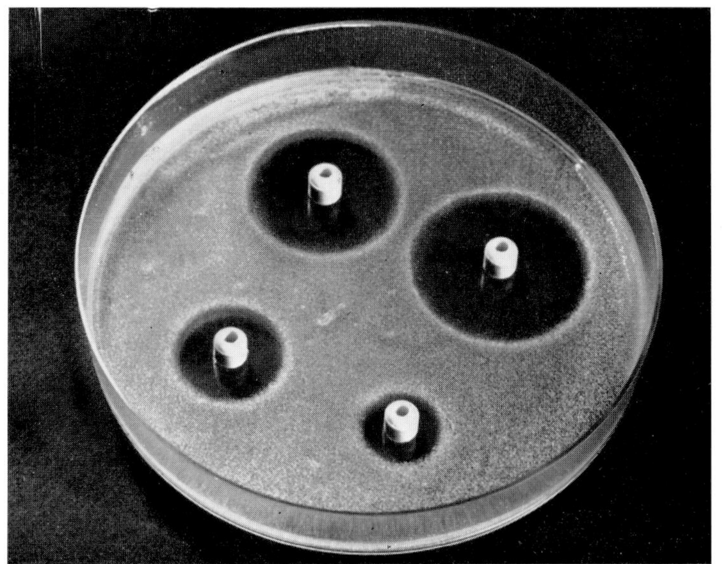

Fig. 38

' Fish-spines ' containing antibiotic solutions on an agar plate seeded with
S. lutea.

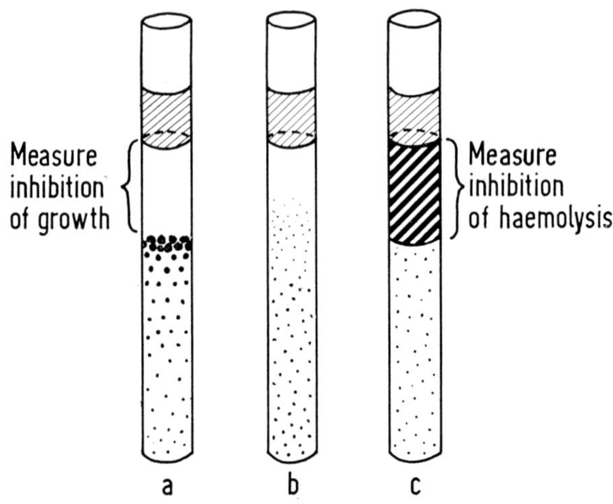

FIG. 39

Diagrammatic illustration of vertical diffusion assays.

a. Streptomycin over assay agar inoculated with *Staph. aureus*. A band of large colonies gives a clear edge to the zone of inhibition.

b. Penicillin over assay agar inoculated with *Staph. aureus*. Colonies gradually increase in size giving no clear definition to the inhibition zone.

c. Penicillin over blood agar inoculated with *Str. pyogenes*. Haemolysis is inhibited through a well-defined zone, the width of which can be measured accurately.

sub-culture. This can be partially overcome by placing a loop-ful of each mixture on a marked area of a plate and allowing the fluid to be absorbed before thoroughly spreading over a wider area. Colonies may then surround a sterile area.

The appearance of such sub-cultures is illustrated in Figure 33.

Velvet Pad Replica Plate

In this method, devised by Elek and Hilson (1954), a wooden block cut to fit into a Petri dish is covered with sterile velvet. The pad so formed is first pressed firmly onto an ordinary disc sensitivity test which has been incubated overnight, and then on to a plate of fresh medium. This is incubated overnight and any colonies appearing within the inhibition zones represent survivors from the original inoculum. Combined action can be studied either by placing discs side by side or by using blotting paper strips set at right angles to each other. The dis-advantage of the method is that the velvet pad transfers only about 0·5 per cent of the cells present.

Cellophane Transfer Method

This method, originally described by Chabbert and his col-leagues and fully described by Garrod and Waterworth (1962) and Chabbert and Waterworth (1965) requires special appara-tus and some practice for its proper execution, but its results are remarkably revealing. A cellophane tambour, inoculated on the inside with the test organism, is placed on a plate into which antibiotics have been pre-diffused from blotting paper strips placed at right angles. Nutrients and antibiotics diffuse through the cellophane to permit growth on the inside of the tambour, the plate remaining sterile. After a period of incubation the tambour is transferred to a plate of normal medium and any bacteria surviving in the inhibition zones will then grow. The final culture will show the bactericidal effect of each drug alone at the ends of each strip and their combined action in the area surrounding the angle where the strips meet.

TECHNIQUE. Immerse 0·5 × 5 cm. strips of sterile blotting paper in anti-biotic solution (Table LII), remove excess fluid by lightly blotting on sterile blotting paper and place at right angles on a plate of suitable medium (Fig. 34A). Allow to diffuse at 37°C. for 5 hours or overnight at 4°C.

Tambours are prepared by stretching cellophane PT 300 (commercially available as jam pot covers) across a pyrex glass ring 8 cm. in diameter and

16

2·5 cm. high* and securing it with a strong rubber band. The cellophane should first be softened to permit stretching; with the present day material it is usually sufficient to wet it in cold water, but if necessary this can be brought to the boil. Tambours must not be allowed to dry before use; they should be placed in glass pots with the cellophane resting on moist filter paper and sterilized by autoclaving for 10 min. at 121°C.

Remove the strips from the plate and apply the tambour to the surface, taking care to avoid trapping any air between the medium and the cellophane. Flood the inside of the tambour with a suspension of the organism containing about 10^7 organisms per ml., removing any surplus with a Pasteur pipette. Place the culture in the incubator with the lid tipped until the surface of the cellophane is dry, then remove the lid and continue incubation overnight with the culture inverted over clean blotting paper (see Figs. 34A-D).

Transfer the tambour to a well-dried plate of suitable medium containing no antibiotic and incubate a further 24 hours.

* Obtainable from Stanmore Surgical Company, 62 Lamorna Grove, Stanmore, Middlesex.

Some antibiotics, particularly those heavily protein-bound, are carried over by the cellophane and if the concentration in the medium is too high, sufficient may be carried over to prevent growth of the surviving organisms. Suitable solutions for preparing the strips are given in Table LII.

TABLE LII

Solutions recommended for preparation of blotting paper strips
(µg. per ml.)

*Ampicillin	50	Kanamycin	1000
Carbenicillin	1000	Lincomycin	200
*Cephaloridine	50	Methicillin	1000
Chloramphenicol	1000	Novobiocin	50
Clindamycin	200	*Penicillin	50
Cloxacillin	200	Rifamide	50
Erythromycin	200	Streptomycin	1000
Fucidin	50	Tetracycline	200
Gentamicin	100	Vancomycin	1000

* Use 500 µg. per ml. if testing enterococci and Gram-negative bacilli.

N.B. Closely related drugs vary and it should not be assumed that the same concentrations will apply.

Based on Chabbert & Waterworth (1965).

Choice of Antibiotics

The tests are made unnecessarily laborious if unsuitable drugs are tested. Table LIII gives the antibiotics most likely to have bactericidal activity against most of the common infections. The bactericidal action of penicillins is always antagonized by the presence of a bacteristatic antibiotic and even

if the organism has been shown to be highly sensitive to tetracycline or chloramphenicol, it is a waste of time to include
either in bactericidal tests with penicillins. On the other hand,
penicillin and streptomycin, gentamicin or kanamycin may act
synergically against streptococci even though the strain is relatively resistant to any or all of them. These combinations
should always be included when testing streptococci (see Fig.

TABLE LIII

COMBINATIONS OF DRUGS LIKELY TO SHOW
BACTERICIDAL SYNERGY

Streptococci

penicillin, cephaloridine or erythromycin	+	streptomycin, kanamycin or vancomycin

Staphylococci

methicillin or cephaloridine	+	streptomycin, gentamicin kanamycin or vancomycin
streptomycin, gentamicin or kanamycin	+	erythromycin or novobiocin
rifamide	+	erythromycin or fucidin

Gram-negative bacilli

ampicillin, carbenicillin or cephaloridine	+	streptomycin gentamicin or kanamycin

35). Penicillin-resistant streptococci other than enterococci may
be sensitive to cephaloridine (Tozer, Boutflower and Gillespie,
1966), and this should be included in tests of such organisms.

It is generally agreed that rifampicin should not be used
indiscriminately because of the risk of unknowingly producing
resistance in tubercle bacilli. Nevertheless, as Peard *et al.*
(1970) have shown, it can be invaluable in life-endangering
staphylococcal infection where other treatment has failed.
Resistant cells are present in most cultures of staphylococci
and if bactericidal tests are done in fluid media, tubes must be
sub-cultivated after 4 or 6 hours as growth of resistant organisms may occur later. Either rifamide or rifampicin can be used
for *in vitro* tests; the former is preferable as it is readily soluble
in water and less carried over by cellophane.

The synergy between penicillin and fucidin and penicillin and erythromycin against some strains of staphylococci is of a different nature (see pp. 168, 208) and cannot be demonstrated by this method. Fucidin and methicillin or cloxacillin are antagonistic. Polymyxin is very heavily carried over by cellophane and must be tested by the tube dilution method.

Interpretation of Results

Combined bactericidal tests can show any of three results:

1. Indifference—the action of the two drugs together is no greater than that of the more active alone.

2. Antagonism—the bactericidal effect of one is reduced by the presence of the other.

3. Synergy—neither drug alone is completely bactericidal but the two together sterilize the inoculum.

Antagonism between penicillin and tetracycline and synergy between penicillin and streptomycin against *Str. faecalis* are demonstrated by the cellophane transfer method in Figure 35. Similar results obtained by the broth dilution method are given in the 'half chess board' illustrated in Figure 32.

Ideally the drugs recommended for the treatment of endocarditis will have been shown to be totally bactericidal *in vitro*. If this has not been achieved other combinations should be tried before finally choosing that which shows the smallest number of survivors.

The cellophane transfer method is a harder test of performance than the broth dilution and it is not uncommon for sub-cultures in the latter to be sterile although there are survivors from the same drug on the tambour. This is probably due mainly to the small amount of the inoculum sub-cultivated from the fluid cultures.

TESTS OF COMBINED BACTERISTATIC ACTION

The combined effects described above cannot be demonstrated by bacteristatic tests: discs containing these mixtures of antibiotics will reflect only the activity of the more active or more diffusible.

The modern practice of testing many discs on a single plate has revealed a number of bacteristatic interactions between drugs placed next to each other. The best known are the synergy between polymyxin and sulphonamides or trimethoprim against *Proteus* spp. and the antagonism between nitrofurantoin and nalidixic acid against various organisms (see p. 272). The synergy between trimethoprim and sulphonamides is of much greater importance and is discussed on page 463 (see Fig. 36). Bacteristatic antagonism is shown in Figure 37.

ANTIBIOTIC ASSAYS IN BODY FLUIDS

These are perhaps less often performed than they should be, and can be useful for two main purposes, apart from studying the absorption, distribution and excretion of a new drug.

1. To verify that adequate concentrations are being attained, as in the blood when absorption from the alimentary tract may be defective, or in the cerebro-spinal fluid during the treatment of meningitis.

2. To guard against excessive blood levels, particularly of antibiotics liable to damage the eighth nerve (streptomycin, gentamicin, kanamycin, vancomycin) in patients with any impairment of renal function.

The interval between the collection of the blood and the last dose is important and should be stated. If the level is being done for the second reason, blood should be taken immediately before the next dose is due. Peak levels vary greatly and when high do not necessarily indicate delayed excretion as does a significant level at the end of the interval between doses (Line, Poole and Waterworth, 1970). It is obviously essential to know whether any other antibiotic is being given, but this information is only too often omitted. It should also be remembered that blood from a patient with impaired renal function may still contain an antibiotic given a week or more earlier.

Assays may be done by tube dilution or diffusion methods. A variety of organisms recommended for different antibiotics are listed in Table LIV. In an emergency any antibiotic can be assayed against either the *Staph. aureus* or *Esch. coli* used as sensitivity test controls.

PREPARATION OF SPORE SUSPENSIONS. Grow cultures on agar, preferably in Roux Bottles, for 1 week at 37°C. (30°C. for *B. cereus*). Suspend the growth in sterile distilled water and heat for 30 minutes at 65°C. Wash the spores in water and resuspend in water. Suspensions will keep at 4°C. indefinitely.

SUSPENSIONS OF VEGETATIVE ORGANISMS can be prepared from broth cultures (if not granular) or by suspending growth from solid medium in broth. They will keep at 4°C. for up to 4 weeks.

TABLE LIV

Appropriate Organisms for Assaying Antibacterial Drugs

Drug	Organism	NCTC Number	Optimum pH
*Penicillins *Cephaloridine	Staph. aureus S. lutea B. subtilis	6571 8340 8236	6·8
‡Carbenicillin	Ps. aeruginosa	10490	
Streptomycin	Staph. aureus Kl. pneumoniae B. subtilis	6571 7242 8236	7·8
Kanamycin Gentamicin	Staph. aureus B. pumilis	6571 8241	
*Tetracyclines	B. cereus Staph. aureus	10320 6571	6·6
*Chloramphenicol	Esch. coli S. lutea	10418 8340	
*Erythromycin *Lincomycin	Staph. aureus B. pumilis	6571 8241	7·8 7·8
*Novobiocin Fucidin	Staph. aureus	6571	6·6
Vancomycin	Staph. aureus B. subtilis	6571 8236	7·8
Polymyxins	Bord. bronchiseptica Esch. coli	8344 10418	7·3
Anti-fungal	Sacch. cerevisiae C. albicans	10716	7·3
Trimethoprim	B. pumilis	8241	7·3

* May be assayed against *Str. pyogenes* by the vertical diffusion method.

‡ Usually contains traces of benzylpenicillin and must therefore be assayed against an organism resistant to this.

Stock solutions may be prepared in water but standards used for assaying serum must be prepared in serum. Ideally pooled human serum should be used, but that collected from blood sent for serological examination is not suitable, as some of the patients concerned may be receiving antibiotics. If human serum of known origin is not available, horse serum should be used.

When assaying urine, the pH of the specimen must first be brought to the optimum for the drug concerned (Table LIV). The standard solutions and any dilutions of the unknown must be prepared in normal urine of the same pH.

The aminoglycosides, vancomycin and chloramphenicol are all very stable and solutions can be kept frozen for several months: other antibiotics must be freshly prepared.

Diffusion Methods

In these methods the size of the inhibition zones produced by the unknown fluid is compared with a graph of the sizes of inhibition zones produced by known concentrations of the antibiotic. A ' standard curve ' is constructed by preparing 5 or 6 two-fold dilutions of the antibiotic, the lowest containing about twice the M.I.C. of the test organism: if the drug is heavily protein-bound, standards in serum should start 4 times higher. The diameters of the resulting zones of inhibition are plotted against the concentration. Alternatively, there is a linear relationship between zone diameter and the log of the concentration (with aminoglycosides the zone diameter must be squared) and only two standard solutions are strictly necessary. In practice a third is an additional check on the method and should always be included with penicillins.

What dilutions of the unknown should be tested depends on the probable antibiotic content. If this is likely to be high as in urine or in serum from patients receiving high dosage penicillin or with gross renal insufficiency, the specimen must be diluted until it falls within the range of the standard curve. With penicillin serum levels, four or five 1 in 5 dilutions may be necessary.

The depth of the medium affects the size of the zones in any test in which the antibiotic is applied to the surface of the medium unless it is more than 8 mm. deep. The thinner the layer of medium, the more sensitive the test. If very thin plates are used for any method, care must be taken to prevent their drying up during incubation. Results will be affected by the size of the inoculum and the sensitivity of the test will be reduced if it is too heavy. It will be increased by allowing a period of pre-diffusion and by incubating cultures at 30°C.

The original diffusion method described by Heatley (1944) for the assay of penicillin employed porcelain cylinders. These have the advantage that the material for assay need not be sterile but considerable skill is required for their use. Cylinders must be heated just sufficiently to form a seal of agar when placed on the plate: if heating is inadequate or excessive they will either leak when filled or sink too far into the medium and interfere with diffusion. They also require a considerable depth of medium, making the test less sensitive and necessitating some means of preventing the lid of the petri dish resting on them. Stainless steel cylinders do not require heating but slide very easily and have been reported to inactivate some antibiotics (Snell and Lewis, 1959).

The method employing fish spine electrical insulating beads (Fig. 38) given below was described by Lightbown and Sulit-zeanu (1957). This has the advantage that beads are filled and placed in position in one operation, they are light and do not move easily and can be used on very thin agar plates.

Holes punched in agar plates are being increasingly used. These can be as little as 4·5 mm. in diameter in plates only 2·5 mm. deep, thus requiring little serum. The surrounding medium must not be lifted when the plug of agar is removed. According to Bennett *et al.* (1966), who give an excellent description of this method, cups must be completely filled, slight overflow not affecting the results. An alternative is to place a measured volume in each. If rather larger holes (8-9 mm.) are used, smaller amounts of antibiotic can be detected by this method than by any other.

Blotting paper discs require little serum and can be used with a thin layer of agar. The disc should be picked up with a needle and dipped into the fluid for assay, excess fluid is drained off by lightly touching the side of the tube with the disc, which is then placed on the seeded agar. If the disc falls off in the tube it must be discarded and a fresh one taken.

Fish Spine Diffusion Assay
PREPARATION OF FISH SPINES (obtainable from electrical engineers—size no. 3).

Boil in 5NHCl. Wash with water until the washings are free from chloride when tested with silver nitrate. Dry at 100°C. overnight. Heat in a muffle furnace at 500°C. for 30 minutes (or roast on asbestos gauze).

PREPARATION OF PLATES. Melt nutrient agar and cool to 48°C. Inoculate to give about 10^5 organisms per ml. Mix well and pipette 10 ml. amounts into flat 9 cm. Petri dishes on a level surface, bursting any bubbles with a hot wire. Allow to dry at room temperature for 1 hour. Alternatively, dry plates containing 10 ml. agar at 37°C. for 30 min. and inoculate by flooding with a suspension of the test organism containing about 10^6 organisms per ml. Drain any excess to the side and remove with a Pasteur pipette. Allow to dry at room temperature.

Prepare standards in serum and if high levels are likely in the specimen, dilute in normal serum. Place all dilutions in shallow wells, as in a suitable blood grouping tile. Fish spines fill by capillarity. Using curved forceps, pick one up as near the top as possible, allow the open end to come in contact with the fluid, lift without tilting and gently place in position on the agar plate without piercing the medium. A ring of fluid appears at the base of the fish spine and does not indicate leakage.

All tests must be done in triplicate.

Incubate overnight, measure zones of inhibition and average the results.

Plot a standard curve and read the concentration corresponding to the diameter of the unknown from this.

Vertical Diffusion Methods

The vertical diffusion method devised by Mitchison and Spicer (1949) for the assay of streptomycin can be used for any aminoglycoside and for vancomycin. Standard solutions and unknown are pipetted into narrow tubes containing a column of agar seeded with *Staph. aureus*. The antibiotic diffuses downwards and the edge of the zone of inhibition is marked by a band of large colonies making it possible to measure the zone microscopically, using a micrometer eye piece and the vernier on the moving stage.

Other antibiotics do not give this band of large colonies; the edge of the zone is ill-defined and impossible to measure microscopically (Fig. 39). This has the advantage that it is at once apparent if a second antibiotic is present, even if this was not suspected.

The method was modified by Fujii, Grossman and Ticknor (1961) who added blood to the medium, used *Str. pyogenes* as the test organism and measured the inhibition of haemolysis in the same way. This method can be used for any antibiotic active against *Str. pyogenes*.

Whilst these tubes take longer to read than plate diffusion methods, they are admirable for routine laboratories where few assays are done, being both quick and easy to set up. The material for assay need not be sterile and very small specimens will suffice. In a recent study on neonates (Davies *et al.*, 1970), kanamycin, penicillin and polymyxin were each assayed separately in specimens of <1 ml. blood by using 3 modifications of the method.

TECHNIQUE. Assay medium. Nutrient agar diluted with an equal amount of 1 per cent peptone in water and brought to pH 7·8. Tube in 19 ml. amounts.

Melt the agar and cool to 48°C. Dilute an overnight broth culture of the Oxford *Staph. aureus* 1 in 100, *shake well* to break up clumps and add 1 ml. to the cooled medium. Mix well. Pipette seeded agar into tubes having an internal diameter of 3 mm. to give a column 2-3 cm. deep. Allow to set at least 5 min. Pipette standards and unknown into at least 3 tubes each: the size of the zone is unaffected by the volume as long as the layer is at least 1 mm. deep. Incubate at 37° C. overnight.

To measure zones lay a tube on a slide and fix in position with plasticine. Place on a microscope with a micrometer eye-piece and using the ⅔ objective and reduced light, move the slide until the line in the eye piece falls across the bottom of the meniscus between the serum and the agar. Record the figure on the vernier on the moving stage. Move the slide across until the large colonies forming the bottom of the zone reach the line; read this measurement and obtain the depth of the zone by subtracting one from the other. The readings for each set of tubes are averaged and a graph constructed from the standards by plotting the log of the concentration against the zone squared (for vancomycin the zone need not be squared). The zone given by the unknown can then be interpreted from this.

BLOOD AGAR MODIFICATION. Melt 17 ml. nutrient agar and cool to 48°C.

Add 2 ml. warmed blood and 1 ml. well shaken overnight culture of *Str. pyogenes* diluted to contain about 10^6 organisms per ml. Mix well and pipette into narrow tubes. Allow to set at least 5 min. Pipette standards and unknown onto at least 3 tubes each and incubate overnight. Measure the zones of inhibition of haemolysis microscopically as in the foregoing method and average the results.

The same standards are used as for other diffusion methods and a straight line is usually obtained by plotting the depth of the zone against the log of the concentration.

Tube Dilution Test

This method is simple to perform and has the advantage that no advance preparations are required, as all drugs can be assayed against either the Oxford staphylococcus or the standard *Esch. coli* (N.C.T.C. 10418), but the dilutions are widely spaced and results are often inexplicably erratic. When serum is assayed it must first be inactivated by heating to 56°C for 20 minutes.

Medium. Aminoglycosides are considerably affected by the composition of the medium. We have recently determined the M.I.C. of streptomycin for the Oxford staphylococcus in 6 commercially available nutrient broths and peptone water, all containing 10 per cent of serum. It was found to vary from 8 μg./ml. in tryptone-soya broth to 1 μg./ml. in peptone water

(2 brands of peptone gave similar results) and there were similar differences with gentamicin and kanamycin. Aminoglycosides should therefore not be assayed in nutrient broth unless that in use is known not to depress their activity. If a special assay medium is kept the addition of 0·5 per cent dextrose and an indicator to 1 per cent peptone water facilitates the reading of the results, but this is not essential and the peptone water usually available is quite adequate. In either case at least 10 per cent serum should be added and if the drug is heavily protein-bound this should be increased to 50 per cent.

TECHNIQUE. Prepare serial two-fold dilutions in serum peptone-water, in volumes of 1 ml. If blow-out pipettes are used, 2 or 3 two-fold dilutions may be made with the same pipette so long as it is rinsed several times in each. Prepare a control series of dilutions in the same medium from a known solution of the antibiotic. Inoculate both sets of tubes with a standard drop of a suspension of the test organism containing about 10^5 organisms per ml.

The amount of antibiotic in the patient's serum is calculated by multiplying the concentration inhibiting growth in the control series by the dilution of the patient's serum inhibiting growth.

Perhaps the greatest advantage of the method is that it can if necessary be made rapid. Dutton and Elmes (1959) describe a modification of it used in controlling dosage of vancomycin in patients with poor renal function. Dilutions of the serum in broth were heavily inoculated with a staphylococcus and placed on a shaker in the incubator: the result could be read by turbidity within five hours. If a shaker is not available, almost equally rapid growth can be obtained in a water-bath, provided the test is set up in wide-bore tubes ($\frac{5}{8}$ in.) containing only 1 ml. of broth.

Assays of Bactericidal Activity

The tube dilution method can be used for estimating the bactericidal activity of the patient's serum during treatment, a proceeding chiefly of interest in cases of bacterial endo-carditis.

A series of two-fold dilutions are made in suitable medium and heavily inoculated with the organism isolated from the patient's blood. As with bactericidal sensitivity tests, the result is greatly influenced by the size of the inoculum: 10^6 organisms per ml. is recommended. Any tubes showing no growth after overnight incubation are subcultivated on suitable solid medium and any growth compared with that from the control tube plated before incubation. The greatest dilution giving no growth (or less than 10 colonies in the convention of some laboratories) is reported, and serum bactericidal in a dilution of 1 in 4 is considered satisfactory. This test is based on that described by Jawetz (1962) who also discusses its interpretation and value.

Polymyxin Assays

Polymyxins diffuse poorly through agar but satisfactory results can be obtained with both plate and vertical diffusion methods using *Bord. bronchiseptica* and a medium consisting of tryptone-soya broth + 1 per cent polysorbate 80 (Tween 80), and 1·2 per cent agar, and incubating at 27°C.

If they are assayed by the dilution methods, results can be much affected by the medium and the most consistent results are obtained using serum-peptone water and a small inoculum (10^5 organisms per ml.). The complications of assaying sulphomethyl polymyxins are discussed on page 194.

Trimethoprim Assays

Trimethoprim is always administered with sulphamethoxazole and whilst it is possible to determine the dilution of the serum which will inhibit growth, this cannot be converted into μg./ml. of the mixture. The trimethoprim content can be assayed by inactivating the sulphonamide with *p*-aminobenzoic acid. In either case 4 per cent lysed horse blood should be added to a medium of low thymidine content (see p. 462) together with 0·005 per cent *p*-aminobenzoic acid if required. A spore suspension of *B. pumilis* is generally used for plate diffusion assays but *Esch. coli* is satisfactory: the inoculum should be light.

Anti-fungal Drugs

The majority of these can be assayed by the plate diffusion method using glucose-peptone agar with *Sacch. cerevisiae* or *C. albicans* as test organism, or, if the levels are high enough, by the tube dilution method with glucose-peptone broth. 5-fluorocytosine is inactivated by these media and that described on page 463 should be used for this drug.

Assays During Combined Treatment

It is often necessary to perform assays on the serum of patients receiving more than one antibiotic. In some cases levels of both drugs may be required (*e.g.* penicillin and streptomycin during the treatment of endocarditis), but more commonly only the aminoglycoside level is required, usually in patients with poor renal function.

Penicillin, ampicillin and carbenicillin can be inactivated by penicillinase; Newsome (1967) suggested that cephaloridine and possibly cloxacillin and methicillin may also be inactivated by commercial penicillinase. It seems that not only different brands but even different batches from the same manufacturer vary in this respect, and none should be relied upon for this purpose without first proving that the batch in use inactivates the drug concerned rapidly. *B. cereus* 569/H has been shown by Kuwabara and Abraham (1967) to produce both a penicillinase and a cephalosporinase (β-lactamases I and II). The crude

TABLE LV

Suitable Organisms for Assaying Streptomycin, Kanamycin or Gentamicin in the Presence of a Second Drug

Second Drug	Test Organism
Penicillin Ampicillin Carbenicillin	*Staph. aureus* after inactivating with penicillinase.
†Cephaloridine	Resistant *Klebsiella**
†Cloxacillin, methicillin Macrolides Lincomycin Fucidin Novobiocin	*Esch. coli.*
Tetracyclines	Resistant *Staph. aureus**
Polymyxins	*Staph. aureus*
Sulphonamides	*Staph. aureus* after the addition of *p*-aminobenzoic acid.
Trimethoprim	*Staph. aureus* in a medium containing thymidine
Isoniazid, PAS, Ethionamide, Ethambutol, Pyrazinamide, Thiacetazone	*Staph. aureus*

* Strain must be sensitive to the aminoglycoside.
† See above concerning the inactivation of these drugs.

supernatant of a culture of this organism in which the cephalosporinase has been stabilized by the addition of zinc (Sabath and Abraham, 1966) can be used to inactivate all penicillins and cephalosporins (Sabath *et al.*, 1968). Such a preparation is not at present available commercially, but the purified β-lactamase II can be obtained from Whatman Biochemicals.

Trimethoprim is neutralized by thymidine; this can be added to the medium (4 μg./ml.) but most nutrient broth and agar already contain sufficient for this purpose. Sulphonamides are inactivated by the addition of 0·005 per cent of p-aminobenzoic acid but this has no action on trimethoprim.

Distinction between other drugs is usually based on their selective bacteristatic activity. Resistant strains of normally sensitive species should not be used for assays unless it is unavoidable, as resistance is frequently unstable whether it is acquired naturally or artificially in the laboratory. It is preferable to use a naturally resistant species. A list of suitable organisms for assaying the streptomycin group in the presence of other antibiotics is given in Table LV.

The greater diffusibility of penicillin and the relative resistance of *Str. pyogenes* to aminoglycosides make it possible to assay penicillin by the blood agar vertical diffusion method despite the presence of streptomycin or kanamycin.

Polymyxins can be assayed in the presence of an aminoglycoside if the pH of the medium is lowered to 6·0. This can be achieved by adding 1 per cent KH_2PO_4 to the medium recommended on page 482.

REFERENCES

ASSOCIATION OF CLINICAL PATHOLOGISTS (1966). Broadsheet No. 55.

ANDERSON, T. G. (1970). In *Manual of Clinical Microbiology*, p. 299. Ed. Blair, J. E., Lenette, E. H. & Truant, J. P. Bethesda, Md., *American Society for Microbiology*, p. 299.

ANNEAR, D. I. (1968). *Med. J. Aust.* **1,** 444.

BARBER, M. (1964). *J. gen. Microbiol.* **35,** 183.

BARRY, A. L., GARCIA, F. & THRUPP, L. D. (1970). *Amer. J. clin. Path.* **53,** 149.

BAUER, A. W., KIRBY, W. M. M., SHERRIS, J. C. & TURCK, M. (1966). *Amer. J. clin. Path.,* **45,** 493.

BECHTLE, R. M. & SCHERR, G. H. (1958). *Antibiot. & Chemother.* **8,** 599.

BENNETT, J. V., BRODIE, J. L., BENNER, E. J. & KIRBY, W. M. M. (1966). *Appl. Microbiol.* **14,** 170.

BULGER, R. J. & NIELSON, K. (1968). *Appl. Microbiol.* **16,** 890.

BUSHBY, S. R. M. (1969). *Postgrad. med. J.* **45** (Suppl. Nov.) 10.

BUSHBY, S. R. M. & HITCHINGS, G. H. (1968). *Brit. J. Pharmacol.* **33,** 72.

CANETTI, G. & 9 others (1963). *Bull. Wld Hlth Org.* **29,** 565.

CHABBERT, Y. A. & WATERWORTH, P. M. (1965). *J. clin. Path.* **18,** 314.

CLARK, J. (1967). *J. med. Lab. Technol.* **24,** 212.

DARRELL, J. H., GARROD, L. P. & WATERWORTH, P. M. (1968). *J. clin. Path.* **21,** 202.

DAVIES, P. A., DARRELL, J. H., CHANDRAN, K. R. & WATERWORTH, P. M. (1970). In *The Control of Chemotherapy,* p. 49. Ed. Watt, P. J. Edinburgh: Livingstone.

DAVIS, I. (1959). *Med. Technicians Bull. Suppl.* to *U.S. armed Forces med. J.* **10,** 131.

DUTTON, A. A. C. & ELMES, P. C. (1959). *Brit. med. J.* **i,** 1144.

ELEK, S. D. & HILSON, G. R. F. (1954). *J. clin. Path.* **7,** 37.

ERICSSON, H. M. (1960). *Scand. J. clin. Lab. Invest.* **12,** Suppl. 50.

ERICSSON, H. M. & SHERRIS, J. C. (1971). *Acta path. microbiol. scand.* Section B Suppl. 217.

FUJII, R., GROSSMAN, M. & TICKNOR, W. (1961). *Pediatrics* **28,** 662.

FUST, B. & BÖHNI, E. (1961). *Pathologia Microbiol. (Basle)* **24,** 378.

GARROD, L. P. & WATERWORTH, P. M. (1962). *J. clin. Path.* **15,** 328.

GARROD, L. P. & WATERWORTH, P. M. (1969). *J. clin. Path.* **22,** 534.

GILLISSEN, G. & BECHER, E. (1957). *Arch. Hyg. (Berl.)* **141,** 403.

GOTS, J. S. (1945). *Science* **102,** 309.

HALLANDER, H. O., LAURELL, G. & DORNBUSCH, K. (1970). *Scand. J. infect. Dis.* **1,** 169.

HANUS, F. J., SANDS, J. G. & BENNETT, E. O. (1967). *Appl. Microbiol.* **15,** 31.

HARPER, G. J. & CAWSTON, W. C. (1945). *J. Path. Bact.* **57,** 59.

HEATLEY, N. G. (1944). *Biochem. J.* **38,** 61.

HEWITT, J. H., COE, A. W. & PARKER, M. T. (1969). *J. med. Microbiol.* **2,** 443.

HOWIE, J. W. (1962). *Lancet* **i,** 1137.

JAWETZ, E. (1962). *Amer. J. Dis. Child.* **103,** 81.

KUNIN, C. M. & EDMONDSON, W. P. (1968). *Proc. Soc. Exp. Biol. (N.Y.)* **129,** 118.

KUWABARA, S. (1970). *Biochem. J.* **118,** 457.

LIGHTBOWN, J. W. & SULITZEANU, D. (1957). *Bull. Wld Hlth Org.* **17,** 553.

LINE, D. H., POOLE, G. W. & WATERWORTH, P. M. (1970). *Tubercle* **51,** 76.

MITCHISON, D. A. & SPICER, C. C. (1949). *J. gen. Microbiol.* **3,** 184.

NEWSOM, S. W. B. (1967). *Brit. med. J.* **3,** 678.

PEARD, M. C., FLECK, D. G., GARROD, L. P. & WATERWORTH, P. M. (1970). *Brit. med J.* In press.

REPORT (1965). 'Report on the antibiotic sensitivity test trial organized by the Bacteriology Committee of the Association of Clinical Pathologists. *J. clin. Path.* **18,** 1.

SABATH, L. D. & ABRAHAM, E. P. (1966). *Biochem. J.* **98,** 11c.

SABATH, L. D., LODER, P. B., GERSTEIN, D. A. & FINLAND, M. (1968). *Appl. Microbiol.* **16,** 877.

SHADOMY, S. (1969). *Appl. Microbiol.* **17,** 871.

SNELL, N. S. & LEWIS, J. C. (1959). *Antibiot. Chemother.* **6,** 609.

STOKES, E. J. (1968). *Clinical Bacteriology,* Third Edition. London: Arnold. p. 179

TOZER, R. A., BOUTFLOWER, S. & GILLESPIE, W. A. (1966). *Lancet* **1,** 686.

WATERWORTH, P. M. (1962). *J. med. Lab. Technol.* **19,** 163.

WATERWORTH, P. M. (1966). *J. med. Lab. Technol.* **23,** 96.

WATERWORTH, P. M. (1969a). *Postgrad. med. J.* **45** (Suppl. Nov.), 21.

WATERWORTH, P. M. (1969b). *J. med. Lab. Technol.* **26,** 106.

WATERWORTH, P. M. (1971). *Postgrad. med. J.* **47** (Suppl. Feb.), 25.

WOLF, D. A. & HAMBURGER, M. (1962). *J. lab. clin. Med.* **59,** 469.

INDEX

ABORTION, septic, 362
Acetazolamide, 373, 387
Achromycin, *see* tetracycline
Acne vulgaris, 306
Acquired resistance, *see* individual drugs and under drug resistance
Actidione, *see* cycloheximide
Actinobacillus actinomycetem comitans, 314
Actinomyces israeli, 266, 313
Actinomycosis, 313
Actinospectacin, 202, 427
Adicillin, 80
Administration, choice of route of, 268
Aerosporin, *see* polymyxin B
Albamycin, *see* novobiocin
Albamycin T, 225
Albomycin, 226
Albucid, *see* sulphacetamide
Alficetyn, *see* chloramphenicol
Amantadines, 443
Amidase, 70
Amidozol, *see* sulphasomizole
p-Aminobenzoic acid, 462
7-Amino-cephalosporanic acid, 70
Aminoglycosides, 115-131
  acquired resistance, 119
  anti-bacterial action, 117
  chemical properties, 116
  clinical application, 122
  cross-resistance, 120
  pH, effect of, 117
  pharmaceutical preparations, 129
  pharmacology, 121
  toxicity, 121
6-Aminopenicillanic acid, 70
Aminosidine, 121
Ammonium chloride, 373
Amoebiasis, 125, 355
Amphomycin, 303
Amphotericin B, **237,** 286, 387
  prophylaxis with, 240
Ampicillin, antibacteral activity, 81
  bacterial inactivation, 81
  bile, passage into, 82, 349
  C.S.F., passage into, 82, 325
  clinical application, 83
  foetal circulation, passage into, 360
  hypersensitivity, 83
  intrathecal, 327
  pharmacology, 81

Ampicillin—*cont.*
  pivaloyloxymethyl ester, 81
  toxicity, 82
  treatment of:
    chronic bronchitis, 341
    typhoid fever, 350
Anaerobic streptococcal infections, 311
Anaflex, *see* polynoxyline
Ancillin, *see* diphenicillin
Antagonism, antibacterial, 40, 170, **271,** 325, 472
Anthrax, 306
Antifungal antibiotics, 235-247
  laboratory control, 463, 482
  pharmaceutical preparations, 248
  prophylaxis with, 240
Antiseptics, local application of, 304
Aristamid, *see* sulphasomidine
Arthritis, septic, 319
Aspergillosis, 237, 239
Assays, 475-484
  anti-fungal, 482
  bactericidal, 481
  combined therapy, 482
  diffusion methods, 477
  fish-spine method, 478
  indications for, 475
  medium, 480
  pH, control of, 477
  polymyxin, 482, 484
  rapid method, 481
  stock solutions, 467, 476
  test organisms, 476, 483
  trimethoprim, 482
  tube dilution method, 480
  vertical diffusion method, 479
Asulfidine, *see* sulphasalazine
Aureomycin, *see* chlortetracycline
Avlosulphon, *see* Dapsone
Azopyrin, *see* sulphasalazine

B663, 416
Bacitracin, antibacterial activity, 185
  clinical application, 186
  eye ointment, 392
  local application, 303
  mode of action, 185
  with neomycin, 303
  source, 8, 185
  Str. pyogenes, identification of by, 186
  toxicity, 186

Bacitracin A, 185
Bacitracin B, 185
Bacitracin C, 185
Bacteriaemic shock, 285, 363
Bactericidal drugs, 271, 288, 472
    and *see* mode of action under
    individual drugs
Bacteriocines, 203
Bacteroides spp., 312, 362
Bactylan, 402
BAY b 5097, *see* clotrimazole
Bejel, 424
Benethamine penicillin, 59, 421
Benzathine penicillin, 59, 421
Benzimidazole derivatives, 441
Berkfurin, *see* nitrofurantoin
Bidizole, *see* sulphasomizole
Bile, passage of drugs into, 349
Biliary tract infections, 348
Blastomycosis, 237
Blood dyscrasias, due to:
    chloramphenicol, 140
    sulphonamides, 24
Boils, 309
Bones, infections of, 316
Bowel flora, suppression of, 124,125,
    356
Breast abscess, 365
Brocillin, *see* propicillin
Bronchiectasis, 342
Bronchitis, acute, 339
    chronic, 339
Bronchopneumonia, 343
Broxil, *see* phenethicillin
Brucellosis, 297
Brulidine, *see* dibromo-propamidine
    isethionate
Burns, 314
4-Butoxy-4-dimethyl-amino diphenyl-
    thiourea, 416

Calcipen V, *see* phenoxymethyl peni-
    cillin
Candicidin, 239
Candida albicans superinfection, 156,
    347, 354
Candidiasis, intestinal, 354
    local treatment, 306
    neonatal, 367
    oral, 347
    septicaemia, 236, 238, 286
    treatment with, amphotericin B,
        237, 286
        nystatin, 236
    vaginal, 365
Capreomycin, 183, 404
Carbenicillin, 84
Carbomycin, 177
Cardelmycin, *see* novobiocin

Carriers, nasal, 309, 336
    typhoid, 352
Catenulin, 117
Catheters, intravenous, 310
Cathocin, *see* novobiocin
Cathomycin, *see* novobiocin
Celbenin, *see* methicillin
Celesticetin, 211
Cellophane transfer sensitivity tests,
    471
Cephalexin, 92
Cephaloglycin, 92
Cephaloridine, 89
    acquired resistance, 93, 461
Cephalosporinase, 93, 483
Cephalosporins, 86-93
    acquired resistance, 93
    pharmaceutical preparations, 94
Cephalosporin C, 86
Cephalosporin N, *see* adicillin
Cephalosporin P, 86, 206
Cephalothin, 87
    acquired resistance, 93
Ceporex, *see* cephalexin
Ceporin, *see* cephaloridine
Cerebrospinal fluid, drugs levels at-
    tained in, 326
    (*see* also individual drugs)
Cetrimide, 304
Chancroid, 433
Chemotherapy, factors governing
    choice, 265, 369
    general principles, 263
Children, dosage in, 267
Chlamydia, 447
Chloramphenicol, 132-145
    absorption, 137
    acquired resistance to, 135, 249
    administration, oral, 137
        parenteral, 138
        local, 303
    antibacterial activity, 133
    aqueous humour, passage into, 138
    bile, passage into, 139, 349
    cerebrospinal fluid, passage into,
        138
    chemistry, 132
    clinical applications, 143
    cross-resistance, 136, 250
    distribution, 138
    dosage, 137, 143, 144
    excretion, 138
    eye ointment, 392
    foetal circulation, passage into,
        138, 361
    inactivation of, bacterial, 135, 249
    infants, excretion in, 143, 276
    mode of action, 135
    optic neuritis, 143

Chloramphenicol—*cont.*
  pharmaceutical preparations, 145
  source of, 132
  toxicity, alimentary tract, 139
    ' grey syndrome ' in infants, 142
    marrow aplasia, 140
  typhoid fever, 144
Chloramphenicol palmitate, 137
Chloramphenicol succinate, 138
Chlorhexidine, 304
Chloromycetin, *see* chloramphenicol
Chloroquin, in amoebic hepatitis, 355
Chlortetracycline, 148
Cholera, 356
Ciba 1906, *see* thiambutosine
Cicatrin, 303
Cidomycin, *see* gentamicin
Clindamycin, 217
Clioquinol, 304
Clomocycline, 159
Clostridium spp., sensitivities, 56, 266, 311
Clotrimazole, 243
Cloxacillin, 76
Coccidioidomycosis, 237
Cold, common, 345
Colicines, 203
Coliform infections, meningitis, 332
  septicaemia, 284
  superficial, 310
Colistin, *see* polymyxin E
Colomycin, *see* polymyxin E
ColyMycin, *see* polymyxin E
Combined sensitivity tests, 469-475
Combined therapy, antagonism, 40, 170, **271**, 325, 474
  brucellosis, 297
  endocarditis, subacute bacterial, 288
  indications for, 270
  synergy, 17, 45, 168, 208, **273**, 289, 463, 474
Commercial combinations, 240, 273
Compocillin VK, *see* phenoxymethyl penicillin
Conjunctivitis, 291
Consulid, *see* sulphachlorpyridazine
Conteben, *see* thiacetazone
Corticosteroids, for Herxheimer reactions, 422
  meningitis, 327, 412
  typhoid fever, 350
Corynebacterium diphtheriae, 338
Cosmetics, antibiotics in, 304
Cross-resistance, 250
  and *see* individual drugs
Croup, 339
Cryptococcosis, 237, 243
Crystalluria, sulphonamide, 22

Crystapen V, *see* phenoxymethyl penicillin
Cycloheximide, 235
Cycloserine, 204, 461
  tuberculosis, 404
  urinary infections, 205, 370
Cylinder plate assays, 478

Dalacin C, *see* clindamycin
Dapsone, 416
Declomycin, *see* demethylchlortetracycline
Demethylchlortetracycline, 157
Dental extractions, cover for, 295
Deodorants, antibiotics in, 304
Desensitization, PAS, 402
  streptomycin, 110
Dialysibility of drugs, 279
Diaminodiphenyl sulphone, 416
Dibromo - propamidine isethianate, 304
Dicloxacillin, 78
Diphenicillin, 79
Diphtheria, 338
Discs, sensitivity test, 452, 455
Distaquaine V, *see* phenoxymethyl penicillin
Ditophal, 416
Dosage 268, 276
  children, 276
  intrathecal, 327
  meningitis, 331
  renal disease, 277
  and *see* individual drugs
Doxycycline, 160
Drug-dependent bacteria, 248
Drug-destroying bacteria, 249
Drug resistance, animals, in, 255
  associated changes in sensitivity, 251
  clinical problem, 257
  combined therapy, 269
  cross-resistance, 250
  episomal transfer of, 254
  Gram-negative bacilli, 260
  infectious, 254
  mode of origin, 251
  Myco. tuberculosis, 403, 413
  nature of, 248
  N. gonorrhoeae, 259, 425
  N. meningitidis, 259
  penicillinase, 249
  prevention of, 270, 274, 410
  stability of, 249
  Staph. aureus, 250, 251, 257
  Str. faecalis, 259
  Str. pneumoniae, 149, 169, 259
  Str. pyogenes, 149, 169, 259
  Str. viridans, 259

Drug resistance—*cont.*
 transduction of, 253
 transfer of, 254
Drug-tolerant bacteria, 248, 252
Durenate, *see* sulphamethoxydiazine
Dysentery, amoebic, 355
 bacillary, 355

E 129, *see* ostreogrycin
Ecomytrin, 303
Elkosin, *see* sulphasomidine
Emetine, in amoebic dysentery, 355
Endocarditis, 286-297
 cause unknown, 293
 combined therapy for, 288
 Coxiella burneti, 293
 Haemophilus spp., 292
 laboratory control, 295, 469, 481
 prophylaxis, 295
 Spitz-Holter valves, 292
 staphylococcal, 291
 Str. faecalis, 288
 Str. viridans, 287
 vancomycin, 232, 294
Entamoeba histolytica, 125, 355
Enteric fever, 350
Enterocolitis, staphylococcal, 353
Erysipeloid of Rosenbach, 306
Erysipelothrix rhusiopathiae, 266, 292
Erythema serpens, 306
Erythrasma, 308
Erythrocin, *see* erythromycin
Erythromycin, 166-175
 absorption, 171
 acquired resistance, 168, 253, 258
 administration, oral, 171
 local instillation, 171
 parenteral, 171
 antagonism with other macrolides, 170
 with lincomycin, 170
 antibacterial activity, 167
 aqueous humour, passage into, 173
 bile, passage into, 173
 cerebrospinal fluid, passage into, 173
 chemistry, 166
 clinical application, 177
 cross-resistance, 136, 170
 dissociated resistance, 170
 distribution, 172
 estolate, 171, 174
 excretion, 173
 glucoheptonate, 171
 lactobionate, 171
 liver damage, caused by, 174
 mode of action, 168

Erythromycin—*cont.*
 pH, effect of, 167
 pharmaceutical preparations, 179
 proprionyl ester, 171
 source of, 166
 stearate, 171
 synergy with penicillin, 168
 toxicity, 174
Escherichia coli, sensitivities, 266, 370
Eskacillin, *see* phenoxymethyl penicillin
Ethambutol, 409
Ethionamide, 408
Etisul, *see* ditophal
Eye, administration:
 dosage, 391
 drops, 391
 intra-ocular penetration of drugs, 385
 ointments, 392
 sub-conjunctival injections, 389
 infections of, fungus, 393
 gonococcal, 392
 herpes simplex, 395, 445
 Koch-Weeks bacillus, 392
 Morax-Axenfeld bacillus, 392
 post-operative, 396
 Ps. aeruginosa, 393, 397
 superficial, 391
 trachoma, 398
 prophylaxis, 396

Famotine, 444
Fanasil, *see* sulfadoxine
Flagyl, *see* metronidazole
Floxapen, *see* flucloxacillin
Flucloxacillin, 78
5-Fluorocytosine, 242, 463, 482
Foetal circulation, passage of drugs through, 361
Folic acid metabolism, 43
Framycetin, administration, 121, 124
 antibacterial activity, 117
 acquired resistance, 119
 chemistry, 116
 clinical applications, 124
 cross-resistance, 120
 nasal carriers, 124
 pharmaceutical preparations, 129
 pharmacology, 121
 source, 116
 toxicity, 121
Framyspray, 304
Fucidin, acquired resistance, 208, 210
 antagonism with other antibiotics, 208
 antibacterial activity, 207
 chemistry, 206

Fucidin—*cont.*
  clinical application, 210
  metabolic effects, 210
  pharmacology, 209
  synergy with penicillin, 208
  toxicity, 209
Fulcin Forte, *see* griseofulvin
Fumagillin, 355
Fungi, antibiotics active against, 235-245
Fungicidin, *see* nystatin
Fungizone, *see* amphotericin **B**
Furadantin, *see* nitrofurantoin
Furan, *see* nitrofurantoin
Furazolidone, 39, 350
Furoxone, *see* furazolidone
Fusidic acid, 206

Gabbromycina, *see* aminosidine
Gantanol, *see* sulphamethoxazole
Gantrisin, *see* sulphafurazole
Garamycin, *see* gentamicin
Gas gangrene, 311
Gastric surgery, antibiotic cover for, 348
Gastro-enteritis, infantile, 353
Gentacin, *see* gentamicin
Gentamicin, acquired resistance, 126
  antibacterial activity, 118, 126
  clinical applications, 127, 285, 316, 332, 393
  cross-resistance, 126
  dosage, 127, 129
  pH, effect of, 127
  pharmaceutical preparations, 129
  pharmacology, 127
  toxicity, 128
Giardiasis, 36
Gonococcal ophthalmia, 392
Gonorrhoea, 425
  proctitis, 430
  re-treatment, 429
Gramicidin, 183
Graneodin, 303
Granuloma inguinale, 434
Grey syndrome, 142
Griseofulvin, 244
Griseovin, *see* griseofulvin

Haemophilus spp., in bronchiectasis, 342
  bronchitis, 339
  drug-resistant, 150
  endocarditis, 292
  eyes, 392
  meningitis, 330
  sensitivities, 43, 266
Haemophilus ducreyi, 433
Hair, fungal infection of, 244, 307

Halquinol, 304
Hamycin, 239
Heart surgery, cover for, 297
Helenine, 9, 442
Helvolic acid, 206
Hepatic failure, 357
Hepatitis, amoebic, 355
Herpes, 395, 445
Herxheimer reaction, in syphilis, 421
Hetacillin, 83
Hexamine, 34
Hexamine mandelate, 35
Histoplasmosis, 237
Humatin, *see* paromomycin
Hydroxymycin, 117
Hyperbaric oxygen, 312, 362
Hypersensitivity reactions, *see* individual drugs

Icipen V, *see* phenoxymethyl penicillin
Idoxuridine, 445
IDU, *see* idoxuridine
5 IDUR, *see* idoxuridine
Ilosone, *see* erythromycin
Ilotycin, *see* erythromycin
Imperacin, *see* oxytetracycline
Impetigo contagiosa, 304
Impetigo neonatorum, 305
Inactivation of antibiotics, bacterial, 249
Incompatibility of drugs, 279
Infectious resistance, 254
Influenza, 345, 443, 444
Interferon, 441
Intra-ocular drug concentrations, 388
Intrathecal injections, 326
Isoniazid, 402
  intrathecal, 412
Isoquinolines, 444

Joints, infection of, 316

Kanamycin, acquired resistance, 119
  administration, 125
  antibacterial activity, 117
  bowel flora, suppression of, 124, 357
  chemistry, 117
  clinical application, 124
  cross-resistance, 104, 120
  dosage, 129
  intraperitoneal, 124
  pH, effect of, 117
  pharmaceutical preparations, 129
  pharmacology, 121
  source, 8, 116
  toxicity, 121
Kannasyn, *see* kanamycin

Kantrex, *see* kanamycin
Keflex, *see* cephalexin
Keflin, *see* cephalothin
Kemicetine, *see* chlorampenicol
Keratitis, herpes, 395, 445
Kirby-Bauer method, 458
Koch-Weeks bacillus, 392
Klebsiella pneumoniae pnuemonia, 343
Klebsiella spp., 266

Laboratory control, 269, 295, 451 *et seq.*
Labour, antibiotics in, 359
Lederkyn, *see* sulphamethoxypyri-dazine
Ledermycin, *see* demethylchlortetra-cycline
Leptospirosis, 435
Leprosy, 415
Leucomycin, 170
Lincocin, *see* lincomycin
Lincomycin, acquired resistance, 213
    antibacterial activity, 212
    chemistry, 211
    7-chlorolincomycin, 217
    clinical application, 216
    C.S.F., passage into, 215
    cross-resistance, 213
    dosage, 217
    mode of action, 214
    pharmacology, 215
    toxicity, 216
Liquor amnii, antibiotics in, 360
Listeria monocytogenes, meningitis due to, 333
    sensitivities, 266
Local application, antiseptics, 304
    burns, 315
    cavities, 281
    choice of drugs, 281, 302
    dangers of, 282
    in infections due to:
        Ps. aeruginosa, 303, 315
        Staph. aureus, 303, 304
Lymecycline, 158
Lymphogranuloma venereum, 433
Lysostaphin, 219

Macrolides, 166, 179
Madribon, *see* sulphadimethoxine
Magmilor, *see* nifuratel
Magnamycin, *see* carbomycin
Malaria, 26
Mandelamine, 35
Mandelic acid, 34
Marboran, *see* methisazone
Marfanil, 31
M and B 693, *see* sulphapyridine

M and B 7714, 447
Megaclor, *see* clomocycline
Meleney's gangrene, 313
Memotine, 444
Meningitis, initial treatment, 327
    coliform, 332
    cryptococcal, 237, 243
    Haemophilus, 330
    Listeria monocytogenes, 333
    meningococcal, 328
    pneumococcal, 330
    Ps. aeruginosa, 332
    staphyloccocal, 333
    streptococcal, 333
    tuberculous, 411
Mercury resistance, 253, 258
Methacycline, 159
Methenamine, *see* hexamine
Methenamine mandelate, *see* hex-amine mandelate
Methicillin, acquired resistance, 75, 460
    antibacterial activity, 74
    chemistry, 74
    hypersensitivity, 76
    mode of action, 57
    pharmacology, 75
    resistant staphylococci, 75, 460
    salt, effect of, 75, 406
    toxicity, 76
Methionine, 373
Methisazone, 446, 447
6-Methyleneoxytetracycline, *see* methacycline
Metronidazole, 35, 432
Microsporum audouini, 244
Midicel, *see* sulphamethoxypyri-dazine
Mikamycin, 187
Minimum inhibitory concentrations, 266
Minocycline, 161
Morax-Axenfeld bacillus, eye infec-tions, 392
Mouth, infections of, 347
Mucoviscidosis, 342
Muramic acid, 57
Myambutol hydrochloride, *see* eth-ambutol
Mycifradin, *see* neomycin
Mycivin, *see* lincomycin
Mycobacterium tuberculosis, ac-quired resistance, 403, 413
    capreomycin, 404
    cycloserine, 404
    ethambutol, 409
    ethionamide, 408
    isoniazid, 402
    kanamycin, 405

Mycobacterium tuberculosis—*cont.*
  PAS, 400
  pyrazinamide, 408
  streptomycin, 112, 400
  tetracyclines, 406
  thioacetazone, 407
  thiocarbanilides, 409
  viomycin, 406
Mycoplasma pneumoniae, 344
Mycoses, amphotericin B, 237
  candicidin, 239
  clotrimazole, 243
  cycloheximide, 235
  5-fluorocytosine, 242
  griseofulvin, 244
  hamycin, 239
  nystatin, 236
  pimaricin, 239
  prophylaxis, 240
  saramycetin, 242
  trichomycin, 240
Mycostatin, *see* nystatin
Myprozine, *see* pimaricin

Nafcillin, 79
Nails, fungus infection of, 244, 308
Nalidixic acid, 36, 370
Nasal carriers, 303, 329, 336
Nasal infections, chronic, 336
Naseptin, 304
Natamycin, *see* pimaricin
Negram, *see* nalidixic acid
Neisseria gonorrhoeae, sensitivities,
    266, 425
  drug-resistant, 259, 425
Neisseria meningitidis, carriers, 329
  drug-resistant, 259
  meningitis, 328
  sensitivities, 266
Neomin, *see* neomycin
Neomycin:
  acquired resistance, 119
  administration:
    aerosol, 123
    intraperitoneal, 124
    intravesical, 124
    local application, 123, 303
    oral, 123
    pH, effect of, 117
    pharmaceutical preparations,
      129, 303
    sub-conjunctival, 391
  antibacterial activity, 117
  bacitracin, with, 123, 303
  bowel flora, suppression of, 123,
    356
  chemistry, 116
  chlorhexidine, with, 123, 304
  clinical application, 122

Neomycin—*cont.*
  cross-resistance, 104, 120
  pharmacology, 121
  source, 8, 115
  toxicity, 121
  treatment of:
    eye infections, 391, 392
    infantile gastro-enteritis, 123, 353
    intestinal infections, 123
    nasal carriers, 123
Neomycin A, 116
Neomycin B, 116
Neomycin C, 116
Neonatal infections, eyes, 392
  generalized, 366
  thrush, 366
Nifuratel, 432
Nitrofurantoin, 40
Nitrofurazone, 38
Nivemycin, *see* neomycin
Nocardiosis, 26
Novobiocin, 220-226
  absorption, 222
  acquired resistance, 222
  administration:
    oral, 222
    parenteral, 223
  antibacterial activity, 221
  bile, passage into, 223, 349
  cerebrospinal fluid, passage into,
    223
  chemistry, 220
  clinical application, 225
  combined with other antibiotics,
    225
  distribution, 223
  excretion, 223
  mode of action, 221
  pH, effect of, 222
  pharmaceutical preparations, 226
  plasma binding, 222
  source, 8, 220
  toxicity, 223
Nystatin, 236
  prophylactic use, 240
  with tetracycline, 240

Oleandomycin, 166, 170, **175**
Oral flora, effect of penicillin on, 55,
    296
Orbenin, *see* cloxacillin
Orisulf, *see* sulphaphenazole
Osteomyelitis, acute, 316
  chronic, 319
Ostreogrycin, 187
Otitis media, 338
Oxacillin, 77
Oxamycin, *see* cycloserine
Oxytetracycline, 147

PAM, 421, 424
Para-aminosalicylic acid, *see* PAS
Paratyphoid fever, 352
Paromomycin, acquired resistance, 119
  amoebiasis, 125
  antibacterial activity, 117
  bowel flora, suppression of, 125, 357
  chemistry, 117
  clinical application, 125
  cross-resistance, 120
  gastro-intestinal infections, 125, 353
  pharmaceutical preparations, 129
  pharmacology, 121
  source, 8, 116
  toxicity, 121
Parotitis, 348
PAS, 400, 410
  enteric-coated, 402
Pasteurella septica, 266, 311
Pecilocin, 308
Penbritin, *see* ampicillin
Penicillins, 53-86
  abnormal resistance to, 55
  absorption:
    benzyl, 58
    phenoxy, 61
  acid-resistant, 61, 71
  acquired resistance:
    drug-destroying, 249, 250
    drug-tolerant, 55, 248
  administration:
    intrathecal, 63
    oral, 61
    parenteral, 58
    snuff, 336
    sub-conjunctival, 390
  amidase, 70
  antagonism with, 271, 325, 472
  antibacterial activity:
    benzyl, 54, 56
    phenoxy, 61, 72
  bactericidal action of, 55, 472
  basophil degranulation test, 66
  benethamine, 59, 421
  benzathine, 59, 421
  bile, passage into, 58, 349
  broad spectrum, 80
  cerebrospinal fluid, passage into, 58, 326
  chemistry, 53, 71
  chewing gum, 347
  clinical application, 62
  comparative activities, 72
  dicloxacillin, 78
  dosage, 62
  excretion, 58
  flucloxacillin, 78

Penicillins—*cont.*
  foetal circulation, passage into, 361
  guinea-pig toxicity, 64
  haemolytic anaemia due to, 64
  hypersensitivity, 64, 294, 423
    tests for, 65
  inactivation of, bacterial, 54, 249
  isoxazolyl, 76
  inoculum size, effect of, 460
  long-acting forms, 59
  methicillin, 74
  mode of action, 55
  nephritis due to, 64
  oral flora, effect on, 55, 296
  penicillinase-resistant, 73 *et seq.*
  penicilloyl-polylysine, 65
  pharmaceutical preparations, 68, 71, 93
  pharmacology, 58
  phenbenicillin, 73
  phenethicillin, 73
  phenoxymethyl penicillin, 61
  phenoxy penicillins, 71
  plasma binding, 73
  procaine, 59
  probenecid, with, 59
  prophylactic, 337
  propicillin, 73
  Purapen G, 66
  sensitization reactions, 64
  snuff, 336
  stability, 54
  synergy with, 168, 208, 273, 473
  synthetic, 70
  toxicity, 63
  unit, definition of, 53
  zone, phenomenon, paradoxical, 55
Penicillin F, 53
Penicillin G, *see* penicillin (benzyl)
Penicillin K, 53
Penicillin V, *see* phenoxymethyl penicillin
Penicillin X, 53
Penicillinase, 483
Penicillinase-producing organisms, 54, 249, 253
Penidural, 60
Penspek, *see* phenbenicillin
Peptide antibiotics, 182-199
Peptolides, 187
Pertussis, 342
pH, effect of, 373, 454
  and *see* individual drugs
Pharyngitis, acute, 336
Phenbenicillin, 73
Phenethicillin, 73
Phenoxymethyl penicillin, 61
Pimaricin, 239

Pimafucin, *see* pimaricin
Pinta, 424
Plasma binding, *see* individual drugs
Pneumonia, broncho-, 343
  Kl. pneumoniae (Friedlander's), 343
  lobar, 343
  Mycoplasma pneumoniae, 344
  pneumococcal, 343
  staphylococcal, 345
Polybactrin, 303
Polyenes, 236
Polymyxins, 187-199
  absorption, 191, 195
  acquired resistance, 191
  administration:
    intrathecal, 197
    local application, 197, 303
    oral, 198
    parenteral, 191
    sub-conjunctival, 391
  antibacterial activity, 189
  bowel flora, suppression of, 198
  cerebrospinal fluid, passage into, 197, 326
  chemistry, 188
  clinical application, 196
  distribution, 191
  dosage, 199
  excretion, 191, 196
  methane sulphonates of, *see* sulphomethyl derivatives
  mode of action, 190
  pharmaceutical preparations, 199
  pharmacological effects, 192
  plasma binding, 190
  selective media, use in, 190
  source, 8, 187
  sulphomethyl derivatives, 193
  synergy with:
    sulphonamides, 45, 191
    trimethoprim, 45, 191
  toxicity, 192, 194
  unit, definition of, 188
  Vibrio cholerae, identification of, 191
Polymyxins, A-E, 188
Polynoxylin, 304
Post-nasal infection, 336
Prasinomycin, 226
Pristinamycin, 187
Probenecid, 59
Prontosil, 3
Prophylaxis, dental, 295
  eye surgery, 396
  gastric surgery, 348
  heart surgery, 297
  N. meningitidis, 329
  with penicillin, 337

Prophylaxis—*cont.*
  Str. pyogenes, 337
  tuberculosis, 413
  urinary tract, 373, 380
Propicillin, 73
Prostaphlin, *see* oxacillin
Proteus spp., choice of drug, 86
  meningitis, 332
  sensitivities, 86, 266
  septicaemia, 285
  superficial infections, 310, 315
  synergy, polymyxin and sulphonamides, 17, 191
    polymyxin and trimethoprim, 46, 191
Pseudomonas aeruginosa:
  burns, 314
  eyes, 393, 397
  meningitis, 332
  sensitivities, 266
  septicaemia, 284
  superficial infections, 314
  wounds, 310
Puerperal fever, 361
Purapen G, 66
Pyopen, *see* carbenicillin
Pyostacine, *see* pristinamycin
Pyrazinamide, 408, 413
Pyrimethamine, 50
Pyrrolidinomethyl tertracycline, *see* rolitetracycline

Q fever, 293
Quinacillin, 79
Quinoderm, *see* quinolines
Quinolines, 304
Quinolor, *see* quinolines

Rat-bite fever, 435
Regression lines, 458
Relapsing fever, 434
Renal failure, 277, 383
Resistance transfer factors, 254
Reverin, *see* rolitetracycline
Rifamide, 227
Rifampicin, 228
  leprosy, 416
  tuberculosis, 405
Rifamycin, 227
Rifandin, *see* rifampicin
Rifocin, *see* rifamide
Rikospray antibiotic, 304
Rimactane, *see* rifampicin
Rimatadine, 444
Ringworm, scalp, 245, 307
Ristocetin, 234
Rolitetracycline, 158
Rondomycin, *see* methacycline
Rovamycin, *see* spiramycin

Salazopyrin, *see* sulphasalazine
Salmonella spp., gastro-intestinal infections, 352
  meningitis, 332
  sensitivities, 266
Saramycetin, 242
Scarlet fever, 337
Sensitization by local treatment, 281
Sensitivity tests, bacterial, 452 *et seq.*
  bactericidal, 469 *et seq.*
  cellophane transfer, 471
  cephaloridine resistance, 461
  choice of drugs, 465, 472
  combined action, bactericidal, 469
    bacteristatic, 463, 474
  control cultures, 457, 458
  diffusion methods, 452
  discs, 455
  ditch plates, 452
  Ericsson method, 459
  factors influencing results, 452 *et seq.*
  fungal, 463
  ' Half Chess Board ', 470
  inoculum size, 454, 462, 470
  interpretation, 457, 474
  Kirby-Bauer method, 458
  mandelamine, 467
  medium, effect of, 452
  methicillin, 460
  Myco. tuberculosis, 468
  penicillinase - forming staphylococci, 454, 460
  pH, effect of, 453
  polymyxins, 462
  pre-diffusion, effect of, 456
  primary culture, 463
  Proteus spp., 461
  rapid methods, 464
  regression lines, 458
  stock solutions, 467, 472
  sulphonamides, 462
  trimethoprim, 462
  tube dilution method, 467, 469
  velvet pad replica plate, 471
Septicaemia, 284-301
  bacteriaemic shock, 285, 363
  coliform, 284
  C. albicans, 238, 243, 286
  Staph. aureus, 284
  Str. pyogenes, 284
Septic shock, 285, 363
Seromycin, *see* cycloserine
Shigella spp., sensitivities, 266
Sigmamycin, 176
Silver nitrate, 315
Sinusitis, acute, 336
Skin infections, 303
Snuff, penicillin, 336

Soframycin, *see* framycetin
Spectinomycin, *see* actinospectacin
Spiramycin, 166, 170, **176**
Spitz-Holter valves, 292
Staphcillin, *see* methicillin
Staphylococcines, 203
Staphylococcus albus, endocarditis, 291
Staphylococcus aureus, in breast abscess, 365
  in burns, 314
  in enterocolitis, 353
  in meningitis, 333
  in neonatal infections, 366
  in septicaemia, 284
  combined therapy against, 270, 291
  drug-resistant, 250, 251, 257
  sensitivities, 266
    bacitracin, 119, 185
    methicillin, 75, 460
Staphylomycin, 187
Statolon, 443
Stevens-Johnson syndrome, 23
Stokes method, 463
Stomach, 348
Stomatitis, 347
Streptobacillus moniliformis, 435
Streptococcus faecalis
  drug-resistance, 259
  endocarditis. 288
  sensitivities, 266, 289
Streptococcus pneumoniae, bronchitis, 339
  drug-resistance, 149, 169, 259
  meningitis, 330
  otitis media, 338
  pneumonia, 343
  sensitivities, 266
Streptococcus pyogenes, bacitracin, sensitivity, 186
  burns, 314
  drug-resistance. 149, 169, 259
  meningitis, 333
  otitis media, 338
  pharyngitis, 336
  prophylaxis, 337
  septicaemia, 284
  sensitivities, 266
Streptococcus viridans, endocarditis, 287
  drug-resistance, 259, 288, 295
Streptogramin, 187
Streptolin, *see* streptomycin
Streptomycin, 98-114
  absorption, 105
  acquired resistance, 103, 252, 254
  administration, 105
    intrathecal, 105
  anaerobiosis, effect of, 100

Streptomycin—*cont.*
  antibacterial activity, 99
  bactericidal activity, 100
  bile, passage into, 107, 349
  cerebrospinal fluid, passage into, 105, 326
  chemistry, 98
  clinical application, 112
  combined treatment with, 112
  cross-resistance, 104
  dependence, bacterial, 103
  desensitization, 110
  dihydrostreptomycin, 112
  distribution, 106
  dosage, 113
  eighth nerve damage caused by, 107
  excretion, 106
  foetal circulation, passage into, 106, 361
  hypersensitivity, 110
  inactivation of, 100
    bacterial, 100
  mode of action, 100
  neuromuscular blockade, 111
  pH, effect of, 100
  pharmaceutical preparations, 113
  source, 98
  toxicity, 107
Streptomycin pantothenate, 110
Streptonivicin, *see* novobiocin
Streptoquaine, *see* streptomycin
Streptothricin, 98
Sulfadoxine, 30, 416
Sulfamylon, 31, 315
Sulfurine, *see* sulphamethizole
Sulphomyxin sodium, *see* polymyxin B
Sulphonamides, 12-33
  absorption, 17
  acquired resistance, 16, 260
  alimentary tract, local action in, 29
  antibacterial action, 12 and Table II *facing* page 14
  bile, passage into, 22
  blood dyscrasias due to, 24
  blood levels, 19
  cerebrospinal fluid, passage into 20, 326
  clinical applications, 25
  comparative activity, 14 and Table II *facing* page 14
  conjugation, 18
  discovery, 3
  dosage, 31
  embryopathy, 25
  excretion, 20
  foetal circulation, passage into, 20
  haemolytic anaemia, caused by, 25

Sulphonamides—*cont.*
  hypersensitivity reactions, 23
  tests for, 24
  inoculum size, effect of, 378, 462
  jaundice, caused by, 25
  local application, 281, 336
  long-acting, 29
  mode of action, 15
  parenteral administration, 17
  pH, effect of, 18
  pharmaceutical preparations, 31
  phthalyl sulphathiazole, 29
  plasma binding, 18
  polyarteritis nodosa, caused by, 23
  renal complications due to, 22
  salicylates, with, 31
  sensitivity tests, 462
  solubilities of, 22
  Stevens-Johnson syndrome, 23
  succinyl sulphathiazole, 29
  sulfadoxine, 30, 416
  sulfamylon, 31
  sulfisoxazole, *see* sulphafurazole
  sulphacetamide, 27
  sulphachlorpyridazine, 29
  sulphadiazine, 27
  sulphadimethoxine, 30
  sulphadimetine, *see* sulphasomidine
  sulphadimidine, 28
  sulphafurazole, 29
  sulphaguanidine, 29
  sulphamerazine, 27
  sulphamethazine, *see* sulphadimidine
  sulphamethizole, 29
  sulphamethoxazole, 29
  sulphamethoxydiazine, 30
  sulphamethoxypyridazine, 30
  sulphamezathine, *see* sulphadimidine
  sulphanilamide, 27
  sulphaphenazole, 30
  sulphapyridine, 27
  sulphasalazine, 31
  sulphasomidine, 29
  sulphasomizole, 29
  sulphasuxidine, *see* succinyl sulphathiazole
  sulphasymazine, 30
  sulphathalidine, *see* phthalyl sulphathiazole
  sulphathiazole, 27
  synergy, polymyxin, 17
    pyrimethamine, 26
    trimethoprim, 17, 463
  toxic effects, 22
  toxoplasmosis, 26
  triple sulphonamide mixture, 28

Sulphones, 415
Sulphormethoxine, *see* sulfadoxine
Sycosis barbae, 305
Symmetrel, 444
Synergy, antibacterial, 17, 45, 168, 208, **273,** 289, 463, 473
Synnematin B, *see* adicillin
Syphilis, 420

T.B.I., *see* thioacetazone
Terramycin, *see* oxytetracycline
Tetracyclines, 147-163
  absorption, 150
  acquired resistance, 149, 250, 253, 254
  administration, oral, 150
    parenteral, 152
  antibacterial activity, 148
  bile, passage into, 152, 349
  bone, deposition in, 152
  calcium binding of, 151
  cerebrospinal fluid, passage into, 152, 326
  chemistry, 148
  chlortetracycline, 148
  clinical applications, 162
  clomocycline, 159
  comparative activity of, 148
  cross-resistance, 250
  demethylchlortetracycline, 157
  α-6-deoxytetracycline, 160
  diarrhoea, caused by, 155
  distribution, 151
  doxycycline, 160
  excretion, 152
  foetal circulation, passage into, 152, 361
  liver damage, caused by, 154
  lymecycline, 158
  methacycline, 159
  6-methylene oxytetracycline, 159
  minocycline, 161
  mode of action, 150
  oxytetracycline, 148
  pH, effect of, 453
  pharmaceutical preparations, 162
  phosphate, addition of, 151
  plasma binding, 151
  pregnancy, use in, 152, 154,
  pyrrolidinomethyl tetracycline, 158
  rolitetracycline, 158
  sources of, 8, 147
  staphylococcal enterocolitis caused by, 156
  superinfections, 155
  teeth, deposition in, 153
  tetracycline-L-methylenelysine, 158
  toxicity, 152
  vitamin B supplements, 157

Tetracycline-L-methylenelysine, 158
Tetracyn, *see* tetracycline
Tetralysal, *see* lymecycline
Thiambutosine, 416
Thioacetazone, 407
Thiocarbanilides, 409
Thioparamizone, see thioacetazone
Thiosemicarbazones, 407
Thiosporin, *see* polymyxin **B**
Thiosulfil, *see* sulphamethizole
Thrush, intestinal, 354
  neonatal, 367
  oral, 347
Tinea capitis, 244, 307
Tinea pedis, 244, 308
Tolnaftate, 308
Toxoplasmosis, 26
Trachoma, 395
Transduction of resistance, 253
Treponema pallidum, erythromycin, 423
  penicillin, 421
  tetracycline, 423
Treponema recurrentis, 434
Trescatyl, *see* ethionamide
Triacetyloleandomycin, 175
Trichomoniasis, 36, 364, 432
Trichomycin, 240
Trichophyton rubrum, 244
Trimethoprim, 42-50
  antibacterial action, 43
  clinical application, 49
  laboratory control, 462, 482
  mode of action, 43
  pharmacology, 47
  toxicity, 48
Trispray, 304
Tube dilution sensitivity tests, 467, 469
Tuberculosis, bone infections, 413
  capreomycin, 404
  chemoprophylaxis, 413
  combined therapy, 410
  corticosteroids, 412
  cycloserine, 404
  drug-resistance, 403, 413
  ethambutol, 409
  ethionamide, 408
  genito-urinary, 412
  isoniazid, 402
  kanamycin, 405
  length of treatment, 411
  meningitis, 411
  PAS, 400
  pharmaceutical preparations, 417
  pulmonary, 410
  pyrazinamide, 408
  rifampicin, 405
  standard treatment, 410

Tuberculosis—*cont.*
  streptomycin, 112, 400
  surgical, 412
  tetracyclines, 406
  thioacetazone, 407
  thiocarbanilides, 409
  viomycin, 406, 413
Tularaemia, 299
Typhoid carriers, 352
Typhoid fever, 350
Tyrocidine, 182, 183
Tyrothricin, 6, 182, 183

Ultrapen, *see* propicillin
Undulant fever, *see* brucellosis
Urethritis, non-specific, 431
Urinary infections, 368-383
  acute, 375
  bacterial sensitivities, 370
  diagnosis, 368
  diuresis, effect of, 378
  drug-resistant, 381
  excretion patterns, 371
  long-term therapy, 381
  pH, control of, 373
  pregnancy, 363
  prophylaxis, 373, 380
  re-infection, 380
  relapse, 377, 379
  renal failure, 277, 383
  specimens, collections of, 368

Urinary infections—*cont.*
  tissue concentrations, 371
  tuberculous, 412
  urinary drug levels, 370
  yeasts, 34
Urolucosil, *see* sulphamethizole

Vaccinia, 447
Vancocin, *see* vancomycin
Vancomycin, acquired resistance, 231
  administration, 232
  antibacterial activity, 230
  clinical application, 232, 354
  pharmacology, 232
  source of, 8, 230
  toxic effects, 233
Variola, 446
Variotin, *see* pecilocin
V-cil-K, *see* phenoxymethyl penicillin
Vibramycin, *see* doxycycline
Vincent's infection, 36, 338, 347
Vioform, *see* quinolines
Viomycin, 406, 413
Viruses, 440
Vitamin B supplements, 139, 157
Vulcamycina, *see* novobiocin

Wounds, aerobic infection, 310
  anaerobic infection, 311

Yaws, 424

Printed at The Central Press (Aberdeen) Ltd., Belmont St., Aberdeen.